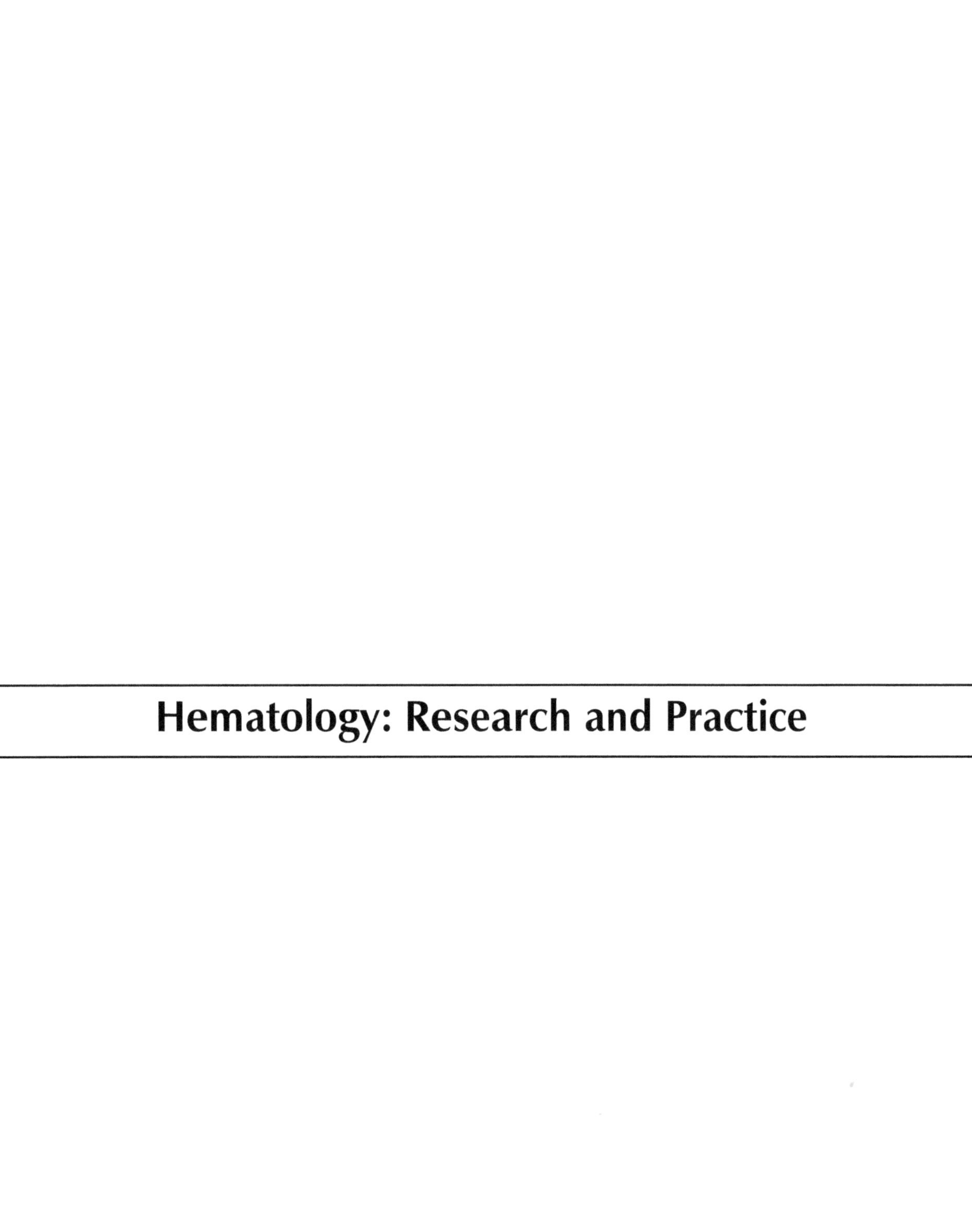

Hematology: Research and Practice

Hematology: Research and Practice

Editor: Rylan Beckham

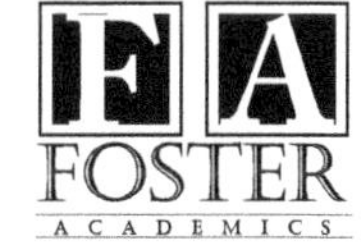

www.fosteracademics.com

www.fosteracademics.com

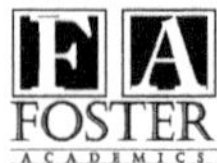

Cataloging-in-Publication Data

Hematology : research and practice / edited by Rylan Beckham.
p. cm.
Includes bibliographical references and index.
ISBN 978-1-63242-675-8
1. Hematology. 2. Hematology--Research. 3. Blood--Diseases. I. Beckham, Rylan.
RC633 .H46 2019
616.15--dc23

Foster Academics,
118-35 Queens Blvd., Suite 400,
Forest Hills, NY 11375, USA

ISBN 978-1-63242-675-8 (Hardback)

Contents

Preface

The branch of medicine that studies the causes, prognosis, treatment and prevention of diseases associated with blood is known as hematology. It is concerned with the treatment of diseases which affect the production of blood, hemoglobin, blood cells, bone marrow, platelets, spleen, blood vessels, etc. Some hematological disorders are hemophilia, blood clots, leukemia, lymphoma and multiple myeloma. These are diagnosed at the hematology laboratory through the examination of bone marrow slides and blood films, along with an analysis of blood clotting test and hematological test results. Hematologists specialize in specific domains, such as in the treatment of hemoglobinopathies, hematological malignancies and bleeding disorders, as well as bone marrow and stem cell transplantation. This book unravels the recent studies in the field of hematology. It presents researches and studies performed by experts across the globe. Those in search of information to further their knowledge will be greatly assisted by this book.

Various studies have approached the subject by analyzing it with a single perspective, but the present book provides diverse methodologies and techniques to address this field. This book contains theories and applications needed for understanding the subject from different perspectives. The aim is to keep the readers informed about the progresses in the field; therefore, the contributions were carefully examined to compile novel researches by specialists from across the globe.

Indeed, the job of the editor is the most crucial and challenging in compiling all chapters into a single book. In the end, I would extend my sincere thanks to the chapter authors for their profound work. I am also thankful for the support provided by my family and colleagues during the compilation of this book.

Editor

1

A quantitative assessment of the content of hematopoietic stem cells in mouse and human endosteal-bone marrow: a simple and rapid method for the isolation of mouse central bone marrow

Maya M. Mahajan[1†], Betty Cheng[1†], Ashley I. Beyer[1†], Usha S. Mulvaney[1], Matt B. Wilkinson[1], Marina E. Fomin[1] and Marcus O. Muench[1,2*]

Abstract

Background: Isolation of bone marrow cells, including hematopoietic stem cells, is a commonly used technique in both the research and clinical settings. A quantitative and qualitative assessment of cell populations isolated from mouse and human bone marrow was undertaken with a focus on the distribution of hematopoietic cells between the central bone marrow (cBM) and endosteal bone marrow (eBM).

Methods: Two approaches to cBM isolation from the hind legs were compared using the C57BL/6J and BALB/cJ strains of laboratory mice. The content of hematopoietic stem cells in eBM was compared to cBM from mice and human fetal bone marrow using flow cytometry. Enzymatic digestion was used to isolate eBM and its effects on antigen expression was evaluated using flow cytometry. Humanized immunodeficient mice were used to evaluate the engraftment of human precursors in the cBM and eBM and the effects of in vivo maturation on the fetal stem cell phenotype were determined.

Results: The two methods of mouse cBM isolation yielded similar numbers of cells from the femur, but the faster single-cut method recovered more cells from the tibia. Isolation of eBM increased the yield of mouse and human stem cells. Enzymatic digestion used to isolate eBM did, however, have a detrimental effect on detecting the expression of the human HSC-antigens CD4, CD90 and CD93, whereas CD34, CD38, CD133 and HLA-DR were unaffected. Human fetal HSCs were capable of engrafting the eBM of immunodeficient mice and their pattern of CD13, CD33 and HLA-DR expression partially changed to an adult pattern of expression about 1 year after transplantation.

Conclusions: A simple, rapid and efficient method for the isolation of cBM from the femora and tibiae of mice is detailed. Harvest of tibial cBM yielded about half as many cells as from the femora, representing 6.4 % and 13 %, respectively, of the total cBM of a mouse based on our analysis and a review of the literature. HSC populations were enriched within the eBM and the yield of HSCs from the mouse and human long bones was increased notably by harvest of eBM.

Keywords: Hematopoietic stem cells, Bone marrow cells, Cell culture techniques, Cell count, Stem cell niche, Flow cytometry, Mice, Humans, Transplantation, Chimera

* Correspondence: mmuench@bloodsystems.org
†Equal contributors
[1]Blood Systems Research Institute, 270 Masonic Ave., San Francisco, CA, USA
[2]Department of Laboratory Medicine, University of California, San Francisco, CA, USA

Background

Collection of bone marrow (BM) from mice is an integral part of a broad range of studies in the fields of hematology and immunology. Murine BM is also a source of other cell types such as mesenchymal stromal cells (MSCs), endothelial cells, osteoblasts, and osteoclasts [1–4]. BM samples are most typically obtained from femora and sometimes tibiae. The method of isolating BM cells typically involves cleaning some degree of soft-tissue from the bone and flushing cells out of the marrow cavity using a syringe with a fine needle [1]. However, based on descriptions in the literature and our own research team's experiences, there are a number of different approaches to the isolation of BM from mouse limb bones. The main difference in approach is whether investigators choose to flush marrow from the bones by removal of one [5] or both epiphyses [1]. Additionally, investigators differ on the degree of soft tissue removal performed prior to flushing the bones. Extensive removal of soft-tissue can be a time-consuming process with an uncertain benefit on the yield of BM cells.

The harvest of BM from human bone samples obtained after surgery from living donors or from cadavers is an important source of tissue for research [6] and may also have clinical use [7]. For instance, BM harvested from the long bones of fetal specimens has been used as a source of hematopoietic stem cells (HSCs) [8] and MSCs [9, 10] for research. These cells have also been proposed as a source of donor cells for clinical transplantation [11–13].

The distribution of cell types within the BM is not homogeneous and, consequently, different harvest techniques may vary in their efficiency in isolating particular cell lineages [14]. Studies of the stem cell niche have shown different types of stem cells and progenitors to reside in different parts of the long-bone marrow. Lord and Hendry were among the first to show an increased density of hematopoietic precursors with distance away from the central axis of the bone – referred to as the central bone marrow (cBM) [15]. Accordingly, higher levels of precursor proliferation are found near the inner wall of the bone, closer to the endosteum, the location of the endosteal bone marrow (eBM) [16].

Recently, Grassinger et al. demonstrated that phenotypically defined HSCs were enriched within the eBM of the mouse [17]. These authors estimated that about a quarter of all $CD48^{-}CD150^{+}CD117^{+}SCA\text{-}1^{+}$ lineage (Lin)-depleted HSCs reside in the endosteum. Likewise, human HSCs are enriched in the trabecular bone found at the ends of the long bones [18]. In chimeric mice, created by the transplantation of human HSCs into immunodeficient mice [19], human HSCs are preferentially localized to the eBM in the metaphysis and epiphysis [18]. Similar to the findings on human bones, transplanted human HSCs were enriched in the trabeculae of the metaphysis/epiphysis of the murine femur. To note, harvest of eBM is technically more time-consuming and costly than simply flushing or rinsing BM from bones as it involves removal of soft tissue, crushing of the bone and enzymatic digestion [20].

One objective in performing this study was to discern the most reliable, simplest and fastest method for the routine isolation of cBM. Two methods were compared: in one method, cBM was flushed from an incision at one end of the bone after only minimal removal of soft tissue and, in a second method, cBM was harvested following removal of the majority of soft tissue and flushing the cBM from one end of the bone and out the other end. These two procedures are referred to simply as the single-cut and double-cut methods, respectively. Both methods were tested on the femora and tibiae of mice and the number of cells obtained and the time required for harvest was compared. In addition, researchers with varying degrees of experience with these procedures were studied to gauge the difficulty in learning the two techniques. Herein, we also quantified the enzymatic harvest of eBM to compare the efficacy of recovering HSCs by this method compared to simple flushing methods used to collect cBM. We not only evaluated the benefit of harvesting eBM for the collection of murine HSCs, but also human HSCs isolated from fetal BM and humanized immunodeficient mice. Lastly, we compared the phenotypic profile of human HSCs isolated from the cBM and eBM from both fetal BM and from transplanted fetal cells recovered from humanized mice.

Methods

Mice

This study was conducted with approval of the Institutional Animal Care and Use Committee at ISIS Services LLC (San Carlos, CA). The C57BL/6J and BALB/cJ strains were purchased from The Jackson Laboratories (Bar Harbor, MN and Sacramento, CA). Breeder pairs of immunodeficient NOD.Cg-*Prkdc*^{scid} *Il2rg*^{tm1Wjl}/SzJ (NSG) mice were also obtained from The Jackson Laboratories and bred at our institute. Additionally, NOD.Cg-*Prkdc*^{scid} *Il2rg*^{tm1Sug} *Tg(Alb-Plau)11-4*/ShiJic (uPA-NOG) mice were bred at our institute by crossing uPA transgene hemizygous X homozygous mice [21].

Male and female mice were obtained through tissue sharing whenever possible and killed by orbital enucleation and exsanguination or by CO_2 asphyxiation and cervical dislocation. All animals were adults (≥8 weeks of age) at the time of sacrifice. Mice were maintained in microisolator cages in a facility free of commonly tested murine pathogens and received humane care according to the criteria outlined by the National Research Council's

Institute of Laboratory Animal Resources in the "Guide for the Care and Use of Laboratory Animals".

Human tissues

Human fetal long-bones and liver were collected from San Francisco General Hospital with consent from the mothers undergoing elective abortions and with approval of the University of California San Francisco's Committee on Human Research. The gestational age of the tissues used was between 20–24 weeks old estimated based on the foot length of the fetus. All specimens were donated anonymously.

Harvest of mouse cBM

The following supplies are required to harvest cBM from mice: 70 % ethanol, phosphate-buffered saline (PBS), 50 ml and 15 ml tubes, sterile gauze pads, a 10 ml syringe, needles, forceps, and scissors. Unless otherwise stated, 27 gauge, 13 mm needles (Becton Dickinson, Franklin Lakes, NJ) were used in this study, but testing of different needle gauges indicate 23 gauge needles offer the best performance. A video has been posted online (see Additional file 1) demonstrating the single-cut method of isolating cBM, which was made following this protocol: Fill a 10 mL syringe with PBS using a 50 ml tube as a reservoir. Attach a 23 gauge, 19 mm needle (Becton Dickinson, Franklin Lakes, NJ) and bend 90° using the plastic cap (Fig. 1a). After sacrifice, spray the mouse with 70 % ethanol to wet the fur to prevent its dispersal before removal of the skin. Make a small incision in the skin above the abdomen of the mouse (Fig. 1b). From this cut, pull the skin apart and gently remove the legs, one at a time, from the skin (Fig. 1c). The legs are removed in the following manner: Bend back the leg dorsally as if to dislocate the joint from the pelvis. While pulling the leg, use scissors to make three cuts to detach the leg from the pelvis (Fig. 1d). The first cut is roughly parallel to the femur towards the pelvis (Fig. 2), thereby removing soft tissue from the femur while severing some of the soft-tissue that connects the femur to the hip. The second cut is made while dislocating the femur to reveal the proximal epiphysis of the femur. The third cut, similar to the first, is made parallel to the femur, towards the knee, to further reduce the soft-tissue around the femur and detach the leg. To collect the cBM from the femur, remove the proximal epiphysis with scissors (Fig. 1e). To reduce the loss of BM, it is important to cut just below the ball joint (Fig. 2). The red BM should be visible. Insert the needle into the opening of the bone (Fig. 1f). Flush the cBM cells into a collection tube by injecting approximately 0.5-3 mL of PBS while holding the bone over the opening of the tube. For the tibia, remove the bulk of the soft tissue by holding the tibia using forceps and cutting roughly parallel towards the knee (Fig. 2). Cut the proximal epiphysis of the tibia by cutting just below the knee joint (Fig. 1). The white ligaments covering the knee provide a landmark and the cut should be immediately below this connective tissue. Flush cells from the tibia as for the femur (Fig. 1g-h).

The double-cut method differed from the single-cut method in that the bone was first cleaned of the majority of soft tissue to allow for visualization of the bones. Complete soft-tissue removal, as is sometimes performed when isolating cBM [1], was not done to allow the duration of the two isolation methods to be more reasonably compared. Then, both the distal and proximal epiphyses were removed and marrow was flushed from the distal out the proximal end of the bones.

For both the single-cut and double-cut methods, the volume of PBS used to harvest the cBM was not fixed. The mean volume used to flush femora was 2.2 ml and 2.0 ml using the single-cut and double-cut methods, respectively ($n = 56$). For the tibiae, an average of 1.8 ml and 1.6 ml were used with the single-cut and double-cut methods, respectively.

The time required to harvest the cBM by the single-cut and double-cut methods was recorded starting at the time of the excision of the leg. Data were collected starting on the left leg and the method of harvest used was alternated between the left and right legs to account for the handedness of the investigators. This approach was used to balance the number of cBM cells recovered and the time required to perform the two procedures. Although the procedure was timed, the investigators were instructed to primarily focus on an accurate collection of the most cells possible with the speed of the procedure being of secondary concern.

Isolation of mouse eBM

Murine eBM was harvested in a manner similar to a previously described method [20]. Briefly, femurs were removed of all soft tissue using scissors and forceps. Bones were cut into smaller fragments and digested with 3 mg/ml collagenase I (Sigma Aldrich, St. Louis, MO) and 4 mg/ml dispase II (Roche Diagnostics Corporation, Indianapolis, IN) at 37 °C for 5 minutes. The eBM was filtered through a 40 μm strainer and washed once by centrifugation.

Isolation of fetal human cBM and eBM

Human cBM was isolated from either a femur or all long bones as previously detailed [12]. Briefly, bones were denuded of all soft tissue, including the fibrous periosteum, using a scalpel and scissors. cBM was

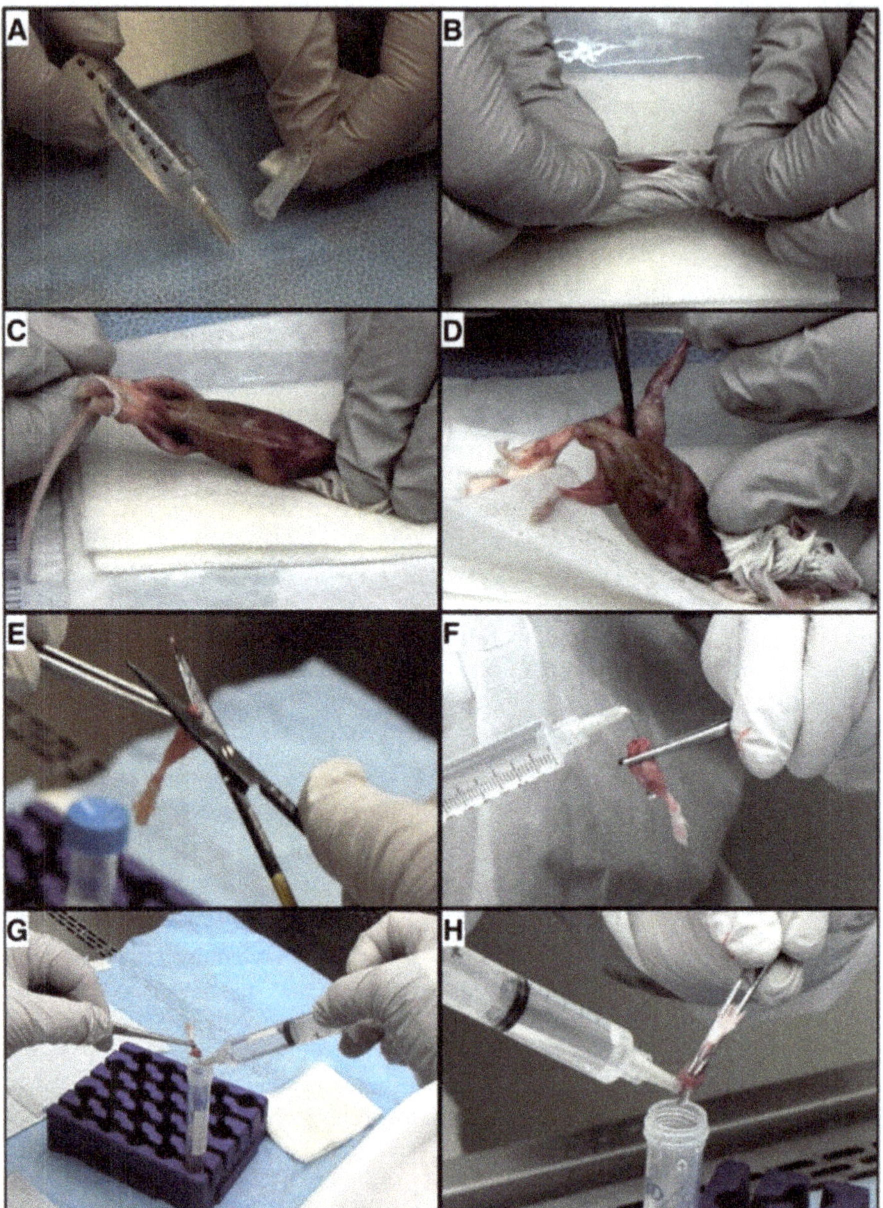

Fig. 1 Stepwise overview of the single-cut method for mouse cBM isolation. Panels (**a**)-(**h**) demonstrate the key steps in the isolation of cBM. Refer to the protocol text for an explanation of the individual steps

flushed with a 19 gauge needle (Becton Dickinson) inserted, often at multiple sites, into both ends of the bone and flushed with PBS until the red-cell content of the marrow was visibly depleted. PBS was used to rinse the bones. Each bone, immersed in fresh PBS, was then cut in half lengthways and the cBM scraped from the bone with a scalpel blade and filtered through a 100 μm cell strainer (Greiner Bio-One, Germany). The cBM was washed once by centrifugation.

The bone fragments that remained after flushing and filtration of the cBM were enzymatically digested to isolate eBM as described for the mouse bones. The eBM was filtered and washed once by centrifugation before flow cytometric analysis.

Construction of humanized mice

Male and female mice were transplanted with human hematopoietic cells to establish hematopoietic chimeras. Immunodeficient uPA-NOG mice [21] were transplanted with fetal liver cells, prepared as described [22]. Cells were transplanted by intra-splenic injection without prior cytoablative irradiation [23]. Additionally, NSG mice were transplanted intravenously with 2×10^6 midgestation light-density cBM cells after 175 cGy X-ray irradiation.

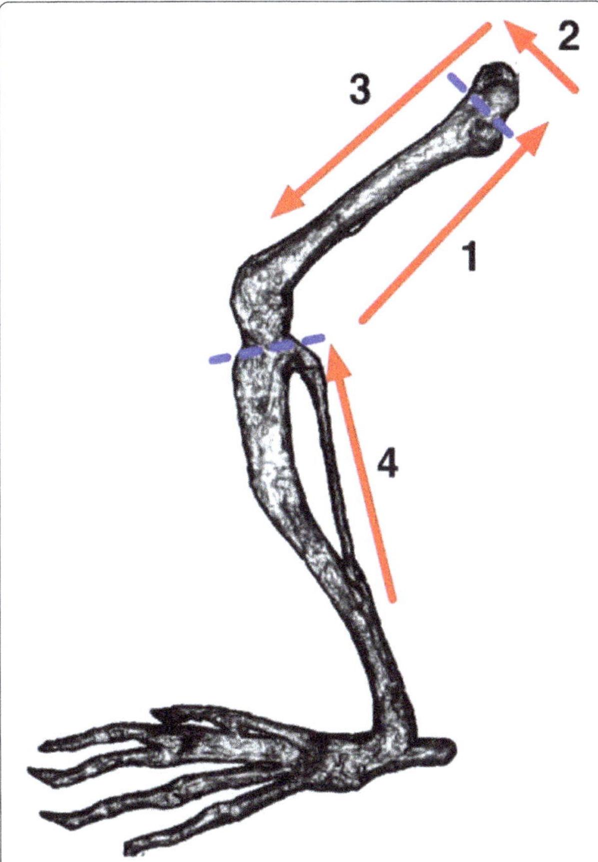

Fig. 2 Stepwise schematic of cuts made in soft-tissue and bone for the isolation of mouse cBM. The direction and numerical sequence of soft-tissue cuts are shown using red arrows. The approximate location of cuts made to remove the bone epiphyses are shown with dashed blue lines

Flow cytometric analysis

Human BM cells were suspended in blocking buffer consisting of PBS with 5 % mouse serum and 0.01 % NaN_3 and, for samples containing mouse BM, the blocking buffer was supplemented with 2 μg/ml rat anti-mouse CD16/CD32 mAb (BioLegend, San Diego, CA). Samples were stained with monoclonal antibodies and live cells, identified using propidium iodide staining, analyzed on a flow cytometer as previously described [24]. Data were analyzed using FlowJo software, version 9.7 (Tree Star, Inc.; Ashland, OR).

The following fluorescein isothiocyanate (FITC)-labelled, phycoerythrin (PE)-labelled, allophycocyanin (APC), PE-cyanine 7 (PE-Cy7), APC-cyanine 7 (APC-Cy7), pacific blue (PB) or Alexa Fluor 700 (AF700) antibodies were purchased from BioLegend or an otherwise stated vendor: mouse IgG1 FITC, mouse IgG1 PE, mouse IgG1 APC, mouse IgG1 PE-Cy7, mouse IgG1 APC-Cy7 and mouse IgG2a PE. The following monoclonal antibodies were used to stain human cells: CD45 FITC (clone HI30), CD45 APC-Cy7 (clone HI30), FITC-labeled mature lineage cocktail (clones UCHT1, HCD14, 3G8, HIB19, 2H7, HCD56), CD133 APC (clone AC133; Miltenyi Biotec, Auburn, CA), CD133 PE (clone AC133; Miltenyi Biotec), CD34 PE-Cy7 (clone 581), CD4 PE (clone L200; BD Pharmingen, San Diego CA), CD13 APC (clone WM15; BD Pharmingen), CD33 (clone WM53), CD38 PE (clone HIT2), CD90 PE (clone 5E10), CD93 PE (clone VIMD2), CD147 (clone TRA-1-85; R&D Systems, Minneapolis, MN), HLA-DR FITC (clone L243; Becton Dickinson) and HLA-DR PE (clone L243). The following monoclonal antibodies were used to stain mouse cells: CD3 (clone17A2), CD11b (clone M1/70), CD45R (clone RA3-6B2), Gr-1 (clone RB6-8C5), TER-119 (clone TER-119), CD45 (clone 30-F11), H-$2K^d$ (clone SF1-1.1) all PB labelled, CD48 PE-Cy7 (clone HM48-1), CD117 (c-kit) FITC (clone 2B8), CD150 (SLAM) PE (clone TC15-12 F12.2) and SCA-1 APC (clone D7).

Cell counts

Live cell counts were performed using a Scepter Handheld Automated Cell Counter with 40 μm sensors (EMD Millipore Corporation, Billerica, MA, USA). Particles >3 μm were counted.

Data presentation and statistical analysis

Statistical analysis and charting was performed using Aabel 3 and Aabel NG software (Gigawiz Ltd. Co. OK, USA). The 2-tailed Wilcoxon Matched-Pairs test was used to determine the significance of differences between cell yields obtained by the single-cut and double-cut methods. The Mann–Whitney U-test was used to determine the significance of differences in cell population frequencies between cBM and eBM. Differences were considered significantly different at $P \leq 0.05$. Notched box and whisker plots are used to display some of the data where the box represents the distribution of the 25th through 75th percentile of the data and the whiskers extend to the extreme data points. Medians are represented by the notch in the box.

Results

Comparison of the single-cut and double-cut methods of mouse cBM isolation

Two methods of mouse cBM isolation were tested. Investigators with differing levels of experience with the procedures performed these experiments to determine which method was best for experienced and novice investigators (Table 1). The two methods were compared to determine which was the most reliable and/or fastest. The median time using the single-cut method was much faster (76 seconds, n = 56) than the

Table 1 Summary of investigator experience and cBM collection times

Investigator	Years experience	Preferred method	Number of harvests	Median time (Seconds) single-cut method	Median time (Seconds) double-cut method
A	≥25 years	Single-cut	18	62	120
B	≥25 years	Double-cut	5	98	187
C	≥5 years	Single-cut	5	68	170
D	<1 year	Novice	12	88	174
E	<1 year	Novice	10	121	149
F	<1 year	Novice	6	75	117

double-cut method (151.5 seconds, n = 56) regardless of experience level of the investigator (Fig. 3a and Table 1). Not surprisingly, investigators experienced with the single-cut method were able to perform their isolations most rapidly (Table 1). Moreover, the single-cut method was the fastest method for isolating cBM from both the femora and tibiae (Fig. 3b).

The median number of cells harvested by the single-cut method was 2.21×10^7, compared to 1.91×10^7 obtained by the double cut method (n = 56, Fig. 3c). The 15.7 % increased yield of cBM obtained by the single-cut method was not significant ($P = 0.057$). When the cell yields were analyzed separately for the two hind-leg bones a modest 8.2 % higher number of femoral cells were recovered using the single-cut method (Fig. 3d), which was not significantly higher than the yield obtained with the double-cut method. However, the 19.4 % increased recovery of cells from the tibia using the single-cut method was significant ($P = 0.043$). Thus, the single-cut method is a favorable method for isolating cBM from both the femur and the tibia.

Given that the murine tibia is a smaller bone than the femur and extra effort is required to harvest cells from it, we sought to determine the quantity of cBM that could be harvested from the tibia. The results were very similar for two strains of mice analyzed (Fig. 3e). For both strains combined, the tibia yielded about 54 % the number of cells obtained from the femur. Stated in another way, about a third of the cBM available for harvest from a hind leg is found in the tibia.

We evaluated the cell yields individually by investigator to gain insight into the effects of experience on performing the two procedures. There was no significant difference in cell yield between the combined results of the 3 experienced investigators and 3 novice investigators (n = 28 harvests each group) for either of the two isolation methods. Investigators A and C, both experienced with the single-cut method, did recover a significantly higher number of cells using this method (Fig. 3f), whereas investigator B, previously experienced with the double-cut method, obtained an insignificantly greater number of cells with their familiar procedure. There was no significant difference in cell yield among the novice investigators comparing the two isolation methods.

Comparison of the yields of hematopoietic precursors found in mouse cBM and eBM

We sought to quantify the number of cells and, more specifically, hematopoietic precursors that remained in the bones after flushing out cBM using the single-cut method. Isolation of eBM recovered 84 % more cells than by flushing alone. The yields of different hematopoietic progenitor compartments were determined using flow cytometric analysis (Fig. 4a). The frequency (Fig. 4b) and total number (Fig. 4c) of Lin^- cells recovered from the femurs of 5 mice were greater from the eBM than the cBM. Recoveries of $Lin^-SCA\text{-}1^+CD117^+$ (LSK) cells, $Lin^-CD48^-CD150^+$ cells and $CD48^-CD150^+$ LSK cells did not differ significantly between the cBM and eBM. These data indicate that approximately equivalent numbers of progenitors and HSCs can be recovered from the cBM and eBM if flushed with a small 27 gauge needle size.

As the size of needle used to flush cBM from the long bones may affect the recovery of cBM and eBM. We compared harvests of cBM, from the femur and tibia, using four needle sizes (Fig. 4d). There were no significant differences in the yield of cBM using the different gauged needles. There was, however, a more varied and decreased median recovery using the largest needles (21 gauge). These needles were too large to easily insert in the marrow cavities of tibiae resulting, sometimes, in fractures. Indeed, there was a significant decrease in the harvest of tibial cBM using 21 gauge needles compared to 25 and 27 gauge needles ($P = 0.016$ and 0.007, respectively), which affected the overall yield of cBM. The recovery of the remaining eBM was less using 23 gauge needles than using the smaller 27 gauge needles (Fig. 4e, $P = 0.025$), which was mirrored by an increased recovery of femoral cBM (not shown, $P = 0.037$). Using 23 gauge needles, the recovery of eBM was only 1.1 % of cBM. Thus, increasing the needle size up to 23 gauge can modestly increase the recovery of cBM and reduce the amount BM cells left in the femur. This affect wasn't apparent using the even larger 21 gauge needles likely because the tight fit of these needles

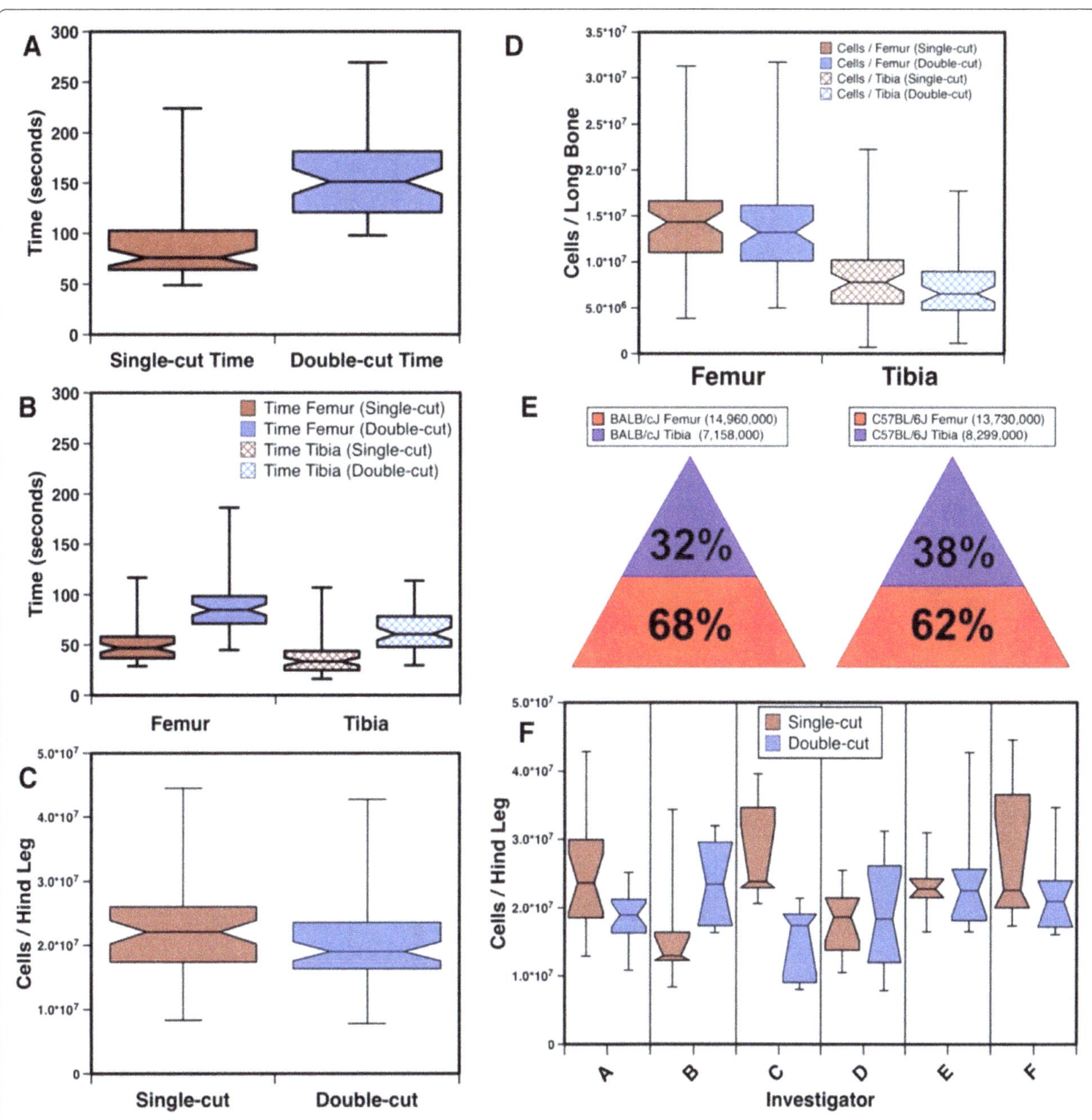

Fig. 3 Comparisons of mouse cBM isolations using the single-cut and double-cut methods. The time required to isolate cBM by the two methods is shown for both the femur and tibia (**a**) and for each of the long bones individually (**b**). The number of cells isolated by the two methods from both long-bones is shown in (**c**) and cell yields for the individual bones are shown in (**d**). The percentages of tibial and femoral BM cells recovered from BALB/cJ (n = 19) and C57BL/6J (n = 37) mice are shown (**e**). The median number of cells recovered from each bone using the single-cut method are indicated in the legends. Cell yields are shown by investigator in (**f**). Refer to Table 1 for the number of harvests performed and the level of experience of the investigator

within the marrow cavity affected the ability to flush the bones.

Comparison of hematopoietic precursors yields from fetal human cBM and eBM

The eBM compartment was also examined in human midgestation long bones. Four specimens of fetal human long-bones were used to isolate cBM and eBM and the recovered cells were analyzed by flow cytometry to determine the yield of HSCs as well as other BM cell populations. In 3 of 4 experiments, eBM cells represented a consistent 7 % of all BM cells recovered (Fig. 5). However, in one experiment, 57 % of cells were recovered from the eBM fraction. We attribute this outlier to the older age of the specimen and the fact that all the long bones found in the legs and arms were processed instead

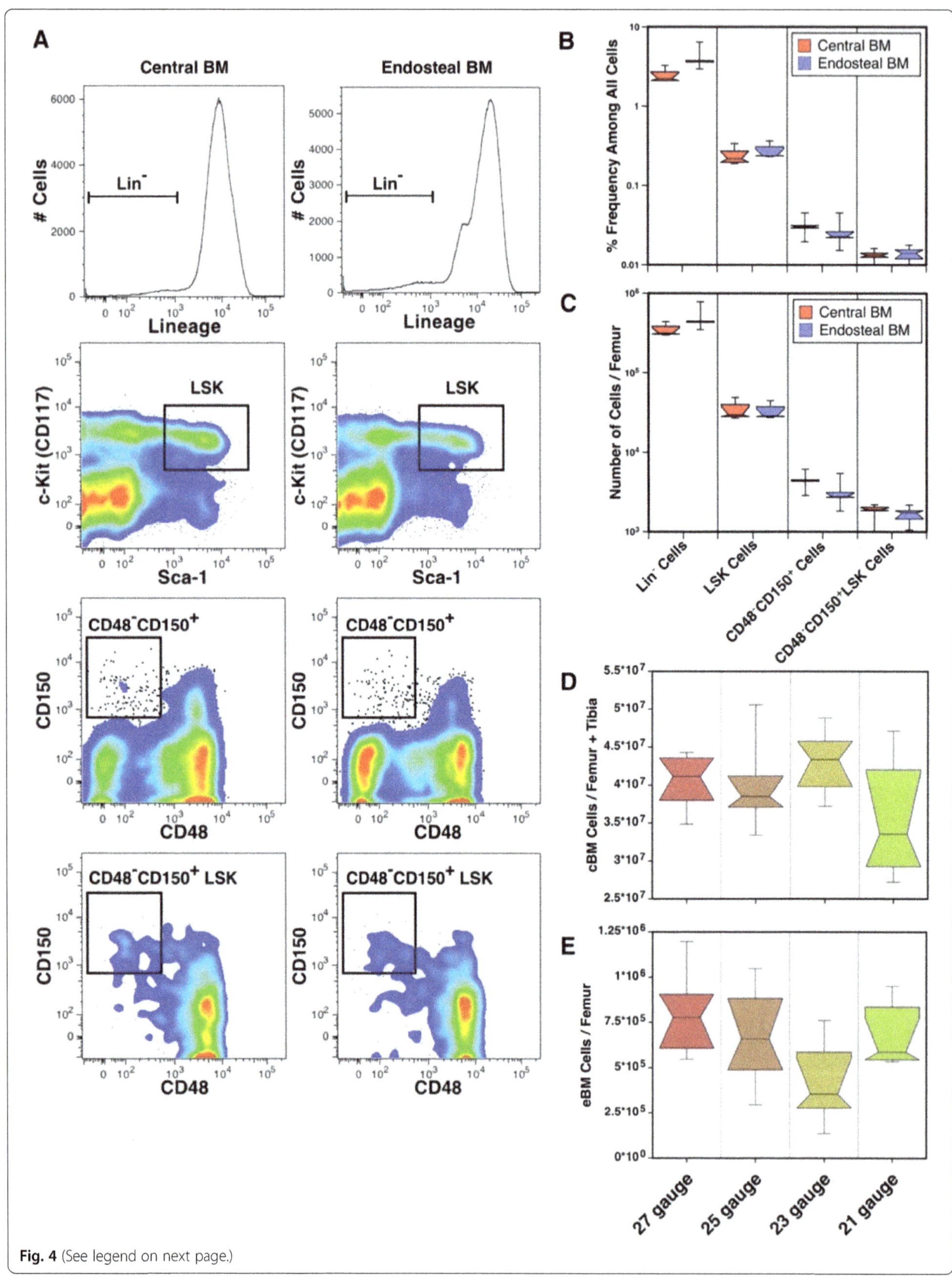

Fig. 4 (See legend on next page.)

(See figure on previous page.)
Fig. 4 The quantities of C57BL/6J mouse hematopoietic precursors from cBM and eBM. Flow cytometric analysis of cBM and eBM was used to identify precursor populations using the gates indicated (**a**). Total cells were defined as live cells – lacking PI staining – from which doublets were excluded by electronic gating (not shown). The median frequencies (**b**) and numbers (**c**) of cells recovered of each precursor population are shown (n = 5). Note, that these data are shown on a logarithmic scale. The effects of needle size on the recovery of cBM (**d**) and eBM (**e**) cells are shown for 6 samples for each group

of a single femur as in the first two experiments. The greater amount of tissue processed and hardness of the bones most likely led to less efficient flushing of the cBM, thereby resulting in a greater yield in the subsequent enzymatic digestion of the tissue.

To estimate the distribution of HSCs between the cBM and eBM compartments of the fetal long bones, two cell populations enriched in HSCs were enumerated from the BM preparations: $CD34^{++}CD133^{+}$ and $CD34^{++}CD38^{low}$ cells (Fig. 5). In all four samples, the frequencies of these primitive progenitors were enriched among eBM cells. $CD34^{++}CD38^{low}$ cells represent a small subset of $CD34^{++}CD133^{+}$ cells and their yield was noticeably lower than for $CD34^{++}CD133^{+}$ cells. A phenotypic profile using a number of markers associated with HSCs further demonstrates the enrichment of HSCs and primitive progenitors among the eBM fraction of BM cells (Fig. 6). The representative analysis shows the enrichment of $CD34^{++}CD133^{+}$ and $CD34^{++}CD38^{low}$ cells found in the eBM fraction. Likewise, $CD34^{++}CD90^{+}$ cells, representing another population enriched in stem cells [25], was also enriched more than 2-fold among eBM cells. In fetal tissues, most primitive progenitors express HLA-DR, although some are HLA-$DR^{low/-}$ [26, 27], whereas adult cells with the properties of HSCs are enriched among HLA-DR^{-} cells [28–30]. $CD34^{++}$HLA-DR^{+} cells were enriched among eBM cells, whereas the frequency of $CD34^{++}$HLA-DR^{-} cells was more or less similar in the two BM preparations. Overall, an enrichment of primitive progenitor populations was observed among eBM cells.

Two cell-surface markers associated with hematopoietic stem cells, CD4 and CD93, were notably absent among eBM cells in contrast to the other markers that were studied (Fig. 6). Since all the gated populations shown in Fig. 6 are largely overlapping populations of primitive hematopoietic cells, the lack of CD4 and CD93 expression was difficult to explain in light of the expression patterns of the other HSC markers. We therefore tested if these antigens were susceptible to enzymatic removal by digestion of cBM under the conditions used to isolate the eBM cells. The panel of Lin markers, used to mark mature cell populations, was modestly affected by enzymatic digestions, whereas CD34 expression was not diminished (Fig. 7). Among the markers used to define hematopoietic stem cells and primitive progenitors, CD4 and CD93 were notably eliminated and CD90 was partially reduced. The other markers were not appreciably affected. Note that the loss of Lin antigen, resulting from enzymatic digestion, did reduce the frequency of gated progenitor populations owing to the greater dilution of these populations by cells that would otherwise be Lin^{+} cells.

Human precursors in the cBM and eBM cells of humanized mice

Humanized mice provide a model for studying human hematopoiesis in an in vivo setting [31]. We evaluated cBM and eBM engraftment by human hematopoietic precursors in uPA-NOG mice. In the first experiment, mice were transplanted with hematopoietic precursors isolated from fetal liver, which is the source of HSCs that seed the BM during development. The first cohort of 5 mice were transplanted without irradiation to avoid the cytoablative treatment that may damage the BM and affect the seeding of the cBM and eBM. Although engraftment varied widely, as is typical of humanized mice, precursors expressing CD34 and CD133 were observed among both the cBM and eBM (Fig. 8a). The frequencies of human hematopoietic precursors are shown among all cBM and eBM cells as well as among only the fraction of human $CD45^{+}$ leukocytes found in the cBM and eBM (Fig. 8b). The median percentage of $CD34^{+/++}$ and $CD133^{+}CD34^{++}$ cells were modestly higher in the eBM, but the increase was not significant given the range of data from different chimeric mice.

Findings with the unirradiated uPA-NOG mice were followed by transplanting NSG mice, after cytoablative irradiation, with human 24 weeks' gestation cBM cells. Engraftment of both the cBM and eBM by $CD133^{+}CD34^{++}$ cells was observed in two mice analyzed 356 days after transplant (Fig. 8c).

The phenotype of fetal HSCs differs somewhat from that of adult HSCs. We hypothesized that long-term engraftment of human fetal cells in the adult environment of immunodeficient mice would result in a switch from a fetal to an adult phenotype. Most fetal HSCs express HLA-DR, CD13 and CD33 in contrast to their adult counterparts [26, 27]. We examined the expression of these antigens after long-term engraftment in mice to determine if the expression of these markers was lost as on adult cells. HLA-DR, CD13 and CD33 were expressed on cBM and eBM cells (Fig. 8c). In Fig. 8d, expression was also compared on enriched HSCs

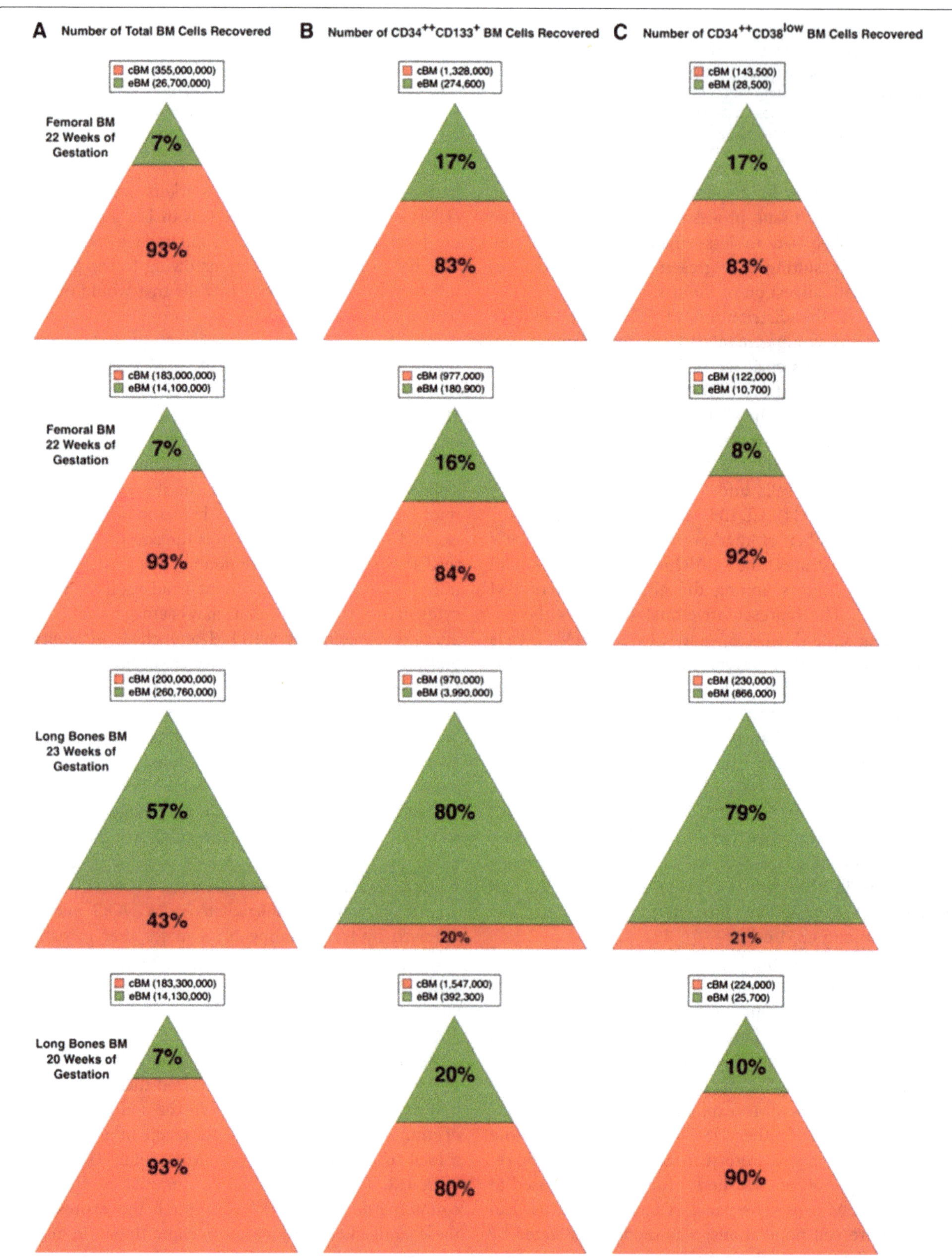

Fig. 5 Isolation of human hematopoietic precursors from cBM and eBM. The relative recovery of total cells (**a**), $CD34^{++}CD133^{+}$ cells (**b**) and $CD34^{++}CD38^{low}$ cells (**c**) from cBM and eBM are shown graphically for 4 samples. The number of cells recovered are indicated in the legends above each triangle

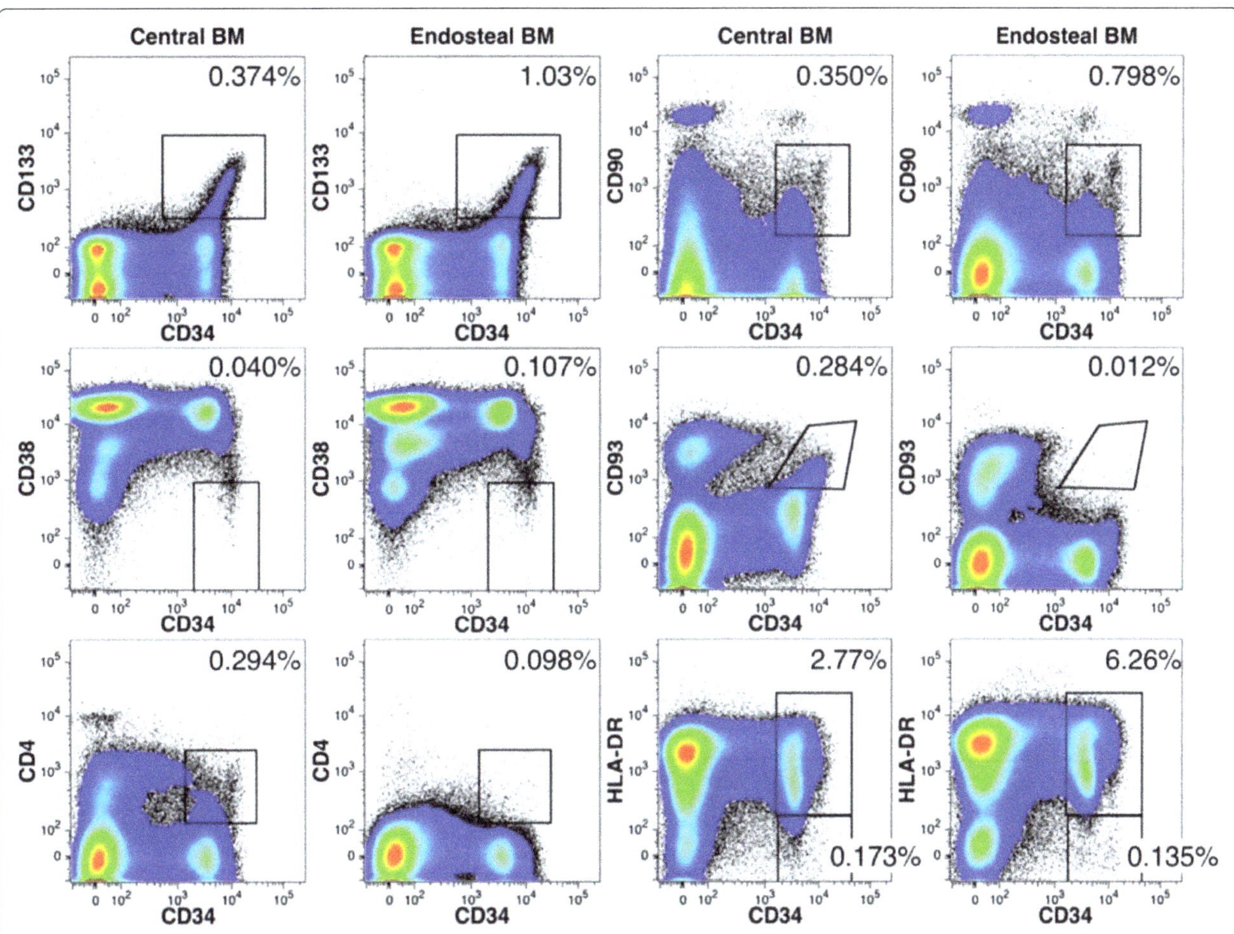

Fig. 6 Flow cytometric analysis of fetal human cBM and eBM. Side-by-side comparisons of cell surface markers on $CD34^{++}$ cells. The frequencies of gated cell populations among live-single cells are indicated in each plot. In addition to the markers shown, hematopoietic precursors were also defined by their expression of CD45 and light-scatter gate that excluded high side-light scatter events (not shown). Femoral cells were obtained from a 22 weeks' gestation fetus

($CD133^{+}CD34^{++}$) and a population of early-stage committed-progenitors ($CD133^{-}CD34^{++}$). HLA-DR was strongly expressed on cells expressing CD133, but had declined on $CD133^{-}CD34^{++}$ cells. The most notable difference found on $CD34^{++}$ precursors from cBM and eBM was a shift towards higher HLA-DR expression on $CD133^{-}$ from the eBM compared to the cBM. CD13 expression was not detected on any $CD34^{++}$ precursors, whereas a very low level of CD33 expression was observed on $CD133^{+}$ cells but not $CD133^{-}$ cells. These data indicate that the fetal HSC phenotype has only partially converted to an adult phenotype after nearly 1 year in vivo.

Discussion

Mice are among the most commonly used laboratory animals in research and the collection of BM from these animals has become a matter of routine. However, somewhat surprisingly, protocols used for the isolation of BM can vary notably from the very simple single-cut method used in this study to the more cumbersome double-cut methods employing varying degrees of soft-tissue removal. This study was performed, in part, to determine if these two methods are comparable in their yield of cBM cells, which they were for harvesting femoral cBM. In the case of the tibia, the single-cut method was found to be superior for maximizing the number of cells that can be harvested. The single-cut method was also notably faster due to its simplicity. Also important, the single-cut method was no more difficult to learn for novice investigators than the double-cut method despite the fact that the latter procedure provides greater visualization of the bone prior to marrow harvest.

A complete harvest of BM is often a requirement for many experiments, either to yield as many cells as possible for analysis or to perform a quantitative analysis of the BM compartment. The higher efficiency of the single-cut method makes it the preferable method to harvest the maximum number of cBM cells. However, the distribution of cell types within the BM is not

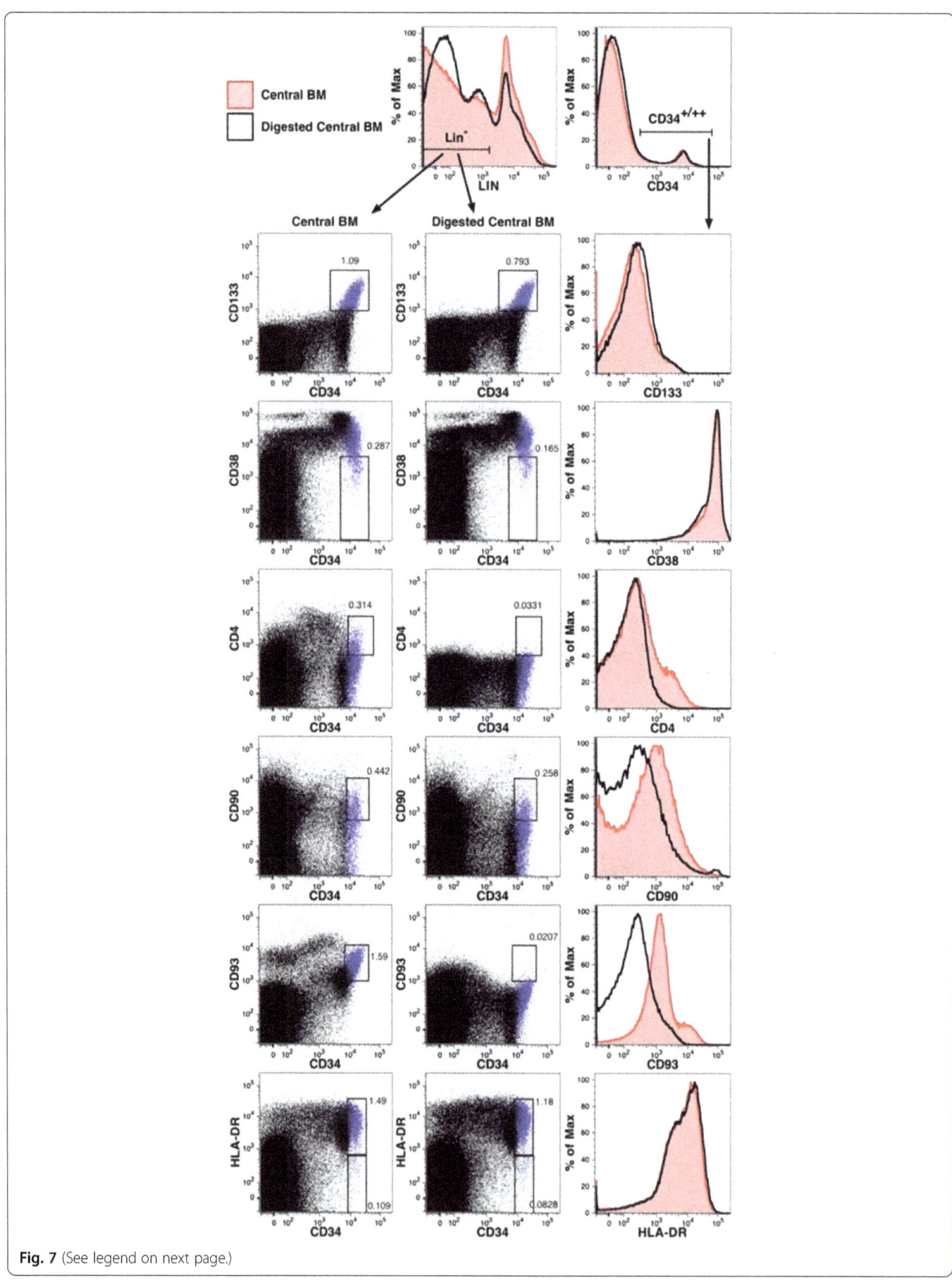

Fig. 7 (See legend on next page.)

(See figure on previous page.)
Fig. 7 Loss of some cell-surface markers on hematopoietic precursors owing to enzymatic digestion. Flow cytometric analysis was performed on cBM before and after enzymatic digestion was performed as for the isolation of eBM. The data shown in the dot plots are gated on live, single, low side-light scatter cells (not shown) as well as Lin$^-$ cells gated as indicated. Expression of CD133 is indicated using blue dots in all dot plots. Numbers represent the frequencies of Lin$^-$ cells represented by the gated populations. Overlay histogram plots show the effects of enzyme digestion on antigen expression. The expression of Lin antigens and CD34 are shown on live, single cells (gating not shown), whereas expression of the remaining antigens are shown on live, single cells expressing CD34 as indicated. BM cells were obtained from a 20 weeks' gestation fetus

homogeneous and, consequently, different harvest techniques may vary in their efficiency in isolating particular cell lineages [14]. Our own experience with the single-cut method shows this method to effectively isolate hematopoietic progenitors and long-term reconstituting HSCs [32, 33]. Nonetheless, studies of the HSC niche have shown different types of HSCs and progenitors to reside in different parts of the long-BM. Lord and Hendry showed an increased density of hematopoietic precursors with distance away from the central axis of the bone [15]. Accordingly, higher levels of precursor proliferation are found near the inner wall of the bone, closer to the endosteum [16]. More recently, Haylock et al. and Grassinger et al. demonstrated that phenotypically-defined HSCs were enriched within the eBM and that the HSCs from eBM have greater proliferative and engraftment potential when compared to those from cBM [17, 20]. These authors estimated that about a third of LSK cells and a quarter of CD48$^-$CD150$^+$ LSK cells reside in the endosteum. Our results yielded somewhat higher recoveries of 49 % of LSK cells and 39 % of CD48$^-$CD150$^+$ LSK cells from the eBM. The higher yields are likely due to subtle differences in methods, techniques and the bones used to isolate cBM and eBM. On of these differences could be the size of the needle used to isolate the cBM. We found 23–27 gauge needles to be similarly effective in harvesting cBM, but would recommend 23 gauge needles to maximize the recovery of cBM and minimize the quantity of eBM remaining in the marrow. Nonetheless, a complete harvest of HSCs requires harvest of the eBM.

Our study also reveals the value of harvesting tibial BM to increase the overall recovery of BM cells. Data on two common strains of mice show that the tibia can provide an additional 54 % of the number of cells collected from the femur alone. Thus, harvesting the tibia is a good option for increasing the yield of BM cells with minimal extra time required for the collection. The quantity of BM in different long bones has been measured by a number of investigators using mice pulsed with ^{59}Fe to radioactively label developing erythroid cells (Table 2). An average femoral BM content from six studies is 6.5 % of total skeletal BM [5, 34–38]. We found only one reported value for tibial BM measured at 3.5 % [34]. However, three other studies measured BM content of both the tibia and fibula at an average 3.1 % [5, 36, 38]. Since the tibia contains nearly all the BM of these two bones, we consider it reasonable to average the tibial measurement made by Chervenick et al. with the other three reported measurements; the average estimate from four studies for tibial BM content is 3.2 %. Based on our calculated averages, harvest of a single femur and tibia should yield 9.7 % of the total skeletal BM (19.4 % for both hind limbs). This estimate is in close agreement with total hind limb measurements made by Boggs and Patrene ranging from 8.4 to 10.75 % [39]. These combined BM measurements are also in agreement with our measurement of an approximate 2:1 ratio of cell content in the femur and tibia.

We evaluated the benefit of enzymatic digestion to isolate fetal human eBM cells. Although the method used for enzymatic digestion of the human BM was that same as for the murine samples, it is important to note that the isolation of human cBM by flushing was prone to more variability. Unlike the single-cut method where insertion of the needle into the BM cavity leaves little room for variability, flushing of the larger human bones requires multiple needle-point entries and physical crushing of the bones to access the cBM throughout the marrow cavity. A simple visual goal employed in cBM isolation was to flush most of the red cells from the bones. Nonetheless, the amount of tissue processed, the size of the bone and the gestational age of the sample can all affect the harvest. We observed eBM to comprise a consistent minimum of 7 % of the total BM content.

We observed an increased frequency of phenotypically defined HSCs in the eBM preparations made from fetal long bones. These results are in agreement with the reported enrichment of HSCs in the trabecular bone area of adult posterior ileac crest by Guezguez et al. [18]. These authors observed a higher frequency of Lin$^-$CD34^{++}CD38$^-$CD45RA$^-$CD49f$^+$ cells in the trabecular bone area, found near the surface of the bone biopsy, compared to the long bone area, defined as being closer to the central core of the biopsy. We observed HSC subsets such as CD34^{++}CD133$^+$, CD34^{++}CD38^{low}, CD34^{++}CD90$^+$ and CD34^{++}HLA-DR$^+$ cells enriched among eBM cells. It was also noted that the enzymatic digestion used to isolate the eBM cells reduced CD4, CD90 and CD93 antigen expression and, consequently, HSCs are best identified using antigens less prone to enzymatic digestion such as CD133, CD38 and HLA-DR.

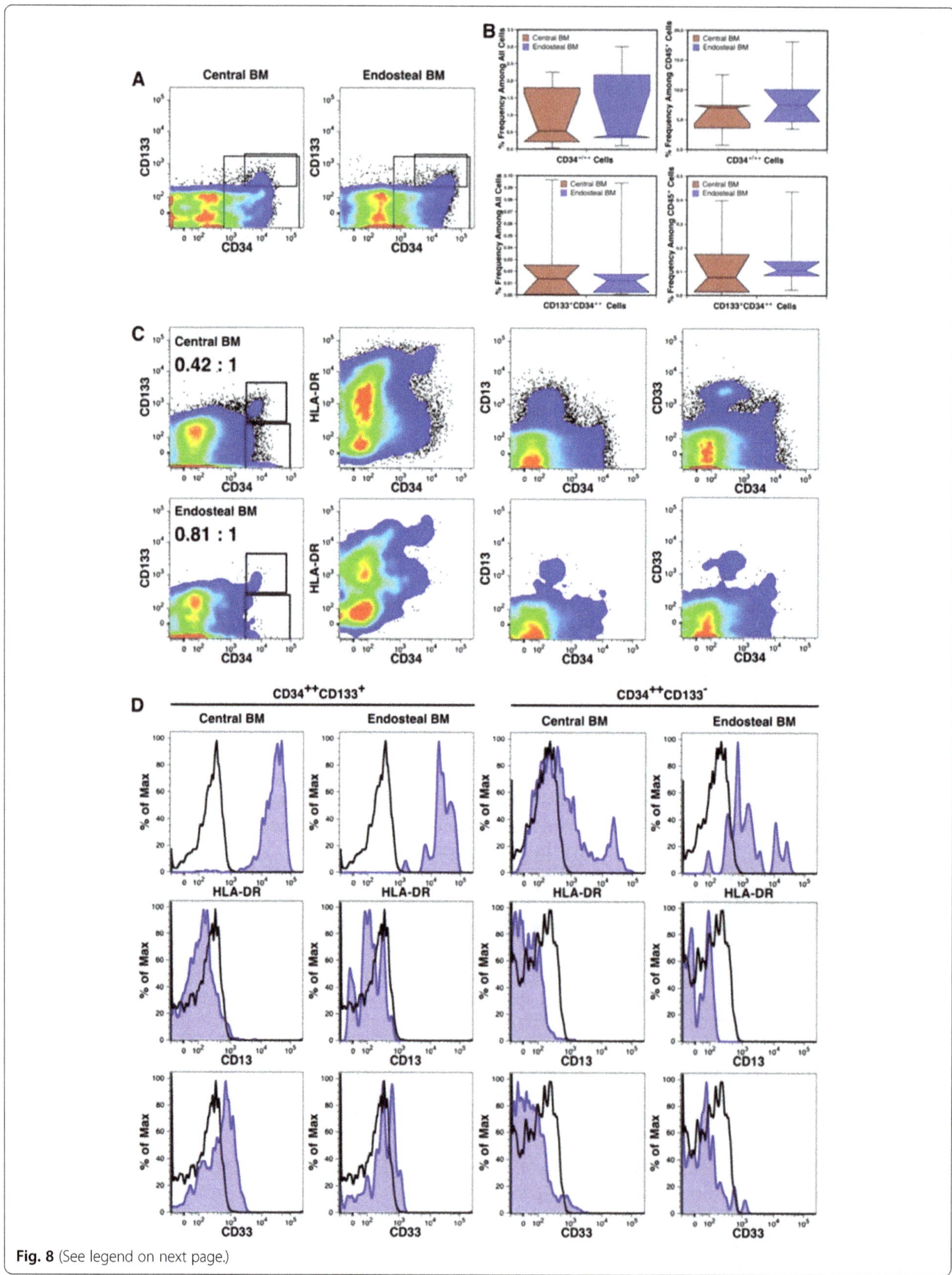

Fig. 8 (See legend on next page.)

(See figure on previous page.)
Fig. 8 Engraftment of the cBM and eBM by human cells in immunodeficient mice. uPA-NOG mice analyzed 308 days after transplant showed engraftment by $CD34^{+/++}$ (large rectangular region) and $CD133^{+}CD34^{++}$ (smaller gated subset) cells in both the cBM and eBM (**a**). The frequencies of these precursor populations found among all live, single cells and human $CD45^{+}$ cells are shown using box plots (n = 5) (**b**). Engraftment of various HSC compartments in irradiated NSG mice is indicated (**c**). Rectangular regions define $CD34^{++}CD133^{+}$ and $CD34^{++}CD133^{-}$ precursors in the cBM (top row) and eBM (bottom row). The ratio of gated $CD133^{+}$ to $CD133^{-}$ cells are indicated for cBM and eBM. The expression HLA-DR, CD13 and CD33 on $CD34^{++}CD133^{+}$ and $CD34^{++}CD133^{-}$ precursors from cBM and eBM is shown in histogram plots (**d**). Staining with the indicated antibody is shown with blue shading, whereas staining with an isotype-matched control antibody is shown in black outline

Human fetal tissue obtained from elective abortions has been used as a source of donor tissue for transplantation and banks of fetal tissue have been established to accommodate such efforts [40–42]. Many of these efforts have centered around the use of fetal donor cells for prenatal transplantation where the patient is also a fetus, thereby matching the developmental stage of the donor cells and the host. Although the fetal liver has been most studied and used as a source of HSCs for transplantation, fetal BM has also been evaluated as a source of HSCs for transplantation [12]. The yield of cells available from the long bones varies significantly with gestational age and only by mid-gestation do these tissues offer an abundant source of hematopoietic cells. At 20 weeks' gestation, we recovered 1.9×10^6 $CD34^{++}CD133^{+}$ and 2.5×10^5 $CD34^{++}CD38^{low}$ cells from the harvest of all long bones, with 10-20 % of the cells coming from the eBM preparation. These values are comparable to the yields of cells from umbilical cord blood [43, 44]. HSC recoveries from fetal BM obtained at 23–24 weeks' gestation can exceed those of a typical umbilical cord blood harvest as demonstrated in this study and previously by Golfier et al. [12]. The increased yield of HSCs offered by harvesting eBM as well as the greater proliferative and engraftment potential of eBM HSCs clearly favors the harvest of eBM for any clinical application.

Humanized mice were created by two methods to test the engraftment of the eBM compartment in mice by human HSCs. In the first model, intra-splenic injection was used in mice that had not been preconditioned with irradiation to preserve the integrity of the normal BM environment. These mice were also transplanted with fetal liver cells, a source of HSCs not compartmentalized into cBM and eBM cells. We observed engraftment of both BM compartments with human donor cells, showing for the first time that human fetal liver cells do engraft the eBM. Similar findings were obtained when mice were transplanted with cBM cells from fetal BM, demonstrating that cBM can engraft the eBM niche. These findings are in agreement with Guezguez et al., who observed that when human cells, engrafted in mice, were isolated from either niche, they could reconstitute both niches in secondary recipients [18]. We have also successfully engrafted human multilineage hematopoiesis in secondary murine hosts using cBM cells isolated by the single-cut method [23]. Despite the capacity of HSCs from cBM to engraft eBM, molecular and functional differences between cBM and eBM have been observed and are believed to be regulated, at least in part, by the differences in the cBM and eBM niches [18].

The phenotypic analysis of fetal human hematopoietic cells engrafted in mice also offered the opportunity to evaluate the expression of several antigens expressed on HSCs only early in ontogeny. We were interested to determine if the fetal HSC phenotype changes to an adult phenotype when cells are transplanted into an adult mouse and analyzed at an age corresponding to about 8 months after a normal term delivery. CD13 and CD33 are generally described as myeloid differentiation

Table 2 Summary of hind limb BM content estimates by ^{59}Fe distribution experiments

Study	Single femur	Single tibia	Single tibia + fibula	Single hind leg	Reference
Chervenick et al.	5.9 %	3.5 %	N.D.[a]	N.D.	[34]
Schofield & Cole	7.0 %	N.D.	N.D.	N.D.	[35]
Briganti et al.	6.1 %	N.D.	3.35 %	N.D.	[36]
Papayannopoulou & Finch	7.4 %	N.D.	N.D.	N.D.	[37]
Lee et al.	6.1 %	N.D.	3.05 %	N.D.	[38]
Boggs et al.	6.7 %	N.D.	2.85 %	N.D.	[5]
Boggs & Patrene	N.D.	N.D.	N.D.	8.4 % & 10.75 %[b]	[39]
Average:	6.5 %	3.5 %	3.1 %	9.6 %	

[a]N.D. = Not Determined
[b]Two different methods of preparation were performed yielding modestly different results

antigens that are not expressed on adult stem cells [45–51], but these antigens are observed on fetal HSCs [26, 27]. Moreover, CD33 expression on fetal peripheral blood HSCs ($CD34^+CD38^-$ and $CD34^+CD117^+$) has been shown to decline with gestational age, with its expression near absent at term birth [52]. Herein, we show that CD13 expression is lost from fetal HSCs maintained in NSG mice, and that CD33 expression also has declined but low level expression remains. The expression of these markers was similar for cBM and eBM. These data show at least a partial shift towards the adult HSC phenotype. HLA-DR expression remained high on engrafted $CD133^+$ HSCs, however, resembling the expression observed in midgestation fetal liver [26, 27]. There was also a shift towards more HLA-DR expression among early progenitors ($CD34^{++}CD133^-$) in the eBM than in the cBM. These findings are in contrast to adult cells for which evidence indicates that the most primitive hematopoietic precursors lack HLA-DR expression [29, 53–55]. Thus, based on HLA-DR expression, transplanted fetal HSCs do not appear to fully acquire an adult phenotype after long-term reconstitution in immunodeficient mice. It should be noted, however, that unavailability of data on the HSC phenotype in children leaves open the possibility that the human HSC phenotype observed in our engrafted mice is actually representative of a hypothetical transitional phenotype that may be observed in neonates and young children.

Conclusions

For most experiments requiring mouse BM cells, the single-cut method offers the simplest, most efficient and fastest method of BM isolation from the femur and tibia. The isolation of HSCs, however, is more complete using enzymatic digestion to harvest the eBM. Enzymatic digestion of human BM also increases the yield of cells and HSCs, but the effects of the digestion on cell-surface antigen expression must be tested to avoid false-negative results. Humanized mice offer an in vivo model to study trafficking of human HSC to the cBM and eBM niches with changes in phenotype noted as fetal HSCs aged in mice.

Abbreviations

AF700: Alexa Fluor 700; APC: Allophycocyanin; APC-Cy7: Allophycocyanin-cyanine 7; BM: Bone marrow; cBM: Central bone marrow; eBM: Endosteal bone marrow; FITC: Fluorescein isothiocyanate; HSC: Hematopoietic stem cell; Lin: Lineage; LSK: $Lin^-SCA\text{-}1^+CD117^+$; MSC: Mesenchymal stromal cell; NSG: NOD.Cg-*Prkdc*^{scid} *Il2rg*^{tm1Wjl}/SzJ; PB: Pacific blue; PBS: Phosphate-buffered saline; PE: Phycoerythrin; PE-Cy7: Phycoerythrin-cyanine 7; uPA-NOG: NOD.Cg-*Prkdc*^{scid} *Il2rg*^{tm1Sug} *Tg(Alb-Plau)11-4/* ShiJic.

Competing interests

The authors declare that they have no competing interests.

Authors' contributions

MMM, BC and AIB contributed equally to the work. MMM collected and analyzed data shown in Figs. 2 and 3. BC collected and analyzed data shown in Figs. 1 and 5–7. AIB collected and analyzed data shown in Figs. 4 and 8. USM helped coordinate and supervise the study of mouse BM collection and contributed to the collection of data for Fig. 3. MBW contributed to the collection of data for Fig. 3. MEF participated to the design and execution of mouse bone marrow isolation experiments and to the construction of humanized mice. MOM conceived of the study, participated in its design and coordination, and contributed to the statistical analysis of the data as well as overall manuscript preparation. All authors contributed to manuscript preparation and approved the final manuscript.

Author's information

Blood Systems Research Institute, 270 Masonic Ave.; San Francisco, CA 94118, USA and the Department of Laboratory Medicine, University of California San Francisco, CA 94143, USA.

Acknowledgements

We thank the staff and faculty at San Francisco General Hospital Women's Options Center for assistance in the collection of human fetal tissues. We thank Dale Hirschkorn for maintenance of the flow cytometry equipment and support in performing the flow cytometric analyses and Guilherme Salles Magalhaes for help processing bone marrow samples. We are also indebted to the administrative staff at our institute for their tireless support. This work was supported by the National Institutes of Health: P01DK088760 from the National Institute Of Diabetes And Digestive And Kidney Diseases. The content is solely the responsibility of the authors and does not necessarily represent the official views of the National Institute Of Diabetes And Digestive And Kidney Diseases or the National Institutes of Health. M.M.M. was supported by Blood Systems Inc. through the Blood Systems Research Institute Summer Internship Program. B.C., U.S.M. and M.B.W. were supported by a Bridges to Stem Cell Training grant TB1-01188 from the California Institute of Regenerative Medicine.

References

1. Soleimani M, Nadri S. A protocol for isolation and culture of mesenchymal stem cells from mouse bone marrow. Nat Protoc. 2009;4:102–6.
2. Fei RG, Penn PE, Wolf NS. A method to establish pure fibroblast and endothelial cell colony cultures from murine bone marrow. Exp Hematol. 1990;18:953–7.
3. Hasthorpe S, Green SL, Rogerson J, Radley JM. A mouse endothelial cell-specific monoclonal antibody: its reactivity with LTMC endothelium. Exp Hematol. 1991;19:166–9.
4. Hattersley G, Chambers TJ. Effects of interleukin 3 and of granulocyte-macrophage and macrophage colony stimulating factors on osteoclast differentiation from mouse hemopoietic tissue. J Cell Physiol. 1990;142:201–9.
5. Boggs DR. The total marrow mass of the mouse: a simplified method of measurement. Am J Hematol. 1984;16:277–86.
6. Lansdorp PM, Dragowska W. Long-term erythropoiesis from constant numbers of CD34+ cells in serum-free cultures initiated with highly purified progenitor cells from human bone marrow. J Exp Med. 1992;175:1501–9.
7. Söderdahl G, Tammik C, Remberger M, Ringdén O. Cadaveric bone marrow and spleen cells for transplantation. Bone Marrow Transplant. 1998;21:79–84.
8. Baum CM, Weissman IL, Tsukamoto AS, Buckle AM, Peault B. Isolation of a candidate human hematopoietic stem-cell population. Proc Natl Acad Sci U S A. 1992;89:2804–8.
9. Slaper-Cortenbach I, Ploemacher R, Löwenberg B. Different stimulative effects of human bone marrow and fetal liver stromal cells on erythropoiesis in long-term culture. Blood. 1987;69:135–9.
10. Brouard N, Chapel A, Thierry D, Charbord P, Péault B. Transplantation of gene-modified human bone marrow stromal cells into mouse-human bone chimeras. J Hematother Stem Cell Res. 2000;9:175–81.

11. Michejda M, Bellanti JA, Mazumder A, Verma UN, Wu AG. Comparative study of hemopoietic precursors from fetal and adult bone marrow: utilization of stem cells derived from miscarriages. Fetal Diagn Ther. 1996;11:373–82.
12. Golfier F, Bárcena A, Harrison MR, Muench MO. Fetal bone marrow as a source of stem cells for in utero or postnatal transplantation. Br J Haematol. 2000;109:173–81.
13. Lee WY, Zhang T, Lau CP, Wang CC, Chan KM, Li G. Immortalized human fetal bone marrow-derived mesenchymal stromal cell expressing suicide gene for anti-tumor therapy in vitro and in vivo. Cytotherapy. 2013;15:1484–97.
14. Lord BI. The architecture of bone marrow cell populations. Int J Cell Cloning. 1990;8:317–31.
15. Lord BI, Hendry JH. The distribution of haemopoietic colony-forming units in the mouse femur, and its modification by x rays. Br J Radiol. 1972;45:110–5.
16. Lord BI, Testa NG, Hendry JH. The relative spatial distributions of CFUs and CFUc in the normal mouse femur. Blood. 1975;46:65–72.
17. Grassinger J, Haylock DN, Williams B, Olsen GH, Nilsson SK. Phenotypically identical hemopoietic stem cells isolated from different regions of bone marrow have different biologic potential. Blood. 2010;116:3185–96.
18. Guezguez B, Campbell CJ, Boyd AL, Karanu F, Casado FL, Di Cresce C, et al. Regional localization within the bone marrow influences the functional capacity of human hscs. Cell Stem Cell. 2013;13:175–89.
19. Shultz LD, Ishikawa F, Greiner DL. Humanized mice in translational biomedical research. Nat Rev Immunol. 2007;7:118–30.
20. Haylock DN, Williams B, Johnston HM, Liu MC, Rutherford KE, Whitty GA, et al. Hemopoietic stem cells with higher hemopoietic potential reside at the bone marrow endosteum. Stem Cells. 2007;25:1062–9.
21. Suemizu H, Hasegawa M, Kawai K, Taniguchi K, Monnai M, Wakui M, et al. Establishment of a humanized model of liver using NOD/Shi-scid IL2Rgnull mice. Biochem Biophys Res Commun. 2008;377:248–52.
22. Fomin ME, Zhou Y, Beyer AI, Publicover J, Baron JL, Muench MO. Production of factor VIII by human liver sinusoidal endothelial cells transplanted in immunodeficient uPA mice. PLoS One. 2013;8:e77255.
23. Muench MO, Beyer AI, Fomin ME, Thakker R, Mulvaney US, Nakamura M, et al. The adult livers of immunodeficient mice support human hematopoiesis: evidence for a hepatic mast cell population that develops early in human ontogeny. PLoS One. 2014;9:e97312.
24. Varga NL, Bárcena A, Fomin ME, Muench MO. Detection of human hematopoietic stem cell engraftment in the livers of adult immunodeficient mice by an optimized flow cytometric method. Stem Cell Stud. 2010;1:e5.
25. Craig W, Kay R, Cutler RL, Lansdorp PM. Expression of Thy-1 on human hematopoietic progenitor cells. J Exp Med. 1993;177:1331–42.
26. Muench MO, Cupp J, Polakoff J, Roncarolo MG. Expression of CD33, CD38, and HLA-DR on CD34+ human fetal liver progenitors with a high proliferative potential. Blood. 1994;83:3170–81.
27. Muench MO, Roncarolo MG, Namikawa R. Phenotypic and functional evidence for the expression of CD4 by hematopoietic stem cells isolated from human fetal liver. Blood. 1997;89:1364–75.
28. Sutherland HJ, Eaves CJ, Eaves AC, Dragowska W, Lansdorp PM. Characterization and partial purification of human marrow cells capable of initiating long-term hematopoiesis in vitro. Blood. 1989;74:1563–70.
29. Verfaillie C, Blakolmer K, McGlave P. Purified primitive human hematopoietic progenitor cells with long-term in vitro repopulating capacity adhere selectively to irradiated bone marrow stroma. J Exp Med. 1990;172:509–2.
30. Srour EF, Brandt JE, Briddell RA, Leemhuis T, van Besien K, Hoffman R. Human CD34+ HLA-DR- bone marrow cells contain progenitor cells capable of self-renewal, multilineage differentiation, and long-term in vitro hematopoiesis. Blood Cells. 1991;17:287–95.
31. Rongvaux A, Takizawa H, Strowig T, Willinger T, Eynon EE, Flavell RA, et al. Human hemato-lymphoid system mice: current use and future potential for medicine. Annu Rev Immunol. 2013;31:635–74.
32. Muench MO, Schneider JG, Moore MA. Interactions among colony-stimulating factors, IL-1 beta, IL-6, and kit-ligand in the regulation of primitive murine hematopoietic cells. Exp Hematol. 1992;20:339–49.
33. Muench MO, Firpo MT, Moore MA. Bone marrow transplantation with interleukin-1 plus kit-ligand ex vivo expanded bone marrow accelerates hematopoietic reconstitution in mice without the loss of stem cell lineage and proliferative potential. Blood. 1993;81:3463–73.
34. Chervenick PA, Boggs DR, Marsh JC, Cartwright GE, Wintrobe MM. Quantitative studies of blood and bone marrow neutrophils in normal mice. Am J Physiol. 1968;215:353–60.
35. Schofield R, Cole LJ. An erythrocyte defect in splenectomized x-irradiated mice restored with spleen colony cells. Br J Haematol. 1968;14:131–40.
36. Briganti G, Covelli V, Silini G, Srivastava PN. The distribution of erythropoietic bone marrow in the mouse. Acta Haematol. 1970;44:355–61.
37. Papayannopoulou T, Finch CA. On the in vivo action of erythropoietin: a quantitative analysis. J Clin Invest. 1972;51:1179–85.
38. Lee M, Durch S, Dale D, Finch C. Kinetics of tumor-induced murine neutrophilia. Blood. 1979;53:619–32.
39. Boggs DR, Patrene KD. Marrow mass and distribution in murine skeletons cleaned by beetles as compared to cut up carcasses and a further simplification of the latter technique. Am J Hematol. 1986;21:49–55.
40. Westgren M, Ek S, Bui TH, Hagenfeldt L, Markling L, Pschera H, et al. Establishment of a tissue bank for fetal stem cell transplantation. Acta Obstet Gynecol Scand. 1994;73:385–8.
41. Jones DR, Anderson EM, Evans AA, Liu DT. Long-term storage of human fetal haematopoietic progenitor cells and their subsequent reconstitution. Implications for in utero transplantation. Bone Marrow Transplant. 1995;16:297–301.
42. Mychaliska GB, Muench MO, Rice HE, Leavitt AD, Cruz J, Harrison MR. The biology and ethics of banking fetal liver hematopoietic stem cells for in utero transplantation. J Pediatr Surg. 1998;33:394–9.
43. Theilgaard-Mönch K, Raaschou-Jensen K, Palm H, Schjødt K, Heilmann C, Vindeløv L, et al. Flow cytometric assessment of lymphocyte subsets, lymphoid progenitors, and hematopoietic stem cells in allogeneic stem cell grafts. Bone Marrow Transplant. 2001;28:1073–82.
44. Cairo MS, Wagner EL, Fraser J, Cohen G, van de Ven C, Carter SL, et al. Characterization of banked umbilical cord blood hematopoietic progenitor cells and lymphocyte subsets and correlation with ethnicity, birth weight, sex, and type of delivery: a Cord Blood Transplantation (COBLT) Study report. Transfusion. 2005;45:856–66.
45. Griffin JD, Ritz J, Nadler LM, Schlossman SF. Expression of myeloid differentiation antigens on normal and malignant myeloid cells. J Clin Invest. 1981;68:932–41.
46. Andrews RG, Torok-Storb B, Bernstein ID. Myeloid-associated differentiation antigens on stem cells and their progeny identified by monoclonal antibodies. Blood. 1983;62:124–32.
47. Andrews RG, Singer JW, Bernstein ID. Precursors of colony-forming cells in humans can be distinguished from colony-forming cells by expression of the CD33 and CD34 antigens and light scatter properties. J Exp Med. 1989;169:1721–31.
48. Litzow MR, Brashem-Stein C, Andrews RG, Bernstein ID. Proliferative responses to interleukin-3 and granulocyte colony-stimulating factor distinguish a minor subpopulation of CD34-positive marrow progenitors that do not express CD33 and a novel antigen, 7B9. Blood. 1991;77:2354–9.
49. Terstappen LW, Huang S, Safford M, Lansdorp PM, Loken MR. Sequential generations of hematopoietic colonies derived from single nonlineage-committed CD34 + CD38- progenitor cells. Blood. 1991;77:1218–27.
50. Robertson MJ, Soiffer RJ, Freedman AS, Rabinowe SL, Anderson KC, Ervin TJ, et al. Human bone marrow depleted of CD33-positive cells mediates delayed but durable reconstitution of hematopoiesis: clinical trial of MY9 monoclonal antibody-purged autografts for the treatment of acute myeloid leukemia. Blood. 1992;79:2229–36.
51. Shipp MA, Look AT. Hematopoietic differentiation antigens that are membrane-associated enzymes: cutting is the key! Blood. 1993;82:1052–70.
52. Jin CH, Takada H, Nomura A, Takahata Y, Nakayama H, Kajiwara M, et al. Immunophenotypic and functional characterization of CD33(+)CD34(+) cells in human cord blood of preterm neonates. Exp Hematol. 2000;28:1174–80.
53. Moore MA, Broxmeyer HE, Sheridan AP, Meyers PA, Jacobsen N, Winchester RJ. Continuous human bone marrow culture: Ia antigen characterization of probable pluripotential stem cells. Blood. 1980;55:682–90.
54. Keating A, Powell J, Takahashi M, Singer JW. The generation of human long-term marrow cultures from marrow depleted of Ia (HLA-DR) positive cells. Blood. 1984;64:1159–62.
55. Prosper F, Stroncek D, Verfaillie CM. Phenotypic and functional characterization of long-term culture-initiating cells present in peripheral blood progenitor collections of normal donors treated with granulocyte colony-stimulating factor. Blood. 1996;88:2033–42.

2

Prevention practices influencing frequency of occurrence of vaso-occlusive crisis among sickle cell patients in Abeokuta South Local Government Area of Ogun State, Nigeria

Olorunfemi Emmanuel Amoran[1*], Ahmed Babatunde Jimoh[2], Omotola Ojo[3] and Temitope Kuponiyi[1]

Abstract

Background: Africa is the most affected continent with 200,000 new born affected by sickle cell anemia annually with of 5% of under five deaths. Nigeria has the largest sickle cell gene pool in the world with about 2% of all babies born to Nigerian parents. This study therefore sets out to assess the prevention practices influencing the frequency of occurrence of vaso-occlusive crisis among patients in Ogun State.

Methods: This study is a descriptive cross-sectional study conducted in Abeokuta South Local Government Area Ogun State. A consecutive non randomized sampling of all the sickle cell patients that attend the selected facilities was recruited into the study. Data were collected with the use of questionnaires which were interviewer administered. A total of 415 patients were recruited into the study. Statistical analyses were conducted using SPSS for Windows version 20.0.

Result: Two- third [64.8%] of study participants have crisis twice or more in a month. The frequency of crisis was statistically significantly associated with the age of the child [$p = 0.006$], use of anti-malaria prophylaxis [$p = 0.006$], analgesics [$p = 0.0001$], taking of plenty fluid [$p = 0.001$] and soothing herbs [$p = 0.0001$]. Lifestyle factors such as giving balance diet [$p = 0.217$], restriction from strenuous activities [$p = 0.08$], and attending Clinic appointments regularly [$p = 0.126$] were not statistically associated with reduction in the frequency of crisis. Logistic regression analysis shows that predictors of frequent crisis were individuals who were using prophylaxis antimalarial drugs [OR = 0.12, CI = 0.05–0.33] and analgesics [OR = 0.15, C.I = 0.06–0.34].

Conclusion: The study reveals that majority of the participants have high frequency of crisis in a month. Drug prophylaxis rather than lifestyle factors may be more important in the prevention of vaso-occlusive crisis among sickle cell patients.

Background

Sickle cell anaemia contributes the equivalent of 5% of under five deaths on the African continent, more than 9% of such deaths in west Africa, and up to 16% of under-five deaths in individual west African countries [1]. Africa is the most affected continent with 200,000 new born affected by sickle cell anemia per year. This constitutes approximately 66.6% of the children born with haemoglobinopathies worldwide [2]. Nigeria has the largest sickle cell gene pool in the world. The sickle cell trait prevalence in Nigeria ranges from 25 to 35%. About 2% of all babies born to Nigerian parents have sickle cell anaemia. Two per hundred births translates to over 150,000 births annually of children with sickle cell anaemia [1]. The prevalence of SCD in Uganda is believed to be the highest in the whole world and it accounts for approximately 16.2% of all pediatric deaths [2].

* Correspondence: drfamoran@yahoo.com
[1]Department of Community Medicine and Primary Care, Olabisi Onabanjo University Teaching Hospital, Sagamu, Nigeria
Full list of author information is available at the end of the article

Appropriate prevention practices and proper management will lead to reduction in the frequency of vaso-occlusive crisis. SCD patients presents with symptoms such as vaso-occlusive pain crises, anemia, dactylitis or hand-foot syndrome, eye damage, splenic sequestration etc. [3–6]. These symptoms occurs in SCD patients as a result of blood cells sticking to the walls of the blood vessels in the brain limiting blood flow [7]. Timely intervention and appropriate prevention practices is essential in the prevention of complications of vaso-occlusive crisis [8–16].

Children with SCD need optimal family support, understanding and care, especially in terms of providing adequate nutrition and health care delivery so as to achieve an optimum and steady state of health. Such favorable family environment and appropriate prevention measures has been shown to be a good prognostic index [17, 18]. The psychosocial burden and stress parents of sickle cell patients undergo could influence their attitude towards the care of their children positively or negatively. This study therefore sets out to assess the prevention practices influencing the frequency of occurrence of vaso-occlusive crisis among patients in Ogun State... Their knowledge and practices towards reducing the frequency and seeking appropriate treatment of vaso-occlusive crisis in their children is inevitable and also help in improving the quality of life of these children.

Methods

Study location and population

Abeokuta South is a Local Government Area in Ogun State, Nigeria. It was established in 1991 and mainly inhabited by the Egbas, who are of Egba Eku, Egba Aarin and Egba Igbeyin. The headquarter of the LGA is at Abeokuta7°09′00″N 3°21′00″E. It has an area of 71 km^2 and a population of 250,278 at the 2006 census. The Local Government shares border with Odede LGA on its North frontier, Obafemi/Owode on the Eastern while Abeokuta North LGA on the Southern part respectively. The Local Government is divided into 15wards for the purpose of electing councilors into the Local Government Council. Each electoral ward has primary health centre, private clinics, laboratories, pharmacy shops, and traditional birth attendants.

Study design

This study is a descriptive cross-sectional study to describe systematically the prevention practices influencing the frequency of occurrence of vaso-occlusive crisis among patients Abeokuta south Local Government Area of Ogun State, Nigeria.

Setting

This study was conducted in State Hospital Sokenu, Abeokuta and Egba Medical Centre, Isabo, Abeokuta both in Abeokuta South Local Government Area. The two hospitals are the two major sickle cell treatment centre in Abeokuta South LGA, Ogun State.

Sampling technique

A consecutive non randomized sampling of all the sickle cell patients that attend the selected facilities was used to recruit participants into the study.

Sample size determination

The minimum number of subjects required for the study is calculated using the formula :

Minimum sample size, n = Z2 p q/d2

Where Z is the standard deviation set at 1.96 at 95% confidence interval, p = prevalence set at 50%, q = 1-p, and d = degree of accuracy set at 0.05

$$n = Z2\,\mathrm{pq}/\mathrm{d2}$$

$$= \frac{1.96\ 2\ \mathrm{x}0.5\mathrm{x}0.5}{0.05^2} = 384.$$

n was calculated to be 384.

A total of 415 participants were recruited.

Data collection method

Data were collected with the use of interviewer administered pre-validated questionnaire. The interviewers were volunteer Doctors, Nurses and Laboratory Scientists. The interviewers were previously briefed on the nature and significance of the study and they were trained on how to administer the questionnaire under supervision. On the clinic days of each selected health facility, the researchers meet the participants, re- explained the purpose of the study and assured them of confidentiality of privileged information and a feedback after the study as told to them in the last meeting. The study was conducted between January and April 2015.

Ethical approval

Ethical approval to conduct the study was obtained from the ethical committee of the Olabisi Onabanjo University Teaching Hospital, Sagamu. Permission was also obtained from the selected health facilities for the study, discussed with the Officers in-charge on the aims and objectives of the study, the procedure and feedback was assured which could contribute to the management of their patients. At the end of each meeting with the hospital management, verbal consent was obtained.

Written consent was obtained from the study participants before the commencement of the study. The participants were met on the day of clinics by the researchers and the purpose, general content and nature of the study were explained and they were given assurance of confidentiality of information offered and feedback at the end of the study.

For participants under the age of 16, written parental consent was obtained. All the patients have their parents or guardians present in the clinic with them to care for them.

Data analysis

Statistical analyses were conducted using SPSS for Windows version 20.0 First, descriptive statistics were generated for each survey measure. Quantitative data collected was checked for errors, cleaned and entered. Data was summarized with proportions and means and presented using frequency tables. Frequency of crisis was categorized as either Once or less monthly (low frequency) and twice or more monthly as high frequency of crisis.

Variables such as plenty fluid was elicited by asking how many glass of cup of water do you take daily- showing them a 500mls cup. Three litres [6 glass of cup daily] was classified as adequate. Balance diet was taken as the description of diet containing carbohydrate, protein and fats for three previous meals. A strenuous activity was described as patient's involvement in additional non routine, high oxygen demanding activities.

Bivariate analyses using the X^2 test were used to compare the socio-demographics of participants with the frequency of sickle cell crisis status of their child. The level of statistical significance was set at 5%. A logistic regression model was produced with low and high frequency of crisis as outcome variable. All explanatory variables that were associated with the outcome variable in bivariate analyses, variables with a P-value of ≤0.05 were included in the logistic models.

Results

Socio-dermographic characteristics of study participants

A total of 415 patients were recruited into the study. About half 42.7% of participants' with SCD age is between 5 and 9 years, 29.4% were under-fives, 22.4% were adolescents aged between 10 and 19 years, 4.8% were young adults between 20 and 24 years and 0.7% of them were 25 years and above. Sex distribution of the children with SCD showed that 53.5% were male and 46.5% females. A third [35.2%] have crisis once or less in a month, 46% have crisis twice in a month, 18.8% have crisis thrice or more in a month (Table 1).

Practice of vaso-occlusive crisis prevention methods

Table 2 shows the distribution on the method of treating SCD crisis, 79% give pain relief drugs at home, 60.7% give anti-malarial, 5.3% patronize local chemist, 2.9% take them to traditional healers/missionary homes while 29.6% more use of herbal remedies, 93.0% parent takes the child to the hospital and 82.4% of participant often meet doctor on duty, 15.9% reasonably often. Table 3 shows the distribution of participants on the method of preventing crisis, 77.3% give plenty of fluids, 73.5% take balance diet, 66.3% use insecticide treated net, 53.7% give prophylaxis drugs, 64.8% dress child in warm clothing, 45.5% restrict child from strenuous oxygen demanding activity, 2.9% sought spiritual means and 42.7% keep clinic appointments whether there's crisis or not.

Table 1 Demographic Characteristics of study Participants

VARIABLES	FREQUENCY (n = 415)	PERCENTAGE (%)
Age of Participants with SCD		
1–4 years	122	29.4
5–9 years	177	42.7
10–14 years	66	15.9
15–19 years	27	6.5
20–24 years	20	4.8
25 years & above	3	0.7
Total	415	100.0
Sex of Participants with SCD		
Male	222	53.5
Female	193	46.5
Total	415	100.0
Number of Siblings lost due to SCD		
One	62	14.9
Two	10	2.4
Three	4	1.0
Four	1	0.2
None	338	81.4
Total	415	100.0

Factors associated with frequency of crisis

The frequency of vaso-occlusive crisis was statistically significantly associated with the age of the participant with SCD [$X^2 = 16.412$, $p = 0.006$] and use of anti-malaria prophylactics [$X^2 = 7.697$, $p = 0.006$], analgesics [$X^2 = 29.186$, $p = 0.0001$], and soothing herbs [$X^2 = 16.918$, $p = 0.0001$]. There was however no statistically significant relationship between frequency of vaso-occlusive crisis and the Sex of the child with SCD [$X^2 = 16.412$, $p = 0.06$], and the number of siblings with SCD [$X^2 = 7.086$, $p = 0.131$].

Lifestyle factors such as giving balance diet [$X^2 = 1.524$, $p = 0.217$], Restriction from strenuous activities [$X^2 = 3.072$, $p = 0.08$], and attending clinic appointments regularly [$X^2 = 2.345$, $p = 0.126$] were not statistically associated with reduction in the frequency of crisis. While taking of plenty of fluid was statistically significantly

Table 2 Practice of vaso-occlusive crisis Prevention Methods

METHODS OF PREVENTING SC CRISIS	FREQUENCY (*n* = 415)	PERCENTAGE (%)
Giving Plenty Fluids		
Yes	321	77.3
No	94	22.7
Total	415	100.0
Giving Balance diet		
Yes	305	73.5
No	110	26.5
Total	415	100.0
Ensure Sleeping Under ITN		
Yes	275	66.3
No	140	33.7
Total	415	100.0
Giving Prophylactic Drugs		
Yes	223	53.7
No	192	46.3
Total	415	100.0
Dressed in Warm Clothing		
Yes	269	64.8
No	146	35.2
Total	415	100.0
Restriction from Strenuous Activity		
Yes	189	45.5
No	226	54.5
Total	415	100.0
Keep Clinic Appointments		
Yes	177	42.7
No	238	57.3
Total	415	100.0
Sought Spiritual Means		
Yes	12	2.9
No	403	97.1
Total	415	100.0

Table 3 Use of Prophylaxis in Prevention of vaso-occlusive crisis

METHOD OF TREATING SC CRISIS	FREQUENCY (*n* = 415)	PERCENTAGE (%)
Give Pain Relieving Drugs at Home		
Yes	328	79.0
No	87	21.0
Total	415	100.0
Give Anti-malaria Drug at Home		
Yes	252	60.7
No	163	39.3
Total	415	100.0
Take Child to Nearby Chemist		
Yes	22	5.3
No	393	94.7
Total	415	100.0
Take Child to Traditional healer/Missionary home		
Yes	12	2.9
No	403	97.1
Total	415	100.0
Give Local Herbal Remedies at Home		
Yes	123	29.6
No	292	70.4
Total	415	100.0
Take Child to The Hospital		
Yes	386	93.0
No	29	7.0
Total	415	100.0
How often they meet Doctor on duty		
Often	342	82.4
Reasonably often	66	15.9
Not often	7	1.7
Total	415	100.0

associated with low frequency of crisis [$X^2 = 13.44$, $p = 0.001$]. This is as shown in Table 4.

In the multiple logistic regression models, two variables were found to be independently associated with frequency of crisis. Predictors of low frequent crisis were individuals who were using prophylaxis antimalarial drugs [OR = 0.12, CI = 0.05–0.33] and analgesics [OR = 0.15, C.I = 0.06–0.34]. Herbs [OR = 3.74, C.I = 0.71–19.73], age of child [OR = 0.063, C.I = 0.001–4.11] and taking plenty of fluid [OR = 1.02, C.I = 0.27–3.78] were not predictors. This is shown in Table 5.

Discussion

The study reveals that majority of the participants have high frequency of crisis in a month despite adequate knowledge in the prevention of crisis and predisposing factors. The high frequency of sickle cell crisis amongst the participants is similar to what has been reported in previous studies [17–19] which reveals that there is overall increase in frequency of vaso occlusive crisis in paediatric SCD that its associated with poorer paediatric quality of life and increases in the psychosocial maladjustment of their caregivers. Obviously, knowledge does not translate to practice, however the prevention of vaso occlusive crisis requires huge financial capability which most of the parents cannot afford.

The age of the participants with SCD shows significant influence in the frequency of crisis, those participants in

Table 4 Factors associated with frequency of vaso-occlusive crisis

GIVING PLENTY FLUIDS	FREQUENCY OF CRISIS IN A MONTH		TOTAL
	LOW	HIGH	
YES	98(67.1%)	223(82.9%)	321(77.3%)
NO	48(32.9%)	46(17.1%)	94(22.7%)
TOTAL	146(100.0%)	269(100.0%)	415(100.0%)
FEEDING WITH BALANCE DIET			
YES	102(69.9%)	203(75.5%)	305(73.5%)
NO	44(30.1%)	66(24.5%)	110(26.5%)
TOTAL	146(100.0%)	269(100.0%)	415(100.0%)
\USE OF ITN			
YES	89(61.0%)	186(69.1%)	275(66.3%) 0.092
NO	57(39.0%)	83(30.9%)	140(33.7%)
TOTAL	146(100.0%)	269(100.0%)	415(100.0%)
USE OF PROPHYLAXIS DRUGS			
YES	65(44.5%)	158(58.7%)	223(53.7%) 0.006
NO	81(55.5%)	111(41.3%)	192(46.3%)
TOTAL	146(100.0%)	269(100.0%)	415(100.0%)
DRESSED IN WARM CLOTHING			
YES	98(67.1%)	171(63.6%)	269(64.8%) 0.479
NO	48(32.9%)	98(36.4%)	146(35.2%)
TOTAL	146(100.0%)	269(100.0%)	415(100.0%)
RESTRICTION FROM STRENOUS ACTIVITY			
YES	58(39.7%)	131(48.7%)	189(45.5%) 0.08
NO	88(60.3%)	138(51.3%)	226(54.5%)
TOTAL	146(100.0%)	269(100.0%)	415(100.0%)
GIVING ANTI-MALARIA DRUGS AT HOME			
YES	69(47.3%)	183(68.0%)	252(60.7%) .0001
NO	77(52.7%)	63(32.0%)	163(39.3%)
TOTAL	146(100.0%)	269(100.0%)	415(100.0%)
TAKEN TO THE HOSPITAL			
YES	132(90.4%)	254(94.4%)	386(93.0%) 0.126
NO	14(9.6%)	15(5.6%)	29(7.0%)
TOTAL	146(100.0%)	269(100.0%)	415(100.0%)
USE OF LOCAL HERBAL REMEDIES			
YES	25(17.1%)	98(36.4%)	123(29.6%) 0.0001
NO	121(82.9%)	171(63.6%)	292(70.4%)
TOTAL	146(100.0)	269(100.0%)	415(100.0%)
USE OF ANALGESICS AT HOME			
YES	94(64.4%)	234(87.0%)	328(79.0%) 0.001
NO	52(35.6%)	35(13.0%)	87(21.0%)
TOTAL	146(100.0%)	269(100.0%)	415(100.0%)

older age group shows significant proportion having low frequency of crisis monthly as they are probably more mature to understand the cause and consequence of the disease, follow rules and regulations,use their drugs when due and show the appropriate attitude towards preventing the frequency of crisis [15, 16]. They are able to detect and complain earlier about the onset of crisis and even seek appropriate treatment before it becomes severe.

Table 5 Multivariate logistic Regression

	Odds Ratio [C.I]
Age of Participants	
Nil	1.00
Primary	0.063 [0.001–4.11]
Secondary	0.11 [0.002–6.63]
Tertiary	0.08 [0.001–5,47]
Antimalarial prophylaxis	
Yes	0.122 [0.05–0.33]
No	1.00
Analgesics	
Yes	0.145 [0.06–0.34]
No	1.00
Herbal use	
Yes	3.74 [0.71–19.73]
No	1.00
Taking Plenty of fluid	
Yes	1.02 [0.27–3.78]
No	1.00

However, more than half of the participants have adequate knowledge of how to prevent vaso-occlusive crisis. In this study majority had the practice of giving balance diet, giving plenty of fluid to prevent dehydration, use of analgesic and taking the patient to the hospital when severe. Over 90% of the participant knows that crisis could not be managed by chemist (road side drug sellers). Several studies have highlighted the fact that in Africa parents and patients have inadequate information on how to prevent vaso-occlusive crisis [1, 20]. This is an indication that parents/caregivers need more information on the disease and there is need for health education to be intensified. A vigorous enlightenment campaign on sickle cell disease should be put in place through appropriate media like print and electronics. National Sickle Cell Centre should be developed to facilitate the development of National control programme, which will be integrated with the National Health Service.

The patronage of traditional healers and missionary homes and the use of local herbs have influence in the frequency of crisis as majority of the participants who use local herbs or seek treatment at the traditional healers have high frequency of sickle cell crisis. This can further worsen the QOL of the SCD child as the herbs given could accelerates the damage to major organs there by leading to increase in morbidity and mortality. The cultural values and believe of the people play a major role in their belief about the cause and form of treatment of diseases generally and SCD is not an exception. Several studies [21–23] have concluded that cultural beliefs have an influence on health and that illness can be caused by natural, preternatural and mystical factors. The preternatural explanation is related to belief in witchcraft where the onset of illness is attributed to the evil machination of an enemy and in most cultures, there is belief that sorcerer, wizard and malevolent human being can cause illness, including sickle cell disease. If parents believe their child is bewitched they are not likely to come to the hospital or follow medical advice if they do.

This study shows that drug prophylaxis rather than lifestyle factors modification may be more important in the reduction of frequency of vaso-occlusive crisis. Several studies have highlighted the importance of both drug prophylaxis and lifestyle modification in the prevention of vaso-occlusive crisis among sickle cell patients [8–14] Further experimental studies will be needed to ascertain which of this is more essential in the prevention of vaso-occlusive crisis but ethical issues in the conduct of such experimental studies will be a serious limitation. However, medical treatment of sickle cell disease should be highly subsidized to make it affordable and accessible for all. Counselling sessions should be encouraged in all treatment centres in order to reduce the burden of the disease.

Conclusion

The high incidence of SCD in Nigeria makes it a public health burden. Overall knowledge about sickle cell disease is poor which makes it difficult to combat the outrageous disease. Health authorities and institutions should adopt measures that have been shown to be effective in the management of sickle cell disorder. More centres should be established for the management of SCD patients and more health personnels should be recruited to these centres for more effective control of the disease.

Acknowledgements

We hereby acknowledge all the research assistants for their participation, encouragement and motivation during the design and conduct of the study.

Funding

The conduct of this research was funded by the contribution of the Authors.

Authors' contributions

JBA participated in the study design and conducted data collection. OEA conceived the study theme, participated in the study design, supervised data collection and prepared the final manuscript. OOO was involved in Data collection and analysis. ALL authors read and approved the final manuscript and gave their consent for publication.

Competing interests

The authors declare that they have no competing interests.

Author details

[1]Department of Community Medicine and Primary Care, Olabisi Onabanjo University Teaching Hospital, Sagamu, Nigeria. [2]State Hospital Ala, Sagamu, Nigeria. [3]Department of Heamatology, College of Health Sciences, Olabisi Onabanjo University Teaching Hospital, Sagamu, Nigeria.

References

1. World Health Organization. Sickle Cell Anaemia Report by the Secretariat. Fifty ninth World Health Assembly [homepage on the internet]. C2006. 2011. Avaible from http://www.afro.who.int/en/nigeria/nigeria-publications/1775-sickle%20cell%20disease.html.
2. Diallo D, Tchernia G. Sickle cell in Africa. Currie Opine Hematol. 2002;9(2): 111–6. doi:10.1097/00062752-200203000-0005.
3. Schatz J, McClellan CB. Sickle cell disease as a neurodevelopmental disorder. Ment Retard Dev Disabil Res Rev. 2006;12:200–7. doi:10.1002/mrdd.20115.
4. Shapiro BS. Management of painful episodes in sickle cell disease. In: Schechter NL, Berde CB, Yaster M, editors. Pain in Infants, Children and Adolescents. Baltimore: Williams and Wikins; 1993.
5. Midence K, Shand P. Family and social issues in sickle cell disease. Health Visit. 1992;65:441–3.
6. Akinyanju OO, Otaigbe AI, Ibidapo MO. Outcome of holistic care in Nigerian patients with sickle cell anaemia. Clin Lab Haematol. 2005;27:195–199. http://dx.doi.org/10.1111/j.1365-2257.2005.00683.x. (Epub 2005/06/09. PubMed PMID:15938726).
7. Aneni EC, Hamer DH, Gill CJ. Systematic review of current and emerging strategies for reducing morbidity from malaria in sickle cell disease. Trop Med Int Health. 2013;18:313–27. (Epub 2013/01/17. PubMed PMID: 23320577).
8. Brown RT, Buchanan I, Doepke K, Eckman JR, Baldwin K, Goonan B, Shoenherr S. Cognitive and academic functioning in children with sickle cell disease. J Clin Child Psychol. 1993;22:207. doi:10.1207/S15374424JCCP2202_740.
9. Brown RT, Kaslow NJ, Doepke K, Buchanan I, Eckman J, Baldwin K, et al. Psychosocial and family functioning in children with sickle cell syndrome and their mothers. J Am Acad Child Adolesc Psychiatry. 1993;32:545–53. doi:10.1097/00004583-19930500-00009.
10. Chapar GN. Chronic diseases of children and neuropsychologicdysfunction. J Dev Behav Paediatr. 1988;9:221–2.
11. Daily BP, Kral MC, Brown RT. Cognitive and academic problems associated with childhood cancers and sickle cell disease. Sch Psychol Q. 2008;23:12. doi:10.1037/1045-3830.23.2.230.
12. Fowler MG, Johnson MP, Atkinson SS. School achievement and absence in children with chronic health conditions. J Paediatr. 1985;106:683–7. doi:10.1016/s0022-3476(85)80103-7.
13. Fowler MG, Whitt JK, Lallinger RR, Nash KB, Atkinson SS, Wells RJ, et al. Neuropsychologic and academic functioning of children with sickle cell anemia. J Dev Behav Paediatr. 1988;9:213–20.
14. Odesina V. Sickle cell pain management in the emergency department: A two phase quality improvement project. Adv Emerg Nurs J. 2010;32:102–11.
15. Balkaran B, Char G, Morris JS, Thomas PW, Serjeant BE, Serjeant GR. Stroke in a cohort of patients with homozygous sickle cell disease. J Paediatr. 1992; 120:360–6. doi:10.1016/S0022-3476(05)80897-2.
16. Ohene-frempong K, Weiner SJ, Sleeper LA, Miller ST, Embury S, Moohr JW, et al. Cerebrovascular accidents in sickle cell disease: rates and risks factors. Blood. 1998;91:288–94.
17. Aliyu ZY, Kato GJ, Taylor Jt, Babadoko A, Mamman AI, Gordeuk VR, et al. Sickle cell disease and pulmonary hypertension in Africa: A global perspective and review of epidemiology, pathophysiology, and management. Am J Hematol. 2008;83:63–70. http://dx.doi.org/10.1002/ajh.21057. (Epub 2007/10/03. PubMed PMID: 17910044).
18. Kral MC, Brown RT, Hynd GW. Neuropsychological aspects of pediatric sickle cell disease. Neuropsychol Rev. 2001;11:179–96. doi:10.1023/A:1012901124088.
19. Welkom JS. Georgia State University. The impact of sickle cell disease on the family: An Examination of the illness intrusiveness framework. 2012.
20. Katibi IA. Anthropometric Profiles of Homozygous Sickle Cell Children in North-western Nigeria. AJOL. 2008;11:2.
21. Jaffer ED, Amrallah KF, Ali MK, Mohammed AN, Hassan AR, Humood MZ. Adult sickle cell disease patient's knowledge and attitude towards preventive measure of sickle cell disease crisis. 2009.
22. Muscari ME. Pediatric nursing. 4th ed. USA: Lippnocott Williams and Wikings; 2005.

3

Endothelial fibrinolytic response onto an evolving matrix of fibrin

O. Castillo[1,2], H. Rojas[3,4], Z. Domínguez[5], E. Anglés-Cano[6,7] and R. Marchi[1*]

Abstract

Background: Fibrin provides a temporary matrix at the site of vascular injury. The aims of the present work were (1) to follow fibrin formation and lysis onto the surface of human dermal microvascular endothelial cells (HMEC-1), and (2) to quantify the secretion of fibrinolytic components in the presence of fibrin.

Methods: Fibrin clots at different fibrinogen concentrations were formed on top of (model 1) or beneath (model 2) the endothelial cells. Fibrin formation or lysis onto the surface of HMEC-1 cells, was followed by turbidity. Clot structure was visualized by laser scanning confocal microscopy (LSCM). The secretion of uPA and PAI-1 by HMEC-1 cells was quantified by ELISA.

Results: The rate of fibrin formation increased approximately 1.5-fold at low fibrinogen content (0.5 and 1 mg/mL; $p < 0.05$) compared to the condition without cells; however, it was decreased at 2 mg/mL fibrinogen ($p < 0.05$) and no differences were found at higher fibrinogen concentrations (3 and 5 mg/mL). HMEC-1 retarded dissolution of clots formed onto their surface at 0.5 to 3 mg/mL fibrinogen ($p < 0.05$). Secretion of uPA was 13×10^{-6} ng/mL *per* cell in the absence of RGD and 8×10^{-6} ng/mL *per* cell in the presence of RGD, when clots were formed on the top of HMEC-1. However, the opposite was found when cells were grown over fibrin: 6×10^{-6} ng/mL *per* cell without RGD vs. 17×10^{-6} ng/mL *per* cell with RGD. The secretion of PAI-1 by HMEC-1 cells was unrelated to the presence of fibrin or RGD, 7×10^{-6} µg/mL *per* cell and 5×10^{-6} µg/mL *per* cell, for the apical (model 1) and basal clots (model 2), respectively.

Conclusions: HMEC-1 cells influence fibrin formation and dissolution as a function of the fibrin content of clots. Clot degradation was accentuated at high fibrin concentrations. The secretion of fibrinolytic components by HMEC-1 cells seemed to be modulated by integrins that bind RGD ligands.

Keywords: Fibrinogen, Fibrin, Fibrinolysis, Urokinase-type plasminogen activator, Plasminogen activator inhibitor type 1, Endothelium, Human dermal microvascular endothelial cells

Background

Fibrinogen is a 340 kDa plasma glycoprotein that circulates at approximately 2–4 mg/mL. The molecule is 45 nm long and comprises a symmetrical dimer consisting of two outer D domains and a central E domain, linked by α- helical coiled-coil rods. The fibrinogen molecule consists of two sets of three different polypeptide chains Aα, Bβ, and γ, joined by disulphide bonds at their N-termini E domain. The C-termini of the Bβ and γ chains are located in the D domain, while that of the Aα chains form a free non well-structured domain, the αC domain [1].

Fibrinogen does not polymerize spontaneously due to negative charges repulsion at the N-termini of the Aα- and Bβ- chains. The removal by thrombin of short peptide sequences at Aα A1-R16 (fibrinopeptide A, FpA) and Bβ Q1-R14 (fibrinopeptide B, FpB) triggers the association between the fibrin monomers (fibrinogen molecules devoid of FpA and FpB) [1, 2]. The release of fibrinopeptides A and B exposes the polymerization sites "A" (knob A) and "B" (knob B), which associate to constitutive polymerization sites located at the C-termini end of the γ chains ("a" or hole a) and β ("b" or hole b). The association of fibrin monomers give rise to protofibrils that have two monomer units of width. The lateral aggregation of protofibrils forms the fibrin fibers. It seems

* Correspondence: rmarchi@ivic.gob.ve
[1]Centro de Medicina Experimental, Laboratorio Biología del Desarrollo de la Hemostasia, Instituto Venezolano de Investigaciones Científicas, Caracas, República Bolivariana de Venezuela
Full list of author information is available at the end of the article

that FpBs release contribute to the lateral aggregation of protofibrils [3–5].

Coagulation and fibrinolysis are activated simultaneously in response to injury. The cross-linked fibrin is deposited in blood vessels and tissues, and plasmin is responsible of the soluble fibrin degradation products [6]. Under physiological conditions, activators, inhibitors, and cofactors finely regulated fibrinolysis. Plasmin is formed from its precursor (plasminogen, Pg) by tissue type plasminogen activator (tPA) at the surface of fibrin [7]. Furthermore, endothelial cells are involved in fibrinolysis regulation by secreting substances, such as tPA and plasminogen activator inhibitor type 1 (PAI-1). Although tPA is a poor plasminogen activator in solution, at the surface of fibrin the reaction is amplified approximately two orders of magnitude [7, 8].

Fibrin network structure depends on the quality and amount of fibrinogen, on thrombin and calcium concentrations, and on ionic strength, among others [9, 10]. The fibrin meshwork structure is characterized by fibrin thickness, fiber density, pores size, and rigidity that reflects fibrin FXIIIa cross-linking and clot structure [11]. It has been found that clots from patients with thrombotic disorders were composed by thin fibers with increased fibrin density and rigidity, and decreased clot lysis rate [12–14]. Endothelial cells (ECs) interact with fibrin at the sites of vascular injury, thrombosis, inflammation and tumour growth, whereas they are quiescent when exposed to circulating fibrinogen [15]. The regulation of fibrinolysis by the endothelium has been widely studied [16–19]; however, the response of ECs to different fibrin structures has not been explored as yet. This knowledge can be relevant in thrombotic or bleeding mechanisms.

In the present work, fibrin clots of different structure were prepared at varying fibrinogen concentrations. Fibrin polymerization and fibrinolysis onto the HMEC-1 surface were followed by turbidity. Furthermore, fibrin association to ECs receptors was visualized by LSCM in the presence and absence of the synthetic disintegrin RGD.

Methods

Materials

The MCDB 131 medium, foetal bovine serum, penicillin, streptomycin, fungizone, L-glutamine were purchased from GIBCO (Grand Island, NY, USA). Epidermal growth factor was from Invitrogen (Nalge Nunc International, Rochester, NY, USA). The 96 well microtiter plates and the 8 wells LabTek® Chamber Slide™ from Nalge Nunc International (Rochester, NY, USA). Lysine-sepharose was purchased from Health Care (Piscataway, NJ, USA). Bovine thrombin and RGD peptide were from Sigma (St Louis, MO. USA). The dyes di-8-anepps and Alexa 488 were from Molecular Probes (Eugene, OR, USA). FluoSpheres size kit # 1 carboxylate modified microspheres red fluorescent was from Molecular Probes (Eugene, OR, USA). The uPA and PAI-1 ELISA kits were purchased from American Diagnostica (Greenwich, Connecticut, USA).

Endothelial cells culture

The human dermal microvascular endothelial cells (HMEC-1) were kindly donated by Dr. Edwin Ades, Department of Health and Human Services Centers for Disease Control and Prevention (CDC, Atlanta USA). The cells were cultivated with MCDB 131 medium supplemented with 10 % foetal bovine serum, penicillin 100 U/mL, streptomycin 100 μg/mL, L-glutamine 200 mM, and epidermal growth factor 10 ng/mL. For polymerization and fibrinolysis experiments, cells were plated in 96 wells microtiter plates, and for confocal microscopy experiments in 8 wells LabTek® Chamber Slide™. Cells were cultivated at 37 °C in a humid atmosphere with 5 % CO_2 until ~80 % confluence. The optimal quantity of thrombin to be used in order to clot fibrinogen without affecting cell morphology and viability was standardized. After cells reached ~80 % confluence, 1 to 5 nM thrombin was incubated on the surface of the cells monolayer during 2 h. The cells' morphology was observed with an optical microscope (unchanged at 1 nM; results not shown). Similarly, the number of cells to be seeded in the microplate wells and confocal microscopy chambers were previously standardized in order to obtain 80 % confluence overnight.

Fibrinogen purification

Fibrinogen was purified from pooled human plasma obtained from healthy donors. The Ethics Committee of the Instituto Venezolano de Investígaciones Científicas (IVIC) approved the project, and all subjects signed an informed consent before blood withdrawal. Blood was collected in citrate (1 volume of 0.13 M trisodium citrate and 9 volumes of blood). Immediately centrifuged at 2500 × g during 20 min, at 4 °C. Fibrinogen was precipitated by salting out using β-alanine, essentially as described elsewhere [20]. The plasminogen was removed from fibrinogen preparation using a lysine-sepharose column, following the manufacturer's instructions. The clottability of the purified fibrinogen was >90 %.

Fibrin polymerization and fibrinolysis on HMEC-1

The HMEC-1 cells (100,000 cells/well) were seeded on 96-well microtiter plate and cultivated overnight. The following day the medium was discarded and the fibrin meshwork was formed on top of the cells. Clots directly formed on the plastic surface of the microtiter plate served as controls. In an Eppendorf tube 143 μL of purified fibrinogen (0.5–5 mg/mL, final), 40 μL MCDB 131 non-supplemented medium and 17.5 μL of bovine thrombin – $CaCl_2$ (1 nM and 2 mM, respectively, final) were mixed and immediately transferred on the top of the cells or directly on the plastic well surface. The optical density (OD) was read every 2 min during 100 min at 350 nm in an Infinite 200 M (Tecan, Vienna, Austria). For each curve it was calculated the slope (mOD/s)×100 and the maximum absorbance (MaxAbs, mOD). Experiments were run at least three times by triplicate. Fibrinolysis was triggered by the addition of 100 nM Pg and 0.145 nM tPA (previously standardized) to fibrinogen solutions (0.5–3 mg/mL) before clotting with thrombin – $CaCl_2$. The OD was recorded every minute until the OD reached baseline values. For each curve it was measured the time needed to decrease by 50 % the maximum absorbance (T50; s), the lysis rate, in the descending part of the curve (LR; mOD/s)×100; and the area under the curve (AUC; mOD × s). Experiments were run at least three times by duplicate.

At the end of each experiment the morphology of the cells was checked with an optical microscope.

Fibrin interaction with HMEC-1

Cells (120,000) were seeded in LabTek glass chamber slide and maintained at 37 °C in a humid atmosphere with 95 % air and 5 % CO_2 and grown-up to 80 % confluence. The culture medium was removed and cells were labelled with 4 μM di-8-anepps for 15 min. The cells were then washed three times with phosphate buffered-saline (PBS). Fibrinogen (0.5, 2, and 5 mg/mL) mixed with 1 mM RGD (or the equivalent volume of buffer) and Alexa Fluor 488-labeled fibrinogen (19 μg/ 206 μL sample volume), was clotted with 1 nM thrombin – 2 mM $CaCl_2$ (final). The clotting mixture was immediately transferred over the cells or directly to the bottom of the glass chamber (control, without cells). Clot formation was allowed to progress for 2 h in a tissue culture incubator. Finally, the clot's surface was covered with supplemented medium without serum. Duplicates of each condition were performed at least in three independent experiments.

In order to discard that the interaction of fibrin with the cells was merely an adsorption phenomenon, 2 μm fluorescent microspheres were included in the reaction mixture before adding thrombin.

The clot structure on the surface of HMEC-1 was visualized using a Nikon Eclipse TE 2000-U laser microscope (with a 488 nm Argon or 543 nm HeNe laser). The objective used was Plan Apo VC 60X in water immersion with a work distance of 0.27. The acquisition pinhole was set to 60 μm. For each clot several fields were examined at random before digital recording. Five areas of 212 × 212 μm (x,y) were selected from each duplicate. A Z- stack was imaged from the bottom of the dish (0 μm) to different distances from the surface of the cells, with step sizes of 0.5 μm. The fibers diameter and density were measured from the volume render obtained with the Olympus FV10-ASW 2.1, and peak analysis from OriginPro 8.

Urokinase-type plasminogen activator (uPA) and plasminogen activator inhibitor 1 (PAI-1) secretion by HMEC-1 in the presence of fibrin

Fibrinogen was polimerized on the top of a HMEC-1 culture (model 1) or the cells were grown on fibrin as substratum (model 2). In model 1, fibrin was formed on HMEC-1 cells (100,000) using different fibrinogen concentration (0.25, 0.5, 1, 1.5, 2, 3, and 5 mg/mL). Clots were allowed to form during 30 min in the incubator and 200 μL of medium without serum was then added. The supernatant was carefully collected after 12 h and stored at −80 °C until use. The following protocol was used with RGD: a cell monolayer was incubated during 3 h with 1 mM RGD prepared in supplemented MCDB 131 medium. The medium was then discarded and the cells washed with PBS. A fibrin reaction mixture with 1 mM RGD was added on the top of the cells. The basal condition consisted of the cell monolayer incubated during 12 h with supplemented MCDB 131 medium.

In order to cultivate the HMEC-1 on a fibrin layer (model 2), thin fibrin films of 30 μL were formed on the bottom of the 96-well microplate, using the same clotting condition as model 1. After 30 min at 37 °C, 100,000 cells/ well supplemented or not with 1 mM RGD were seeded on the top of the fibrin and the plate left overnight in the incubator. The following day fresh medium without serum was added, and incubated for 12 h. The supernatant was collected and kept at −80 °C until use. Experiments were performed in triplicate and uPA and PAI-1 concentrations were measured in the cell supernatant by ELISA. The basal condition consisted of the cells monolayer incubated during 12 h with supplemented MCDB 131 medium.

The quantity of uPA and PAI-1 secreted was normalized to the number of cells *per* well.

Statistical analysis

Statistical analysis was performed with OriginPro version 8.1. Descriptive statistics: mean, standard deviation (SD) or the standard error of the mean (SEM) were calculated. Normality was assessed by Shapiro-Wilk Test. Means were compared by one-way-ANOVA. A significance level of 0.05 was used.

Results

Fibrin polymerization and fibrinolysis on the top of HMEC-1

The slope and MaxAbs increase steadily from 0.5 to 5 mg/mL both when fibrin was formed on the top of HMEC monolayer or without cells (Table 1). Figure 1 shows the time course of fibrin formation at 3 different

Table 1 Summary of the kinetics of fibrin polymerization on the top of HMEC-1 at different fibrinogen concentrations

	Fibrin + Cells		Fibrin	
Fg (mg/mL)	Slope (mOD/s)×100	MaxAbs (mOD)	Slope (mOD/s)×100	MaxAbs (mOD)
0.5	50 ± 7*	305 ± 20*	33 ± 4	221 ± 14
1	83 ± 3*	494 ± 16*	61 ± 2	406 ± 10
2	111 ± 5*	976 ± 45	132 ± 11	1019 ± 58
3	519 ± 59	1715 ± 42	668 ± 154	1543 ± 179
5	710 ± 37	1890 ± 113*	710 ± 103	1657 ± 82

Results are expressed as the mean (± SD)
Fg fibrinogen, *MaxAbs* maximum absorbance
*$p < 0.05$ Comparison between fibrin polymerization parameters of clots formed on the top of the cells with those performed in its absence

fibrinogen concentrations (1, 3 and 5 mg/mL). The influence of fibrinogen concentration on the kinetics of fibrin polymerization is clearly evidenced. In the presence of cells MaxAbs was higher compared to the condition without cells. Fibrinolysis results are summarized in Table 2. The lysis rate (LR) was slightly but significantly decreased in the presence of cells at the fibrinogen concentrations tested (0.5 to 3 mg/mL). However, the time needed for 50 % of clot lysis (T50%) was similar. In Fig. 2 are shown the time course of fibrinolysis at 1, 2, and 3 mg/mL fibrinogen.

Fibrin interaction with HMEC-1

Fibrin network formed at three different fibrinogen concentrations (0.5, 2, and 5 mg/mL) on the top of HMEC-1 monolayers were digitized near the cell surface and at 15 μm, both in the presence and absence of 1 mM of the synthetic peptide RGD that competes with fibrinogen for integrin-ligand binding. In Fig. 3 it is clearly seen that at 0.5 and 2 mg/mL the fibrin fibers interacted profoundly with the cell surface, the fibers looked radially stressed and the colocalization (in yellow) of the fibrin (green) with the cells membrane (red) is evidenced. However, at 5 mg/mL the interaction with the cell surface was rather decreased. This peculiar fibrin fibers distribution disappears with distance from the cell surface. At approximately 15 μm, the fibers looked uniformly distributed. When RGD was added to the fibrinogen solutions, the interaction between fibrin and cells decreased.

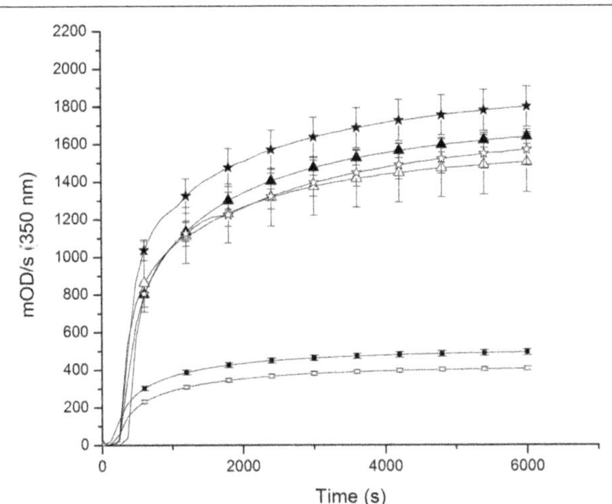

Fig. 1 Fibrin polymerization on the top of HMEC-1 at different fibrinogen concentrations. Filled symbols represent the condition of fibrin formed on the top of the cells and empty symbols clots formed directly on the plastic dish. (■, □): 1 mg/mL, (▲, △): 3 mg/mL and (★, ☆): 5 mg/mL

In order to rule out that the fibrin association to the cells was merely an adsorption phenomenon, fluorescent microspheres of 2 μm were incorporated into the clotting mixture. The fibrin fibers did not interact with the beads nor looked stressed, confirming that fibrin fibers are interacting with specific receptors on the cell membrane (Fig. 4).

The fibrin network was characterized by measuring fibrin fiber diameter and fibrin density near the cell surface and at 15 μm (Table 3). Fibrin fibers were thicker near the cell surface compared to that observed at 15 μm at all fibrinogen concentrations tested without RGD. In contrast, in the presence of RGD there was not such relationship. Apparently, only at 5 mg/mL the fibrin fibers diameter did not change. Fibrin density was greater near the cell surface both in the presence or absence of RGD, except at 0.5 mg/mL in the presence of RGD ($p > 0.05$).

Changes in fluorescence intensity as a function of the distance from the cell surface at 2 mg/mL of fibrinogen is shown in Fig. 5.

HMEC-1 secretion of uPA and PAI-1 in the presence of fibrin

The basal secretion of uPA was $7.0 \pm 0.5\times10^{-6}$ ng/mL *per* cell and that of PAI-1 $6.7 \pm 0.5\times10^{-6}$ μg/mL *per* cell. Since the secretion of uPA and PAI-1 was almost similar at the different fibrinogen concentrations tested in the presence or not of RGD, these values were averaged and reported in Table 4. In model 1, when fibrin was formed on the top of the cells monolayer, uPA secretion in the absence of RGD was ~2-fold higher than in its presence ($p < 0.05$). However, the opposite was found for model 2.

Table 2 Summary of the fibrin degradation on the top of HMEC-1

	Fibrin + Cells			Fibrin		
Fg (mg/mL)	T50% (s)	LR (mOD/s) ×100	AUC (mODxs) ×10^6	T50% (s)	LR (mOD/s) ×100	AUC (mODxs) ×10^6
0.5	870 ± 79	41 ± 4*	0.3230 ± 0.0204	820 ± 17	48 ± 2	0.2946 ± 0.0147
1	1790 ± 173	58 ± 0.8*	1.5004 ± 0.1617	1650 ± 60	77 ± 2	1.4120 ± 0.0843
2	4330 ± 466	54 ± 2.3*	7.5957 ± 0.0927*	4150 ± 69	68 ± 1.4	6.8737 ± 0.2645
3	5860 ± 259	77 ± 21*	19.6071 ± 1.0103*	5690 ± 193	135 ± 1.4	16.1075 ± 1.0519

Results are expressed as the mean (± SD)
Fg fibrinogen, *T50%* time required to decrease the MaxAbs 50 %, *LR* lysis rate, *AUC* area under the curve
*$p < 0.05$ Comparison between fibrin degradation parameters of clots formed on the top of the cells with those performed in its absence

When cells were grown on the top of the fibrin network the secretion of uPA in the absence of RGD was decreased 2-fold ($p < 0.05$). The secretion of PAI-1 in model 1 was 1.3-fold higher compared to model 2 ($p < 0.05$). The PAI-1 concentration in the presence of fibrin was comprised in the 95 % CI of HMEC-1 basal secretion.

Discussion

The aims of the present work were (1) to study fibrin formation and lysis onto the surface of HMEC-1 cells, and (2) to quantify uPA and PAI-1 secretion in the presence of fibrin. We also analyzed the fibrin meshwork formed on the top of HMEC-1 cells by laser scanning confocal microscopy. The structure of fibrin was modulated by modifying the concentration of fibrinogen.

Fibrin is pro inflammatory, pro-angiogenic and may contribute to the development of inflammatory disease processes and tumorigenesis [21–23]. Atherogenesis is a multifactorial process and the atherosclerotic lesions may be initiated by the interaction of fibrin with the endothelium [24]. In normal physiologic conditions, the endothelium displays antiplatelet, anticoagulant and fibrinolytic properties [25].

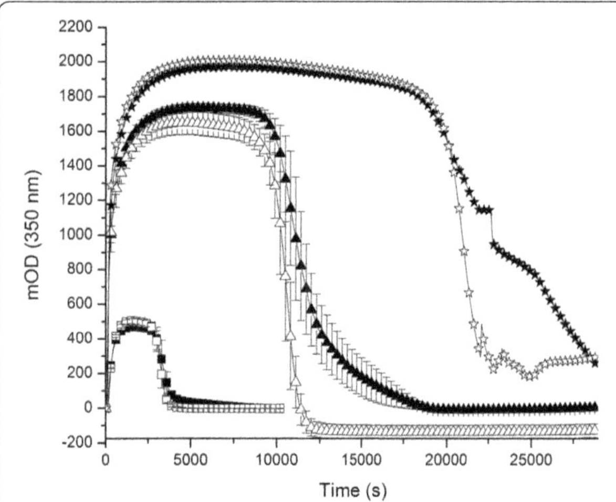

Fig. 2 Fibrin degradation on the top of HMEC-1 at different fibrinogen concentrations followed by turbidity. (■, □): 1 mg/mL, (▲, △): 2 mg/mL and (★, ☆): 3 mg/mL. Filled symbols: fibrin formed on the top of the cells; empty symbols: clots formed directly on the plastic dish

In order to measure the secretion of fibrinolytic components from HMEC-1 we have used an adhesion model, where HMEC-1 cells were seeded directly on the plastic surface and after reaching 80 % of confluence fibrin was formed on their top (model 1) or cells were grown on a fibrin film (model 2).

The type of plasminogen activator secreted by HMEC-1 has been differently reported in the literature [26–28]. However, a majority of reports [29–31], including those from the group of Angles-Cano [26, 32, 33], have clearly demonstrated, using methods that identify either the molecular mass (Western blot) or the activity of the molecular mass (fibrin or casein zymography) that only uPA (54 kDa) is detected in culture media or lysates from HMEC-1. We have verified that the HMEC-1 line used in these studies secretes uPA (lysis band at 54 kDa by zymography).

Similar to what has been found for other ECs cultured in vitro, HMEC-1 basal PAI-1 secretion was higher than uPA, approximately 1000-fold [34–36]. In model 1, without RGD, the amount of uPA secreted to the medium was 2-fold higher compared to the basal secretion and to model 2. This difference was attributed to the availability of thrombin. In model 1, at the beginning of fibrin formation, thrombin is in solution and directly in contact with the cells, while in model 2 fibrin was already gelled, and less thrombin was accessible to the cells. The response of the ECs to thrombin depends on their origin, in human umbilical vein endothelial cells (HUVEC) the quantity of tPA and PAI-1 is dose-dependent on thrombin concentration, but not in human omental tissue microvascular endothelial cells (HOTMC) [35].

During fibrin formation from 0.5, 1, and 5 mg/mL fibrinogen the OD increased faster in the presence of HMEC-1 than without it ($p < 0.05$). Tietze et al. found similar results with human mesothelial cells (HOMC) but at constant fibrinogen concentration [34]. This "catalytic" cell effect at low fibrinogen concentration may be an advantage for patients with hypofibrinogenemia, which could contribute to stop faster blood extravasation. The rate of fibrin degradation in the presence of HMEC-1 was significantly decreased at all fibrin concentration (0.5 to 3 mg/mL), reaching a maximum value at 3 mg/mL (2-fold less). These results were attributed to several factors. The

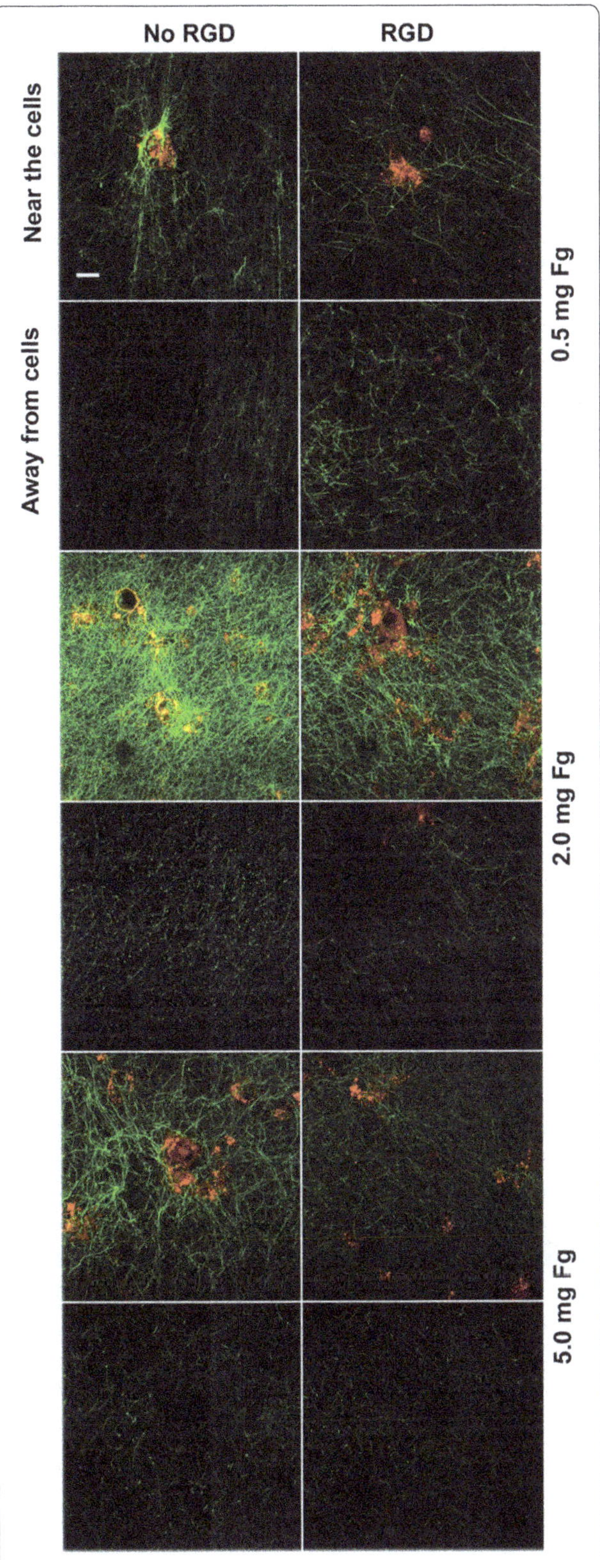

Fig. 3 Laser scanning confocal microscopy images of clots formed on the top of HMEC-1 at different fibrinogen concentrations. The fibrin fibers were visualized with Alexa 488 and the cell membrane with di-8-anepps. The pictures show the fibrin fibers arrangements of clots supplemented or not with 1 mM RGD near the cell surface at 0.5, 2 and 5 mg/mL fibrinogen, and at 15 μm away. The tool bar represents 20 μm

presence of PAI-1 (basal secretion ~ 6.7×10^{-6} μg/mL *per* cell) could decrease both the functional availability of uPA and tPA (externally added tPA), although the tPA bound to fibrin is less susceptible to PAI-1 inactivation [7, 37]. The peculiar fibrin structure observed near the cell surface could impair clot dissolution. In general, fibrin network with increased fibers density are digested slower [38]. However, opposite results were found with HOMC, where the T50% was decreased in the presence of cells [34]. The results reported by these authors were intriguing, since clots formed without cells were totally degraded earlier than those in the presence of cells.

It was previously found that fibrin fibers forms clumps near the surface of HUVEC culture; however, at 50 μm this pattern disappear and they distributed homogeneously [39]. The integrin involved in this interaction was the $\alpha v\beta_3$ [39]. This integrin binds the ligand at specific RGD sequences of different adhesive proteins such as fibronectin, vitronectin, fibrinogen, among others [40]. In the present work the fibrin network structure formed at different fibrinogen concentrations was analyzed by LSCM. As expected, increasing the fibrinogen concentration increases the fibrin density [41], and the fibers associated to the cell surface looked

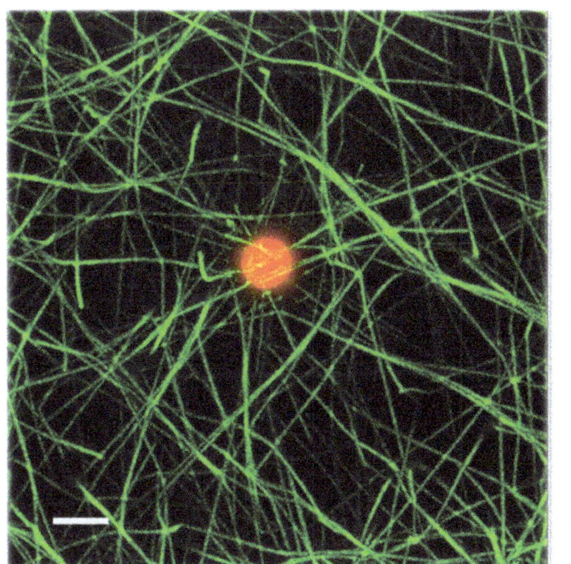

Fig. 4 Fibrin network formed with fluorescent microspheres. A field with only one bead was magnified in order to appreciate that these particles did not interact with fibers. The tool bar represents 2 μm

Table 3 Characterization of fibrin networks formed on the surface of HMEC-1 culture by laser scanning confocal microscopy (LSCM)

Fibers diameter (μm)				
Fg (mg/mL)	- RGD Near	- RGD Far	+ RGD Near	+ RGD Far
0.5	2.02 ± 0.05*	1.65 ± 0.05	1.49 ± 0.09*	1.72 ± 0.07
2	1.98 ± 0.12*	1.76 ± 0.12	1.99 ± 0.06*	1.62 ± 0.07
5	2.03 ± 0.65*	1.52 ± 0.33	2.00 ± 0.10	1.95 ± 0.33
Fibrin density (peaks/μm)				
Fg (mg/mL)	- RGD Near	- RGD Far	+ RGD Near	+ RGD Far
0.5	0.192 ± 0.052*	0.099 ± 0.045	0.205 ± 0.051	0.160 ± 0.054
2	0.299 ± 0.029*	0.135 ± 0.035	0.270 ± 0.023*	0.152 ± 0.030
5	0.254 ± 0.030*	0.141 ± 0.057	0.282 ± 0.022*	0.138 ± 0.056

Fibrin fibers diameter and density were quantified from LSCM images
Values are expressed as mean (± SEM) of 3 experiments performed in duplicate
*$p < 0.05$. Comparisons are between near the cells surface vs. far, without (−) and with (+) RGD

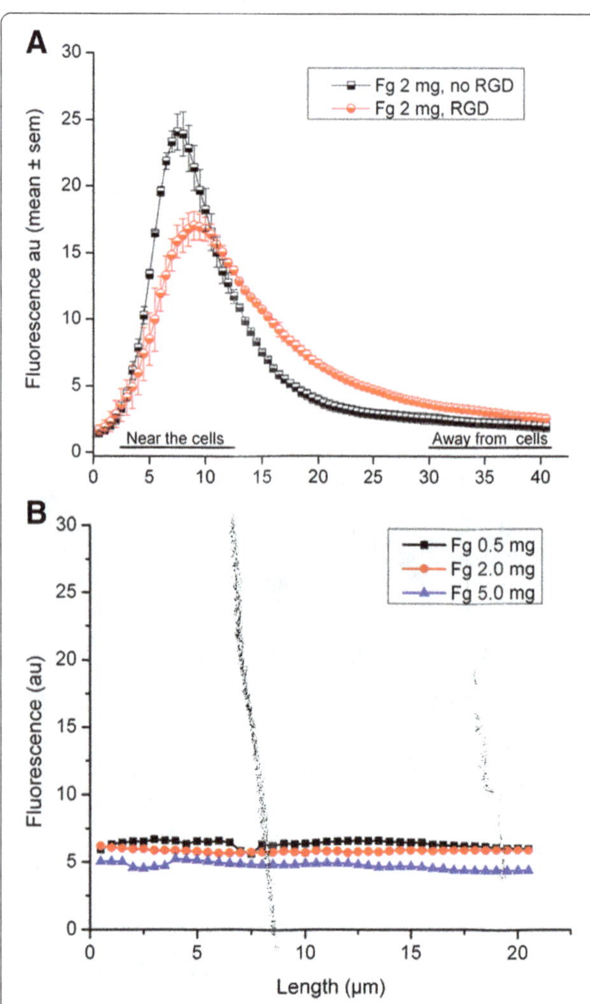

Fig. 5 Representation of the changes of the mean fluorescence intensity according to the distance from the bottom of the dish up to 40 μm. **a** Without and with RGD at 2 mg/mL fibrinogen. **b** Without cells at 0.5, 2 and 5 mg/mL fibrinogen

Table 4 HMEC-1 cells secrete urokinase-type plasminogen activator and plasminogen activator inhibitor type 1

μg/mL *per* cell	Model 1	Model 2
uPA×10^{-9} (−RGD)	12.7*,** (11.2–14.1)	6.2* (5.0–7.4)
uPA×10^{-9} (+RGD)	7.5** (5.9–9.1)	17.3 (15.0–19.6)
PAI-1×10^{-6} (−RGD)	7.87** (6.65–9.10)	5.97 (4.50–7.44)
PAI-1×10^{-6} (+RGD)	7.38** (6.54–8.23)	5.08 (3.01–7.16)

Urokinase and PAI-1 were quantified by ELISA in HMEC conditioned-medium obtained in the presence of fibrin. Fibrin was formed on the top of the cells monolayer (model 1) or cells were seeded on the top of fibrin film (model 2). The basal secretion of uPA was 7.0 ± 0.5 × 10^{-9} μg/mL *per* cell, and that of PAI-1 6.7 ± 0.5 × 10^{-6} μg/mL *per* cell. The quantity of uPA and PAI-1 secreted was normalized to the number of cells. Results are expressed as the mean and the 95 % confidence interval (CI) in brackets
*$p < 0.05$ uPA secretion without RGD (−RGD) compared to that with RGD (+RGD) for model 1
**$p < 0.05$ uPA secretion without RGD of model 1 compared to that of model 2, and with RGD in model 1 compared to that in model 2

stressed (Fig. 3), as has already been observed in other works at a given fibrinogen concentration [39, 42, 43]. Interestingly, at high fibrinogen concentration (5 mg/mL) the interaction of fibrin with the cells was decreased. Indeed, at increasing fibrin content, the number of protofibrils *per* fiber are greater [44], probably diminishing the accessibility of the RGD sites on the fibrin fibers (Aα 572–575) to integrins [40, 45].

The changes in fibrin fiber diameter at varying fibrinogen concentrations were not clearly appreciated by LSCM in spite of the low thrombin concentration used. This is probably due to the lower resolution limit of LSCM (~200–400 nm).

Conclusions

We demonstrated that HMEC-1 influenced fibrin formation as a function of the fibrinogen input. However, the rate of fibrin degradation in the presence of HMEC-1 was significantly decreased at all fibrin concentrations. Impairment of fibrin binding to its cell receptor by RGD influenced the secretion of fibrinolytic components thus suggesting a role for fibrin binding in this mechanism. The next step would be to investigate the signalling pathway involved in the $\alpha v\beta_3$ integrin activation, probably coupled to thrombin. A limitation of our study is that the results were obtained using HMEC-1 cells and may therefore be pertinent only to this cell line.

Abbreviations

ECs: endothelial cells; ELISA: enzyme-linked immunosorbent assay; Fg: fibrinogen; FXIIIa: activated factor XIII; HMEC: human dermal microvascular endothelial cells; HOMC: human mesothelial cells; HOTMC: human omental tissue microvascular endothelial cells; HUVEC: human umbilical vein endothelial cell; LR: lysis rate; LSCM: laser scanning confocal microscopy; MaxAbs: maximum absorbance; OD: optical density; PAI-1: plasminogen activator inhibitor type 1; PBS: phosphate buffered-saline; Pg: plasminogen; RGD: arginyl glycyl aspartic acid; SEM: standard error of the mean; tPA: tissue type plasminogen activator; uPA: urokinase-type plasminogen activator.

Competing interests
The authors declare that they have no competing interests.

Authors' contributions
CO has performed the experiments, standardization of most of the techniques, and contributed to experiments design and data discussion. RH handled the LSCM, and quantified and analyzed LSCM images. DZ participated in cells culture. A-CE participated in the fibrinolysis experiments and interpretation of data, and manuscript writing. MR: designed the project, participated in data analysis and wrote the manuscript. All authors have read and approved the final manuscript.

Acknowledgements
The authors are grateful to Drs. Peter Taylor and Reinaldo Di Polo of IVIC (Caracas, República Bolivariana de Venezuela), for cell culture and confocal microscopy facility, respectively. The human microvascular endothelial cells (HMEC-1) were kindly donated by Dr. Edwin Ades and Mr. Francisco J. Candal of the Centers for Disease Control and Prevention (CDC) (Atlanta, GA, USA) and Dr. Thomas Lawley of Emory University (Atlanta, GA, USA). Dr. Eduardo Anglés-Cano is supported by Inserm.
This work was partially financed by Oficina de Planificación del Sector Universitario (OPSU).

Author details
[1]Centro de Medicina Experimental, Laboratorio Biología del Desarrollo de la Hemostasia, Instituto Venezolano de Investigaciones Científicas, Caracas, República Bolivariana de Venezuela. [2]Universidad de Carabobo, Escuela de Bioanálisis (Sede Aragua), Maracay, República Bolivariana de Venezuela. [3]Instituto de Inmunología, Universidad Central de Venezuela, Caracas, República Bolivariana de Venezuela. [4]Laboratorio de Fisiología Celular, Centro de Biofísica y Bioquímica, Instituto Venezolano de Investigaciones Científicas, Caracas, República Bolivariana de Venezuela. [5]Instituto de Medicina Experimental, Universidad Central de Venezuela, Caracas, República Bolivariana de Venezuela. [6]Inserm UMR_S 1140, Faculté de Pharmacie, Paris, France. [7]Université Paris Descartes, Sorbonne Paris Cité, Paris, France.

References

1. Weisel JW. Fibrinogen and fibrin. Adv Protein Chem. 2005;70:247–99.
2. Blomback B, Hessel B, Hogg D, Therkildsen L. A two-step fibrinogen–fibrin transition in blood coagulation. Nature. 1978;275:501–5.
3. Weisel JW, Veklich Y, Gorkun O. The sequence of cleavage of fibrinopeptides from fibrinogen is important for protofibril formation and enhancement of lateral aggregation in fibrin clots. J Mol Biol. 1993;232:285–97.
4. Medved L, Weisel JW. Recommendations for nomenclature on fibrinogen and fibrin. J Thromb Haemost. 2009;7:355–9.
5. Okumura N, Terasawa F, Haneishi A, Fujihara N, Hirota-Kawadobora M, Yamauchi K, et al. B:b interactions are essential for polymerization of variant fibrinogens with impaired holes 'a'. J Thromb Haemost. 2007;5:2352–9.
6. Cesarman-Maus G, Hajjar KA. Molecular mechanisms of fibrinolysis. Br J Haematol. 2005;129:307–21.
7. Hoylaerts M, Rijken DC, Lijnen HR, Collen D. Kinetics of the activation of plasminogen by human tissue plasminogen activator. Role of fibrin. J Biol Chem. 1982;257:2912–9.
8. Diamond SL, Eskin SG, McIntire LV. Fluid flow stimulates tissue plasminogen activator secretion by cultured human endothelial cells. Science. 1989;243:1483–5.
9. Blomback B, Banerjee D, Carlsson K, Hamsten A, Hessel B, Procyk R, et al. Native fibrin gel networks and factors influencing their formation in health and disease. Adv Exp Med Biol. 1990;281:1–23.
10. Wolberg AS, Monroe DM, Roberts HR, Hoffman M. Elevated prothrombin results in clots with an altered fiber structure: a possible mechanism of the increased thrombotic risk. Blood. 2003;101:3008–13.
11. Ryan EA, Mockros LF, Weisel JW, Lorand L. Structural origins of fibrin clot rheology. Biophys J. 1999;77:2813–26.
12. Mills JD, Ariens RA, Mansfield MW, Grant PJ. Altered fibrin clot structure in the healthy relatives of patients with premature coronary artery disease. Circulation. 2002;106:1938–42.
13. Collet JP, Allali Y, Lesty C, Tanguy ML, Silvain J, Ankri A, et al. Altered fibrin architecture is associated with hypofibrinolysis and premature coronary atherothrombosis. Arterioscler Thromb Vasc Biol. 2006;26:2567–73.
14. Undas A, Kaczmarek P, Sladek K, Stepien E, Skucha W, Rzeszutko M, et al. Fibrin clot properties are altered in patients with chronic obstructive pulmonary disease. Beneficial effects of simvastatin treatment. Thromb Haemost. 2009;102:1176–82.
15. Francis CW, Bunce LA, Sporn LA. Endothelial cell responses to fibrin mediated by FPB cleavage and the amino terminus of the beta chain. Blood Cells. 1993;19:291–306.
16. Michiels C. Endothelial cell functions. J Cell Physiol. 2003;196:430–43.
17. Libby P, Aikawa M, Jain MK. Vascular endothelium and atherosclerosis. Handb Exp Pharmacol. 2006;176(Pt 2):285–306.
18. van Hinsbergh VW. Endothelium–role in regulation of coagulation and inflammation. Semin Immunopathol. 2012;34:93–106.
19. Suzuki Y, Yasui H, Brzoska T, Mogami H, Urano T. Surface-retained tPA is essential for effective fibrinolysis on vascular endothelial cells. Blood. 2011;118:3182–5.
20. Jakobsen E, Kierulf P. A modified beta-alanine precipitation procedure to preparefibrinogen free of antithrombin-III and plasminogen. Thromb Res. 1973;3:145–59.
21. Tang L, Eaton JW. Fibrin(ogen) mediates acute inflammatory responses to biomaterials. J Exp Med. 1993;178:2147–56.
22. Varisco PA, Peclat V, van Ness K, Bischof-Delaloye A, So A, Busso N. Effect of thrombin inhibition on synovial inflammation in antigen induced arthritis. Ann Rheum Dis. 2000;59:781–7.
23. van Hinsbergh VW, Engelse MA, Quax PH. Pericellular proteases in angiogenesis and vasculogenesis. Arterioscler Thromb Vasc Biol. 2006;26:716–28.
24. Zacharowski K, Zacharowski P, Reingruber S, Petzelbauer P. Fibrin(ogen) and its fragments in the pathophysiology and treatment of myocardial infarction. J Mol Med (Berl). 2006;84(6):469–77.
25. De Caterina R, Massaro M, Libby P. Endothelial functions and dysfunctions. In: De Caterina R, Libby P, editors. Endothelial dysfunctions and vascular disease. Oxford, UK: Blackwell Futura; 2007. p. 3–25.
26. Lacroix R, Sabatier F, Mialhe A, Basire A, Pannell R, Borghi H, et al. Activation of plasminogen into plasmin at the surface of endothelial microparticles: a mechanism that modulates angiogenic properties of endothelial progenitor cells in vitro. Blood. 2007;110:2432–9.
27. Fiuza C, Bustin M, Talwar S, Tropea M, Gerstenberger E, Shelhamer JH, et al. Inflammation-promoting activity of HMGB1 on human microvascular endothelial cells. Blood. 2003;101:2652–60.
28. Jiang SJ, Lin TM, Wu HL, Han HS, Shi GY. Decrease of fibrinolytic activity in human endothelial cells by arsenite. Thromb Res. 2002;105:55–62.
29. Michaud-Levesque J, Rolland Y, Demeule M, Bertrand Y, Beliveau R. Inhibition of endothelial cell movement and tubulogenesis by human recombinant soluble melanotransferrin: involvement of the u-PAR/LRP plasminolytic system. Biochim Biophys Acta. 2005;1743:243–53.
30. Quemener C, Gabison EE, Naimi B, Lescaille G, Bougatef F, Podgorniak MP, et al. Extracellular matrix metalloproteinase inducer up-regulates the urokinase-type plasminogen activator system promoting tumor cell invasion. Cancer Res. 2007;67:9–15.
31. Senchenko VN, Anedchenko EA, Kondratieva TT, Krasnov GS, Dmitriev AA, Zabarovska VI, et al. Simultaneous down-regulation of tumor suppressor genes RBSP3/CTDSPL, NPRL2/G21 and RASSF1A in primary non-small cell lung cancer. BMC Cancer. 2010;10:75.
32. Doeuvre L, Plawinski L, Goux D, Vivien D, Angles-Cano E. Plasmin on adherent cells: from microvesiculation to apoptosis. Biochem J. 2010;432:365–73.
33. Lacroix R, Plawinski L, Robert S, Doeuvre L, Sabatier F, Martinez De Lizarrondo S, et al. Leukocyte- and endothelial-derived microparticles: a circulating source for fibrinolysis. Haematologica. 2012;97:1864–72.
34. Tietze L, Elbrecht A, Schauerte C, Klosterhalfen B, Amo-Takyi B, Gehlen J, et al. Modulation of pro- and antifibrinolytic properties of human peritoneal mesothelial cells by transforming growth factor beta1 (TGF-beta1), tumor necrosis factor alpha (TNF-alpha) and interleukin 1beta (IL-1beta). Thromb Haemost. 1998;79:362–70.
35. Speiser W, Anders E, Binder BR, Muller-Berghaus G. Clot lysis mediated by cultured human microvascular endothelial cells. Thromb Haemost. 1988;60:463–7.
36. Van Hinsbergh VW, Sprengers ED, Kooistra T. Effect of thrombin on the production of plasminogen activators and PA inhibitor-1 by human foreskin microvascular endothelial cells. Thromb Haemost. 1987;57:148–53.

37. Wun TC, Capuano A. Initiation and regulation of fibrinolysis in human plasma at the plasminogen activator level. Blood. 1987;69:1354–62.
38. Weisel JW, Litvinov RI. The biochemical and physical process of fibrinolysis and effects of clot structure and stability on the lysis rate. Cardiovasc Hematol Agents Med Chem. 2008;6:161–80.
39. Jerome WG, Handt S, Hantgan RR. Endothelial cells organize fibrin clots into structures that are more resistant to lysis. Microsc Microanal. 2005;11:268–77.
40. Cheresh DA, Berliner SA, Vicente V, Ruggeri ZM. Recognition of distinct adhesive sites on fibrinogen by related integrins on platelets and endothelial cells. Cell. 1989;58:945–53.
41. Blomback B, Carlsson K, Hessel B, Liljeborg A, Procyk R, Aslund N. Native fibrin gel networks observed by 3D microscopy, permeation and turbidity. Biochim Biophys Acta. 1989;997:96–110.
42. Marchi R, Rojas H, Castillo O, Kanzler D. Structure of fibrin network of two abnormal fibrinogens with mutations in the alphaC domain on the human dermal microvascular endothelial cells 1. Blood Coagul Fibrinolysis. 2011;22:706–11.
43. Campbell RA, Overmyer KA, Selzman CH, Sheridan BC, Wolberg AS. Contributions of extravascular and intravascular cells to fibrin network formation, structure, and stability. Blood. 2009;114:4886–96.
44. Weisel JW, Nagaswami C. Computer modeling of fibrin polymerization kinetics correlated with electron microscope and turbidity observations: clot structure and assembly are kinetically controlled. Biophys J. 1992;63:111–28.
45. Suehiro K, Mizuguchi J, Nishiyama K, Iwanaga S, Farrell DH, Ohtaki S. Fibrinogen binds to integrin alpha(5)beta(1) via the carboxyl-terminal RGD site of the Aalpha-chain. J Biochem. 2000;128:705–10.

4

Generic and disease-specific quality of life among youth and young men with Hemophilia in Canada

J. St-Louis[1,2*], D. J. Urajnik[3], F. Ménard[1], S. Cloutier[4], R. J. Klaassen[6], B. Ritchie[5], G. E. Rivard[1], M. Warner[7], V. Blanchette[8,9] and N. L. Young[3,9]

Abstract

Background: This study was undertaken to explore the longitudinal patterns of health-related quality of life (HRQoL) among youth and young adults with Hemophilia A (HA) over a 3-year period. This report presents the baseline characteristics of the study cohort.

Methods: Males, 14 to 29 years of age, with predominantly severe HA were recruited from six treatment centres in Canada. Subjects completed a comprehensive survey. HRQoL was measured using: the CHO-KLAT$_{2.0}$ (youth), Haemo-QoL-A (young adults) and the SF-36v2 (all).

Results: 13 youth (mean age = 15.7, range = 12.9-17.9 years) and 33 young adults (mean age = 23.6; range = 18.4 -28.7 years) with moderate (7 %) and severe (93 %) HA were enrolled. All were on a prophylactic regimen with antihemophilic factor (Helixate FS®) during the study. The youth had minimal joint damage (mean HJHS = 5.2) compared to young adults (mean HJHS = 13.3). The mean HRQoL scores for youth were: 79.2 (SD = 11.9) for the CHO-KLAT, and 53.0 (5.5) and 52.3 (6.8) for the SF-36 Physical Component Summary (PCS) and Mental Component Summary (MCS) scores respectively. The mean HRQoL scores for young adults were: 85.8 (9.5) for the Haemo-Qol-A, and 50.8 (6.4) and 50.9 (8.8) for PCS and MCS respectively. PCS and MCS scores were comparable to published Canadian norms, however significant differences were found for the domains of Physical Functioning and Bodily Pain. The disease-specific HRQoL scores were weakly correlated with the PCS for youth (CHO-KLAT vs. PCS $r = 0.28$, $p = 0.35$); and moderately correlated for the MCS ($r = 0.39$, $p = 0.19$). Haemo-QoL-A scores for young adults were strongly correlated with the PCS ($r = 0.53$, $p = 0.001$); and weakly correlated with the MCS ($r = 0.26$, $p = 0.13$). Joint status as assessed by HJHS was correlated with PCS scores. A history of lifelong prophylaxis resulted in better PCS but worse MCS scores.

Conclusion: Despite having hemophilia, the youth in this cohort have minimal joint disease and good HRQoL. The young adults demonstrated more joint disease and slightly worse HRQoL in the domains of physical functioning and pain. The data presented here provide new information to inform the selection of Health Related Quality of Life (HRQoL) instruments for use in future clinical trials involving persons with hemophilia.

Keywords: Hemophilia, Health-related quality of life, Canadian population, Prophylaxis

* Correspondence: jean.st-louis.1@umontreal.ca
[1]CHU Sainte-Justine, Montréal, Canada
[2]Hôpital Maisonneuve-Rosemont, Montreal, Canada
Full list of author information is available at the end of the article

Background

Hemophilia A is a hereditary disorder resulting in deficient levels of plasma coagulation factor VIII (FVIII) and lifelong bleeding manifestations, particularly repeated hemarthroses leading to permanent joint damage. Major progress has been demonstrated in preventing bleeding and disability when intensive factor replacement therapy is administered prophylactically from an early age [1]. The objective assessment of the outcome of different treatment strategies in hemophilia is multidimensional and includes the measurement of bleeding rates, joint and musculoskeletal status, pain, physical functioning and social functioning based on holistic models of health as recommended by the WHO [2]. Health-related quality of life (HRQoL) tools are self-administered questionnaires developed in order to measure the perceived impact of a medical condition and its treatment on a person's physical, emotional and social well-being.

In hemophilia both generic and disease-specific HRQoL questionnaires have been used in recent years although seldom simultaneously in the same subjects. Recent clinical trials have incorporated the measurement of HRQoL scores before and after an intervention such as the introduction of a prophylactic factor replacement regimen. However, there is very little published data on long term longitudinal trends of HRQoL in hemophilia. Significant variations in HRQoL may not be determined only by change in physical status but may be influenced by common social events such as educational, vocational or relational changes associated with transition from adolescence to adulthood.

We initiated a study in which HRQoL was assessed and described prospectively every 6 months over a 3-year period in a cohort of youth and young adults with severe or moderate hemophilia A receiving routine care. This study will enable the assessment of the relationship between changes in HRQoL scores and changes in physical health as evaluated by clinical assessments (bleeding frequency, product utilization and joint scores). It will also enable us to examine the sensitivity of the main HRQoL measures to significant life events in patients with hemophilia. We present in this report the baseline information on HRQoL for the cohort of Canadian youth and young adults with HA that were followed prospectively over a 3-year period.

Methods

Recruitment/Sample

To be included in the study subjects were required to be males 14 to 29 years of age with moderate (FVIII level 0.02 – 0.05 U/ml) or severe HA (FVIII level < 0.02 U/ml) treated with the recombinant antihemophilic factor Helixate FS® either on a prophylactic or "on-demand" regimen. Subjects were identified from the clinical records at six hemophilia treatment centres in Canada, three in the province of Quebec (Montreal and Quebec City) and three outside (Edmonton, Toronto, Ottawa). Potential subjects were excluded if they had a current inhibitor to FVIII defined as an inhibitor level of equal to or greater than 0.6 Bethesda Units/mL, human immunodeficiency virus (HIV) infection or symptomatic hepatitis C virus (HCV) infection. Information on ethics approval and consent is provided in the Declarations section below. Study funding was provided by CSL Behring Canada. The study was registered in the ClinicalTrials.gov database on December 17, 2009 under the trial number: NCT01034904.

Measures/Manoeuvre

Chart review and demographic survey

The following baseline data was obtained by chart review: severity of haemophilia, history of target joints in the preceding year (defined as a joint with 3 or more bleeds in 3-month period), history of prior major bleeding events requiring hospital admission (e.g. an intracranial hemorr hage), previous surgery, current treatment program, and any concomitant medical condition. Definitions of a target joint and prophylaxis as stated in the protocol were based on published Canadian consensus definitions [3]. Subjects also completed a comprehensive demographic survey relating to educational and professional experience.

Health- related quality of life assessment

All subjects completed a generic and a disease-specific HRQoL questionnaire at baseline.

The same generic questionnaire was used for all subjects. The Medical Outcomes Study 36-item Short Form health survey (SF-36) is an instrument that has been validated for a variety of diseases and has been widely used in hemophilia. It has been normed for populations in several countries and therefore allows comparisons with both normal and diseased populations [4]. The 36 questions are grouped to assess 8 domains of HRQoL with scores ranging from 0 (worse) to 100 (best): Physical Functioning (PF), Role Physical (RP), Bodily Pain (BP), General Health (GH), Vitality (VT), Social Functioning (SF), Role Emotion (RE) and Mental Health (MH). Furthermore, the Physical Component Summary (PCS) and Mental Component Summary (MSC) scores are derived from the 8 domains. These are reported using norm-referenced scoring with a mean of 50 and standard deviation of 10 points [5].

Subjects completed a different disease-specific HRQoL questionnaire depending on their age. Youth aged 14 to 17 years completed the Canadian Haemophilia Outcomes – Kids Life Assessment Tool (CHO-KLAT) version 2.0 [6–9], which was developed and validated for children and adolescents with hemophilia. It consists of 35 questions and is scored from 0 to 100.

In subjects 18 years and above the Haemo-QoL-A, developed by Rentz et al, was used [10]. It comprises 41 items grouped into 6 subscales, each scored from 0 (worst) to 100 (best): Physical Functioning, Role Functioning, Worry, Consequences of Bleeding, Emotional Impact and Treatment Concerns. This disease-specific instrument has also been demonstrated to be reliable and valid for assessing HRQoL in adult patients in hemophilia clinical trials [10].

Joint status assessment

A standardized physical examination of the joints most commonly affected by hemophilia (the elbows, knees and ankles) was performed by a trained physiotherapist using the Hemophilia Joint Health Score (HJHS) version 2.0 [11–13]. This comprises an assessment of each of these 6 joints with regards to swelling, muscle atrophy, crepitus, range of motion, joint pain, strength, and global gait. The score for each joint is summed to obtain a total score ranging from 0 to 124, where no joint damage is indicated by a score of 0. A total score above 10 has been considered indicative of significant joint disease in a published study of young adults [14].

Statistical analysis

Descriptive statistics were generated for the demographic, clinical, and HRQoL measures. Frequencies and/or percentages (%) are reported for categorical data. Means and standard deviations (SD) are presented for continuous measures that are normally distributed. Medians and ranges are presented for skewed data (skew or kurtosis ratio > ±3.0). Benchmarks from the literature were included to enable comparisons.

The scores from generic and disease specific HRQoL measures were compared using Pearson correlations. Pearson correlations were also used to examine the relationship between HRQoL and joint status as measured by the HJHS. We interpreted the strength of each correlation as recommended by Cohen, with a correlation of 0.1 indicating a weak relationship, 0.3 to 0.5 indicating a moderate relationship, and above 0.5 indicating a large or strong relationship [15].

The relationships between disease characteristics, treatment program, joint status and HRQoL were explored using independent sample t-tests and analysis of variance (ANOVA). The incremental impact of age on the PCS and MCS SF-36 summary scores was tested via linear multiple regression controlling for joint status as measured by the HJHS. The minimally important difference (MID) threshold for the SF-36 was used as the criterion for clinical significance on this generic measure. MID's are reported for the PCS (2–3), MCS (3), PF (2–3), RP (2), BP (2–3), GH (2–3), VT (2–3), SF (3), RE (4), and MH (3) [5]. Score differences above the MID are considered meaningful. Minimal thresholds for changes in scores that are clinically relevant have not been defined for CHO-KLAT and Haemo-QoL-A. Stata® version 13.0 was used to perform all analyses.

Results

Forty-eight subjects were enrolled into this longitudinal study however two subjects were excluded from the analysis due to incomplete data and withdrawal of consent. The sample reported here included: 13 youth (mean age = 15.7, range = 12.9–17.9 years) and 33 young adults (mean age = 23.6; range = 18.4–28.7 years). One 12.9 year-old subject was included in the analysis. His recruitment was a protocol deviation allowed by the investigators due to the small number of youth in this study. The group included 43 patients with severe disease (93 %); as well as 2 youth and one adult with moderate disease.

At recruitment, 15 % of the youth and 27 % of the young adults were considered to have had an active target joint in the prior year. Of these, 2 young adults had more than one target joint. HJHS scores ranged from 0 to 17 in the youth (mean = 5.2, standard deviation, SD = 5.61) and 0 to 34 in the young adults (mean = 13.3, SD = 8.93), where no joint damage is indicated by a score of 0. Significant joint disease (HJHS scores >10) was more common among young adults (64 %) as compared to youth (23 %).

All subjects were on some form of prophylaxis at the time of recruitment, which was defined as the regular infusion of FVIII at least once weekly with the aim of preventing clinically significant bleeding [3]. Although eligible, no subjects on an "on demand" regimen were recruited because of the paucity of patients on such a regimen in the specified age group at the study sites. Ten subjects (8 youth and 2 adults) were considered by the investigators to have been on lifelong primary prophylaxis from early childhood until the time they were recruited to the study. For the purpose of this study, primary prophylaxis was defined as prophylaxis that was started in a patient with no established joint disease, usually in the first or second year of life, before a third bleed but usually after a first bleed [3]. In our sample, 8 subjects (17.4 %) were currently on prophylaxis one to two times per week, 21 (45.6 %) were on 3x/week or alternate day prophylaxis and 17 (36.9 %) were on daily prophylaxis. These details are summarized in Table 1.

The subjects were predominantly (83 %) from three centres in Quebec, a province where Helixate FS® was preferentially prescribed for public tender contractual reasons. Treatment protocols in this region do not differ in any meaningful way from protocols elsewhere in Canada.

Subjects had a mean body mass index (BMI) of 25.1 (SD = 4.80) with a range of 18.4 to 37.9, which is similar to the Canadian norm of 26.1 [16]. Based on 45 subjects with complete BMI data, none of the subjects were underweight, 56 % of the subjects were of normal weight, 24 % of them were overweight (BMI of 25 to 34.9) and 20 % of study subjects were obese (BMI ≥ 35).

The group was diverse in terms of occupation. Of 46 subjects, 9 (20 %) were in occupations that were physically demanding, 9 (20 %) were in jobs of relatively low physical

Table 1 Baseline sample characteristics

	Study cohort youth	Study cohort young adults
Sample Size	13	33
Ages (years)	Mean = 15.6	Mean = 23.6
	SD = 1.4	SD = 2.9
	Range: 12.9 to 17.9	Range: 18.4 to 28.7
Proportion with Severe Haemophilia	85 %	97 %
Proportion with a Target Joint	15 %	27 %
Proportion on Prophylaxis	100 %	100 %
Prophylaxis Frequency	Once or Twice a week = 15 %	Once or Twice a week = 18 %
	Alternate Days = 54 %	Alternate Days = 42 %
	Daily = 31 %	Daily = 39 %
HJHS	Mean = 5.2	Mean = 13.3
	SD = 5.6	SD = 8.9
	Range: 0 to 17	Range: 0 to 34

demand, and 27 (60 %) were students. Among the students, 14 were in secondary school, 9 were attending college or a vocational school and 4 were attending university.

There were no major comorbidities in the study cohort. Seven patients had asymptomatic HCV. All other concomitant medical conditions were of mild severity (2 patients had asthma, and one each with hypertension, hypothyroidism and angioedema). One patient had a major depression more than 5 years prior, and 7 were considered to have suffered from attention deficit/hyperactivity disorder during childhood.

HRQoL scores

Generic HRQoL scores (as measured by the SF36) were available for the whole cohort of 46 subjects, including the Component Summary scores (PCS and MCS), and scores for the 8 domains. Disease specific HRQoL scores were also available for the 13 youth (as measured by the CHO-KLAT) and 33 young adults (as measured by the Haemo-QoL-A).

In the combined cohort of 46 youth and young adults all core variables met the distributional assumptions necessary for parametric analyses. The PCS scores ranged from 35 to 63 with a mean of 51.4 (SD = 6.20), and MCS scores ranged from 32 to 64 with a mean of 51.3 (SD = 8.23). Details for the SF-36 results for youth and young adults are provided in Table 2. This table shows the distributions of scores for each group. Scores were slightly better in youth than in young adults on all scales, as would be expected based on the prevalence of target joints and arthropathy, with the exception of Social Functioning. In order to compare to published Canadian norms [17], we computed SF-36 scores for the sub-set of 27 subjects who were between the ages of 16 to 24.9 years at recruitment. These are presented on the right side of Table 2; mean differences between this group and the Canadian norms are also shown. When we examined the results in comparison to the Canadian norms, Physical Functioning and Bodily Pain scores were significantly worse in our hemophilia sample.

The CHO-KLAT scores for the youth ranged from 57.9 to 97.9 with a mean of 79.2 (SD = 11.86). The Haemo-QoL-A scores for the young adults ranged from 65.9 to 98.1 with a mean of 85.8 (SD = 9.54). Additional details of the Haemo-QoL-A scores in our adult cohort are presented in Table 3. This table also includes median scores from Manco-Johnson et al. [18], who reported results for a sample with a similar age range (all of whom were on prophylaxis) from the United States, and mean scores from Rentz et al. [10] based on an international sample of older patients with a range of disease severity and comorbidity. The overall Haemo-QoL-A scores in our cohort are similar to the US cohort with the exception of higher (better) scores for Treatment Concerns in the Canadians, and all of our scale scores were significantly higher than those reported by Rentz ($p < 0.0001$).

Relationships between HRQoL measures

The relationships between the generic and disease-specific HRQoL scores were modest. The CHOK-LAT scores for the 13 youth had a weak correlation with the PCS ($r = 0.28$, $p = 0.35$), and moderate correlation with the MCS ($r = 0.39$, $p = 0.19$). The Haemo-QoL-A scores for the 33 young adults had a strong correlation with the PCS ($r = 0.53$, $p = 0.001$) and a weak correlation with the MCS ($r = 0.26$, $p = 0.13$). The lack of statistical significance for some of these observed relationships may be due in part to the small sample.

Relationships between target joints and HRQoL

The interpretation of HRQoL scores may be aided by an understanding of how scores vary in relation to key clinical characteristics. Therefore, we explored the relationship between HRQoL scores and the presence of a target joint.

There was a clinically meaningful difference in PCS scores in the 11 subjects with one or more target joints (mean = 49.1; SD = 6.32) compared to those without a target joint (mean = 52.1; SD = 6.08). The MCS scores were minimally lower in the 11 subjects with a target joint (mean = 50.3; SD = 2.37) compared to those without a target joint (mean = 51.6; SD = 1.43). A difference of 3 points is considered clinically meaningful for the component scores [5] Neither of these differences were statistically significant ($p = 0.18$ and $p = 0.66$ respectively).

The Haemo-QoL-A scores did not reveal clinically meaningful or statistically significant differences between those with or without active target joints. We also explored the

Table 2 SF36 score distributions and comparisons to Canadian Norms

Means (standard deviations)	Study Cohort Youth	Study cohort young adults	Study cohort comparative sub-set (selected to match the age range for published Canadian Norms [17])	Canadian Norms for Males [17]	Mean Difference
Ages (years)	12.9 to 17.9	18.4 to 28.7	16 to 24.9	16 to 24.9	
Sample Size	13	33	27	474	
PCS (norm-referenced scoring)	53.00	50.79	51.74	53.9	2.16
	(5.5)	(6.4)	(6.5)	(6.9)	
MCS (norm-referenced scoring)	52.3	50.9	51.1	49.3	-1.79
	(6.8)	(8.8)	(8.6)	(9.7)	
Physical Functioning	90.0	87.1	87.9	93.6	5.64*
	(10.4)	(13.2)	(13.7)	(13.3)	
Role Physical	86.1	84.1	84.5	89.9	5.41
	(17.2)	(13.9)	(14.9)	(27.1)	
Bodily Pain	75.9	66.2	69.2	79.1	9.9*
	(11.1)	(19.4)	(20.3)	(19.4)	
General Health	82.6	75.4	79.6	78.7	-0.93
	(13.6)	(15.5)	(13.9)	(14.7)	
Vitality	71.2	64.9	65.7	64.0	-1.74
	(10.4)	(16.4)	(16.9)	(16.5)	
Social Functioning	83.7	86.4	86.6	86.5	-0.07
	(16.4)	(12.6)	(14.3)	(18.7)	
Role Emotional	89.7	85.1	86.7	82.7	-4.03
	(14.5)	(18.9)	(17.5)	(32.8)	
Mental Health	80.4	77.1	77.2	74.3	-2.92
	(9.9)	(15.5)	(15.2)	(16.6)	

MID's definitions: PCS =2-3; MCS = 3; PF = 2-3; RP = 2; BP = 2-3; GH = 2-3; VT = 2-3; SF = 3; RE = 4; and MH = 3 [5]
$^*p < 0.05$

Physical Functioning sub-scale of the Haemo-QoL-A and found no difference. We were unable to assess the difference in CHO-KLAT scores associated with target joints, as there were only 2 youth with target joints.

Relationships between joint status and HRQoL

Next, we explored the relationship between HRQoL scores relative to joint damage as measured by the HJHS. PCS scores were strongly correlated with HJHS scores ($r = -0.62$, $p < 0.0001$) in the combined sample (note: the correlations were similar for both the youth and adult groups). MCS scores had a weak correlation with HJHS scores ($r = 0.12$, $p = 0.42$). HJHS total scores were weakly correlated with both the CHO-KLAT scores in youth ($r = -0.20$, $p = 0.52$) and the Haemo-QoL-A scores in adults ($r = -0.19$, $p = 0.28$).

Relationships between treatment and HRQoL

Finally, we explored the HRQoL scores in groups with different treatments. We began by looking specifically at the 10 subjects (including 8 youth) who had been on primary prophylaxis from early childhood compared to the 36 subjects who had not. The PCS scores for the 8 youth on primary prophylaxis (mean = 53.5; SD = 5.54) were only slightly higher than those for the 5 remaining youth (mean = 52.3 SD = 5.91). However, the MCS scores were worse for the youth on primary prophylaxis (mean = 49.9; SD = 7.70) when compared to the others (mean = 56.2; SD = 1.85). A similar trend was found for the two adults on primary prophylaxis (mean PCS = 53.8 SD = 9.79 and mean MCS = 36.6 SD = 4.29) compared to the 31 others (mean PCS = 50.6 SD = 6.35 and mean MCS = 51.8 SD = 8.23).

When we combined youth and adult groups the mean PCS for the primary prophylaxis group was 53.5 (SD = 5.87) vs. 50.83 (SD = 6.24) for the others, and the mean MCS score for the primary prophylaxis group was 47.2 (SD = 8.90) vs 52.4 (SD = 7.80). Data for the combined sample are shown in Fig. 1, and may suggest that primary prophylaxis is associated with better physical scores but worse mental scores. It is worth noting that the group on primary prophylaxis were younger by approximately 5 years,

Table 3 Haemo-QoL-A score distributions and comparisons published results

	Study cohort young adults	United States Cohort Manco-Johnson Prophylaxis Group [18]	International Cohort Rentz [10]
Age (years)	Mean age23.6 (SD = 2.87) [range 18.4–28.7]	Median age 19.5 [range 14–29]	mean age 38.9 (SD = 14.7)
Proportion with Severe Haemophilia	93 %	100 %	52 %
Sample Size	$n = 33$	$n = 21$	$n = 221$
Total Score	85.8	85.6	73.1
	(9.53)	(10.7)	(16.96)
Physical Functioning	82.1	88.4	66.8
	(12.4)	(11.9)	(23.9)
Role Functioning	86.4	86.0	79.4
	(10.4)	(10.3)	(17.3)
Worry	82.4	85.5	73.6
	(17.1)	(15.3)	(24.2)
Consequences of Bleeding	87.5	86.7	72.2
	(10.9)	(9.4)	(21.9)
Emotional Impact	85.1	89.8	76.9
	(12.8)	(11.8)	(18.1)
Treatment Concerns	91.1	77.5	60.1
	(13.4)	(20.9)	(30.6)

were less likely to have a target joint, had lower (better) HJHS scores and all had severe hemophilia. We were not able to examine the relationship between those on primary prophylaxis with the disease-specific HRQoL scores because of small sample sizes.

SF-36 component summary scores were also examined according to weekly frequency of prophylactic regimen at the time of recruitment. In the combined cohort, the mean PCS score for the 8 subjects on prophylaxis one to two times per week was 53.6 (SD = 4.78). The 21 subjects on prophylaxis 3 times per week or alternate days had a mean PCS score of 52.4 (SD = 6.73). The 17 subjects receiving daily prophylaxis had a mean PCS score of 49.1 (SD = 5.66). Mean MCS scores for these same groups were 48.3 (SD = 9.9), 52.6 (SD = 8.0), and 51.0 (SD = 7.83) respectively.

Impact of age

It is known that in the general population HRQoL diminishes as a function of age [5]. We found a reduction of 0.31 points per year of age ($p = 0.14$) in the PCS scores, and a decline by 0.33 per year ($p = 0.25$) in the MCS, but neither reached statistical significance. The reduction of scores as a function of age was also observed with the disease-specific measures: CHO-KLAT scores decreased by 0.73 points per year of age among the 13 youth ($p = 0.78$); and Haemo-QoL-A scores decreased 1.01 points per year of age ($p = 0.09$) among the 33 young adults.

Discussion

This paper reports the baseline data of a study with a primary objective to describe the patterns of QoL over a 3-year period in Canadian youth and young adults who have moderate or severe hemophilia A and who are using Helixate FS®.

Forty-six subjects were recruited from 6 centres in 3 Canadian provinces but were predominantly from Quebec because Helixate FS® is preferentially used in that province for reasons of public tender contract. Although limited to one brand of recombinant factor concentrate, there is no reason to suspect that the product brand would have a significant impact on HRQoL. This cohort comprised subjects 12.9 to 28.7 years of age who were free from HIV or other significant comorbid conditions.

We had a relatively small group of youth, most of whom had been on prophylaxis from an early age, and a larger group of young adults most of whom had not been introduced to prophylaxis at an early age as is typical in Canada for these age groups. While very frequently used in Canada, prophylaxis is not universal in this age group and our findings may not be applicable to patients who are “on-demand”. There are no other recruitment criteria that would differentiate this cohort, and it is therefore a small but representative sample of Canadians with moderate or severe HA. The subjects were unremarkable in terms of their BMI scores. In our sample (mean age of 21.4 years), 52 % had significant joint disease (HJHS > 10) which compares to the slightly older Dutch cohort (mean age of 24.8 years) described by Fischer et al. [14], in which 46 % had significant joint disease.

Generic HRQoL scores

The main focus of this study was on the HRQoL of youth and young adults with hemophilia which was captured using both a generic (SF-36) and two disease-specific questionnaires; one for youth (CHO-KLAT) and one for adults (Haemo-QoL-A). We began with an examination of the SF36 component scores. When we compared the results of our study subjects, between the ages of 16 to 24.9 years, to published normative data for healthy Canadian males in the same age range, we found that our mean scores were similar to the PCS and MCS norms. However, we found several notable differences when we examined the 8 domains within the SF-36 (see Table 2). Our cohort reported lower scores compared to Canadian normative data in the following domains: Physical Functioning (mean difference = 5.6), Role Physical (5.4), and Bodily Pain (9.9). The differences for Physical Functioning and Bodily Pain were clinically

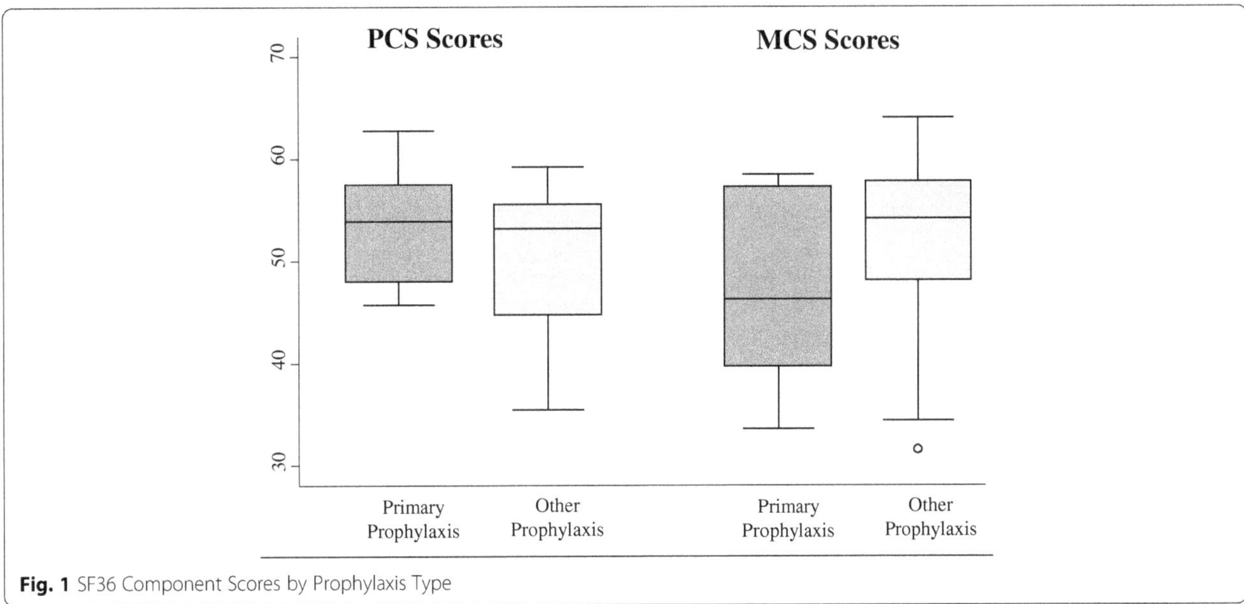

Fig. 1 SF36 Component Scores by Prophylaxis Type

meaningful (exceeded the MIDs) and statistically significant. These results are consistent with what one would expect based on clinical experience. We also identified areas of strengths in our cohort, with higher scores than the norms in the following domains: Role Emotional (mean difference = 4.0) and Mental Health (2.9). These differences were not statistically significant.

Similar comparative analysis was conducted in Sweden, by Lindvall et al. [19], who reported on a cross-sectional study of severe HA subjects aged 15–34 years from a single treatment center. They found that SF-36 PCS and MCS scores were not statistically different than the national norms, which is consistent with our findings. However, they found significantly impaired HRQoL based on some of the SF-36 domains (PF and PR), and for PCS scores only in their older subjects (35 to 64 years). More intensive prophylaxis in Sweden than in Canada may explain the delay in decline of HRQoL in that country.

We found significant differences in PCS but not MCS scores related to joint status (HJHS) in our Canadian cohort. However, PCS and MCS were not worse in those reporting an active target joint in the preceding year, suggesting that functional joint status more than bleed frequency impacts HRQoL.

To explore the relationship of HRQoL to treatment history we first compared the PCS and MCS scores in those who had been on lifelong primary prophylaxis versus the others. We found better PCS scores but worse MCS scores in the primary prophylaxis group. These results should be interpreted with caution given the small number of subjects involved and the difference in age between the two categories of subjects. They are intriguing given that we identified Role Emotional and Mental Health domains as areas of strength in our hemophilia cohort compared to Canadian norms. The exploration of HRQoL in relation to prophylaxis frequency found an inverse relationship, in that those receiving the most frequent treatment (daily) had the lowest PCS scores. However, there was no clear relationship between frequency of treatment and MCS scores. These mental health findings warrant investigation in future larger studies.

When we explored age-related differences in the cross-sectional cohort, we found that PCS and MCS scores declined as a function of age in a similar fashion. However, clinical experience suggests that the PCS scores should decline to a greater extent than MCS, given the contributions of both the natural aging process and cumulative joint damage associated with hemophilia. This requires further examination in longitudinal studies.

Disease specific HRQoL scores

The analysis of the disease-specific results from this study is limited due to the small sample sizes, particularly for youth. The mean CHO-KLAT score in this cohort (79.2) was somewhat higher than reported in previous studies such as: the Canadian validation study 74.6 [9]; Quebec validation study 71.9 [8]; and recent Toronto study 75.4 [20]. However, the scores are very close to the mean of 78.0 for a subset of 19 patients from the Toronto study who were 14 years of age or older [20].

Although the mean Haemo-QoL-A total score found in our young adults (85.8) appears high compared to the Rentz et al. results [10], our adult cohort was much younger, had less viral co-morbidity and did not include a significant proportion of subjects treated "on demand" (see Table 3). Similarly, Ingerslev found much higher Haemo-QoL-A total scores for Danish patients on prophylaxis (median score = 86.5) than in Russian patients that had been mostly treated on-demand (median score = 71.0). Manco-Johnson et al. [18] studied prospectively a cohort of severe HA subjects also age 14-29 years who had mostly been on prophylaxis. She reported a mean Haemo-QoL-A total score of 85.6 (SD = 10.7) for a group of 22 subjects (with a median age of 17 years) who had been on uninterrupted prophylaxis at the time of study entry. The results from the latter study are very similar to ours (Table 3).

Our data revealed modest correlations between disease specific scores and the generic SF36. The CHO-KLAT demonstrated a better relationship with the MCS than PCS and the Haemo-QoL-A demonstrated a better relationship with the PCS than MCS indicating again that they are not assessing the same aspects of quality of life.

We have found that global scores are less sensitive than subdomains in understanding HRQoL in severe hemophilia as a decline in physical scales may be offset by mental scores higher than normative data in this condition. The areas of bodily pain and physical functioning deserve particular attention when assessing differences in cohorts or treatment approach. The lack of statistical correlation between joint status and disease specific HRQoL scores (CHO-KLAT and Haemo-QoL-A) may reflect differences in the nature of the items included in these tools which focus more on emotional health.

We were not surprised to see the subtle decline in HRQoL as a function of age; this should be kept in mind when comparing SF-36 and other instruments' scores between studies involving cohorts of different age groups. The small sample size did not allow us to perform more sophisticated analyses, therefore the relationship between age, HJHS and HRQoL could not be fully assessed.

Conclusions

Despite having mostly severe hemophilia, the youth in this cohort had minimal joint disease and good HRQoL. The young adults demonstrated more joint disease and slightly worse HRQoL – but were almost comparable to healthy populations of the same age. These findings confirm those of other investigators studying cohorts in developed countries and should now be expected in patients with access to adequate levels of prophylaxis.

We also identified that primary prophylaxis was associated with better PCS scores, which is consistent with their younger age, lower prevalence of target joints and better HJHS scores. However, this group also had lower MCS scores which were atypical for their age group. This requires further examination and potentially warrants more emotional health related questions be asked of youth with a history of primary prophylaxis in clinical practice.

Comparatively little is known about factors that might influence longitudinal patterns of HRQoL in patients on a stable treatment regimen. The current results form the foundation for a longitudinal study to examine the impact of biological factors and life events on the HRQoL of youth and young adults with haemophilia followed prospectively for 3 years.

Abbreviations

BP: Bodily Pain; CHO-KLAT: Canadian Haemophilia Outcomes – Kids Life Assessment Tool; ERB: Ethics Review Board; FVIII: Factor VIII; GH: General Health; HA: Hemophilia A; HCV: Hepatitis C virus; HIV: Human immunodeficiency virus; HJHS: Hemophilia Joint Health Score (HJHS) version 2.0; HRQoL: Health-related quality of life; MCS: Mental Component Summary; MH: Mental Health; PCS: Physical Component Summary; PF: Physical Functioning; RF: Role Emotion; RP: Role Physical; SD: Standard Deviation; SF: Social Functioning; SF-36: Short Form 36; VT: Vitality.

Competing interests

The authors declare that they have no competing interests which might be perceived as posing a conflict or bias.

Authors' contributions

JSL was the Principal Investigator on this grant and made a substantive contribution to all aspects of the work; DJU was the primary analyst and assisted in the writing of the manuscript; FM recruited patients and administered study questionnaires; SC, RK, BR, GER and MW enrolled patients in the study and critically reviewed the manuscript; VB and NL Young were the Co-PI on this grant and assisted in developing all aspects of the manuscript. All authors approved the final version of the manuscript.

Authors' information

No other relevant information.

Acknowledgements

NL Young was supported by a Canada Research Chair from CIHR. GE Rivard was supported by a Grant for Center of Excellence in Hemostasis from Bayer Canada. We thank the patients and their families for participating in this study as well as the research personnel and physiotherapists of the recruiting sites for their important contribution.

Funding

Funding for this research was provided by CSL Behring Canada. The funder contributed to the design of the study but had no role in the analysis and interpretation of the data or in the writing of the manuscript or the decision to submit the manuscript to publication.

Author details

[1]CHU Sainte-Justine, Montréal, Canada. [2]Hôpital Maisonneuve-Rosemont, Montreal, Canada. [3]Laurentian University, Sudbury, Canada. [4]Hôpital de l'Enfant-Jésus, Quebec city, Canada. [5]University of Alberta, Edmonton, Canada. [6]Children's Hospital of Eastern Ontario, Ottawa, Canada. [7]McGill University Health Centre, Montréal, Canada. [8]University of Toronto, Toronto, Canada. [9]Hospital for Sick Children, Toronto, Canada.

References

1. Franchini M, Mannucci PM. Hemophilia a in the third millennium. Blood Rev. 2013;27:179–84.
2. Organization WH. World health organization. International classification of functioning, disability and health, children and youth version. 2014 [cited 2015 August 15, 2015].
3. Ota S, McLimont M, Carcao MD, Blanchette VS, Graham N, Paradis E, et al. Definitions for haemophilia prophylaxis and its outcomes: The Canadian consensus study. Haemophilia. 2007;13:12–20.
4. Ware JE, Sherbourne CD. The mos 36-item short-form health survey (sf-36): I. Conceptual framework and item selection. Med Care Res Rev. 1992;30:473–83.
5. Ware JE, Kosinsk IM, Bjorner JB, Turner-Bowker DM, Gandek B, Maruish ME. User's manual for the sf-36v2tm health survey. 2nd ed. Lincoln: QualityMetric Incorporated; 2007.

6. Young NL, Bradley CS, Blanchette V, Wakefield CD, Barnard D, Wu JKM, et al. Development of a health-related quality of life measure for boys with haemophilia: The Canadian haemophilia outcomes - kids' life assessment tool (CHO-KLAT). Haemophilia. 2004;10:34–43.
7. Young NL, Bradley CS, Wakefield CD, Barnard D, Blanchette VS, McCusker PJ. How well does the Canadian haemophilia outcomes-kids' life assessment tool (CHO-KLAT) measure the quality of life of boys with haemophilia? Pediatr Blood Cancer. 2006;47:305–11.
8. Young NL, St-Louis J, Burke TA, Hershon L, Blanchette V. Cross-cultural validation of the CHO-KLAT and haemo-QoL-a in Canadian French. Haemophilia. 2012;18:353–7.
9. McCusker PJ, Burke TA, Holzhauer S, Fischer K, Altisent C, Grainger JD, et al. International cross cultural validation study of the Canadian hemophilia outcomes – kids life assessment tool (CHO-KLAT). Haemophilia. 2015;21:351–7.
10. Rentz A, Flood E, Altisent C, Bullinger M, Klamroth R, Garrido RP, et al. Cross-cultural development and psychometric evaluation of a patient-reported health-related quality of life questionnaire for adults with haemophilia. Haemophilia. 2008;14:1023–34.
11. Feldman BM, Funk S, Lundin B, Doria AS, Ljung R, Blanchette V. Musculoskeletal measurement tools from the international prophylaxis study group (ipsg). Haemophilia. 2008;14:162–9.
12. Feldman BM, Funk SM, Bergstrom BM, Zourikian N, Hilliard P, van der Net J, et al. Validation of a new pediatric joint scoring system from the international hemophilia prophylaxis study group: Validity of the hemophilia joint health score. Arthritis Care Res. 2011;63:223–30.
13. Fischer K, Kleijn P. Using the haemophilia joint health score for assessment of teenagers and young adults: Exploring reliability and validity. Haemophilia. 2013;19:944–50.
14. Fischer K, Carlsson KS, Petrini P, Holmström M, Ljung R, van den Berg HM, et al. Intermediate-dose versus high-dose prophylaxis for severe hemophilia: Comparing outcome and costs since the 1970s. Blood. 2013;122:1129–36.
15. Cohen J. Statistical power analysis for the behavioral sciences. New York: Academic press; 2013.
16. Ross NA, Tremblay S, Khan S, Crouse D, Tremblay M, Berthelot J-M. Body mass index in urban Canada: Neighborhood and metropolitan area effect. Am J Public Health Nations Health. 2007;97:500–8.
17. Hopman WM, Berger C, Joseph L, Towheed T, Prior JC, Anastassiades T, et al. Health-related quality of life in Canadian adolescents and young adults: Normative data using the sf-36. Can J Public Health. 2009;100:449–52.
18. Manco-Johnson M, Sanders J, Ewing N, Rodriguez N, Tarantino M, Humphries T. Consequences of switching from prophylactic treatment to on-demand treatment in late teens and early adults with severe haemophilia a: The teen/twen study. Haemophilia. 2013;19:727–35.
19. Lindvall K, Von Mackensen S, Berntorp E. Quality of life in adult patients with haemophilia–a single centre experience from sweden. Haemophilia. 2012;18:527–31.
20. Young NL, Wakefield C, Burke TA, Ray R, McCusker PJ, Blanchette V. Updating the Canadian hemophilia outcomes–kids life assessment tool (CHO-KLAT version2.0). Value Health. 2013;16:837–41.

5

Ferumoxytol versus iron sucrose treatment: a post-hoc analysis of randomized controlled trials in patients with varying renal function and iron deficiency anemia

William E. Strauss*, Naomi V. Dahl, Zhu Li, Gloria Lau and Lee F. Allen

Abstract

Background: Iron deficiency anemia is highly prevalent in patients with chronic kidney disease and is often treated with intravenous iron. There are few trials directly comparing the safety and efficacy of different intravenous iron products.

Methods: This post-hoc analysis pooled data from 767 patients enrolled in two randomized, controlled, open-label trials of similar design comparing the treatment of iron deficiency anemia with ferumoxytol and iron sucrose across patients with all stages of renal function. One trial was conducted in adults with CKD either on or not on dialysis and the second in adults with IDA of any underlying cause and a history of unsatisfactory oral iron therapy or in whom oral iron could not be used who had normal to no worse than moderately impaired renal function. Patients were categorized by chronic kidney disease stage (i.e., estimated glomerular filtration rate), and the primary efficacy endpoint was the mean change in hemoglobin from Baseline to Week 5.

Results: The overall incidence of adverse events was numerically lower in ferumoxytol-treated patients compared to those treated with iron sucrose (42.4 vs. 50.2 %, respectively); the incidence of treatment-related adverse events was generally similar between the two treatment groups (13.6 vs. 16.0 %, respectively). Adverse events of Special Interest (i.e., hypotension, hypersensitivity) occurred at lower rates in those treated with ferumoxytol compared to those treated with iron sucrose (2.5 vs. 5.3 %, respectively). Overall, mean hemoglobin increased in both treatment groups, regardless of degree of renal insufficiency, although greater increases were seen among those with less severe kidney damage. Mean increases in hemoglobin from Baseline to Week 5 were significantly greater with ferumoxytol than with iron sucrose treatment in the subgroup with an estimated glomerular filtration rate ≥90 mL/min (Least Squares mean difference = 0.53 g/dL; $p < 0.001$). There were no other consistent, significant differences in hemoglobin levels between treatment groups for the other chronic kidney disease categories except for isolated instances favoring ferumoxytol.

Conclusions: The efficacy and safety of ferumoxytol is at least comparable to iron sucrose in patients with varying degrees of renal function.

Trial registration: (**CKD-201**; ClinicalTrials.gov identifier: NCT01052779; registered 15 January, 2010), (**IDA-302**; ClinicalTrials.gov identifier: NCT01114204; registered 29 April, 2010).

Keywords: Ferumoxytol, Hemoglobin, Iron deficiency anemia, Iron sucrose, Chronic kidney disease

* Correspondence: wstrauss@amagpharma.com
AMAG Pharmaceuticals, Inc., 1100 Winter Street, Waltham, MA 02451, USA

Background

Iron deficiency anemia (IDA) is the leading cause of anemia worldwide [1]. In the United States, IDA affects approximately 1 to 2 % of men and 2 to 5 % of women [2]. IDA is particularly common in patients with chronic kidney disease (CKD) [3–5].

Correction of the underlying cause of IDA and repletion of depleted iron stores are fundamental approaches to the treatment and management of IDA [6]. Intravenous (IV) iron plays a major role in the treatment of IDA across all degrees of renal function, and in particular for those with CKD, including dialysis-dependent CKD patients, and non-CKD patients unable to tolerate oral iron or in whom oral iron is either ineffective or contraindicated. According to the 2012 Kidney Disease Improving Global Outcomes clinical practice guidelines, a trial of IV iron is recommended in all adult CKD dialysis patients with anemia not on iron or erythropoiesis-stimulating agent therapy and in non-dialysis patients with CKD after a failed trial of oral iron [7].

The efficacy of IV iron supplementation in the treatment of IDA has been studied in patients with a variety of underlying conditions, including CKD, abnormal uterine bleeding, pregnancy, postpartum anemia, cancer, and gastrointestinal (GI) disorders, including inflammatory bowel disease and GI blood loss. However, few randomized head-to-head studies specifically comparing the relative safety and efficacy of IV iron products have been conducted [8–12].

Ferumoxytol, a colloidal iron oxide, is an IV iron product approved for the treatment of IDA in adult patients with CKD in the US and Canada as Feraheme® (ferumoxytol) Injection and, at the time of this analysis, was marketed in the US as Feraheme and in the European Union and Switzerland as Rienso® (ferumoxytol) [13]. Ferumoxytol has been investigated for the broad indication of IDA in those who have failed or who are intolerant to oral iron therapy. Unlike most other IV iron products, a full course of ferumoxytol therapy (1.02 g) requires only two IV administrations of 510 mg, delivered between 3 and 8 days apart. Iron sucrose (Venofer®) is approved in the US as an iron replacement product for the treatment of IDA in patients with CKD. Iron sucrose is administered in small doses as a slow IV injection or longer infusion and requires the administration of multiple doses. At the time of this publication, there were little data on the efficacy and safety of iron replacement therapy in patients with various stages of renal function. Thus, the primary objective of this analysis was to provide a deeper understanding of the comparative safety and efficacy of ferumoxytol and iron sucrose across all stages of renal function, from normal kidney function to end-stage CKD.

Methods

Two recently completed clinical trials compared the efficacy and safety of ferumoxytol with iron sucrose for the treatment of IDA in adults with CKD either on or not on dialysis (**CKD-201**; ClinicalTrials.gov identifier: NCT01052779), and in adults with IDA of any underlying cause and a history of unsatisfactory oral iron therapy or in whom oral iron could not be used (**IDA-302**; ClinicalTrials.gov identifier: NCT01114204). Here, we report the pooled safety and efficacy results of these two randomized, controlled studies with similar study designs to better characterize the safety and efficacy of these IV iron products across all stages of renal function, from normal kidney function to end-stage CKD, as categorized by estimated glomerular filtration rate (eGFR) levels of ≥90, 60 to <90, 30 to <60, 15 to <30, and <15 mL/min.

This post-hoc analysis included pooled data from all patients in the Intent-to-Treat (ITT) populations of two randomized, open-label, controlled clinical trials (**CKD-201** and **IDA-302**) of similar design ($N = 767$). Full details of the study designs and results for the overall patient populations were presented separately in the original two papers [14, 15]. Both studies were conducted in accordance with the ethical principles of Good Clinical Practice and in compliance with the Declaration of Helsinki. The study protocols were reviewed and approved by the institutional review boards or ethics committees at each study site (Additional file 1). Ethical approval for the current study was not required, as it is a post-hoc analysis of pooled data from two previously published clinical trials. All patients provided written informed consent prior to study entry.

The **CKD-201** study included adults aged ≥18 years with CKD on or not on hemodialysis. Patients were required to have a serum hemoglobin (Hgb) <11.0 and ≥7 g/dL and a transferrin saturation (TSAT) <30 % [14]. The **IDA-302** study included patients who had various primary underlying conditions associated with IDA (e.g., abnormal uterine bleeding, cancer, GI disorders, postpartum anemia, and other conditions) with normal (eGFR >90 mL/min), mild (eGFR of 60–90 mL/min), and moderate (eGFR of 30–59 mL/min) decreased renal function, but excluded those with severe (eGFR < 30 mL/min) kidney disease. Patients in **IDA-302** included adults aged ≥18 years with a Baseline Hgb >7 to <10 g/dL and a TSAT <20 % who had either failed oral iron therapy or were intolerant to oral iron [15].

There were a total of 162 patients from the **CKD-201** study and 605 patients from the **IDA-302** study. Overall, 486 patients received ferumoxytol and 281 received iron sucrose. Both studies included a 14-day screening period. Patients in the Ferumoxytol Treatment Group received a 510-mg IV dose at the Baseline visit (Day 1) followed by a second IV dose 2 to 8 days later (Week 1) as a rapid IV injection of 17 mL at a rate not to exceed 1 mL/sec. Patients were observed weekly until the end of the 5-week treatment period (Weeks 2–5). Patients randomized to the Iron Sucrose Treatment Group received a cumulative dose of 1 g as 10 IV doses of 100 mg (hemodialysis patients, **CKD-201**) within 3 weeks or five IV doses of 200 mg on five non-consecutive days over a 14-day period (non-dialysis CKD patients, **CKD-201**; all patients, **IDA-302**). Iron Sucrose was given as an infusion or slow injection. Infusions were given at 25 mg for the first 15 min; if no adverse events (AEs) occurred, the remaining dose was given at a rate not exceeding 100 mg over 15 min. Slow injections were given at 1 mL (20 mg) over 1–2 min; if no AEs occurred, the remaining dose was given. Blood samples were collected at Screening, Baseline, and weekly Visits 2 to 5 to assess efficacy (Hgb, TSAT, other iron measures).

The safety population included all randomized patients who had any exposure to study drug and was based on actual treatment received. The ITT population included any randomized patient who had any exposure to study drug (IV ferumoxytol or IV iron sucrose) and was based upon randomized treatment assignment. The safety and ITT populations were identical in this analysis.

The safety analysis included descriptive summaries of overall AEs, serious AEs (SAEs), study drug-related AEs, AEs resulting in study drug discontinuation, and AEs of Special Interest (AESIs; predefined as moderate-to-severe hypotension occurring on the day of dosing and moderate-to-severe hypersensitivity reactions) and Composite Cardiovascular AEs (predefined as nonfatal myocardial infarction, heart failure, moderate-to-severe hypertension, and hospitalization due to any cardiovascular event). The efficacy analysis focused on mean change

Table 1 Demographic and baseline characteristics of pooled treatment groups (total study population - safety population)[a]

	Ferumoxytol Treatment Group (*n* = 486)	Iron Sucrose Treatment Group (*n* = 281)	Total (*N* = 767)
Mean age, years (SD)	50.1 (15.75)	52.8 (16.06)	51.1 (15.90)
Mean weight, kg (SD)	70.9 (16.07)	76.0 (20.29)	72.8 (17.89)
Mean height, cm (SD)	165.8 (8.17)	166.5 (8.18)	166.0 (8.18)
Sex, n (%)			
Female	383 (78.8)	199 (70.8)	582 (75.9)
Male	103 (21.2)	82 (29.2)	185 (24.1)
Race, n (%)			
American Indian/Alaskan Native	0 (0.0)	1 (0.4)	1 (0.1)
Asian	51 (10.5)	18 (6.4)	69 (9.0)
Black/African American	27 (5.6)	16 (5.7)	43 (5.6)
Native Hawaiian/other Pacific Islander	2 (0.4)	1 (0.4)	3 (0.4)
White	390 (80.2)	234 (83.3)	624 (81.4)
Other/multiracial	16 (3.3)	11 (3.9)	27 (3.5)
Ethnicity, n (%)			
Hispanic/Latino	12 (2.5)	13 (4.6)	25 (3.3)
Not Hispanic/Latino	474 (97.5)	268 (95.4)	742 (96.7)
CKD stage, n (%)			
Stage 1 (eGFR ≥90 mL/min)	280 (57.6)	126 (44.8)	406 (52.9)
Stage 2 (eGFR 60 to <90 mL/min)	104 (21.4)	59 (21.0)	163 (21.3)
Stage 3 (eGFR 30 to <60 mL/min)	41 (8.4)	33 (11.7)	74 (9.6)
Stage 4 (eGFR 15 to <30 mL/min)	23 (4.7)	20 (7.1)	43 (5.6)
Stage 5 (eGFR <15 mL/min)	38 (7.8)	42 (14.9)	80 (10.4)
Unknown	0 (0.0)	1 (0.4)	1 (0.1)
Dialysis status, n			
Hemodialysis	34	36	70
ESA use, n (%)	45 (9.3)	40 (14.2)	85 (11.1)

ESA erythropoiesis-stimulating agent, *eGFR* estimated glomerular filtration rate, *Hgb* hemoglobin, *SD* standard deviation
[a]Baseline values obtained Day 1 prior to injection of study drug

Table 2 Baseline laboratory values by CKD stage, mean (SD)

CKD Stage	Hgb, g/dL		TSAT, %		Ferritin, μg/L	
	Ferumoxytol Treatment Group	Iron Sucrose Treatment Group	Ferumoxytol Treatment Group	Iron Sucrose Treatment Group	Ferumoxytol Treatment Group	Iron Sucrose Treatment Group
All stages	9.1 (1.04) (*n* = 486)	9.2 (1.11) (*n* = 280)	8.7 (12.93) (*n* = 486)	9.4 (12.40) (*n* = 280)	68.8 (170.04) (*n* = 481)	88.6 (184.48) (*n* = 279)
Stage 1 (eGFR ≥90 mL/min)	8.8 (0.95) (*n* = 280)	8.8 (0.98) (*n* = 126)	5.8 (11.25) (*n* = 280)	4.3 (5.21) (*n* = 126)	14.1 (39.76) (*n* = 276)	15.4 (53.11) (*n* = 125)
Stage 2 (eGFR 60 to <90 mL/min)	9.1 (1.0) (*n* = 104)	8.9 (0.89) (*n* = 59)	6.6 (5.7) (*n* = 104)	5.1 (3.47) (*n* = 59)	55.4 (138.26) (*n* = 103)	22.7 (80.21) (*n* = 59)
Stage 3 (eGFR 30 to <60 mL/min)	9.3 (0.86) (*n* = 41)	9.5 (0.88) (*n* = 33)	13.4 (18.31) (*n* = 41)	16.1 (22.18) (*n* = 33)	106.6 (168.37) (*n* = 41)	106.5 (157.15) (*n* = 33)
Stage 4 (eGFR 15 to <30 mL/min)	9.8 (0.84) (*n* = 23)	10.0 (0.76) (*n* = 20)	21.7 (19.41) (*n* = 23)	17.0 (6.49) (*n* = 20)	152.3 (123.03) (*n* = 23)	141.4 (158.16) (*n* = 20)
Stage 5 (eGFR <15 mL/min)	10.2 (1.09) (*n* = 38)	10.2 (1.10) (*n* = 42)	22.3 (12.91) (*n* = 38)	21.7 (14.76) (*n* = 42)	411.3 (348.97) (*n* = 38)	359.7 (287.65) (*n* = 42)

eGFR estimated glomerular filtration rate, *Hgb* hemoglobin, *SD* standard deviation, *TSAT* transferrin saturation

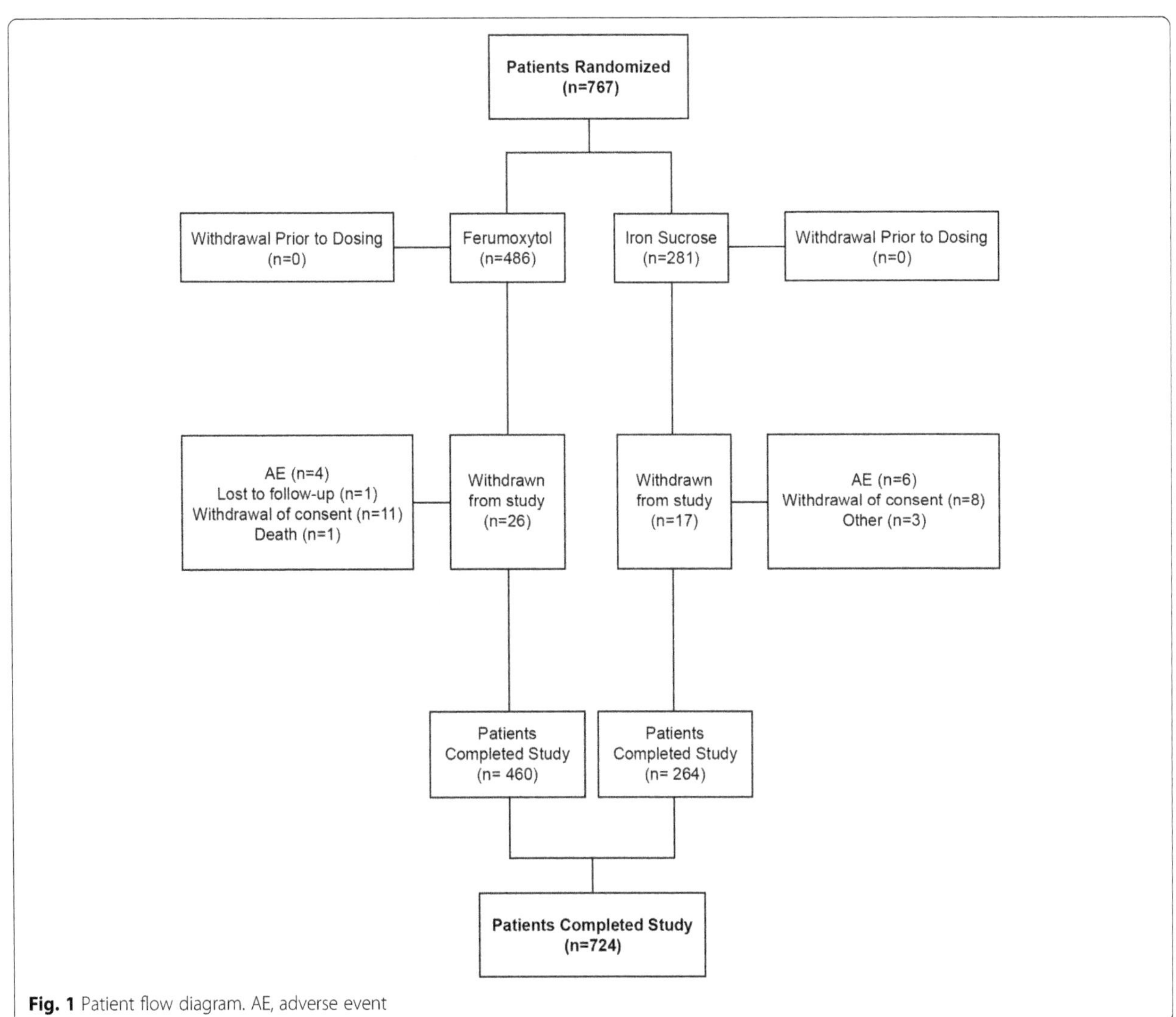

Fig. 1 Patient flow diagram. AE, adverse event

in Hgb from Baseline to Week 5, which was the primary efficacy endpoint in both individual studies. The treatment difference in the Hgb change was analyzed using an analysis of covariance model adjusting for Baseline Hgb, primary underlying conditions, and dialysis status.

Results

Baseline characteristics and patient disposition

The demographic and baseline characteristics for the Ferumoxytol and Iron Sucrose Treatment Groups were comparable (Table 1). The majority of the study population was comprised of women (75.9 %). The mean (± standard deviation [SD]) age was 51.1 ± 15.9 years and most patients were white (81.4 %). The following differences were noted in the characteristics between the two study populations: The mean age of patients in **CKD-201** was 14.4 years greater and the mean weight was 16.3 kg greater. More patients in CKD-201 were receiving treatment with an erythropoiesis-stimulating agent than those from **IDA-302** (52 % of patients in **CKD-201** vs. 1 patient of 605 in **IDA-302**). In addition, a greater percentage of patients from **IDA-302** had more severe anemia on study entry with 33 % having a Baseline Hgb value ≤8.5 g/dL, while only 13 % of patients from **CKD-201** had a Baseline Hgb ≤9 g/dL. Approximately one-half of the study population (52.9 %) had normal renal function (eGFR >90 mL/min), and the distribution of patients classified by eGFR category (i.e., eGFR ≥90, 60 to <90, 30 to <60, 15 to <30, and <15 mL/min) is summarized in Table 1. Mean Baseline values for iron parameters by Baseline CKD stage are summarized in Table 2, with an overall Baseline mean Hgb of 9.1 (±1.04) g/dL in the Ferumoxytol Treatment Group and 9.2 (±1.11) g/dL in the Iron Sucrose treatment group. Patient disposition is illustrated in Fig. 1.

Approximately 94 % of patients in each treatment group completed the study. The mean total cumulative doses of IV iron (mg) in the Ferumoxytol and Iron Sucrose Treatment Groups were comparable (1005.0 ± 85.61 and 966.0 ± 142.6 mg, respectively).

Safety

The pooled safety population (i.e., ITT population) included 486 patients in the Ferumoxytol Treatment

Table 3 Treatment-emergent AEs and incidence of Treatment-emergent AEs occurring in ≥2 % of patients (safety population)

	Ferumoxytol Treatment Group (n = 486)	Iron Sucrose Treatment Group (n = 281)	Total (N = 767)
AE Summary			
All AEs	206 (42.4)	141 (50.2)	347 (45.2)
Treatment-related AEs	66 (13.6)	45 (16.0)	111 (14.5)
SAEs	24 (4.9)	11 (3.9)	35 (4.6)
Treatment-related SAEs	3 (0.6)	1 (0.4)	4 (0.5)
AEs of Special Interest[a]	12 (2.5)	15 (5.3)	27 (3.5)
Cardiovascular AEs[b]	6 (1.2)	3 (1.1)	9 (1.2)
AEs resulting in temporary discontinuation of study drug	3 (0.6)	4 (1.4)	7 (0.9)
AEs resulting in permanent discontinuation of study drug	7 (1.4)	9 (3.2)	16 (2.1)
AEs resulting in study discontinuation	4 (0.8)	6 (2.1)	10 (1.3)
Death	1 (0.2)	0 (0.0)	1 (0.1)
Treatment-emergent AEs occurring in ≥2 % of patients in any treatment group by decreasing incidence in the Ferumoxytol Treatment Group			
Headache	22 (4.5)	13 (4.6)	35 (4.6)
Nausea	17 (3.5)	10 (3.6)	27 (3.5)
Dizziness	10 (2.1)	5 (1.5)	15 (2.0)
Dysgeusia	10 (2.1)	14 (5.0)	24 (3.1)
Peripheral edema	5 (1.0)	8 (2.8)	13 (1.7)
Urinary tract infection	5 (1.0)	9 (3.2)	14 (1.8)
Muscle spasms	5 (1.0)	6 (2.1)	11 (1.4)
Vomiting	4 (0.8)	6 (2.1)	10 (1.3)
Hypotension	3 (0.6)	10 (3.6)	13 (1.7)
Pyrexia	2 (0.4)	7 (2.5)	9 (1.2)

Data are presented as n (%). AE: adverse event; SAE: serious adverse event
[a]Includes hypotension and hypersensitivity
[b]Includes myocardial infarction, heart failure, moderate to severe hypertension, and hospitalization due to any cardiovascular cause

Group and 281 in the Iron Sucrose Treatment Group. The overall incidence of all AEs was 42.4 % in the Ferumoxytol Treatment Group and 50.2 % in the Iron Sucrose Treatment Group. The incidence of treatment-related AEs was similar (13.6 and 16.0 % for ferumoxytol and iron sucrose, respectively; Table 3). The most frequent AEs were headache (4.5 %) and nausea (3.5 %) in the Ferumoxytol Treatment Group, and dysgeusia (5.0 %) and headache (4.6 %) in the Iron Sucrose Treatment Group (Table 3). Overall AEs and treatment-related AEs occurring within 24 h of each dose are summarized in Fig. 2. Frequencies of AEs were generally similar between the Ferumoxytol and Iron Sucrose Treatment Groups during Weeks 1 and 2, although the Iron Sucrose Treatment Group continued to experience AEs with subsequent administrations.

Discontinuation due to AEs occurred at comparable rates in the Ferumoxytol (0.8 %) and Iron Sucrose (2.1 %) Treatment Groups. Similarly, the proportion of patients experiencing AESIs (i.e., hypotension and hypersensitivity) was comparable between treatment groups (ferumoxytol, 2.5 %; iron sucrose, 5.3 %; Table 3). Five of the AESIs in the Iron Sucrose Treatment Group occurred at Weeks 3 through 10 (i.e., after all ferumoxytol administrations had been completed). One patient death occurred in the Ferumoxytol Treatment Group. The patient had a pancreatic tumor causing duodenal obstruction and died postoperatively; this was considered unrelated by the Investigator. Composite Cardiovascular AEs occurred at a similar incidence in both treatment groups (ferumoxytol, 1.2 %; iron sucrose, 1.1 %). Similarly, rates of SAEs and treatment-related SAEs were comparable between treatment groups (ferumoxytol, 4.9 and 0.6 %; iron sucrose 3.9 and 0.4 %, respectively). Four patients (0.5 %) experienced an SAE within 24 h of the first dose of IV iron (ferumoxytol, $n = 1$ [0.2 %]; iron sucrose, $n = 3$ [1.1 %]). SAEs occurring within 24 h of the first dose of IV iron were considered treatment-related in one patient in each group (ferumoxytol, 0.2 %-moderate intensity anaphylactic-type reaction that resolved on the day of dosing; iron sucrose, 0.4 %-moderate intensity hypotension treated with volume and Trendelenburg positioning).

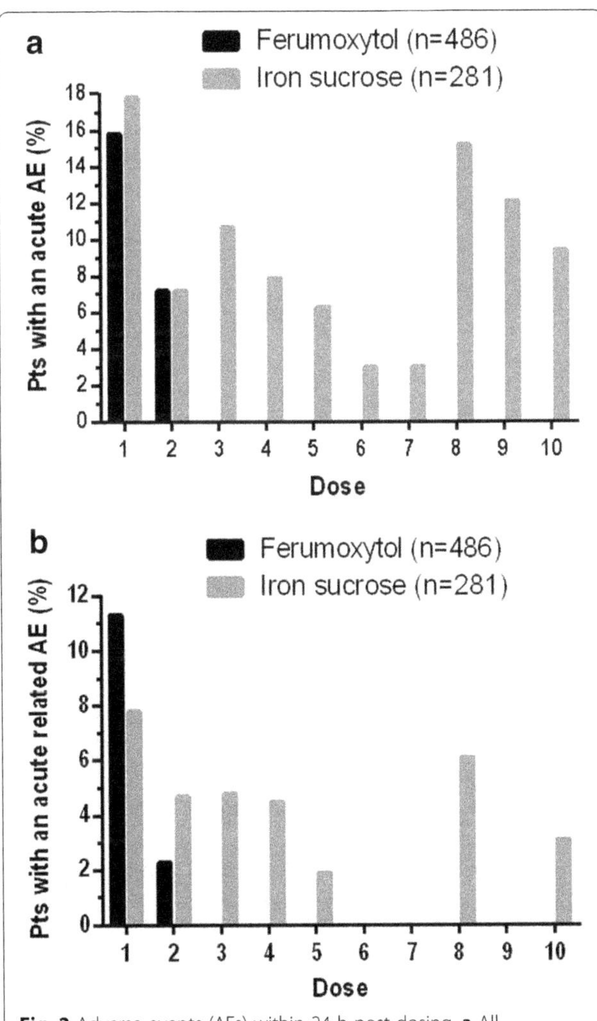

Fig. 2 Adverse events (AEs) within 24 h post-dosing. **a** All treatment-emergent AEs by treatment and dose number. **b** All treatment-related AEs by treatment and dose number. Pts, patients

Efficacy

Hgb levels increased from Baseline until the end of the study in both treatment groups; Fig. 3 summarizes mean Hgb levels over time by CKD stage. For patients with an eGFR ≥90 mL/min (normal renal function), mean (± SD) Hgb increased from 8.8 (±0.95) mg/dL at Baseline to 12.1 (±1.3) mg/dL at Week 5 (a change of 3.3 g/dL) in the Ferumoxytol Treatment Group, while mean Hgb increased from 8.8 (±0.98) mg/dL to 11.6 (±1.33) mg/dL (a change of 2.8 g/dL) for those in the Iron Sucrose Treatment Group. For patients with normal renal function, ferumoxytol treatment resulted in significantly greater increases in mean Hgb levels compared with iron sucrose treatment at Weeks 2, 3, 4, and 5 ($p < 0.001$ vs. iron sucrose for all; Fig. 3a). Least Squares (LS) mean treatment differences between the Ferumoxytol and Iron Sucrose Treatment Groups for Hgb levels ranged from 0.50 to 0.76 g/dL. Mean Hgb values over time for the other CKD categories are illustrated in Fig. 3b–e. Ferumoxytol-treated patients with eGFRs of 60 to <90 mL/min and <15 mL/min at Week 2 also had a significantly greater increase in Hgb levels compared with iron sucrose-treated patients ($p = 0.009$ and $p = 0.012$, respectively, vs. iron sucrose); there were no significant treatment differences in Hgb levels between treatment groups in the other categories of renal function (Fig. 3b).

Mean Baseline TSAT increased with declining renal function (Table 2). Treatment with both ferumoxytol

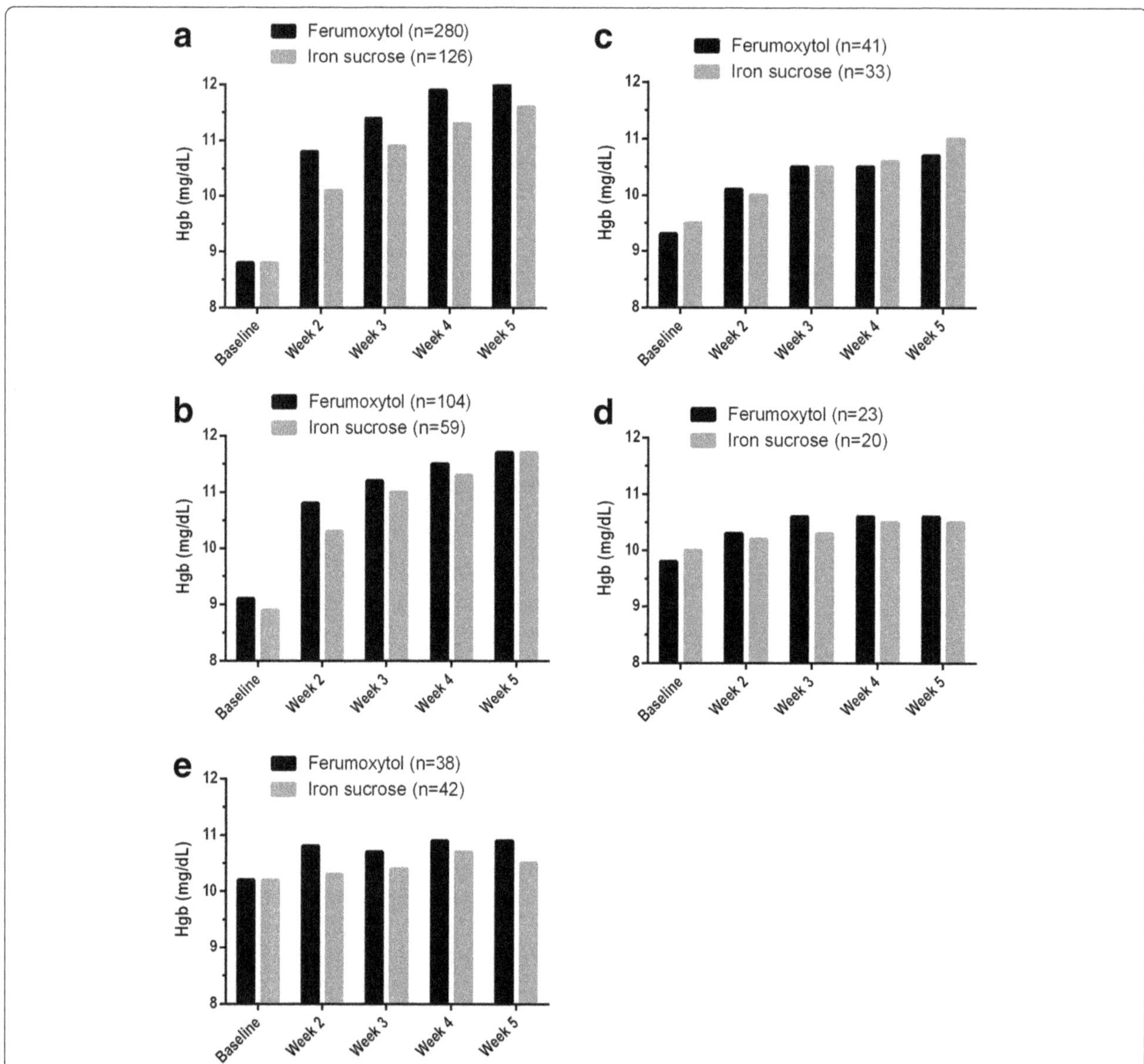

Fig. 3 Mean hemoglobin (Hgb) levels across renal functions. **a** eGFR ≥90 mL/min; (**b**) eGFR 60 to <90 mL/min; (**c**) eGFR 30 to <60 mL/min; (**d**) eGFR 15 to <30 mL/min; and (**e**) eGFR <15 mL/min at Weeks 2, 3, 4, and 5 in patients receiving ferumoxytol or iron sucrose therapy (Intent-to-Treat population). eGFR, estimated glomerular filtration rate

and iron sucrose resulted in increased mean TSAT values over the 5-week study period (Table 4). LS mean increases in TSAT from Baseline to Week 5 were significantly greater for those receiving ferumoxytol compared with those receiving iron sucrose for the eGFR category of 60 to <90 mL/min (15.9 vs. 11.3 %; $p = 0.001$). There were no significant differences between Ferumoxytol and Iron Sucrose Treatment Groups at Week 5 for any of the other CKD categories.

Low serum ferritin is a marker for IDA, but an elevated serum ferritin can be a marker of either increased iron levels or inflammation, the latter of which can mask the presence of IDA [7]. Overall, mean Baseline values for ferritin levels in the Ferumoxytol and Iron Sucrose Treatment Groups were similar with increasing Baseline ferritin levels with declining renal function (Table 2). As for other iron parameters, treatment with either ferumoxytol or iron sucrose was associated with increased ferritin levels over time in all eGFR categories (Table 4).

Discussion

The current analysis pooled data from two randomized, controlled clinical studies of IV iron treatment in adults with IDA, which provided the opportunity to more thoroughly analyze a larger number of patients

Table 4 Mean change in TSAT and serum ferritin over time by CKD stage

CKD Stage	TSAT, % (SD)		Ferritin, µg/L (SD)	
	Ferumoxytol Treatment Group	Iron Sucrose Treatment Group	Ferumoxytol Treatment Group	Iron Sucrose Treatment Group
Stage 1 (eGFR ≥90 mL/min)	(*n* = 280)	(*n* = 126)	(*n* = 280)	(*n* = 126)
Baseline	5.8 (11.25)	4.3 (5.21)	14.1 (39.76)	15.4 (53.11)
Week 2	26.1 (19.59)	15.8 (11.90)	291.1 (192.69)	172.5 (245.93)
Week 3	24.1 (11.54)	19.8 (15.38)	179.7 (157.02)	157.3 (211.08)
Week 4	22.7 (10.95)	19.2 (13.81)	123.7 (124.20)	124.0 (211.93)
Week 5	22.9 (21.75)	19.1 (14.77)	98.3 (118.96)	96.4 (185.27)
Stage 2 (eGFR 60 to <90 mL/min)	(*n* = 104)	(*n* = 59)	(*n* = 104)	(*n* = 59)
Baseline	6.6 (5.7)	5.1 (3.47)	55.4 (138.26)	22.7 (80.21)
Week 2	26.2 (11.41)	25.8 (51.56)	442.0 (398.63)	215.0 (226.93)
Week 3	24.3 (10.39)	17.2 (7.81)	325.6 (385.93)	196.6 (212.70)
Week 4	23.9 (11.17)	18.9 (12.46)	277.9 (394.82)	166.2 (254.32)
Week 5	22.5 (10.35)	16.5 (6.66)	247.2 (471.24)	127.5 (214.99)
Stage 3 (eGFR 30 to <60 mL/min)	(*n* = 41)	(*n* = 33)	(*n* = 41)	(*n* = 33)
Baseline	13.4 (18.31)	16.1 (22.18)	106.6 (168.37)	106.5 (157.15)
Week 2	26.6 (13.27)	21.8 (22.81)	629.3 (507.21)	338.6 (296.76)
Week 3	25.0 (11.45)	18.9 (8.16)	518.1 (425.74)	373.0 (321.68)
Week 4	23.2 (11.01)	19.2 (7.78)	452.5 (443.14)	314.8 (284.35)
Week 5	23.1 (12.15)	19.4 (7.86)	426.0 (433.68)	312.0 (284.41)
Stage 4 (eGFR 15 to <30 mL/min)	(*n* = 23)	(*n* = 20)	(*n* = 23)	(*n* = 20)
Baseline	21.7 (19.41)	17.0 (6.49)	152.3 (123.03)	141.4 (158.16)
Week 2	30.6 (9.71)	24.3 (7.14)	720.7 (280.38)	520.2 (244.56)
Week 3	28.6 (13.22)	24.0 (5.85)	632.8 (324.78)	529.6 (244.92)
Week 4	32.2 (15.81)	25.7 (7.18)	552.4 (327.53)	440.5 (228.45)
Week 5	26.3 (6.34)	23.1 (5.79)	514.6 (285.12)	407.0 (231.30)
Stage 5 (eGFR <15 mL/min)	(*n* = 38)	(*n* = 42)	(*n* = 38)	(*n* = 42)
Baseline	22.3 (12.91)	21.7 (14.76)	411.3 (348.97)	359.7 (287.65)
Week 2	34.6 (16.18)	25.4 (12.87)	915.8 (372.92)	603.4 (338.87)
Week 3	32.2 (12.81)	24.7 (7.44)	959.0 (605.92)	675.2 (339.54)
Week 4	30.4 (12.57)	27.7 (13.27)	831.7 (452.94)	682.2 (391.21)
Week 5	28.7 (8.82)	27.9 (15.80)	788.4 (427.21)	618.9 (355.47)

CKD chronic kidney disease, *GFR* glomerular filtration rate, *SD* standard deviation, *TSAT* transferrin saturation

across the full range of Baseline renal function. It also allowed for a comparative analysis of the Hgb response to IV iron treatment based on underlying renal function. Across all stages of renal function—from normal to end-stage CKD—the comparison of the safety and efficacy of ferumoxytol versus iron sucrose treatment demonstrated consistent findings. Overall, the incidences of all AEs were numerically lower in the Ferumoxytol Treatment Group compared to those treated with iron sucrose. This may be related to the risk of AEs associated with each instance of an IV administration, as suggested by the continued occurrence of AEs (including AESIs) after each dose in patients in the Iron Sucrose Treatment Group who received up to 10 individual doses. The frequencies of drug-related AEs and AE-related treatment discontinuations were slightly lower in the Ferumoxytol Treatment Group compared with the Iron Sucrose Treatment Group, while SAEs and treatment-related SAEs were slightly higher with ferumoxytol than iron sucrose. It is important to emphasize that, given the low overall rates, no statistical comparisons were appropriate. Overall, both agents had a comparable rate of SAEs, treatment-related SAEs, and cardiovascular AEs, and no new safety signals were identified. These results are consistent with those observed in the original Phase 3 studies [14, 15].

Hgb levels were increased in both the Ferumoxytol and Iron Sucrose Treatment Groups at the end of the study. Patients in all of the CKD categories were shown to benefit from iron therapy, although those with the most severe renal dysfunction achieved somewhat less of an Hgb response. Compared with iron sucrose, ferumoxytol treatment resulted in a significantly greater increase in Hgb at all time points assessed in those with an eGFR ≥90 mL/min. Statistically significant differences between treatment groups were not observed for patients with decreased levels of renal function for the majority of time points.

A low serum ferritin is indicative of iron deficiency, and elevated levels may be indicative of increased iron stores or iron overload. However, since ferritin is also an acute phase reactant, it is also a surrogate marker for inflammation and may be elevated due to chronic inflammation even in the presence of IDA [7]. Thus, while ferritin levels can be used to assess iron levels and the efficacy of active therapies, they must be used with caution in patients with CKD, especially with those on dialysis [7]. In this study, Baseline levels were increased in patients with reduced renal function. Treatment with either ferumoxytol or iron sucrose was shown to produce increases in serum ferritin across all CKD categories. The increases in TSAT levels were significantly greater with ferumoxytol than with iron sucrose in all CKD categories as early as Week 2 and/or 3 following the start of treatment, indicating that ferumoxytol is associated with a faster replenishment of iron stores available for erythropoiesis.

A limitation of this study is the retrospective nature of the analysis. Another limitation of this pooled analysis is that data were pooled across different populations. In particular, patients in **CKD-201** were older and heavier compared with those from study **IDA-302**. Patients in **CKD-201** were also less likely to have more severe anemia than those in **IDA-302**, most likely because CKD patients routinely receive aggressive therapy for anemia (e.g., iron therapy, erythropoiesis-stimulating agents).

Conclusions

This pooled analysis of two randomized, controlled clinical trials of IV iron treatment provides the opportunity to compare the safety and efficacy of two IV iron replacement products in a large population of patients with IDA and varying degrees of renal function. Overall, the efficacy of ferumoxytol was shown to be comparable, and at times greater, to that of iron sucrose for increasing Hgb across the spectrum of renal function, from normal to patients with CKD on dialysis. Overall, mean Hgb increased in both treatment groups, regardless of degree of renal insufficiency. Although patients with worse renal function did not respond as well to IV iron therapy with either drug compared to those with normal renal function, patients in all CKD categories experienced improved iron parameters. In this pooled analysis, both ferumoxytol and iron sucrose were shown to have comparable safety profiles consistent with those observed in the original studies.

Abbreviations

AE, adverse event; AESI, adverse event of special interest; CKD, chronic kidney disease; eGFR, estimated glomerular filtration rate; ESA, erythropoiesis-stimulating agent; GI, gastrointestinal; Hgb, hemoglobin; IDA, iron deficiency anemia; ITT, intent to treat; IV, intravenous; LS, least squares; SAE, serious adverse event; SD, standard deviation; TSAT, transferrin saturation

Acknowledgements

Maria McGill, RPh, CMPP, and Alan Klopp, PhD, CMPP, of inScience Communications, Springer Healthcare, and Bret Fulton, RPh, provided medical writing support funded by AMAG Pharmaceuticals.
Carol Jasuta of in Science Communications, Springer Healthcare provided administrative assistance.

Funding

The design of the study, data collection, analysis, and interpretation of data were funded by AMAG Pharmaceuticals, Inc. Both the primary study and the writing of the secondary analysis were supported financially by AMAG Pharmaceuticals, Inc.

Authors' contributions

WES designed and oversaw the execution of the trial; analyzed the data; wrote, edited, and proofread the manuscript; and agreed upon the data presented. NVD analyzed the data; wrote, edited and proofread the manuscript; and agreed upon the data presented. GL designed and oversaw the execution of the trial; analyzed the data; wrote, edited and proofread the manuscript; and agreed upon the data presented. ZL designed and oversaw the execution of the trial; analyzed the data; performed statistical analysis; wrote, edited, and proofread the manuscript; and agreed upon the data presented. LFA designed and oversaw the execution of the trial; analyzed the data; wrote, edited, and proofread the manuscript; and agreed upon the data presented. All authors read and approved the final manuscript.

Authors' information

Not applicable.

Competing interests

William E. Strauss, Naomi V. Dahl, and Zhu Li are employees of AMAG Pharmaceuticals, Inc. and hold equity in the company. Gloria Lau and Lee F. Allen were employees of AMAG at the time of the study and writing of the manuscript.

References

1. World Health Organization. Worldwide prevalence of anaemia 1993–2005: WHO global database on anaemia. World Health Organization, Geneva. 2008. http://whqlibdoc.who.int/publications/2008/9789241596657_eng.pdf. Accessed 15 Mar 2013.
2. Looker AC, Dallman PR, Carroll MD, Gunter EW, Johnson CL. Prevalence of iron deficiency in the United States. JAMA. 1997;277(12):973–6.
3. Fishbane S, Pollack S, Feldman HI, Joffe MM. Iron indices in chronic kidney disease in the National Health and Nutritional Examination Survey 1988–2004. Clin J Am Soc Nephrol. 2009;4(1):57–61.
4. Valderrabano F, Horl WH, Macdougall IC, Rossert J, Rutkowski B, Wauters JP. PRE-dialysis survey on anaemia management. Nephrol Dial Transplant. 2003;18(1):89–100.
5. Kazmi WH, Kausz AT, Khan S, Abichandani R, Ruthazer R, Obrador GT, et al. Anemia: an early complication of chronic renal insufficiency. Am J Kidney Dis. 2001;38(4):803–12.
6. Liu K, Kaffes AJ. Iron deficiency anaemia: a review of diagnosis, investigation and management. Eur J Gastroenterol Hepatol. 2012;24(2):109–16.
7. Kidney Disease Improving Global Outcomes (KDIGO). KDIGO Clinical practice guideline for anemia in chronic kidney disease. Kidney Int Suppl. 2012;2:282–7.
8. Bisbe E, Garcia-Erce JA, Diez-Lobo AI, Munoz M. A multicentre comparative study on the efficacy of intravenous ferric carboxymaltose and iron sucrose for correcting preoperative anaemia in patients undergoing major elective surgery. Br J Anaesth. 2011;107(3):477–8.
9. Evstatiev R, Marteau P, Iqbal T, Khalif IL, Stein J, Bokemeyer B, et al. FERGIcor, a randomized controlled trial on ferric carboxymaltose for iron deficiency anemia in inflammatory bowel disease. Gastroenterology. 2011;141(3):846–53 e1–2.
10. Onken JE, Bregman DB, Harrington RA, Morris D, Buerkert J, Hamerski D, et al. Ferric carboxymaltose in patients with iron-deficiency anemia and impaired renal function: the REPAIR-IDA trial. Nephrol Dial Transplant. 2014;29(4):833–42.
11. Barish CF, Koch T, Butcher A, Morris D, Bregman DB. Safety and efficacy of intravenous ferric carboxymaltose (750 mg) in the treatment of iron deficiency anemia: two randomized, controlled trials. Anemia. 2012;2012:172104.
12. Hussain I, Bhoyroo J, Butcher A, Koch TA, He A, Bregman DB. Direct comparison of the safety and efficacy of ferric carboxymaltose versus iron dextran in patients with iron deficiency anemia. Anemia. 2013;2013:169107.
13. Feraheme (ferumoxytol) Injection for Intravenous (IV) use: prescribing information. AMAG Pharmaceuticals, Inc.: Waltham, MA. 2015. http://www.amagpharma.com/documents/feraheme-productinsert.pdf. Accessed 4 Jun 2015.
14. Macdougall IC, Strauss WE, McLaughlin J, Li Z, Dellanna F, Hertel J. A randomized comparison of ferumoxytol and iron sucrose for treating iron deficiency anemia in patients with CKD. Clin J Am Soc Nephrol. 2014;9(4):705–12.
15. Hetzel D, Strauss WE, Bernard K, Li Z, Urboniene A, Allen LF. A phase III, randomized, open-label trial of ferumoxytol compared with iron sucrose for the treatment of iron deficiency anemia in patients with a history of unsatisfactory oral iron therapy. Am J Hematol. 2014;89(6):646–50.

6

Bleeding complications from the direct oral anticoagulants

Michelle Sholzberg[1*], Katerina Pavenski[2], Nadine Shehata[3], Christine Cserti-Gazdewich[4] and Yulia Lin[5]

Abstract

Background: Direct oral anticoagulants (DOACs) are now standard of care for the management of thromboembolic risk. A prevalent issue of concern is how to manage direct oral anticoagulant (DOAC)-associated bleeding for which there is no specific antidote available for clinical use. We conducted a retrospective case series to describe the Toronto, Canada multicenter experience with bleeding from dabigatran or rivaroxaban.

Methods: Retrospective chart review of DOAC bleeding necessitating referral to hematology and/or transfusion medicine services at five large University of Toronto affiliated academic hospitals from January 2011 to December 2013.

Results: Twenty-six patients with DOAC bleeding were reviewed; 42 % bleeds intracranial and 50 %, gastrointestinal. All patients had at least one risk factor associated with DOAC bleeding reported in previous studies. Inconsistent bleed management strategies were evident. Median length of hospital stay was 11 days (1–90). Five thromboembolic events occurred after transfusion based-hemostatic therapy and there were six deaths.

Conclusions: Management of DOAC bleeding is variable. Clinical trial data regarding DOAC reversal is needed to facilitate optimization and standardization of bleeding treatment algorithms.

Keywords: Anticoagulants, Blood transfusion, Dabigatran, Hemorrhage, Rivaroxaban

Background

Vitamin K antagonists have long been the mainstay of prophylactic or therapeutic anticoagulation for thromboembolism. The cumbersome disadvantages of warfarin from both the patient and physician perspective have led to the development, and now standard use, of direct oral anticoagulants (DOACs) that do not require laboratory monitoring and have fewer food and drug interactions.

Large clinical trials comparing the DOACs to vitamin K antagonists have demonstrated similar efficacy in the management and prevention of thromboembolism and similar or reduced major bleeding rates [1–3]. As indications for DOACs expand, an issue of concern is how to manage real-world DOAC-associated bleeding for which no antidote is currently available. Guidelines and reviews have extrapolated bleeding management principles from results of animal and human volunteer studies with laboratory, not clinical, parameters as primary outcomes [4–7]. Since no evidence-based, standard therapeutic algorithm for DOAC bleeding is available, the primary objective of our study was to determine how patients are currently being managed in this setting. We focused on the experience with hemorrhage from dabigatran, a direct thrombin inhibitor, and rivaroxaban, a direct factor Xa inhibitor, as apixaban, a direct factor Xa inhibitor, was not yet approved for use in Canada.

Methods

We conducted a retrospective chart review of DOAC bleeding necessitating referral to hematology and/or transfusion medicine services at five large University of Toronto affiliated academic hospitals (St. Michael's Hospital, Toronto General Hospital, Toronto Western Hospital, Sunnybrook Health Sciences Centre, Mount Sinai Hospital) from January 2011 to December 2013. Patients were included if they were: over the age of 18 years, documented to have a DOAC associated hemorrhage and

* Correspondence: sholzbergm@smh.ca
[1]Division of Hematology, Department of Medicine and Department of Laboratory Medicine and Pathobiology, St. Michael's Hospital, University of Toronto, 30 Bond Street, Room 2-007G Core Lab, Carter Wing, Toronto, ON M5B-1 W8, Canada
Full list of author information is available at the end of the article

identified to hematology and/or transfusion medicine services.

The following data were abstracted from medical records: age and sex; body weight; DOAC type; indication for DOAC; duration of time on DOAC therapy until bleeding event (days); concomitant medication use; initial blood work (including complete blood cell count, activated partial thromboplastin time (aPTT), prothrombin time (PT), fibrinogen (Claus method), liver enzymes (aspartate aminotransferase [AST], alanine transaminase [ALT], alkaline phosphatase [ALP]), albumin, bilirubin, estimated creatinine clearance (Cockcroft-Gault formula); description of bleeding episode (site, date/time documented, red blood cell (RBC) transfusion, severity of bleed – major or minor). Major bleeding was defined according to the International Society on Thrombosis and Haemostasis (ISTH)'s recommendations [8] as either involvement of a critical organ, fall in haemoglobin of more than 20 g/L or requirement of greater than two RBC transfusions. Of note, aforementioned data points included those known to be associated with increased risk of DOAC bleeding.

Additional data collected included: management of bleeding (DOAC held, site compression, surgical management, fluids/adequate urine output, charcoal, haemodialysis, transfusion [activated prothrombin complex concentrate (aPCC), prothrombin complex concentrate (PCC), activated recombinant factor VII, frozen plasma, platelets, cryoprecipitate, fibrinogen concentrate] and non-transfusion based [tranexamic acid, desmopressin, vitamin K] hemostatic support; coagulation based test results post-transfusion therapy; bleeding outcome (decrease, increase, no change, cessation); venous or arterial thromboembolic (TE) event (with supportive imaging results and/or blood work); length of hospital stay; and hospital discharge status (alive, dead).

Data were analyzed using descriptive statistics (mean, median, range and standard deviation) and inferential statistics (confidence interval). All analyses were performed using SAS statistical software, version 9.2 (SAS Institute Inc). Approval to perform this study and to report the results was obtained from St Michael's Hospital Research Ethics Board, University Health Network Research Ethics Board associated with Toronto General Hospital and Toronto Western Hospital, the Human Research Protections Program associated with Sunnybrook Health Sciences Centre, and Mount Sinai Hospital Research Ethics Board. The aforementioned list of research ethics committees approved this study and granted access to medical records and databases at their respective hospital sites. Approval to publicize the data set was not obtained by the hospital Research Ethics Boards. Hospitals are required to protect the privacy of citizens whose information they collect. The hospitals strive to comply with the Personal Health Information Protection Act (PHIPA). Therefore data supporting the study findings are unavailable.

Results

Twenty-seven bleeding events were captured upon retrospective review; one patient had two events hence a total of 26 patients were reviewed. Nine bleeding events occurred with rivaroxaban while 18 occurred with dabigatran. All except four patients were over the age of 70 years with a median age of 78 years (range 52–91 years). Approximately 69 % (18/26) of patients were male. Three individuals were underweight (less than 60 kilograms) while the median weight was 78.3 (range 50–150) kilograms. The median time taking the DOAC prior to bleeding was 120 days (range 5–810). The indications for DOAC therapy included the following: atrial fibrillation ($n = 24$), deep vein thrombosis ($n = 1$), and two patients (7 %) treated for an off-label indication (one for cancer associated pulmonary embolism and the other for prophylaxis for an automated implantable cardioverter-defibrillator. Of the nine rivaroxaban associated bleeds, five occurred at a dosage of 20 mg daily and four at 15 mg daily. Of the 18 dabigatran bleeds, eight occurred at a dosage of 150 mg twice per day and ten at 110 mg twice per day. The median number of concomitant medications was 7 (range 1–16). Five bleeding events occurred while the patient was taking concomitant aspirin therapy, five events with non-steroidal anti-inflammatory drugs (NSAIDs) and three occurred with concomitant P-glycoprotein (P-gp) inhibitors.

Eighty-nine percent of the bleeding events were classified as a major hemorrhage with 50 % requiring RBC transfusion. Of those who were transfused with RBCs, a median of 2.5 units (range 1–9) was required. Half of the dabigatran patients were transfused with RBCs (median 3 units, range 1–3) compared to 44 % treated with rivaroxaban (median 2 units, range 1–4).

Eleven (42 %) bleeding events were intracranial (ICH) and 13 (50 %) were gastrointestinal (GI) in origin. Of note, two of these events were combined ICH and GI hemorrhages. Of the 13 GI hemorrhages, nine were associated with dabigatran use and four with rivaroxaban. There were 11 ICH events, six occurred in dabigatran users and five in rivaroxaban users. There was no statistically significant association between dabigatran versus rivaroxaban use and type of hemorrhage using a two-tailed Fischer's exact test ($p = 0.68$). More patients with GI bleeds received RBC transfusion (62 %), as compared to ICH (27 %).

The remaining four bleeds involved the following sites: vaginal, pulmonary, subcutaneous or musculoskeletal with

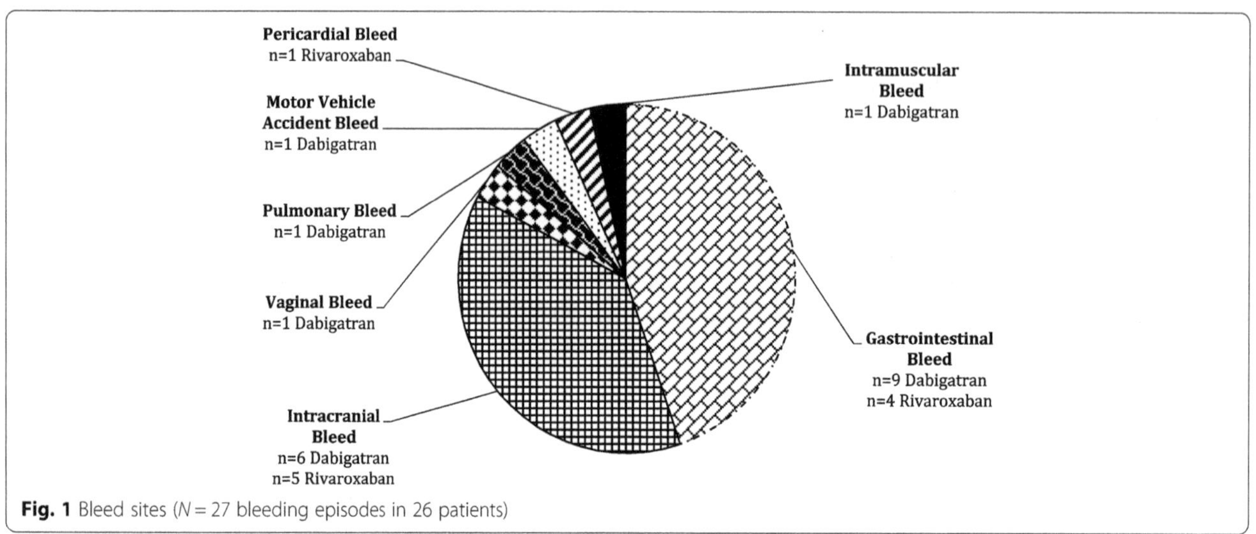

Fig. 1 Bleed sites ($N = 27$ bleeding episodes in 26 patients)

some occurring in combination. One of these events was associated with a motor vehicle collision (Fig. 1).

Data were reviewed for risk factors (found in previous observational studies) associated with DOAC bleeding. In this study, all bleeding events occurred in the context of at least one previously identified associating factor and 63 % occurred with more than one. Specifically, 50 % of subjects were above 80 years of age and 33 % of cases occurred with severe (<30 ml/min) or moderate (30–50 ml/min) impairment in creatinine clearance at time of bleeding. Five subjects had comorbid diabetes mellitus, five were on concomitant aspirin and another 19 % were taking a NSAID (Table 1). Of the 26 patients, 14 were on a reduced dose of dabigatran (110 mg) or rivaroxaban (15 mg). All of those patients were either of older age or had impaired renal function. Fifty percent of those on standard dose DOAC were older or had abnormal kidney function.

Table 1 Risk factors associated with direct oral anticoagulant bleeding

Clinical Variable	Number of patients
>80 years of age	12
Weight < 63 kg	4
Severe (<30 ml/min) or moderate (30–50 ml/min) impairment in creatinine clearance	9
Diabetes mellitus	5
Concomitant aspirin	5
Concomitant NSAID[a]	5
Concomitant strong P-gp[b] inhibitors	3
Higher than recommended dose of dabigatran	1

[a]non-steroidal anti-inflammatory drug
[b]p-glycoprotein

Of the 18 dabigatran related bleed events (in 17 patients), five (28 %) received aPCC alone, two (11 %) received aPCC and PCC, 13 (72 %) received at least one hemostatic support of any kind and five (28 %) did not receive any hemostatic therapy. Of the nine rivaroxaban related bleeding events, six (67 %) received at least one hemostatic support (two (22 %) received aPCC, two (22 %) received PCC) and three (33 %) did not receive any hemostatic therapy.

APCC tended to be administered to a larger number of patients with ICH - six (54 %) - compared with isolated GI hemorrhage - one (8 %). However, a similar proportion of individuals received hemostatic therapy of any kind (63 % for ICH and 69 % for GI bleed) (Table 2).

Hemostatic response to aPCC and/or PCC seemed to differ according to the DOAC. Of the nine total patients that received aPCC, three (all dabigatran related) had resolution of bleeding within 12 to 24 h of administration. Of the five total patients that received PCC, one bleed (rivaroxaban related) had resolution of bleeding at 24 h and there was no abnormal intra-operative bleeding in another rivaroxaban related case. CBC, PT and aPTT

Table 2 Hemostatic therapy according to bleed site

Intracranial Hemorrhage (ICH) Events (N = 11) 2 combined ICH and GIB	Gastrointestinal Bleed (GIB) Events (N = 12) 2 combined ICH and GIB
6 (54 %) received aPCC[a]	1 (8 %) received aPCC
0 (0 %) received PCC[b]	2 (17 %) received PCC
	2 (17 %) received both aPCC and PCC
7 (64 %) received hemostatic support of any kind	9 (75 %) received hemostatic support of any kind
4 (36 %) did not receive hemostatic therapy	3 (25 %) did not receive hemostatic therapy

[a]activated prothrombin complex concentrate
[b]prothrombin complex concentrate

were the most commonly ordered initial laboratory tests. However, the frequency of repeated testing was highly variable. Concise summarization of laboratory data was not possible. Furthermore, we cannot comment on the pattern of coagulation study normalization due to inconsistencies within the dataset.

There were five TE events in subjects who received transfusion based hemostatic therapy (i.e. aPCC, PCC, FP and/or platelets). All of the events were arterial in nature involving either myocardial infarction or bowel ischemia. A single arterial TE event occurred within 24 h of hemostatic transfusion (aPCC). There were no TE events in patients who did not receive transfusion based hemostatic therapy.

The median length of hospital stay was 11 days (range 1–90). There were six deaths (four dabigatran and two rivaroxaban) (23 % of cases). The cause of death was ICH in five patients and one death occurred secondary to multi-organ failure and myocardial infarction. The proportion of ICH resulting in death was 45 %.

Discussion

We found, in this case series, that the management of DOAC bleeding is highly variable. A large proportion of patients in this study required prolonged hospitalization and experienced TE complications. Additionally, a substantial proportion of patients died. Of interest, 33 % of the patients in this case series would not have qualified for enrolment in the studies on the respective drugs.

This study is limited by the lack of control and denominator data, however, it highlights the importance of 'risk' factors for major DOAC related bleeding namely, advanced age, renal impairment, diabetes mellitus and concomitant treatment with aspirin and NSAIDs [9–12]. Despite reassuring recent evidence from a meta-analysis reviewing the bleeding rates in the elderly from published randomized controlled trials comparing DOACs with standard anticoagulant therapy, this study suggests that careful patient selection for treatment with DOACs remains paramount [12]. Interestingly, data from this case series is in contrast to the recently published data on rivaroxaban bleeding from the Dresden registry [13]. Most notably, this case series confirms that a high proportion of patients who experience anticoagulant associated ICH die [14].

Conclusion

In summary, this case series shows that there is considerable variation in the treatment used to control DOAC associated bleeding. This study also highlights the importance of proper patient selection for DOAC therapy. In conclusion, management of DOAC bleeding needs to be optimized and standardized once clinical trial data regarding reversal becomes available.

Abbreviations

ALP: Alkaline phosphatase; ALT: Alanine transaminase; AST: Aspartate aminotransferase; aPCC: Activated prothrombin complex concentrate; aPTT: Activated partial thromboplastin time; DOAC: Direct oral anticoagulants; GI: Gastrointestinal; ICH: Intracranial hemorrhage; ISTH: International society of thrombosis and haemostasis; NSAID: Non-steroidal anti-inflammatory drug; PCC: Prothrombin complex concentrate; P-gp: P-glycoprotein; PT: Prothrombin time; RBC: Red blood cell; TE: Thromboembolic.

Competing interests

The conduct of this multicenter case series was supported by unrestricted research/educational grants from the following pharmaceutical sponsors: Baxter, Octapharma, Boehringer-Ingelheim and CSL Behring. Research assistant salary support was provided in part by a grant from Boehringer-Ingelheim (Canada) Ltd.

Authors' contributions

MS participated in the study design, data collection, analysis, analysis interpretation, and manuscript preparation. KP participated in study design, data collection, analysis interpretation, and manuscript editing. NS participated in study design, data collection, analysis interpretation, and manuscript editing. CCG participated in study design, data collection, analysis interpretation, and manuscript editing. YL participated in study design, data collection, analysis interpretation, and manuscript editing. All authors read and approved the final manuscript.

Acknowledgements

We would like to acknowledge the unrestricted research/educational grant support from Baxter, Octapharma and CSL Behring. Research assistant salary support was provided in part by a grant from Boehringer-Ingelheim (Canada) Ltd. We would also like to acknowledge support from our research coordinators, Ms. Daisy Dastur, Mr. Aziz Jiwajee, Ms. Jessica Petrucci, Ms. Lorna Sampson, Ms. Nusrat Zaffar, Ms. Cassandra Ottawa, Mr. Syed Mahamad, Ms. Natalya O'Neill and Mr. Joshua Tseng.

Author details

[1]Division of Hematology, Department of Medicine and Department of Laboratory Medicine and Pathobiology, St. Michael's Hospital, University of Toronto, 30 Bond Street, Room 2-007G Core Lab, Carter Wing, Toronto, ON M5B-1 W8, Canada. [2]Division of Hematology, Department of Medicine and Department of Laboratory Medicine and Pathobiology St. Michael's Hospital, University of Toronto, Toronto, Ontario, Canada. [3]Departments of Medicine and Laboratory Medicine and Pathobiology, Mount Sinai Hospital, University of Toronto, Toronto, ON, Canada. [4]Department of Laboratory Medicine and Pathobiology, University Health Network, University of Toronto, Toronto, ON, Canada. [5]Department of Clinical Pathology, Sunnybrook Health Sciences Centre; and Department of Laboratory Medicine and Pathobiology, University of Toronto, Toronto, ON, Canada.

References

1. Dentali F, Riva N, Crowther M, Turpie AG, Lip GY,Ageno W. Efficacy and safety of the novel oral anticoagulants in atrial fibrillation: a systematic review and meta-analysis of the literature. Circulation. 2012;126(20):2381–91
2. Fox BD, Kahn SR, Langleben D, Eisenberg MJ, Shimony A. Efficacy and safety of novel oral anticoagulants for treatment of acute venous thromboembolism: direct and adjusted indirect meta-analysis of randomised controlled trials. 2012.
3. Chai-Adisaksopha C, Crowther M, Isayama T, Lim W. The impact of bleeding complications in patients receiving target-specific oral anticoagulants: a systematic review and meta-analysis. Blood. 2014;124(15):2450–8.
4. Eerenberg ES, Kamphuisen PW, Sijpkens MK, Meijers JC, Buller HR, Levi M. Reversal of rivaroxaban and dabigatran by prothrombin complex concentrate: a randomized, placebo-controlled, crossover study in healthy subjects. Circulation. 2011;124(14):1573–9. doi:10.1161/circulationaha.111.029017.

5. Heidbuchel H, Verhamme P, Alings M, Antz M, Hacke W, Oldgren J, et al. EHRA Practical guide on the use of new oral anticoagulants in patients with non-valvular atrial fibrillation: executive summary. Eur Heart J. 2013;27:2094–106.
6. Pernod G, Albaladejo P, Godier A, Samama CM, Susen S, Gruel Yet al. Management of major bleeding complications and emergency surgery in patients on long-term treatment with direct oral anticoagulants, thrombin or factor-Xa inhibitors: Proposals of the Working Group on Perioperative Haemostasis (GIHP) – March 2013. Archives of Cardiovascular Diseases. 2013; 106(6–7):382–93. doi:http://dx.doi.org/10.1016/j.acvd.2013.04.009.
7. Levy JH, Spyropoulos AC, Samama CM,Douketis J. Direct Oral Anticoagulants: New Drugs and New Concepts. JACC: Cardiovascular Interventions. 2014;7(12):1333–51. doi:http://dx.doi.org/10.1016/j.jcin.2014.06.014.
8. Schulman S, Kearon C. Definition of major bleeding in clinical investigations of antihemostatic medicinal products in non-surgical patients. Thromb Haemost. 2005;3(4):692–4.
9. Deedwania PC. New oral anticoagulants in elderly patients with atrial fibrillation. Am J Med. 2013;126(4):289–96.
10. Harper P, Young L, Merriman E. Bleeding risk with dabigatran in the frail elderly. N Engl J Med. 2012;366(9):864–6.
11. Jacobs JM, Stessman J. New anticoagulant drugs among elderly patients is caution necessary? Comment on "The use of dabigatran in elderly patients". Arch Intern Med. 2011;171(14):1287–8.
12. Sardar P, Chatterjee S, Chaudhari S, Lip GY. New oral anticoagulants in elderly adults: evidence from a meta-Analysis of randomized trials. J Am Geriatr Soc. 2014;62(5):857–64.
13. Beyer-Westendorf J, Förster K, Pannach S, Ebertz F, Gelbricht V, Thieme C, et al. Rates, management, and outcome of rivaroxaban bleeding in daily care: results from the Dresden NOAC registry. Blood. 2014;6:955–62.
14. Alonso A, Bengtson LGS, MacLehose RF, Lutsey PL, Chen LY, Lakshminarayan K. Intracranial hemorrhage mortality in atrial fibrillation patients treated with dabigatran or warfarin. Stroke. 2014;45(8):2286–91. doi:10.1161/strokeaha.114.006016.

7

Chronic complications and quality of life of patients living with sickle cell disease and receiving care in three hospitals in Cameroon

Anne M. Andong[1,2], Eveline D. T. Ngouadjeu[3,4], Cavin E. Bekolo[5], Vincent S. Verla[1], Daniel Nebongo[2], Yannick Mboue-Djieka[2] and Simeon-Pierre Choukem[1,2,4*]

Abstract

Background: Sickle Cell Disease (SCD) is associated with chronic multisystem complications that significantly influence the quality of life (QOL) of patients early in their life. Although sub-Saharan Africa bears 75% of the global burden of SCD, there is a paucity of data on these complications and their effects on the QOL. We aimed to record these chronic complications, to estimate the QOL, and to identify the corresponding risk factors in patients with SCD receiving care in three hospitals in Cameroon.

Methods: In this cross-sectional study, a questionnaire was used to collect data from consecutive consenting patients. Information recorded included data on the yearly frequency of painful crisis, the types of SCD, and the occurrence of chronic complications. A 36-Item Short Form (SF-36) standard questionnaire that examines the level of physical and mental well-being, was administered to all eligible participants. Data were analyzed with STATA® software.

Results: Of 175 participants included, 93 (53.1%) were female and 111 (aged ≥14 years) were eligible for QOL assessment. The median (interquartile range, IQR) age at diagnosis was 4.0 (2.0-8.0) years and the median (IQR) number of yearly painful crisis was 3.0 (1.0–7.0). The most frequent chronic complications reported were: nocturnal enuresis, chronic leg ulcers, osteomyelitis and priapism (30.9%, 24.6%, 19.4%, and 18.3% respectively). The prevalence of stroke and avascular necrosis of the hip were 8.0% and 13.1% respectively. The median (IQR) physical and mental scores were 47.3 (43.9–58.5) and 41.0 (38.8–44.6) respectively. Age and chronic complications such as stroke and avascular necrosis were independently associated with poor QOL.

Conclusions: In this population of patients living with SCD, chronic complications are frequent and their QOL is consequently poor. Our results highlight the need for national guidelines for SCD control, which should include new-born screening programs and strategies to prevent chronic complications.

Keywords: Sickle cell disease, Chronic complications, Prevalence, Quality of life, Cameroon

* Correspondence: schoukem@gmail.com
[1]Department of Internal Medicine and Pediatrics, Faculty of Health Sciences, University of Buea, Buea, Cameroon
[2]Health and Human Development (2HD) Research Network, P.O. Box 4856, Douala, Cameroon
Full list of author information is available at the end of the article

Background

Sickle cell disease (SCD) is often associated with chronic complications in the long term [1]. These complications include consequences of chronic anemia and susceptibility to infections owing to functional splenectomy, and may lead to a poor quality of life (QOL) [2]. The World Health Organization (WHO) estimates that 300,000 children are born with SCD each year, 75% of whom are in sub-Saharan Africa (SSA); they also state that the burden of the disease could be reduced by simple careful management and prevention programs [3, 4].

The WHO also recommends that a global management be put in place to reduce SCD morbidity (chronic complications) and mortality, and to improve on the QOL [3]. The disease morbidity and mortality improved in two small samples of patients in Nigeria and Angola using these simple but cost-effective interventions recommended by the WHO [5, 6]. However, data especially those focusing on QOL are still scanty or inexistent in most SSA countries.

To the best of our knowledge, chronic complications that have been reported in Cameroon –a SCD endemic country- are stroke (6.7%) [7] and gall stone diseases (30%) [8]. The aim our study was to assess a group of children and adults living with SCD, with particular reference to the types and determinants of the QOL and complications of SCD, in order to inform the actions that could be undertaken to reduce the burden of the disease and to improve the QOL.

Methods

Study design, setting and participants

We carried out a cross-sectional study over a period of five months, from November 2014 to March 2015, in three hospitals in Cameroon: the Douala General Hospital, a country reference hospital, the Douala Laquintinie Hospital, which has a sickle cell care center in Douala, and the Buea Regional Hospital, which is the reference hospital for the South-West Region of the country. The first two hospitals are located in the Littoral Region and the third in South-West Region. The two regions are at the coastal area of the country and serve as university teaching hospitals for our Faculty of Health Sciences of The University of Buea. Recruitment of participants was done at the inpatient and outpatient units and during their monthly visits at the Laquintinie Hospital. All the centers had comprehensive medical records. All patients with SCD confirmed by a hemoglobin electrophoresis were consecutively included if they gave their informed written consent or assent to participate. Patients in sickle cell crises at the time of the study were not considered (for QOL assessment), until they completely recovered from the crises as indicated by their caring physician.

All patients above the age of 5 years were included in the assessment of chronic complications because complications such as stroke have been shown to occur as early as the age of 5 years in children with sickle cell disease [9]. Only patients above 14 years were included in the assessment of the QOL, because the short form 36 questionnaire has been validated in sickle cell population at or above this age [10].

Definition of terms and variables

Sickle cell disease had been diagnosed by haemoglobin electrophoresis. Painful sickle cell crises were defined as any bony painful event in the absence of any recent trauma, for which a medical consultation was done or not. Chronic leg ulcers were defined as any leg wound that had lasted longer than three months. Stroke was defined as any sudden onset neurological dysfunction (mainly one side body weakness) in the absence of trauma, that resolved or not. Avascular necrosis of the hip was self-reported or collected from medical records. Immunization status relating to pneumococcal vaccine, meningococcal vaccine, Typhim Vi (against typhoid fever) and Hepatitis B vaccine) was also recorded.

Data collection and score calculation

All participants underwent a comprehensive multisystem physical examination. Data on chronic complications were collected by use of a questionnaire (Additional file 1) that contained information on the history obtained from the participant and/or the guardian. Additional clinical data were retrieved from the patient's medical record.

The Short Form (SF)-36 either self-administered or interviewer-administered was used to collect data on the QOL (Additional file 1). This questionnaire reviewed both physical and mental aspect of health comprising eight scored scales each belonging to the two main scores known as Physical and Mental health component scores. The SF 36 form was clearly explained and self-administered except for participants who did not understand the questions. All the 8 components were assessed through 11 questions. An overall score, physical component score and mental component score were computed. Individual scores for all 8 components were also given. The scores were then standardized using the online newborn screening (NBS) calculator so that the values could be compared to other populations, both the healthy and sickle cell populations. Only one investigator administered the questionnaire to all participants.

Data analysis

The data set was checked for logical inconsistencies, invalid codes, omissions and improbable data by tabulating, summarizing, describing and plotting variables, depending on their nature. Missing observations were systematically excluded. Summary statistics were presented as proportions for categorical variables, as mean and standard deviation for normally distributed continuous variables and as median and interquartile range (IQR) for continuous variables with a skewed distribution. Associations between QOL scores and exposure variables were evaluated by a linear regression model. Variables associated with Total SF-36 score, PCS and MCS in separate univariate analyses at the 5% significance level were included in respective multivariate linear regression models. Backward elimination based on a p-value lower than 0.05 was used to retain variables that were independently associated with each QOL scores. Adjusted regression and correlation coefficients with their p-values and 95% confidence intervals (CI) were obtained. The goodness of model fit was assessed by post-estimation of homoscedasticity of residuals.

Results

In this study 182 participants met the inclusion criteria of which 175 finally took part in the study giving a response rate of 96.2% (Fig. 1). Of these, 94 (54.9%) were recruited at Laquintinie Hospital, 72 (41.1%) at Douala General Hospital and 9 (5.1%) at Buea Regional Hospital.

General characteristics of the participants

Of the 175 participants, 93 (53.1%) were females. The median (IQR) age at which the diagnosis of SCD was confirmed was 4.0 years (2.0–8.5); 113 (64.6%) participants were below the age of 21 and therefore needed consent by proxy, 21 being the age of majority in Cameroon. The median (IQR) age was 16.0 years (9.0–24.0). Concerning ongoing treatment, 122 (69.7%) patients were on folic acid alone, 1 (0.6%) on a vasodilator only, 17 (9.7%) on both folic acid and hydroxyurea, 21 (12.0%) on both folic acid and a vasodilator, 1 (0.6%) were on all three medications and 13 (7.4%) were not taking any medication. Most of the participants 103 (58.9%) did not have their vaccines up-to-date. Only 75(42.9%) had regular medical follow-up at the time of the study, 45(25.7%) being seen by pediatricians. Hemoglobin electrophoresis results were available for 58 (33.1%) participants and distributed as follow: 28 (48.3%) $SSFA_2$, 16 (27.6%) SSA_2, 10 (17.2%) SSF, 3 (5.2%) SS, and 1 (1.7%) SSC. The median number of yearly painful sickle cell crisis was 3.0 (IQR: 1.0–7.0). Details of other characteristics are shown in Table 1.

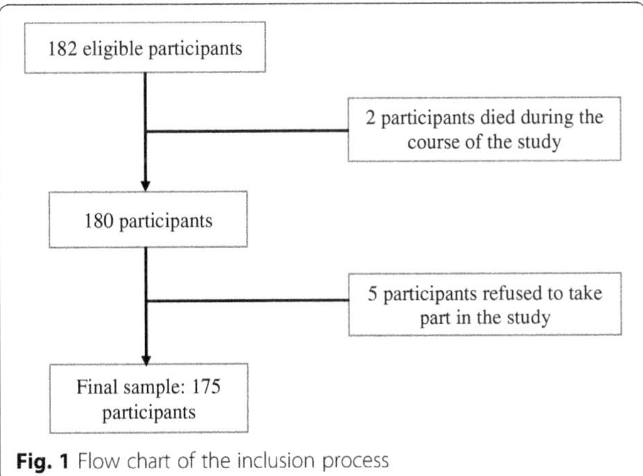

Fig. 1 Flow chart of the inclusion process

Chronic complications

Details of chronic complications found in participants are depicted in Table 2. The mean (SD) age at first stroke was 12.6 (7.3) years. The majority (52.2%) of cases of avascular necrosis were on the right hip. The mean age at which participants had their first leg ulcer was 18.6 ± 7.9 years. Forty (22.9%) patients had a systolic murmur. The prevalence of enuresis was similar between children and adults. Eight (4.6%) participants had opioid tolerance.

Quality of life

All 111 participants aged 14 years and above were included in the QOL study; their median (IQR) physical component score (PCS) and mental component score (MCS) were 47.3 (43.9–58.5) and 41.0 (38.8–44.6), respectively. The median (IQR) total SF-36 score was 62 (57–66) (Fig. 2). The total score strongly correlated with both the PCS ($r = 0.88$, $p = 0.01$) and the MCS (0.71, $p = 0.04$) (Fig. 3).

Independent associations of QOL scores are shown in Table 3. Holding everything else constant, on average: every one year increase in age was associated with a decrease in the total QOL score by 0.15 point; urban dwellers had a total score that was about 8 points above that of patients living in rural areas; stroke was associated

Table 1 General characteristics of the study participants

Characteristics		Number	Percent
Gender	Females	93	53.1
	Males	82	46.9
Age (years)	5–15	81	46.3
	≥16	94	53.7
Education	None	4	2.3
	Primary	65	37.1
	Secondary	73	41.7
	Tertiary	33	18.9
Marital status	Single	168	96.0
	Married	7	4.0
Residence	Rural	9	5.1
	Urban	166	94.9
Employment Status	Unemployed	155	88.6
	Employed	19	10.9

Table 2 Chronic complications of sickle cell disease

Complications	Number (*n*)	Prevalence (%)
Ischemic complications		
Refractive eye disorders	47	26.9
Avascular necrosis of the hip	23	13.1
Priapism	15	18.3[a]
Stroke	14	8.0
Anemic complications		
Heart disease	46	26.2
Chronic leg ulcers	43	24.6
Gall stones	12	6.9
Infectious complications		
Osteomyelitis	34	19.4
Septic arthritis	24	13.7
Tuberculosis	9	5.1
Others		
Enuresis	54	30.9
Sleep apnoea	10	5.4

[a]The denominator included males only ($n = 82$)

with about a 5-point reduction in the total score while ANH was associated with a 3-point reduction in the total QOL score. Factors associated with poor PCS were ageing, stroke, ANH and chronic leg ulcer. The MCS was higher in urban residents but was lower in females and in patients who had gall stones. Other coefficients were not significantly different from zero.

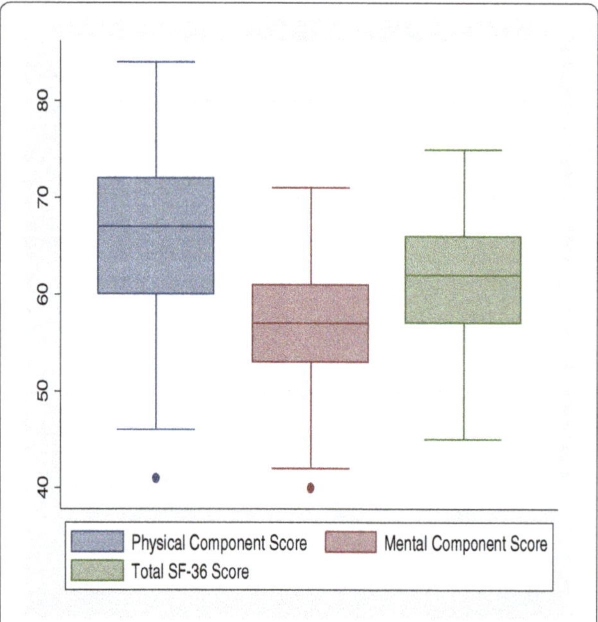

Fig. 2 Box plot summarizing quality of life scores. Blue: physical component scores; Red mental component scores; Green: total SF-36 scores. Isolated points are outliers

Discussion

We found in this study that our participants living with SCD are diagnosed late (median of 4 years) contrary to WHO recommendations of new-born screening and diagnosis. With a median age of 16 years, they presented frequent and multiple chronic complications of which 8% of stroke. The level of care is globally below the standards, and consequently the QOL is poor with the severity associated with age and the presence of chronic complications.

Though late, the diagnosis was however done earlier than was reported by Wonkam et al. in Yaoundé (8.3 years), the capital of Cameroon, in 2014 [11]. Countries that have instituted newborn screening such as Belgium have their diagnosis done earlier (median 0.7 years) have improved the mortality and morbidity of the disease and therefore a better quality of life [12]. Late diagnosis in Cameroon potentially affects the health status and quality of life of the individual, as well as the whole family's economic and psychological wellbeing.

The participants of this study had more frequent painful crises per year than that reported in nearby Nigeria [13] which has adopted systematic follow-up of patients. In addition, only 57% of our sickle cell population have had some kind of medical follow-up compared to SCD populations in the USA where more than 9 out of 10 do have regular follow up [14].

The prevalence of stroke in this study (8.0%), was similar to that reported by Njamnshi et al. in 2006 in Yaoundé (6.67%) [7]. About two fifth of our male study population suffered from priapism (18.3%), compared to other sickle cell populations in Africa like in Nigeria, where the prevalence was 39.1% in adults [15]. This probably reflects differences in the age groups studied, as we found that increasing age was significantly associated with priapism. The same reason may explain the lower prevalence of avascular necrosis (AVN) of the hip in our study (13.1%) compared with reports from the USA in 2014 (29%) [16].

The high prevalence of leg ulcers (24.6%) is a good indicator of lack of medical follow-up in our study population [17, 18]. The prevalence of osteomyelitis in this study (19.4%) was similar to that obtained from other sickle cell populations [19]. Nocturnal enuresis was the chronic complication with the highest prevalence affecting about one in three persons of our study population (30.1%). This prevalence was comparable to what has been reported from other studies [20, 21].

All median SF-36 scores in our study were lower than the USA norms studied and implemented in 1998 [10]. This indicates a globally low QOL in our population. The median PCS and MCS we report here (47.3 and 41.0 respectively) suggest that our study population had below normal physical and mental health.

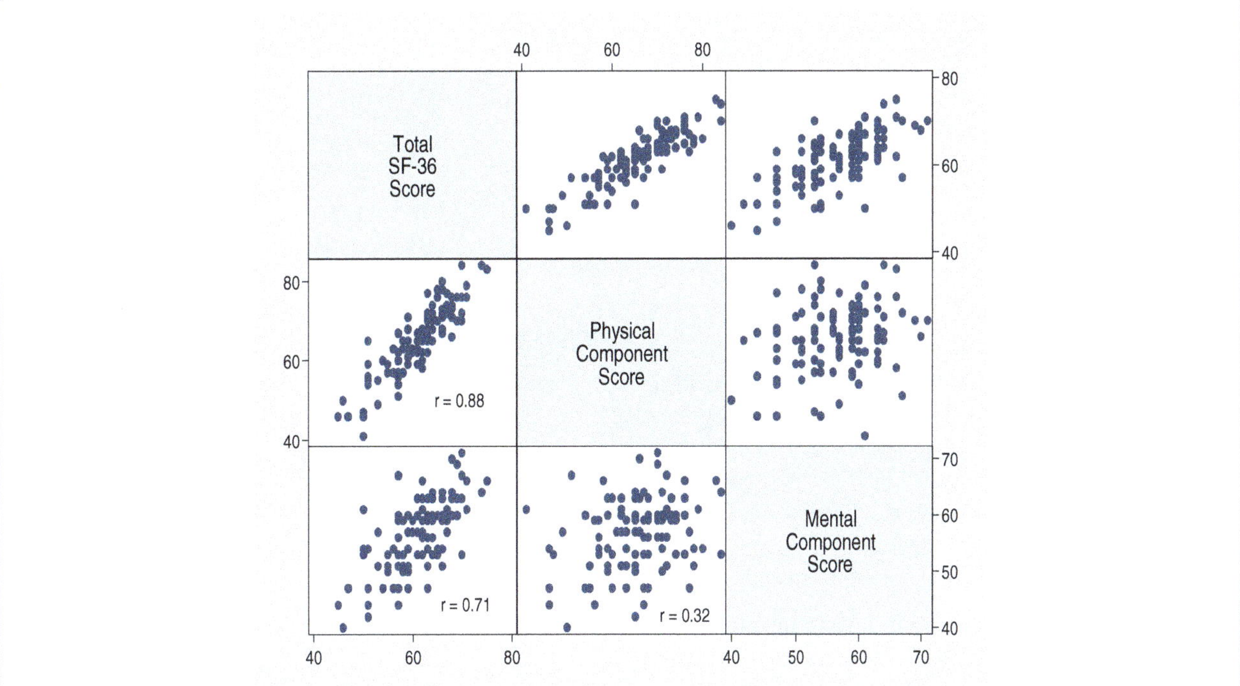

Fig. 3 Correlation matrix between the SF-36 components of quality of life score. The squares with scattered plots represent the areas and directions of correlation of the total scores and the specific scores

Considering the study of Abdel-Monhem Amr et al. conducted in Saudi Arabia in 2011, all the median SF-36 scores in our study were higher than those of their sickle cell population but lower than that of their healthy population [22]. They used a narrower age group (14–18 years) and their questionnaire was administered even during painful episodes.

Our study has potential limitations. Being conducted in the hospital rather than the community, we have probably lost some information like lifestyle factors which can influence patients' outcome. Though all patients had had a confirmed diagnosis of SCD by electrophoresis, we could access only 33% of results, which did not allow a strong assessment of a potential association

Table 3 Multiple Linear regression models of factors associated with quality of life scores

Factor	*Regression coefficient (ß)*	*95% confidence interval*	*P-value*
Total SF-36 Score, F(4, 105)			
Age	−0.15	−0.28 to −0.02	0.025
Urban residence	7.92	2.86 to 13.00	0.002
Stroke	−4.85	−8.76 to −0.94	0.015
Avascular necrosis of the hip	−3.35	−6.11 to −0.60	0.018
Physical Component Score, F(4, 105)			
Age	−0.25	−0.43 to −0.07	0.007
Stroke	−8.68	−14.12 to −3.24	0.002
Avascular necrosis of the hip	−4.63	−8.45 to −0.80	0.018
Chronic leg ulcer	−3.70	−6.75 to −0.65	0.018
Mental Component Score, F(4, 105)			
Females	−2.46	−4.78 to −0.14	0.038
Urban residence	8.29	2.76 to 13.80	0.004
Gall stones	−4.02	−7.70 to −0.34	0.033

SF Short form, *F* regression analysis significance

between genotype and QOL. Also, self-reporting of chronic complications may have caused potential report bias. Finally, some files did not have all information required. However, we have provided accurate data on the current standards of care and QOL of individuals living with SCD that may probably guide stakeholders to improve on policies on screening and follow up of these patients in Cameroon.

Conclusions

The prevalence of chronic complications in sickle cell patients in Cameroon is higher than in most other Sickle cell populations worldwide, probably due to late diagnosis. Chronic complications are also common and are the main drivers of low QOL. Our results highlight the need for national guidelines for SCD control, which should include early or newborn screening programs.

Abbreviations

ANH: Avascular necrosis of the hip; IQR: Interquartile range; MCS: Mental component score; NBS: New-born screening; PCS: Physical component score; QOL: Quality of life; SCA: Sickle cell anemia; SCD: Sickle cell disease; SD: Standard deviation; SF-36: Short Form-36; WHO: World Health Organization

Acknowledgements

The authors are grateful to all participants to this study. We also thank members of the 2HD Research Network for their contribution in improving the proposal, and the pediatric team of the Douala Laquintinie Hospital for their contribution. The 2HD Research Network is supported by a Cruddas Link Fellowship to SPC (Tseu Medical Institute, Harris Manchester College, University of Oxford, UK).

Funding

This work did not receive any funding.

Authors' contributions

AMA: conception and design of the study, data collection, data interpretation, drafting and review of the manuscript. EDTN: conception and design of the study, data collection, review of the manuscript. CEB: data analysis, data interpretation, drafting and review of the manuscript. VSV: data interpretation, drafting and review of the manuscript. DN: data interpretation, drafting and review of the manuscript. YMD: data interpretation, drafting and review of the manuscript. SPC: conception and design of the study, data collection, data interpretation, drafting and review of the manuscript. All authors revised and approved the final version of the manuscript.

Authors' information

Not applicable.

Competing interests

The authors declare that they have no competing interests.

Author details

[1]Department of Internal Medicine and Pediatrics, Faculty of Health Sciences, University of Buea, Buea, Cameroon. [2]Health and Human Development (2HD) Research Network, P.O. Box 4856, Douala, Cameroon. [3]Faculty of Medicine and Pharmaceutical Sciences, University of Douala, Douala, Cameroon. [4]Department of Internal Medicine, Douala General Hospital, P.O. Box 4856, Douala, Cameroon. [5]Ministry of Public Health, Centre Medical d'Arrondissement de Bare, Nkongsamba, Cameroon.

References

1. Ballas SK, Kesen MR, Goldberg MF, Lutty GA, Dampier C, Osunkwo I, et al. Beyond the Definitions of the Phenotypic Complications of Sickle Cell Disease: An Update on Management. Sci World J. 2012;2012:949535.
2. Asnani MR, Reid ME, Ali SB, Lipps G, Williams-Green P. Quality of life in patients with sickle cell disease in Jamaica: rural–urban differences. Rural Remote Health. 2008;8:890.
3. World Health Organization. Sickle-cell disease and other haemoglobin disorders: Fact sheet N°308. 2011. http://www.who.int/mediacentre/factsheets/fs308/en/. Accessed 4 Sept 2016.
4. Makani J, Cox SE, Soka D, Komba AN, Oruo J, Mwamtemi H, et al. Mortality in Sickle Cell Anemia in Africa: A Prospective Cohort Study in Tanzania. PLoS One. 2011;6:e14699.
5. Akinyanju OO, Otaigbe AI, Ibidapo MOO. Outcome of holistic care in Nigerian patients with sickle cell anaemia. Clin Lab Haematol. 2005;27:195–9.
6. McGann P, Muhongo M, McGann E, Oliveira V de, Santos B, Ware RE. Successful Outcomes Of An Infant Sickle Cell Clinic In Luanda, Angola. Blood 2013;122:2934–2934.
7. Njamnshi AK, Mbong EN, Wonkam A, Ongolo-Zogo P, Djientcheu VD, Sunjoh FL, et al. The epidemiology of stroke in sickle cell patients in Yaounde, Cameroon. J Neurol Sci. 2006;250:79–84.
8. Billa RF, Biwole MS, Juimo AG, Bejanga BI, Blackett K. Gall stone disease in African patients with sickle cell anaemia: a preliminary report from Yaounde, Cameroon. Gut. 1991;32:539–41.
9. Ohene-Frempong K, Weiner SJ, Sleeper LA, Miller ST, Embury S, Moohr JW, et al. Cerebrovascular accidents in sickle cell disease: rates and risk factors. Blood. 1998;91:288–94.
10. Ware JE Jr, Sherbourne CD. The MOS 36-item short-form health survey (SF-36). I. Conceptual framework and item selection. Med Care. 1992;30:473–83.
11. Wonkam A, Mba CZ, Mbanya D, Ngogang J, Ramesar R, Angwafo 3rd FF. Psychosocial Stressors of Sickle Cell Disease on Adult Patients in Cameroon. J Genet Couns. 2014;23:948–56.
12. Lê PQ, Dedeken L, Gulbis B, Vermylen C, Vanderfaeillie A, Heijmans C, et al. Low Sickle Cell Disease Mortality In Belgium and Benefit From Hydroxyurea Therapy. Blood. 2013;122:2231.
13. Adegoke SA, Adeodu OO, Adekile AD. Sickle cell disease clinical phenotypes in children from South-Western, Nigeria. Niger J Clin Pract. 2015;18:95–101.
14. Barnes M, French K, Rogers C, Berger W. Outpatient Opioid Use In Adult Patients With Sickle Cell Disease. Blood. 2013;122:4699.
15. Adediran A, Wright K, Akinbami A, Dosunmu A, Oshinaike O, Osikomaiya B, et al. Prevalence of Priapism and Its Awareness amongst Male Homozygous Sickle Cell Patients in Lagos, Nigeria. Adv Urol. 2013;2013:890328.
16. Blinder MA, Russel S, Barnes M. Prevalence of Symptomatic Avascular Necrosis and the Operative Treatment in Adult Patients with Sickle Cell Disease. Blood. 2014;124:1379.
17. Dampier C, LeBeau P, Rhee S, Lieff S, Kesler K, Ballas S, et al. Health-related quality of life in adults with sickle cell disease (SCD): a report from the comprehensive sickle cell centers clinical trial consortium. Am J Hematol. 2011;86:203–5.
18. Delaney KM, Axelrod KC, Buscetta A, Hassell KL, Adams-Graves PE, Seamon C, et al. Leg ulcers in sickle cell disease: current patterns and practices. Hemoglobin. 2013;37:325–32.
19. Menadi A, Chaise F, Bellemere P, Mehalleg M, Atia R. Contribution to the study of bone and joint infections in sickle-cell anemia children: Orthopaedic Proceedings.Bone & Joint 2008. http://www.bjjprocs.boneandjoint.org.uk/content/90-B/SUPP_II/264.2. Accessed 4 Sept 2016.

20. Ali M, Chakravorty S. Prevalence of nocturnal enuresis and proteinuria in children with sickle cell disease and its relation to severity of painful crises. Arch Dis Child. 2014;99 Suppl 1:A101–2.
21. Lehmann GC, Bell TR, Kirkham FJ, Gavlak JC, Ferguson TF, Strunk RC, et al. Enuresis Associated with Sleep Disordered Breathing in Children with Sickle Cell Anemia. J Urol. 2012;188:1572–6.
22. Abdel-Monhem Amr M, Tawfik AT, Al-Omair AO. Health related quality of life among adolescents with sickle cell disease in Saudi Arabia. Pan Afr Med J. 2011;8:10.

8

Challenges in achieving a target international normalized ratio for deep vein thrombosis among HIV-infected patients with tuberculosis

C Sekaggya[1*], D Nalwanga[1], A Von Braun[1], R Nakijoba[1], A Kambugu[1], J Fehr[2], M Lamorde[1] and B Castelnuovo[1]

Abstract

Background: Tuberculosis (TB) and HIV are among the risk factors for deep vein thrombosis (DVT). There are several challenges in the management of DVT patients with TB-HIV co-infection including drug-drug interactions and non-adherence due to pill burden.

Methods: HIV infected patients starting treatment for TB were identified and followed up two weekly. Cases of DVT were diagnosed with Doppler ultrasound and patients were initiated on oral anticoagulation with warfarin and followed up with repeated INR measurements and warfarin dose adjustment.

Results: We describe 7 cases of TB and HIV-infected patients in Uganda diagnosed with DVT and started on anticoagulation therapy. Their median age was 30 (IQR: 27–39) years and 86 % were male. All patients had co-medication with cotrimoxazole, tenofovir, lamivudine and efavirenz and some were on fluconazole. The therapeutic range of the International Normalization Ratio (INR) was difficult to attain and unpredictable with some patients being under-anticoagulated and others over-anticoagulated. The mean Time in Therapeutic Range (TTR) for patients who had all scheduled INR measurements in the first 12 weeks was 33.3 %. Only one patient among those with all the scheduled INR measurements had achieved a therapeutic INR by 2 weeks. Four out of seven (57 %) of the patients had at least one INR above the therapeutic range which required treatment interruption. None of the patients had major bleeding.

Conclusion: We recommend more frequent monitoring and timely dose adjustment of the INR, as well as studies on alternative strategies for the treatment of DVT in TB-HIV co-infected patients.

Keywords: Tuberculosis, HIV, Thrombosis, Monitoring

Background

The risk of deep vein thrombosis (DVT) is one and a half times higher among patients with tuberculosis (TB) compared to those without TB [1] due to a hypercoagulable state which occurs among patients with TB resulting from endothelial dysfunction due to the mycobacteria, increased fibrinogen, fibrin, tissue plasminogen activator, decreased anti-thrombin III [2, 3] and use of rifampicin especially in the first two weeks following TB treatment initiation [4]. Furthermore HIV infection, which is the highest risk factor for TB, is also considered a pro-thrombotic condition occurring most commonly in those with a low CD4 cell count [5, 6]. The mechanism leading to DVT in HIV is thought to be multifactorial including Protein C, S and antithrombin deficiency and increased antiphospholipid and antilupus antibodies [7, 8].

Several challenges due to drug-drug interactions occur during the management of DVT in patients co-infected with HIV and TB. Warfarin is metabolized by CYP450 pathway. Therefore drugs which induce this pathway (rifampicin and nevirapine) or inhibit them (isoniazid and efavirenz) could lead to under-anticoagulation or over-

* Correspondence: csekaggya@idi.co.ug
[1]Infectious Diseases Institute, College of Health Sciences, Makerere University, P.O. Box 22418, Kampala, Uganda
Full list of author information is available at the end of the article

anticoagulation respectively. These interactions influence the ability to attain the therapeutic target required for adequate anticoagulation [9]. Table 1 demonstrates drug interactions that may occur in patients with HIV and TB.

Several case series have discussed the occurrence of thrombosis in patients with TB [10, 11] and in those with HIV [12, 13], however, in this case series we demonstrate the challenges encountered when trying to achieve an International Normalized Ratio (INR) within the therapeutic window with warfarin in this population of TB-HIV co-infected patients.

Methods

The cases described are from patients enrolled in the "Study of Outcomes in TB-HIV co-infected patients" (SOUTH), a study conducted at the integrated HIV and TB clinic at the Infectious Diseases Institute in Kampala [14]. The SOUTH study aims to investigate the relationship between anti-TB drug concentrations and treatment outcomes in HIV infected patients treated for pulmonary TB (PTB). Patients are reviewed by a clinician every two weeks during the first two months of their treatment and monthly subsequently. Patients with clinical symptoms of TB are investigated using chest x-ray, sputum smear microscopy, sputum culture for *Mycobacterium tuberculosis* and Xpert MTB/RIF. Patients were followed up starting from the day TB treatment was initiated. TB treatment included a fixed dose regimen consisting of two months of rifampicin, isoniazid, pyrazinamide and ethambutol followed by four months of rifampicin and isoniazid. CD4 counts were measured within two weeks prior to or after TB diagnosis. Patients were initiated on antiretroviral therapy (ART) after the second week of anti-TB treatment according to WHO guidelines [15, 16] and included tenofovir, lamivudine and efavirenz. Patients remained on this ART regimen throughout the follow-up period. All patients were on cotrimoxazole before the start of the study and also remained on it throughout follow-up. Cases of DVT were identified by clinical history and physical examination between May 2013 and June 2015; all patients who reported or were observed to have limb swelling were referred for Doppler ultrasound scan to confirm the clinical diagnosis. Patients diagnosed with DVT were initiated on warfarin tablets (Bristol®) at an initial dose of 2.5 - 5 mg once daily, as well as low molecular heparin (LMWH), Enoxaparin (Clexane®) 1 mg/kg for five days and subsequently continued on warfarin alone. The INR was monitored weekly and dose adjustment was made at the discretion of the clinician depending on the INR results. Adherence to warfarin was assessed through self-report and the number of days that warfarin doses were missed were recorded in the patient's file. Patients who missed a visit were called on the same day and rescheduled for the closest opportunity within the same week. Time in therapeutic range (TTR) was calculated as the number of therapeutic INR values during the first 12 weeks of anticoagulation as a percentage of all the INR values measured during this same period.

Table 1 Drug interactions in patients with HIV and TB

DRUG	EFFECT ON CYTOCHROME P450	
	Induce Cytochrome P450 (Decrease effect of warfarin)	Inhibit Cytochrome P450 (Increase effect of warfarin)
Rifampicin	X	
Ritonavir (protease inhibitor)	X	
Nevirapine	X	
Isoniazid		X
Efavirenz[a]	X	X
Fluconazole		X
Cotrimoxazole		X

[a]Efavirenz may induce or inhibit cytochrome P450 through its action on CYP3A4 and CYP2C9 respectively

Informed consent was obtained from all patients prior to involvement in the study.

The study was reviewed and approved by the Joint Clinical Research Centre Research and Ethics Committee and the Uganda National Council for Science and Technology (HS 1303).

Results

During this review period, 7/268 (2.6 %) patients with confirmed PTB presented with pain and swelling of the lower limb and were diagnosed with DVT through Doppler ultrasound scan. All patients were HIV positive. Individual patients' characteristics are displayed in Table 2. Six (86 %) were male with a median age of 30 (interquartile range (IQR): 27–39) years and a median CD4 count at the time of TB diagnosis of 72cells/μl (19–78). All patients were not on ART at the time of anti-TB treatment initiation and started on tenofovir, lamivudine and efavirenz after two weeks of TB treatment. The median time from initiation of anti-TB treatment to DVT diagnosis was 2 (IQR: 2–4) weeks. From their clinical history, none of the patients was bedridden at the time of DVT diagnosis.

Three patients were on 600-800 mg of fluconazole before the diagnosis of DVT was made (patients 1, 5 and 7) due to cryptococcal antigenemia. Figure 1 below shows the trend of INR values for each patient while Table 3 shows the corresponding warfarin doses.

Patient 1 was started on the standard ART mentioned ten days after the diagnosis of DVT was made. He had only one therapeutic INR during the first 12 weeks of anticoagulation with a TTR of 8.3 %. Three of his INR measurements were supratherapeutic with no major bleeding while taking 7.5 mg and 5 mg respectively which

Table 2 Patient baseline characteristics

Patient number	Age (years)	Gender	Baseline CD4 (cells/μL)	Week of TB treatment when DVT diagnosed	Symptoms of bleeding	Co-medication[a]
1	30	M	6	1.5	No	CTX, Fluconazole
2	26	M	73	4	No	CTX
3	40	F	40	2	Epistaxis	CTX
4	39	M	72	10	No	CTX
5	27	M	78	2	Epistaxis	CTX, fluconazole
6	31	M	19	4	No	CTX
7	28	M	180	2	No	CTX, fluconazole

M male, *F* female, *CTX* cotrimoxazole
[a]All patients were on tenofovir, lamivudine and efavirenz

were initially leading to sub-therapeutic INR values. His maximum dose during this period was 10 mg. He was on fluconazole throughout the follow-up period.

Patient 2, who had started ART two weeks prior to the diagnosis of DVT had a supratherapeutic INR after 3 weeks of anticoagulation while on 10 mg of warfarin with no major bleeding episode. From 8 weeks onwards, his INR was maintained within the therapeutic range on 10 mg. His TTR was 41.7 %.

Patient 3 had a therapeutic INR at the earliest time point compared to the other patients (1 week) and had the best INR control. She developed DVT two weeks into her TB treatment and ART and warfarin were started at the same time. She had a supratherapeutic INR while on 10 mg of warfarin with epistaxis. She later had a therapeutic INR initially on 5 mg and later 7.5 mg of warfarin. She had the highest TTR of 58.3 %.

Patient 4 had a history of alcohol abuse and had five intermittent INR measurements (1.53 at week one, 2.10 at week two, 1.29 at week six, 1.04 at week ten and 1.29 at week twelve) He missed visits at weeks 3, 4, 5, 7, 8, 9, 11 despite phone call reminders to come to the clinic. He admitted to poor adherence whenever he run out of pills.

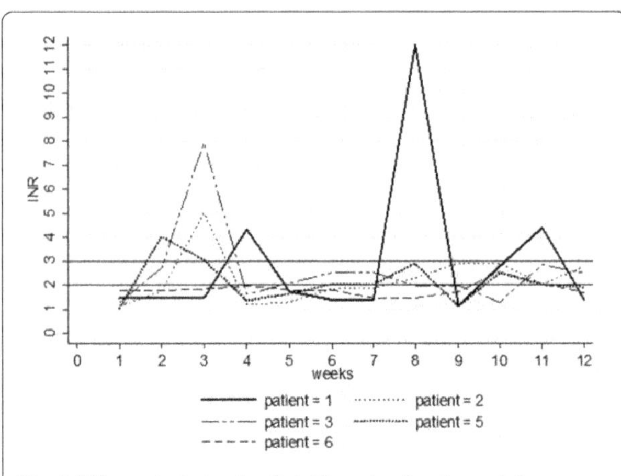

Fig. 1 INR trends during the first 12 weeks of anticoagulation

Patient 5 started on ART on the day DVT was diagnosed, and was also on fluconazole. He had supratherapeutic INR on a dose of 5 mg of warfarin. This same dose subsequently kept him within the therapeutic range for most of the time after week 6 even while he was still on fluconazole and his TTR was 41.7 %.

Patient 6 was diagnosed with DVT a week after starting ART. He had dose escalation up to 12.5 mg, the highest dose used among these patients, and only attained a therapeutic INR at two time points. He attained the lowest TTR of 16.7 %.

Patient 7 had only 2 INR measurements after 1 and 3 weeks (1.15 and 2.21 respectively) and there after requested to be transferred to another center.

The mean TTR for patients who had all scheduled INR measurements in the first 12 weeks was 33.3 %. Only one patient (patient 3) among those with all the scheduled INR measurements had achieved a therapeutic INR by 2 weeks.

Four out of seven (57 %) of the patients (cases 1, 2, 3 and 5) had at least one INR above the therapeutic range which required treatment interruption. Two patients developed epistaxis (patient 5 and 3); however none of them experienced severe bleeding. Patient 1 had supratherapeutic INR values at weeks 4, 8 and 11 and the INR only reached the therapeutic range once during the first 12 weeks of treatment despite several dose adjustments each week as shown in the graph below.

Of the remaining two patients, one (patient 7) missed several clinic visits and subsequently asked to be transferred to another health care center and patient 4 frequently missed clinic visits and achieved therapeutic ranges only at time point (week 4). All patients reported 100 % adherence except patients 4 and 7 who missed over 60 % of their warfarin doses during the follow-up period.

Discussion

Achieving a target INR was challenging in our TB-HIV co-infected population, and we supposed that drug-drug interactions and unreported non-adherence could have

Table 3 Warfarin doses adjustments per week

Patient number	Dose of warfarin (mg)											
	Week 1	Week 2	Week 3	Week 4	Week 5	Week 6	Week 7	Week 8	Week 9	Week 10	Week 11	Week 12
Patient 1	5	7.5	7.5	7.5	0	5	7.5	10	0	5	5	0
Patient 2	5	7.5	10	0	5	7.5	7.5	10	10	10	10	10
Patient 3	5	10	10	0	2.5	5	5	5	7.5	7.5	7.5	7.5
Patient 5	2.5	5	0	0	5	5	5	5	5	5	5	5
Patient 6	2.5	5	5	7.5	7.5	10	10	12.5	12.5	12.5	12.5	12.5

played a role. Several dose adjustments occurred which resulted in supratherapeutic or subtherapeutic INR values. On some occasions, the same dose of warfarin that kept a patient within the therapeutic range would also lead to a subtherapeutic or supratherapeutic INR later as in the case of patients 1 and 2 which could be due to drug interactions or non-adherence that was not reported.

Warfarin prescriptions increase the pill burden in TB-HIV co-infected patients who are already taking up to 9 tablets per day. Pill burden has been shown to enhance non-adherence [17] and therefore contribute to difficulty in attaining a target INR.

Drug interactions with fluconazole, which increases the effect of warfarin through inhibition of CYP2C9 and CYP3A4, may explain the low daily warfarin requirement for patients 1 and 5 compared to the other patients. Patient 1 also had several supratherapeutic INR values due to the increased effect of warfarin. Drug-drug interactions between warfarin and fluconazole has also been reported by others [18].

All patients were on rifampicn, isoniazid and efavirenz, making it difficult to ascertain which of these drugs contributed to the subtherapeutic or supratherapeutic INR values; however, the challenge of drug-drug interactions is evident. Lee et al. reported that a 233 % increase in warfarin dosage over 4 months was insufficient to attain an INR within the therapeutic range in a patient on rifampicin [19].

Where there are drug interactions, a switch to a more suitable option is necessary, however we recognize that there are not many alternative therapies for treatment of DVT; therefore this may not be practical. Newer drugs like factor Xa inhibitors also pose a challenge due to drug-drug interactions in patients on TB treatment and ART as is the case of warfarin. LMWH which is the recommended anticoagulation therapy in patients with cancer, may be suitable for this patient population, an area that also needs to be explored further considering the similar mechanisms of thrombosis involving an increase in inflammatory markers.

Most INR values measured in these patients were outside the therapeutic range and the mean time in the therapeutic range for all the patients with regular follow-up was only 33.3 %. Although we did not have a direct measure of clinical improvement, TTR has been shown to correlate with DVT treatment outcome and is used in the assessment of the management of DVT [20]. There are however many methods of measurement of TTR which may limit its utility in day to day practice. Time in therapeutic range has been reported to be higher in other studies (56 %–75 %) [21] in comparison to our patients.

Our time in therapeutic range may have implications on the duration of treatment that is adequate to achieve actual resolution of symptoms and resorption of the thrombus. Further studies need to evaluate if prolonging treatment in patients with low TTR values affects DVT treatment outcomes.

Conclusion

The course of INR in this population was unpredictable in any individual patient. This could be due to a number of reasons including non-adherence and changing dose requirements due to drug interactions.

More frequent monitoring of INR with timely dose adjustments is required in TB-HIV patients. Studies on alternative medication for example long term LMWH in TB-HIV infected patients should be considered.

Abbreviations

ART, Antiretroviral therapy; CD4, Cluster of Differentiation; CTX, Cotrimoxazole; DVT, Deep vein thrombosis; HIV, Human Immunodeficiency virus; INR, International Normalized Ratio; IQR, Interquartile range; MTB/Rif, Mycobacteria tuberculosis/Rifampicin; TB, Tuberculosis; TTR, Time in therapeutic range.

Acknowledgements

We would like to acknowledge and thank the staff of the Infectious Diseases Institute integrated tuberculosis clinic for their efforts in ensuring patients get the best care as well as the patients and their families for supporting this work.

Funding

This study was funded by a collaboration between the University of Zurich in Switzerland and the Infectious Diseases Institute in Kampala.

Authors' contributions

CS, DN and AB contributed to the collection of data and writing of this case report. ML and BC contributed to its revision and all authors read and approved the final version.

Author's information
CS and AvB are physicians and research fellows at the Infectious Diseases Institute in Kampala. DN and RN are clinicians at the Infectious Diseases Institute. AK, ML and BC are physicians and senior researchers at the Infectious Diseases Institute and JF is a physician in University Hospital of Zurich in Switzerland.

Competing interests
The authors declare that they have no competing interests.

Author details
[1]Infectious Diseases Institute, College of Health Sciences, Makerere University, P.O. Box 22418, Kampala, Uganda. [2]Division of Infectious Diseases and Infection Control, University Hospital Zurich, University of Zurich, Zurich, Switzerland.

References
1. Dentan C, Epaulard O, Seynaeve D, Genty C, Bosson JL. Active tuberculosis and venous thromboembolism: association according to international classification of diseases, ninth revision hospital discharge diagnosis codes. Clin Infect Dis. 2014;58(4):495–501.
2. Robson SC, White NW, Aronson I, Woollgar R, Goodman H, Jacobs P. Acute-phase response and the hypercoagulable state in pulmonary tuberculosis. Br J Haematol. 1996;93(4):943–9.
3. Kager LM, Blok DC, Lede IO, Rahman W, Afroz R, Bresser P, et al. Pulmonary tuberculosis induces a systemic hypercoagulable state. J Infect. 2015; 70(4):324–34.
4. White NW. Venous thrombosis and rifampicin. Lancet. 1989;2(8660):434–5.
5. Sullivan PS, Dworkin MS, Jones JL, Hooper WC. Epidemiology of thrombosis in HIV-infected individuals. The Adult/Adolescent Spectrum of HIV Disease Project. AIDS. 2000;14(3):321–4.
6. Rasmussen LD, Dybdal M, Gerstoft J, Kronborg G, Larsen CS, Pedersen C, et al. HIV and risk of venous thromboembolism: a Danish nationwide population-based cohort study. HIV Med. 2011;12(4):202–10.
7. Leder AN, Flansbaum B, Zandman-Goddard G, Asherson R, Shoenfeld Y. Antiphospholipid syndrome induced by HIV. Lupus. 2001;10(5):370–4.
8. Majluf-Cruz A, Silva-Estrada M, Sanchez-Barboza R, Montiel-Manzano G, Trevino-Perez S, Santoscoy-Gomez M, et al. Venous thrombosis among patients with AIDS. Clin Appl Thromb Hemost. 2004;10(1):19–25.
9. Liedtke MD, Rathbun RC. Warfarin-antiretroviral interactions. Ann Pharmacother. 2009;43(2):322–8.
10. Goncalves IM, Alves DC, Carvalho A, Do Ceu Brito M, Calvario F, Duarte R. Tuberculosis and Venous Thromboembolism: a case series. Cases J. 2009;2:9333.
11. Kumarihamy KW, Ralapanawa DM, Jayalath WA. A rare complication of pulmonary tuberculosis: a case report. BMC Res Notes. 2015;8:39.
12. Jacobson MC, Dezube BJ, Aboulafia DM. Thrombotic complications in patients infected with HIV in the era of highly active antiretroviral therapy: a case series. Clin Infect Dis. 2004;39(8):1214–22.
13. Konin C, Anzouan-Kacou JB, Essam N'I A. Arterial thrombosis in patients with human immunodeficiency virus: two-case reports and review of the literature. Case Rep Vasc Med. 2011;2011:847241.
14. Hermans SM, Castelnuovo B, Katabira C, Mbidde P, Lange JM, Hoepelman AI, et al. Integration of HIV and TB services results in improved TB treatment outcomes and earlier prioritized ART initiation in a large urban HIV clinic in Uganda. J Acquir Immune Defic Syndr. 1999;60(2):e29–35.
15. Padayatchi N, Abdool Karim SS, Naidoo K, Grobler A, Friedland G. Improved survival in multidrug-resistant tuberculosis patients receiving integrated tuberculosis and antiretroviral treatment in the SAPiT Trial. Int J Tuberc Lung Dis. 2014;18(2):147–54.
16. WHO Policy on Collaborative TB/HIV Activities: Guidelines for National Programmes and Other Stakeholders. Geneva: World Health Organization; 2012.
17. Kneeland PP, Fang MC. Current issues in patient adherence and persistence: focus on anticoagulants for the treatment and prevention of thromboembolism. Patient Preference Adherence. 2010;4:51–60.
18. Gericke KR. Possible interaction between warfarin and fluconazole. Pharmacotherapy. 1993;13(5):508–9.
19. Lee CR, Thrasher KA. Difficulties in anticoagulation management during coadministration of warfarin and rifampin. Pharmacotherapy. 2001; 21(10):1240–6.
20. Phillips KW, Ansell J. Outpatient management of oral vitamin K antagonist therapy: defining and measuring high-quality management. Expert Rev Cardiovasc Ther. 2008;6(1):57–70.
21. Erkens PM, Ten Cate H, Buller HR, Prins MH. Benchmark for time in therapeutic range in venous thromboembolism: a systematic review and meta-analysis. PLoS One. 2012;7(9), e42269.

9

Prevalence of Anaemia and Associated Risk Factors among Children in North-western Uganda: A Cross Sectional Study

Ismail Dragon Legason[1], Alex Atiku[2], Ronald Ssenyonga[3], Peter Olupot-Olupot[4] and John Banson Barugahare[1,5*]

Abstract

Background: Despite the public health significance of anaemia in African children, its broader and often preventable risk factors remain largely under described. This study investigated, for the first time, the prevalence of childhood anaemia and its risk factors in an urban setting in Uganda.

Methods: A total of 342 children were enrolled. Venous blood samples were collected in EDTA tubes and analyzed using Symex 500i (Symex Corp. Japan). Stool and urine samples were analyzed according to established standard methods. Anthropometric indicators were calculated according to the CDC/WHO 1978 references. Ethical approval was granted.

Results: Categorically, the prevalence of anaemia was; 37.2, 33.3 and 11.8% among children aged 1–5 years, 6–11 years and 12–14 years respectively. Overall anaemia prevalence was 34.4%. The risk of anaemia was higher among males than females [(OR = 1.3, 95% CI = 0.8, 2.1), *P* = .22]. Malaria was associated with a 1.5 times risk of anaemia though not statistically significant in the multivariate analysis (*P* = *.19*). Maternal parity <5 (*P* = .002), and stunting [(OR = 2.5, 95% CI = 1.3, 4.7), *P* = .004] were positively associated with anaemia. There was a positive correlation between household size and income (*Pearson* X^2 *= 22.96; P = .001)*, implying that large families were of higher socioeconomic status.

Conclusions: This study demonstrates that anaemia is more prevalent in the under-5 age. The risk factors are stunting and low maternal parity. Interventions that address nutritional deficiencies in both pre-school and school children are recommended. Malaria and helminthiasis control measures counter the risk of anaemia. Further studies are required to investigate the association between maternal parity and anaemia found in this study.

Keywords: Prevalence, Anaemia, Risk factors, Children, North-western Uganda

Background

Anaemia remains a major public health problem in young children particularly in the developing world [1]. Over 273 million children under – five, suffer from anaemia worldwide [2]. The Sub-Saharan Africa is one of the most affected regions - with more than half (53.8%) of children under - 5 years old suffering from anaemia [2]. In Uganda, some hospital-based data is available, however, there is a paucity of data on anaemia in school children and community based surveys. Nevertheless, in a few of the studies, anaemia prevalence ranges from 38 to 46% [3, 4]. In a more recent community pilot survey conducted in Arua district (same study area) hemoglobin <11.0 g/dl was observed in nearly half of the children less than 16 years enrolled (unpublished data).

Recent descriptions have shown that the aetiology of anaemia is multi-factorial with severe micronutrient deficiencies playing a major role [5], as opposed to earlier data describing the condition as being caused mainly by infectious agents, folate and iron deficiencies [2]. This calls for new approaches in prevention and management of childhood anaemia. Among the well described consequences are impaired physical growth [6], immune alterations and increased susceptibility to infections [7], impaired motor development leading to reduced cognitive ability [8–10], poor school performance [11] and short or long term mortality in acute severe cases [5].

* Correspondence: barugahare@gmail.com; banbarugahare@sci.busitema.ac.ug
[1]School of Postgraduate Studies, Uganda Christian University, Mukono, Uganda
[5]Faculty of Science and Education, Busitema University, Tororo, Uganda
Full list of author information is available at the end of the article

Significant in the pathogenesis of anaemia is the fact that it is detrimental even before symptoms become apparent hence, the need to identify the risk factors for timely and effective management strategies.

In malaria endemic areas, the risk of anaemia is particularly important [12, 13]. Moreover, asymptomatic malaria infections often labelled carrier states, contribute to substantial development of anaemia even though mortality in this category is <1% [14, 15]. Infections with gastrointestinal helminthes and Schistosomes have also been shown to significantly contribute to the risk of childhood anaemia in the East African region [16, 17]. Despite the public health significance of anaemia in African children, its broader and often preventable risk factors remain largely under described. The aim of the study was to determine the prevalence of anaemia and associated risk factors among children aged 1–14 years in an urban setting.

Methods

Study design and setting

We conducted a cross sectional study among children aged 1–14 years in 20 local administrative units (villages) of Arua municipality in Arua district, North-western Uganda. The study was conducted between March and May 2016. A two-stage cluster-sampling was used in the survey. The first stage involved selection of villages. A probability proportional-to-number was applied to select the villages from each cluster. The second stage involved selection of households using Village health Team (VHT) registers.

Inclusion/exclusion criteria

Children were eligible if they; were at least 1 year old but not more than 14 years old and had been living in the study area for at least 3 months prior to the study. Children were excluded if they had a history of anti malarial or helminthes treatment 2 weeks prior to the study, were not usual residents and their parents did not consent.

Data collection

The data collection tool was developed based on the national survey questionnaire and was administered to the consenting parents/caregivers of the prospective enrolees. Height was measured using Charder HM200P-portable stadiometer (precision 0.1 cm) with child head positioned according to the Frankfurt plane. Weight was measured using Taylor digital floor scale with the child standing. Children who were unable to stand on their own were held on the scale and then difference in weight subtracted. Nutritional status was assessed and stratified by age and sex.

Up to 4 ml of venous blood was collected into EDTA vacutainer for complete blood count (CBC) performed on a 5-Diff automated analyzer, Symex 500i, Symex Corp. Japan. Typing of anaemia was by morphological examination of peripheral blood films and results were compared with MCV, MCHC and RDW values obtained on an automated analyzer. Reference data published by Lugada et al., was used to interpret the red cell indices [18]. Anaemia status was defined, adjusted for altitude as recommended by WHO [19]; Hb < 11.0 g/dl for age 6 months to 5 years, Hb < 11.5 g/dl for age 6 to 11 years and Hb < 12.0 g/dl for age 12 to 14 years. The severity of anaemia was classified based on the WHO scheme as mild (Hb ≥ 11 but less than normal), moderate (Hb between 8 and 10.9 g/dl) and severe (Hb < 8).

Thick and thin blood slides were prepared, stained with Giemsa and examined microscopically for malaria parasites. Malaria was excluded when thick smears were reported negative after examining 100 fields under ×100 oil immersion objective. The species of infecting *Plasmodium* parasite was determined using the thin blood film. Where it was not possible, a rapid malaria test kit with multiple species detection was used to identify the species. Children were provided with a pair of universal containers, a plastic bag, a clean non-disinfectant impregnated disposable towel and tissue paper in order to collect good quality stool samples and urine. Children above 7 years of age were instructed to lay the disposal kitchen towel and defecate on it. With the applicator stick or spoon attached to the cap of the stool container, pick about 2 g of sample and put into the container and deliver immediately to the laboratory. For younger children parents were given the same instructions above to collect stool samples. Intestinal helminthes were detected microscopically by wet preparation and Kato-Katz technique [20]. Urine specimens were first centrifuged at 1000 g for 5 min and sediment examined microscopically for Schistosome eggs. HIV screening was done in accordance to Uganda ministry of health guidelines. Plasma obtained from centrifuged whole blood was then used for testing HIV infection.

Statistical analysis

The data was entered in EPi Info software version 3.3.2 (Centre for Diseases Control and prevention, USA) and analysed using Stata version 12 (Stata Corp., Texas). Proportions, means and medians were computed for the demographic characteristics. Pearson chi-square or Fisher's test and analysis of variance (ANOVA) were calculated at bivariate analysis. Multivariate analysis was performed using a logistic regression model utilizing odds ratios to quantify the association and two-sided *P*-values to determine statistical significance. Interaction and confounding at a 10% cut off was assessed during the model fitting. The 95% confidence interval was determined and factors with a P-value <0.05 were considered significant.

Nutritional status was assessed and stratified by age and sex. Weight-for-age, height-for-age, and weight-for-height Z-scores were calculated based on CDC/WHO 1978 reference data using Epi Info version 3.3.2. Z-scores <−2 SD were indicative of underweight, stunting and wasting respectively [20].

Results

Out of the 342 children enrolled, 183 (53.5%) were males and 159 (46.5%) females. Pre-school children (1-5 years) comprised 57.3% of the overall sample size. The mean age was 5.6 years and median age was 5.1 years. Children lived in households with an average of 7.3 members. The homes had an average of two rooms dedicated for sleeping. Business (commercial units) is the most common occupation (37.7%). Most homesteads (98%) had either a latrine or toilet for family use and this level of sanitation is above the average reported nationally [19]. Only 9.4% of the households were less than 0.25 km from a perennial water source. Mosquito bed net usage was reported by 93.9% of the households and 95.3% of the children reported having slept under bed net throughout the week before the study. Nearly all children (98.8%) lived in households that had access to an "improved" drinking water source (tap water, borehole, protected well or spring, bottled water). Primary school education is most common level of the children's mothers (N = 195, 57.0%). Whereas, a majority of the children's fathers (N = 209, 61.1%) had at least a secondary school education, only 110 (32.2%) females had attained similar levels of education. Only 12.6% of the households had difficulty satisfying their food needs and 88.8% reported having at least three meals per day. 23.7% (N = 81) of the households did not consume meat regularly. The baseline characteristics of the study population are included in Table 1.

Blood samples were collected from 332 (97.1%), stool from 291 (85.1%) and urine samples from 317 (92.7%). The urine sediments were microscopically examined for Schistosome eggs. Complete blood counts including hemoglobin measurement were available for 329 (96.2%) children. Overall, 14.2% of the children tested positive for malaria, 0.3% HIV positive and 15.5% had stool

Table 1 Showing some baseline characteristics of the study population

Variable	Age group in Years n = 342			Overall
	1–5 196 (57.3)	6–11 129 (37.7)	12–14 17 (5.0)	
Sex				
Male	111 (60.7)	66 (36.1)	6 (3.3)	183
Female	85 (53.5)	63 (39.6)	11 (6.9)	159
Age: mean (SD)	3.4 (1.4)	8.0 (1.6)	12.9 (0.9)	5.6 (3.1)
Religion				
Protestant	27 (51.9)	20 (38.5)	5 (9.6)	52
Islam	130 (63.4)	67 (32.7)	8 (3.9)	205
Catholic	39 (45.9)	42 (49.4)	4 (4.7)	85
Mother's level of education				
No formal education	16 (43.2)	20 (54.1)	1 (2.7)	37
Primary	108 (55.4)	76 (39.0)	11 (5.6)	195
Secondary or above	72 (65.4)	33 (30.0)	5 (4.6)	110
Household size: mean (SD)	6.8 (3.4)	7.8 (4.6)	9.1 (2.9)	7.3 (4.0)
Household's main source of income				
Employment/Salary	40 (50.6)	33 (41.8)	6 (7.6)	79
Agriculture related	6 (60.0)	4 (40.0)	0 (0)	10
Property income	19 (73.1)	6 (23.1)	1 (3.9)	26
Business enterprise	73 (56.6)	51 (39.5)	5 (3.9)	129
Other	58 (59.2)	35 (35.7	5 (5.1)	98
Monthly household income'000				
Median(IQR)	233.5 (150–300)	240(150–300)	300 (210–450)	240 (150–300)

parasites detected in their samples. Malaria was higher (17.8%) among the school age group (6–14 years) compared to pre-school age (11.4%). Stool parasites detected included: *Entamoeba histolytica* (24/291, 8.2%), *Giardia lamblia* (13/291, 4.5%), *Hymenolepsis nana* (4/291, 1.4%), Schistosomes (3/291, 1.0%) and hookworm (1/291, 0.3%). The prevalence of malaria, HIV, helminthes and intestinal protozoa are summarised in Table 2.

Overall, anaemia prevalence was 34.4%. Anaemia was more prevalent in the age group 1–5 years (37.2%, Hb < 11.0 g/dl) compared to age group 6–11 years (33.3%, Hb < 11.5 g/dl). The lowest prevalence was found in the age group 12–14 years (11.8%, Hb < 12.0 g/dl). Some of the children, 65/329 (19.8%) had mild anaemia (Hb 10.0–10.9 g/dl) compared to 48/329 (14.6%) with moderate anaemia (Hb 8.0–9.9 g/dl). There were no cases of severe anaemia (Hb < 7.0 g/dL) in the asymptomatic children of the study population. All the nutritional deficiencies observed in this study were more common among males. This result is summarised in Table 3.

Children who were stunted had 2.5 times risk of anaemia than non-stunted children (95% CI = 1.3, 4.7). The risk of anaemia was 2.6 times among underweight children (95% CI = 1.2, 5.6). Anaemia was also observed to decrease with increasing maternal age. Children whose mothers were between 30 and 33 years had the least risk of anaemia (OR = 0.4, 95% CI = 0.2, 0.9). Maternal parity ≥5 was negatively associated with anaemia in the offspring (OR = 0.5, 95% CI = 0.3, 0.8). Though not of statistical significance (*P = .16),* the risk of anaemia was observed to decrease with increasing age and the least risk of anaemia was among children aged 12–14 years (OR =0.3, 95% CI = 0.1, 1.1). Boys were 1.3 times more likely to be anaemic than girls (95% CI =0.8, 2.1). Children with only one parent surviving were 1.5 times more likely to be anaemic (95% CI = 0.6, 3.9) compared to those with both parents. The risk of anaemia was 1.5 times (95% CI = 0.8, 2.9) higher among malaria positive children compared to malaria negative. Distance of the child's home from a perennial water source (X^2 *= 1.3900, P = .24*), access to safe water (Fisher's exact = .55), presence of toilet/latrine for family use and helminthes infection were not associated with anaemia in the bivariate analysis. The risk of anaemia decreased with increase in household income, and household size. There was a positive correlation between household size and income (*Pearson* X^2 *= 22.96; P = .001)*, implying that large families were of higher socioeconomic status. It is important to note that this community has a reasonable percentage of Muslims – with small businesses but also characterised by large families. Though, not of statistical significance *(P = .61)*, the risk of anaemia was found to be low among children who lived in households that reported bed net use (OR = 0.8, 95% CI = 0.3, 2.0). Anaemia was prevalent in households that consumed fewer meals per day and, without meat and fish. These results are shown in the Table 4.

Table 2 Prevalence of malaria, HIV, helminthes and intestinal protozoa

Variable	Preschool (1–5 years)	School (6–14 years)	Overall
Malaria[a]			
Positive	21 (11.4)	26 (17.8)	47 (14.2)
Negative	164 (88.6)	120 (82.2)	284 (85.8)
HIV[b]			
Positive	0 (0)	1 (0.7)	1 (0.3)
Negative	186(100)	145 (99.3))	331 (99.7)
Parasites[c]			
Helminthes			
Hookworm	0 (0)	1 (0.7)	1 (0.3)
H. nana	1 (0.7)	3 (2.1)	4 (1.4)
Schistosome	1 (0.7)	2 (1.4)	3 (1.0)
Protozoa			
Giardia lamblia	9 (6.0)	4 (2.8)	13 (4.5)
Entamoeba histolytica	13 (8.7)	11 (7.7)	24 (8.2)

Note: [a]11, [b]10, [c]45 reported

Table 3 Prevalence of under - nutrition

	Underweight	Stunting	Wasting
Age			
Pre-school: 1–5	21 (10.7)	32 (16.3)	10 (5.1)
School: 6–14	9 (6.2)	18 (12.3)	3 (2.6)
Sex			
Male	20 (10.9)	29 (15.9)	10 (5.8)
Female	10 (6.3)	21 (13.2)	3 (2.2)

Stunting [(OR = 2.5, 95% CI = 1.3, 4.7), *P = .004*], household size [(OR = 0.4, 95% CI = 0.2, 0.8), *P = .021*] and maternal parity [(OR = 0.4, 95% CI = 0.3, 0.7), *P = .002]* were significantly associated with risk of anaemia. Children who were stunted were 2.5 times likely to have anaemia compared to normal children. Households with family members exceeding three had less risk of anaemia. Similarly, maternal parity ≥5 was associated with a lower risk of anaemia in the offspring. Table 5 shows the multivariate analysis of the factors associated with anaemia.

Discussion

Our study to the best of our knowledge was the first to describe prevalence of childhood anaemia and it is risk factors in an urban setting in the North-western part of Uganda. In these settings, the overall prevalence of anaemia was 34.4%, which was higher than previously

Table 4 Bivariate Analysis of factors associated with anaemia

Variables	Have anaemia		Odds ratio (95% CI)	P-value
	Yes	No		
Sex				
Female[a]	48 (31.0)	107 (69.0)	1	0.224
Male	65 (37.4)	109 (62.6)	1.3 (0.8,2.1)	
Age group				
1–5[a]	68 (37.2)	128 (62.8)	1	0.156
6–11	43 (33.3)	86 (66.7)	0.9 (0.6,1.5)	
12–14	2 (11.8)	15 (88.2)	0.3 (0.1,1,1)	
Malaria				
Negative[a]	93 (32.8)	191 (67.2)	1	0.190
Positive	20 (42.6)	27 (57.4)	1.5 (0.8,2.9)	
Bed net				
No[a]	8 (38.1)	13 (61.9)	1	0.612
Yes	105 (32.7)	216 (67.3)	0.8 (0.3,2.0)	
Meat				
Never[a]	28 (34.6)	53 (65.4)	1	0.943
Once/week	44 (32.3)	92 (67.7)	0.9 (0.5,1.6)	
> 1 per week	41 (32.8)	84 (67.2)	0.9 (0.5,1.7)	
Fish				
Never[a]	18 (41.9)	25 (58.1)	1	0.336
Once/week	43 (29.9)	101 (70.1)	0.6 (0.3,1.2)	
> 1 per week	52 (33.6)	103 (66.4)	0.7 (0.3,1.4)	
Meals				
once/twice[a]	15 (36.6)	26 (63.4)	1	0.608
Thrice	98 (32.6)	203 (67.4)	0.8 (0.4,1.7)	
Survival				
Both alive[a]	105 (32.5)	218 (67.5)	1	0.388
One parent	8 (42.1)	11 (57.9)	1.5 (0.6,3.9)	
HH size (members)				
1–3[a]	19 (55.9)	15 (44.1)	1	0.021
4–6	44 (31.9)	94 (68.1)	0.4 (0.2,0.8)	
6 or more	50 (31.9)	107 (68.1)	0.4 (0.2,0.8)	
Income				
10 k–149 k[a]	31 (44.3)	39 (55.7)	1	0.136
150 k–299 k	35 (31.0)	78 (69.0)	0.6 (0.3,1.1)	
300 k–599 k	40 (30.8)	90 (69.2)	0.6 (0.3,1.0)	
600 k +	7 (24.1)	22 (75.9)	0.4 (0.1,1.1)	
Maternal parity				
1–4[a]	89 (37.9)	146 (62.1)	1	0.005
5 +	24 (22.4)	83 (77.6)	0.5 (0.3,0.8)	
Maternal age				
16–23[a]	34 (42.0)	47 (58.0)	1	0.040
24–29	39 (37.9)	64 (62.1)	0.8 (0.5,1.5)	
30–33	17 (24.3)	53 (75.7)	0.4 (0.2,0.9)	
34–58	23 (26.1)	65 (73.9)	0.5 (0.3,0.9)	
Underweight (Weight for age Z scores)				
No[a]	97 (32.2)	203 (67.7)	1	0.014
Yes	16 (55.2)	13 (44.8)	2.6 (1.2,5.6)	
Stunting (Height for age Z scores)				
No[a]	87 (31.1)	193 (68.9)	1	0.003
Yes	26 (53.1)	23 (46.9)	2.5 (1.3,4.7)	
Wasting (Weight for Height Z scores)				
No[a]	105 (36.6)	182 (63.4)	1	0.670
Yes	4 (30.8)	9 (69.2)	0.8 (0.2,2.6)	
Mother's Highest Level of education				
No formal education[a]	12 (32.4)	25 (67.6)	1	0.576
Primary	70 (36.7)	121 (63.4)	1.2 (0.6,2.6)	
Secondary and above	31 (30.7)	70 (69.3)	0.9 (0.4,2.1)	
Father's Highest Level of education				
No formal education[a]	4 (33.3)	8 (66.7)	1	0.926
Primary	39 (33.0)	79 (67.0)	1.0 (0.3,3.5)	
Secondary and above	70 (35.2)	129 (64.8)	1.1 (0.3,3.7)	
Presence of worms				
Yes[a]	1 (12.5)	7 (87.5)	1	0.193
No	179 (65.3)	95 (34.7)	0.27 (0.03,2.24)	

Note:[a] (Reference group)

reported in similar studies conducted in East Africa [13, 17]. The prevalence of anaemia was 37.2 and 30.8% among children 1–5 and 6–14 years respectively, suggesting unmet nutritional supplements among males and young children with increased activity and growth demands, respectively. Most of the children had mild anaemia 65 (19.8%), while 48 (14.6%) had moderate anaemia. There was no case of severe anaemia in this study, which was expected especially that this was a community and not hospital based study. The 37.2% anaemia prevalence among children 1–5 years is lower than previous findings elsewhere in Uganda [16], possibly because of differences in the settings and malaria seasonality. We found lower prevalence of malaria (14.2%), compared to 60.6 and 47.5% reported by Green et al. [16] among children living along shores of Lake Albert and in the Islands of Lake Victoria where prevalence of anaemia was 68.9 and 27.3% respectively. In the same report, the prevalence of Schistosomiasis was 45.9 and 40.7% respectively [16], confirming that malaria, helminthiasis and the co-infections thereof, are key risk factors for anaemia, possibly by virtue of haemolysis, nutrient depletion, bone marrow suppression or chronic disease, or various combinations of underlying mechanisms. Nevertheless, a higher

Table 5 Multivariate analysis of factors associated with anaemia

Variables	Have anaemia		Unadjusted Odd ratio (95% CI)	*P*-value	Adjusted Odd ratio (95% CI)	*P*-value
	Yes	No				
Sex						
Female[a]	48 (31.0)	107 (69.0)	1	0.224		
Male	65 (37.4)	109 (62.6)	1.3 (0.8,2.1)			
Age group						
1–5[a]	68 (37.2)	128 (62.8)	1	0.156		
6–11	43 (33.3)	86 (66.7)	0.9 (0.6,1.5)			
12–14	2 (11.8)	15 (88.2)	0.3 (0.1,1,1)			
Malaria						
Negative[a]	93 (32.8)	191 (67.2)	1	0.190		
Positive	20 (42.6)	27 (57.4)	1.5 (0.8,2.9)			
HH size (members)						
1–3[a]	19 (55.9)	15 (44.1)	1	0.021		
4–6	44 (31.9)	94 (68.1)	0.4 (0.2,0.8)			
6 or more	50 (31.9)	107 (68.1)	0.4 (0.2,0.8)			
Income						
10 k–149 k[a]	31 (44.3)	39 (55.7)	1	0.136		
150 k–299 k	35 (31.0)	78 (69.0)	0.6 (0.3,1.1)			
300 k–599 k	40 (30.8)	90 (69.2)	0.6 (0.3,1.0)			
600 k +	7 (24.1)	22 (75.9)	0.4 (0.1,1.1)			
Maternal parity						
1–4[a]	89 (37.9)	146 (62.1)	1	0.005	1	0.002
5 +	24 (22.4)	83 (77.6)	0.5 (0.3,0.8)		0.4 (0.3,0.7)	
Maternal age						
16–23[a]	34 (42.0)	47 (58.0)	1	0.040	1	0.321
24–29	39 (37.9)	64 (62.1)	0.8 (0.5,1.5)		1.0 (0.9,1.0)	
30–33	17 (24.3)	53 (75.7)	0.4 (0.2,0.9)			
34–58	23 (26.1)	65 (73.9)	0.5 (0.3,0.9)			
Underweight (Weight for age Z scores)						
No[a]	97 (32.2)	203 (67.7)	1	0.014	1	0.352
Yes	16 (55.2)	13 (44.8)	2.6 (1.2,5.6)		1.6 (0.6,4.2)	
Stunting (Height for age Z scores)						
No[a]	87 (31.1)	193 (68.9)	1	0.003	1	0.004
Yes	26 (53.1)	23 (46.9)	2.5 (1.3,4.7)		2.5 (1.3,4.7)	
Presence of worms						
No[a]	179 (65.3)	95 (34.7)	1	0.193	1	0.167
Yes	1 (12.5)	7 (87.5)	0.27(0.03,2.24)		0.22 (0.26,1.88)	

Note:[a] (Reference group)

prevalence of anaemia than in our study was previously reported among school children (age 6–14 years) in two Ugandan studies [3, 4]. The discrepancy may be attributed to the difference in the study settings where by the latter were carried out in rural areas and the timing of these studies in which ours was conducted at the time when there was increased use of insecticide-treated bed nets and regular use of antihelminthes.

Malaria has been shown to cause anaemia in several studies [17, 21–24]. In our study, the prevalence of malaria is 14.2% lower than reported by Marcelline et al., [17] among Rwandan children aged 1–15 years. Our study also revealed that children who had malaria were 1.5 times more likely to have anaemia compared to those who tested negative (OR = 1.5, 95% CI = 0.8, 2.9). However, this association was not statistically significant (*P = .19)* in the multivariate analysis possibly due to the low prevalence of malaria.

Helminthiasis has been shown to significantly contribute to the problem of anaemia [17, 25–27]. In our study, we did not find statistical relationship between helminthes infections and anaemia (*P = .17)* possibly due to the extremely low prevalence. Generally, Uganda has recorded tremendous progress in eliminating neglected tropical diseases over the past decade. The prevalence of Schistosomiasis declined from 42.4 to 17.9% in 2005, while hookworm prevalence reduced from 50.9 to 10.7% during the same period [28]. Other helminthes infections that showed decline were Ascariasis and Trichuriasis from 2.8 and 2.2% in 2003, to very undetectable levels in 2005 [28]. Therefore, the very low prevalence of helminthiasis in our study is not surprising.

Similarly, HIV infection in our study was very low (0.3%) and insignificant to assess the relationship with anaemia. Elsewhere, HIV infection has been associated with risk of anaemia. In two studies conducted in Uganda, the prevalence of anaemia among HIV infected children ranged from 85 to 91.7% and HIV was independently associated with anaemia [29, 30]. However, another study in Uganda found no significant difference in the prevalence of anaemia among HIV infected and uninfected children [31]. There have been pronounced improvements in the HIV care and these have reduced new HIV infections tremendously, particularly mother-to-child transmissions. The current HIV prevalence among children aged 5 years and below is less than 1% [32] and with the current strategy of EMTCT, this is likely to shrink further in the coming years.

In our study, older children (6–11 and 12–14 years) were less likely to be anaemic than younger children (1–5 years) [(OR = 0.3, 95% CI =0.1, 1.1), *P = .16*]. This finding is consistent with the previous reports that anaemia is common among children around the time of the growth spurt [33, 34]. During this period, children's physical development is rapid, and the blood volume is largely expanded, whereas the iron storage from the maternal source has usually been depleted; diet becomes a vital source for iron as a result [35]. In a more recent community pilot survey conducted in Arua district (same study area) hemoglobin <11.0 g/dl was observed in nearly half of the children less than 16 years enrolled (unpublished data).

Anaemia was also found to be more common among male children compared to females, though, not significant [(OR = 1.3, 95% CI = 0.8, 2.4), *P = .22*]. This result is comparable with one reported by Ngesa and Mwambi [13], where the risk of anaemia was 1.2 times higher among boys than girls. The higher prevalence of anaemia in males is related to the higher growth rate in boys, resulting in greater need for iron by the body, not supplied by the diet [36].

In our study, higher maternal parity (≥5 child births) was negatively associated with anaemia (*P = .002)* contrary to the finding by Cardoso et al., [37]. Elsewhere, early motherhood has also been shown to increase the risk of anaemia in the offspring [38]. The risk of anaemia in children of teenage mothers suggests that they are less prepared to meet the nutritional needs of their children and to perform the duties of motherhood. It is interesting to report that the risk of anaemia decreased with increasing household size (*P = .02*) contrary to the previous report [39]. We therefore concluded that this finding was a factor of household income rather than actual household size. In addition to the household size, we observed that the risk of anaemia declined with increasing household income. This finding is consistent with the previous reports that high socioeconomic status is associated with better nutrition, education and life [40].

The association between mother's education level and the care provided for children has been greatly discussed in the literature, given that education has a relationship with the capacity to grasp the knowledge needed for adequate healthcare and nutrition for children, just as it provides a chance to enter the labor market and probably better socioeconomic conditions [39, 41, 42]. The results from the current study reflect this relationship, though, not significant in the bivariate analysis (*P = .58).* The findings of this study indicate that promoting maternal health and providing mothers with anaemia - related information may help with controlling anaemia incidence. Children with a single parent surviving were 1.5 times more likely to be anaemic compared to those with both parents though this association was not statistically significant (*P = .39).* This result is consistent with that of a study carried out in India [43].

Stunting, a proxy for chronic under-nutrition, was significantly associated with anaemia (*P – .004).* This finding is consistent with reports elsewhere [44, 45]. Children who were stunted had 2.5 times risk of anaemia (95% CI = 1.3, 4.7). Therefore, stunting which is a consequence of malnutrition is a significant risk factor for anaemia. In our study, prevalence of underweight, stunting and wasting among children aged 1–5 years were 10.7, 16.3 and 5.1% respectively. Among children aged 6–14 years, underweight was 6.2%, stunting 12.3% and wasting 2.6%. By WHO classification [46] of public health importance of prevalence of malnutrition, our findings can be described as acceptable.

We acknowledge that resources limited the scope of this study to one geographical region, and, thus recommend similar studies in other geographical regions to confirm our findings about the changing context of nutrition, hygiene, and maternal wealth. Limited laboratory resources precluded examination of factors like hemoglobinopathies or lead intoxication, however, these factors are likely to be more important for a hospital-based study of children with severe anemia than a community-based study.

Conclusions

Our study demonstrates that anaemia is more prevalent in under - 5 year old children. Factors independently associated with the risk of anaemia included child stunting and low maternal parity. The lower prevalence of malaria and helminthiasis in this study population suggest increased protection from the risk of anaemia in the community. Further studies are required to investigate the association between maternal parity and anaemia found in this study.

Acknowledgements

We are very grateful to the Arua municipal authorities for granting us the permission to carry out this study in their area. Special thanks to the office of town clerk, municipal health officer and senior medical officer, Oli HC IV for the cooperation shown. We wish to thank the management of Kuluva hospital for the laboratory equipment, reagents and other support rendered to us during this study. We also thank the data collectors, children and their parents/caregivers who participated in this research.

Funding

This study was locally supported by the management of Kuluva hospital, Arua.

Authors' contributions

This work was collaboratively carried out. Authors IDL, AA and BJB were involved in the conception, design, data collection, analysis and interpretation. Author IDL was involved in data collection and processing. Authors SR and IDL were involved in data analysis and interpretation, Author POO was involved in manuscript editing and interpretation of findings. All authors were involved in the manuscript preparation and approval of the final version submitted.

Competing interests

The authors declare that they have no competing interests.

Author details

[1]School of Postgraduate Studies, Uganda Christian University, Mukono, Uganda. [2]Kuluva Hospital, Arua, Uganda. [3]School of Public Health, Makerere College of Health Sciences, Kampala, Uganda. [4]Faculty of Health Sciences, Busitema University, Mbale, Uganda. [5]Faculty of Science and Education, Busitema University, Tororo, Uganda.

References

1. Kassebaum NJ, Jasrasaria R, Naghavi M, Wulf SK, Johns N, Lozano R, et al. A systematic analysis of global anemia burden from 1990 to 2010. Blood. 2014;123(5):615–24.
2. WHO. The global prevalence of anemia in 2011. Geneva: World Health Organization; 2015.
3. Turyashemererwa FM, Kikafunda J, Annan R, Tumuhimbise GA. Dietary patterns, anthropometric status, prevalence and risk factors for anaemia among school children aged 5–11 years in Central Uganda; 2013. doi:10.1111/jhn.12069.
4. Barugahara EI, Kikafunda J, Gakenia WM. Prevalence and risk factors of nutritional anaemia among female school children in Masindi District, Western Uganda. Afr J Food Agric Nutr Dev. 2013;13(3):7679–92.
5. Phiri KS, et al. Long term outcome of severe anaemia in Malawian children. PLoS One. 2008;3(8):e2903.
6. Sachdev HPS, Gera T, Nestel P. Effect of iron supplementation on physical growth in children: systematic review of randomised controlled trials. Public Health Nutr. 2006;9(07):904–20.
7. Oppenheimer SJ. Iron and its relation to immunity and infectious disease. J Nutr. 2001;131(2):616S–35S.
8. Grein J. The cognitive effects of iron deficiency in non-anemic children. Nutr Noteworthy. 2001;4(1):1556–1895.
9. Halterman JS, Kaczorowski JM, Aligne CA, Auinger P, Szilagyi PG. Iron deficiency and cognitive achievement among school-aged children and adolescents in the United States. Pediatrics. 2001;107(6):1381–6.
10. Santos JN, Rates SPM, Lemos SMA, Lamounier JA. Consequences of anemia on language development of children from a public day care center. Revista Paulista de Pediatria. 2009;27(1):67–73.
11. Bobonis GJ, Miguel E, Puri-Sharma C. Anemia and school participation. J Hum Resour. 2006;41(4):692–721.
12. Menon MP, Yoon SS. Prevalence and factors associated with anemia among children under 5 years of age—Uganda, 2009. Am J Trop Med Hyg. 2015; 93(3):521–6.
13. Ngesa O, Mwambi H. Prevalence and risk factors of anaemia among children aged between 6 months and 14 years in Kenya. PLoS One. 2014;9(11):e113756.
14. English M, et al. Blood transfusion for severe anaemia in children in a Kenyan hospital. Lancet. 2002;359(9305):494–5.
15. Marsh K, et al. Indicators of life-threatening malaria in African children. N Engl J Med. 1995;332(21):1399–404.
16. Green HK, Jose C, Sousa F, Basáñez MG, Betson M, Kabatereine NB, et al. Anaemia in Ugandan preschool-aged children: the relative contribution of intestinal parasites and malaria. Parasitology. 2011;138:1534–45.
17. Marcelline, U., Umulisa, N., Munyaneza, T., Karema, C., Maniga, J., and Barugahare, J. B.. The impact of malaria and Gastointestinal Helminthiasis co-infection on Aneamia and severe malaria among children in Bugesera District, Rwanda. Inter J Trop Dis Health. 2015;13(4):1–7, 2016, Article no. IJTDH.23241 *DOI:* 10.9734/IJTDH/2016/23241.
18. Lugada ES, Mermin J, Kaharuza F, Ulvestad E, Were W, Langeland N, et al. Population-based hematologic and immunologic reference values for a healthy Ugandan population. Clin Diagn Lab Immunol. 2004;11(1):29–34.
19. Ministry of Water and Environment. Water and environment sector performance report 2015. Uganda: Kampala; 2016.
20. WHO. Bench aids for the diagnosis of intestinal parasites. Geneva: World Health Organization; 1994.
21. McElroy PD, ter Kuile FO, Lal AA, Bloland PB, Hawley WA, Oloo AJ, et al. Effect of plasmodium falciparum parasitemia density on hemoglobin concentrations among full-term, normal birth weight children in western Kenya, IV. The Asembo Bay cohort project. Am J Trop Med Hyg. 2000;62(4):504–12.
22. Hotez PJ, Molyneux DH, Fenwick A, Ottesen E, Sachs SE, Sachs JD. Incorporating a rapid-impact package for neglected tropical diseases with programs for HIV/AIDS, tuberculosis, and malaria. PLoS Med. 2006;3(5):e102.
23. Tolentino K, Friedman JF. An update on anemia in less developed countries. Am J Trop Med Hyg. 2007;77(1):44–51.
24. De Mast Q, Syafruddin D, Keijmel S, Riekerink TO, Deky O, Asih PB, et al. Increased serum hepcidin and alterations in blood iron parameters associated with asymptomatic P. Falciparum and *P. vivax* malaria. Haematologica. 2010;95(7):1068–74.

25. Brooker S, Peshu N, Warn PA, Mosobo M, Guyatt HL, Marsh K, et al. The epidemiology of hookworm infection and its contribution to anaemia among pre-school children on the Kenyan coast. Trans R Soc Trop Med Hyg. 1999;93(3):240–6.
26. Hotez JP, Brooker S, Bethony MJ, Bottazzi ME, Louka A, Shuhua X. Hookworm infection. N Engl J Med. 2004;351:799–807. doi:10.1056/NEJMra032492.
27. Standley CJ, Adriko M, Alinaitwe M, Kazibwe F, Kabatereine NB, Stothard JR. Intestinal schistosomiasis and soil-transmitted helminthiasis in Ugandan schoolchildren: a rapid mapping assessment. Geospat Health. 2009;4(1):39–53.
28. Kabatereine NB, Brooker S, Koukounari A, Kazibwe F, Tukahebwa EM, Fleming FM, et al. Impact of a national helminth control programme on infection and morbidity in Ugandan schoolchildren. Bull World Health Organ. 2007;85(2):91–9.
29. Clark TD, Mimiro F, Ndugwa C. Risk factors and cumulative incidence of anaemia among human immunodeficiency virus-infected children in Uganda. Ann Trop Paediatr. 2002;22:11–7.
30. Munyagwa, M., 2007. Prevalence and factors associated with moderate to severe anaemia among HIV infected children admitted at Mulago hospital (doctoral dissertation, Makerere University).
31. Totin D, Ndugwa C, Mmiro F, Perry RT, Brooks J, Semba RD. Iron deficiency anemia is highly prevalent in HIV-infected and uninfected infants in Uganda. J Nutr. 2002;132(3):423–9.
32. MoH. The 2014 Uganda HIV and AIDS country progress report: Uganda AIDS commission, Ministry of Health, Kampala, Uganda; 2015. p. 8.
33. Ewusie JE, Ahiadeke C, Beyene J, Hamid JS. Prevalence of anemia among under-5 children in the Ghanaian population: estimates from the Ghana demographic and health survey. BMC Public Health. 2014;14(1):1. doi:10.1186/1471-2458-14-626.
34. Mesfin F, Berhane Y, Worku A. Anemia among Primary school children in eastern Ethiopia. PLoS One. 2015;10(4):e0123615.
35. Kotecha PV. Nutritional anemia in young children with focus on Asia and India. Indian J Community Med. 2011;36(1):8.
36. Spinelli MGN, Marchioni DML, Souza JMP, Souza SBD, Szarfarc SC. Risk factors for anemia among 6-to 12-month-old children in Brazil. Revista Panamericana de Salud Publica. 2005;17(2):84–91.
37. Cardoso MA, Scopel KK, Muniz PT, Villamor E, Ferreira MU. Underlying factors associated with anemia in Amazonian children: a population-based, cross-sectional study. PLoS One. 2012;7(5):e36341. doi:10.1371/journal.pone.0036341.
38. Najati N, Gojazadeh M. Maternal and neonatal complications in mothers aged under 18 years. Patient Prefer Adherence. 2010;4:219–22.
39. Ngnie-Teta I, Receveur O, Kuate-Defo B. Risk factors for moderate to severe anemia among children in Benin and Mali: insights from a multilevel analysis. Food Nutr Bull. 2007;28(1):76–89.
40. Al-Zain BF. Impact of socioeconomic conditions and parasitic infection on hemoglobin level among children in um-Unnasser Village, Gaza strip. Turkish J Med Sci. 2009;39(1):53–8.
41. Provan D. Mechanisms and management of iron deficiency anemia. Br J Haematol. 1999;105:19–26.
42. Kemmer TM, Bovill ME, Kongsomboon W, Hansch SJ, Geisler KL, Cheney C, et al. Iron deficiency is unacceptably high in refugee children from Burma. J Nutr. 2003;133(12):4143–9.
43. Senthamarai M, Shankar JARP, Majeed NA. Prevalence of anemia and malnutrition in children and adolescent in selected orphanages in rural areas of Salem district, Rural medicine Indian journal of rural health care; 2015. p. 91.
44. Magalhães RJS, Clements AC. Mapping the risk of anaemia in preschool-age children: the contribution of malnutrition, malaria, and helminth infections in West Africa. PLoS Med. 2011;8(6):e1000438.
45. Awasthi S, Das R, Verma T, Vir S. Anemia and under nutrition among preschool children in Uttar Pradesh, India. Indian Pediatr. 2003;40(10):985–90.
46. WHO. Physical status: the use and interpretation of anthropometry. Report of an expert WHO Committee. Technical report series no 854. Geneva: WHO; 1995.

Kinetics of Langerhans cell chimerism in the skin of dogs following 2 Gy TBI allogeneic hematopoietic stem cell transplantation

Sabrina Peters[1†], Christian Junghanss[1*†], Anne Knueppel[1], Hugo Murua Escobar[1], Catrin Roolf[1], Gudrun Knuebel[1], Anett Sekora[1], Iris Lindner[2], Ludwig Jonas[3], Mathias Freund[1] and Sandra Lange[1]

Abstract

Background: Langerhans cells (LC) are bone marrow-derived cells in the skin. The LC donor/recipient chimerism is assumed to influence the incidence and severity of graft-versus-host disease (GVHD) after hematopoietic stem cell transplantation (HSCT). In nonmyeloablative (NM) HSCT the appearance of acute GVHD is delayed when compared with myeloablative conditioning. Therefore, we examined the development of LC chimerism in a NM canine HSCT model.

Methods: 2 Gy conditioned dogs received bone marrow from dog leukocyte antigen identical littermates. Skin biopsies were obtained pre- and post-transplant. LC isolation was performed by immunomagnetic separation and chimerism analysis by PCR analyzing variable-number-of-tandem-repeat markers with subsequent capillary electrophoresis.

Results: All dogs engrafted. Compared to peripheral blood chimerism the development of LC chimerism was delayed (earliest at day +56). None of the dogs achieved complete donor LC chimerism, although two dogs manifested a 100 % donor chimerism in peripheral blood at days +91 and +77. Of interest, one dog remained LC chimeric despite loss of donor chimerism in the peripheral blood cells.

Conclusion: Our study indicates that LC donor chimerism correlates with chimerism development in the peripheral blood but occurs delayed following NM-HSCT.

Keywords: Langerhans cells, Dogs, Stem cell transplantation, Chimerism, Nonmyeloablative

Background

Haematopoietic stem cell transplantation (HSCT) is an essential option for therapeutic treatment of malignant haematopoietic diseases. Nonmyeloablative (NM) HSCT is characterized by reduced intensity and toxicity [1, 2] and is therefore a treatment option for patients with contraindications (e.g. old age) who are not eligible candidates for conventional myeloablative (M)-HSCT [3]. The success of NM-HSCT in donor engraftment is (yet) associated with acute graft-versus-host disease (GVHD) rates affecting up to 50 % of the patients causing post therapeutic morbidity, mortality and decrease in quality of life [1, 4]. Acute GVHD typically develops within the first 3 months after M-HSCT and mainly affects the skin, but also the liver and the gastrointestinal tract [5]. Following NM-HSCT the signs and symptoms of acute GVHD are usually delayed and arise beyond day +100 [6].

Langerhans cells (LC) are CD1a positive bone marrow-derived dendritic cells located in the epidermis and mucous membrane [7, 8]. They are characterised by the presence of cytoplasmatic Birbeck granules [9]. LC are able to deliver antigenic information of their environment to the draining lymph nodes for presentation to the T lymphocytes [10]. In addition, LC might play an important role in skin GVHD [11, 12].

* Correspondence: christian.junghanss@med.uni-rostock.de
†Equal contributors
[1]Department of Hematology, Oncology, Palliative Medicine, Division of Medicine, University of Rostock, Ernst-Heydemann-Str. 6, 18057 Rostock, Germany
Full list of author information is available at the end of the article

The origin of LC (donor or recipient) appears to be of importance in GVHD development [11, 13]. The engraftment kinetic of donor LC is influenced by the conditioning. In conventional M-HSCT the majority of LC are of donor origin as soon as day +40. After reduced intensity conditioning the engraftment of donor LC is delayed and full donor LC chimerism is not detected before day +100 [12]. However, data regarding LC kinetics after NM-HSCT are rare and the correlation between LC chimerism and development of GVHD remains to be investigated.

For preclinical studies, especially in the field of HSCT, the dog has proven as unique model organism for decades due to high transferability potential of the gained results to humans [2, 14]. Canines and humans show common similarities in physiology, metabolism and lifespan of blood cells [15]. The clinical application of NM-HSCT in humans is based on a meanwhile well-established canine NM-HSCT model using 2 Gy total body irradiation for conditioning [14].

Lowering the intensity of the conditioning appears to increase the incidence of graft rejection [16]. Therefore, the development of new NM-HSCT regimens, e.g. application of new immunosuppressive drugs, is required. Hence, our present study was initially designed to assess the impact of the new immunosuppressant everolimus in the canine NM-HSCT model. In general occurrence of GVHD in the canine matched-sibling NM-HSCT model is rare, and thus the herein used experimental setting is not suitable for methodical GVHD studies. However, the development of donor LC chimerism following NM-HSCT is an observed phenomenon providing an important issue in transplantation LC biology that can be adequately investigated with this model.

In this study we therefore described the kinetics of LC number and chimerism in a canine 2 Gy NM-HSCT model to give a first insight into the role of LC in NM-HSCT.

Methods

Laboratory animals

Experiments were approved by the regional review board of the state Mecklenburg-Vorpommern (State Institute for Agriculture, Food Safety and Fishery Mecklenburg-Vorpommern, Germany; AZ: 7221.3-1.2-039/06) under advice of the regional animal ethics committee (§15 committee). Litters of beagles were obtained from commercial kennels licensed by the German Department of Agriculture. All dogs were dewormed and immunized against rabies, parainfluenca, leptospirosis, distemper, hepatitis, and parvovirus. Dog leukocyte antigen (DLA)-identical donor/recipient sibling pairs were selected on the basis of matching for highly polymorphic DLA class I and class II microsatellite markers [17, 18].

Haematopoietic stem cell transplantation

Animals were treated according to a protocol evaluating everolimus as new immunosuppressant in a NM-HSCT setting [19]. Briefly, dogs were conditioned at day -1 with 2 Gy total body irradiation and received unmodified bone marrow from DLA-identical littermates at day 0. Marrow grafts contained a median of 3.7×10^8 (range 1.9–11.8×10^8) total nucleated cells/kg, 6.7×10^6 (2.6–18.2×10^6) CD34+ cells/kg and a median of 2.0×10^7 (range 0.9–7.9×10^7) $CD3^+$ cells/kg (Table 2). Immunosuppression consisted of cyclosporin A (15 mg/kg BID) from day -1 to +35 and everolimus (0.25 mg BID) from day 0 to +27.

Preparation of Langerhans cells

Tissue samples of the skin were obtained from the neck of 9 dogs before and after HSCT on days +28, +56 and +105 under general anaesthesia (punch biopsies, 2×50.5 mm^2). In long-term chimeras specimen of dermal tissue were also taken after day +105. Tissue samples were disinfected in povidone-iodine (Mundipharma, Limburg/Lahn, Germany), bleached with sodium thiosulfate (0.05 %, Sigma Aldrich, Hamburg, Germany) and washed in phosphate buffered saline (PBS, Biochrom AG, Berlin, Germany). The epidermis was separated from the dermis by digestion with dispase (2.24 U/ml, Roche, Mannheim, Germany) at 4 °C overnight and at 37 °C (water bath) for one additional hour. Subsequently the epidermis was incubated at 37 °C for 30 min in trypsin (0.25 %, Biochrom AG) with DNase (10 μl/ml, Roche) to obtain a single cell suspension.

Single cells were labelled with a monoclonal mouse anti-canine CD1a antibody (clone CA9.AG5; kindly provided by Dr. P.F. Moore, School of Veterinary Medicine, University of California). Afterwards cell suspension was incubated with a goat-anti-mouse MicroBead (Miltenyi Biotec, Bergisch Gladbach, Germany). The labelled LC were enriched by MiniMACS device using large cell columns (Miltenyi Biotec).

Blood preparation and chimerism analyses

Before and after HSCT peripheral blood of the recipients was taken weekly up to day +77 and in larger intervals thereafter for analyses of the donor/recipient haematopoietic chimerism. Granulocytes and peripheral blood mononuclear cell (PBMC) fractions were separated by standard Ficoll-Hypaque density gradient centrifugation (density 1.074 g/ml).

Genomic DNA of LC was isolated using *Genomic DNA from Tissue-Kit* (Macherey-Nagel, Düren, Germany). Genomic DNA of granulocytes and PBMC was isolated using *Nucleobond CB 100-Kit* (Macherey-Nagel). Subsequently, polymorphic tetranucleotide repeats were amplified by PCR using commercially fluorescein-labelled primers (BioTez Berlin-Buch GmbH, Berlin, Germany) according to standard protocols. PCR-products were analysed by capillary electrophoresis as described elsewhere [20].

Statistics

The Mann-Whitney *U*-Test was performed to compare LC cell counts between dogs that rejected the graft and long-term chimeras. Data of LC chimerism versus chimerism in the peripheral blood were analysed by the Wilcoxon test. Correlations between LC chimerism and chimerism in the peripheral blood compartments were evaluated using the Spearman's rank correlation coefficient. Probability of $p < 0.05$ was considered significant.

Results

Cell purity and yield

Punch biopsies of the skin from 9 dogs were obtained before and on days +28, +56 and +105 after NM-HSCT. Flow cytometric analyses of isolated LC revealed a purity of CDla positive cells of median 91 % (range 28–97 %) (Fig. 1). Absolute LC cell counts showing a median of 3.0×10^4 (range $0.8–13.5 \times 10^4$) per 100 mm^2 biopsy were obtained before HSCT. After transplantation a decrease in LC to a median of 1.5×10^4 (range $0.3–5.6 \times 10^4$) was detected at day +28. Normal counts of 3.0×10^4 could be reached at day +56 after HSCT (Table 1). Differences in LC counts between dogs that rejected the graft and long-term chimeras were not observed.

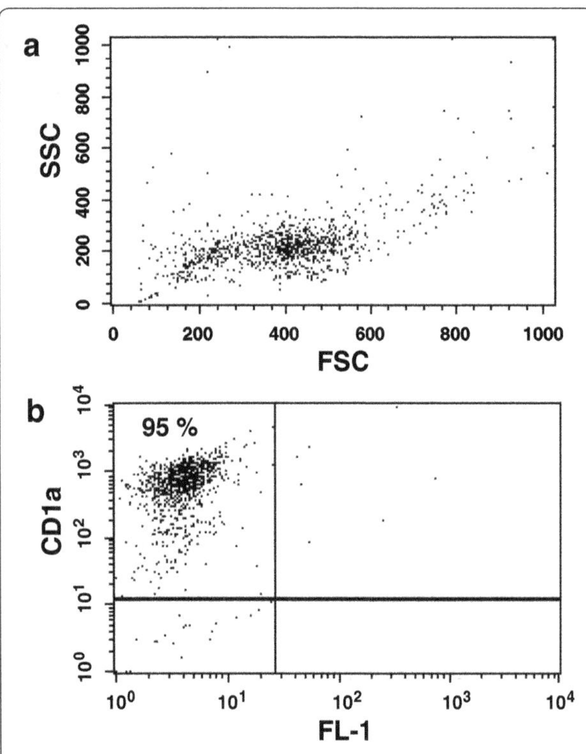

Fig. 1 Representative flow cytometric analysis of CD1a expressing epidermal canine Langerhans cells (LC). **a** Forward scatter (FSC) and side scatter (SSC) characteristics of canine LC. **b** FACS dot plot showing a purity of 95 % CD1a expressing LC after isolation with MiniMACS technology

To verify that the enriched CDla positive cells were true LC, electron microscopic identification of LC-characteristic Birbeck granules were performed (Fig. 2).

Chimerism

All dogs initially engrafted (Table 2). Three dogs (No. 1, 8, 9) rejected their grafts before day +100 (days +70, +70, +91). Dog no. 6 had a late rejection more than 1 year after HSCT (day +391). One animal (No. 2) died at day +60 due to an infection. At day +28 the donor chimerisms in the granulocyte and PBMC compartments were median 55 % (24–100 %) and 26 % (14–58 %) in all dogs, respectively. In none of the animals LC donor chimerism could be demonstrated at that time.

First LC donor chimerism was detected by day +56 in the dogs (No. 3, 4, 5, 7) that experienced a stable long-term chimerism in the granulocytes and PBMC compartments as well as in the dog that died. The median LC donor percentage of these five animals amounted to 6 % (2–42 %) at that time. Subsequently, a gradual increase in donor LC chimerism over the time was observed (exemplified by dog No.3 in Fig. 3a). The two dogs (No. 3, 4) that developed a full donor chimerism in the peripheral blood by days +77 and +91 also achieved the highest level of donor LC chimerism. Dog No. 4 showed the most rapid increase in donor LC percentage, and suffered as the only one from acute GVHD starting by day +70.

The dog (No. 6) that experienced late rejection showed first detectable LC chimerism not until day +112 although a donor chimerism in granulocytes and PBMC of 58 % and 40 % was already present at day +56. Interestingly, despite a subsequent decline in donor chimerism in the peripheral blood to 0 %, a constantly increasing LC donor chimerism up to 36 % (day +469) was observed (Fig. 3b). In contrast, in the dogs that rejected their grafts before day +100 LC of donor type could not be detected during the complete observation period.

In summary, donor LC chimerism was significantly lower than donor chimerism in the PBMC or granulocytes compartments (day +56: $p = 0.011$ each). Furthermore, there was a strong correlation between the PBMC donor chimerism and the donor chimerism in LC (day +56: $r = 0.7$, $p = 0.038$). Dogs that showed PBMC donor chimerism < 11 % at day +56 experienced early graft rejection and had no donor-derived LC at any time point. However, PBMC donor chimerism of 20–40 % at day +56 resulted subsequently in increasing LC donor chimerism despite decreasing PBMC chimerism. Only PBMC donor chimerism ≥ 50 % at day +56 correlated to high-level long-term engraftment in the peripheral blood and in the LC.

Table 1 Langerhans cell counts and purity following isolation and enrichment

	before HSCT		d +28		d +56		d +104-112		d +140-280		d > +280	
	cells [x10^4][a]	purity [%][b]	cells [x10^4]	purity [%]	cells [x10^4]	purity [%]	cells [x10^4]	purity [%]	cells [x10^4]	purity [%]	cells [x10^4]	purity [%]
No. 1	2.3	69.4	1.5	81.2	0.8	82.2	0.4	80.5	n.d.	n.d.	n.d.	n.d.
No. 2[c]	1.9	93.2	0.8	79.2	3.8	87.5	c		c		c	
No. 3	2.0	41.5	0.3	69.0	1.5	68.6	1.9	68.2	4.1	84.1	6.4	92.7
No. 4	0.8	82.4	1.5	73.2	1.1	71.9	4.3	78.4	7.1	88.7	10.5	94.3
No. 5	13.5	92.0	5.6	89.8	11.6	92.7	9.7	96.7	n.d.	n.d.	9.0	94.2
No. 6	3.0	27.7	2.0	34.0	3.0	66.8	1.5	67.0	1.1	86.7	6.4	93.2
No. 7	4.5	96.7	3.4	72.9	7.2	87.5	0.3	78.1	4.5	93.3	4.1	92.2
No. 8	5.3	97.3	0.8	79.1	5.3	90.9	6.0	87.5	8.6	92.1	1.9	87.2
No. 9	4.1	91.2	1.9	87.2	2.6	93.5	3.4	89.2	6.0	90.0	n.d.	n.d.
Median	3.0	91.2	1.5	79.1	3.0	87.5	2.7	79.5	5.3	89.4	6.4	93.0

[a]cell counts per 100 mm^2; [b]purity = % of CD1a + cells; [c]died day +60; n.d. not determined

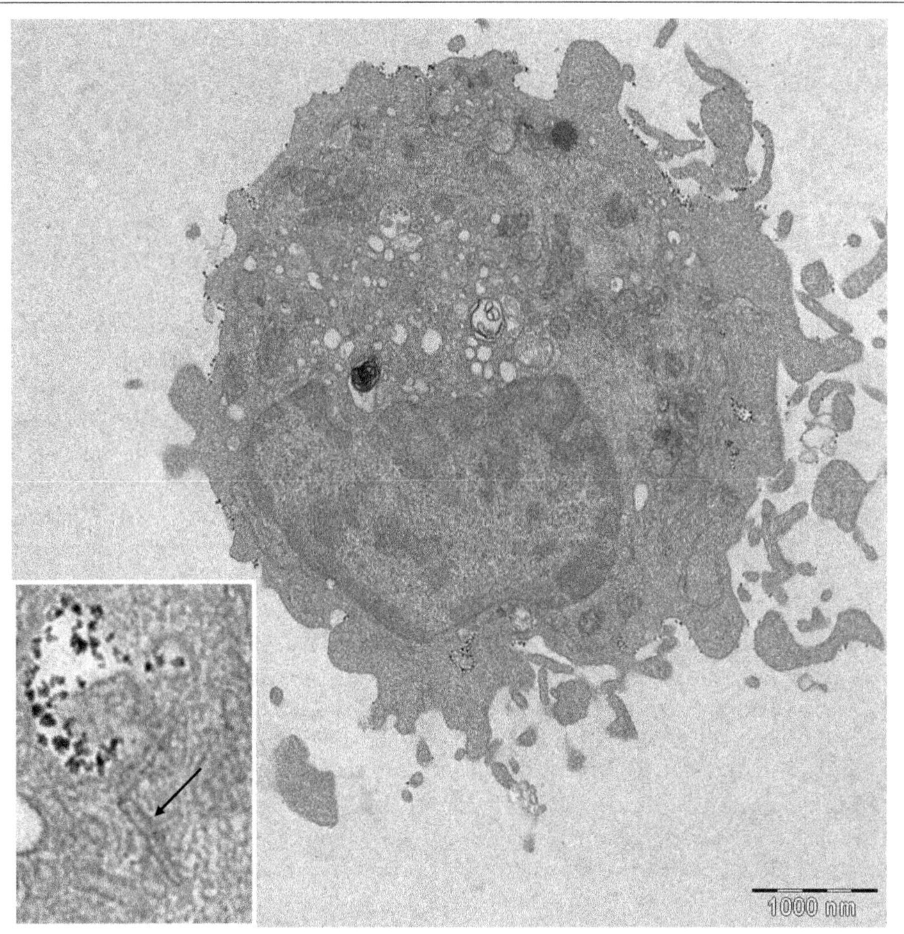

Fig. 2 Electron microscopic image of a Langerhans cell. The figure insert shows a characteristic Birbeck granule (*black arrow*)

Table 2 Graft composition and donor percentages of mononuclear cells of the peripheral blood (PBMC) and Langerhans cells (LC) after transplantation

Dog	Graft composition			Donor chimerism [%]										
				d +28		d +56		d +104-112		d +140-280		d > +280		rejection
	TNC [x10^8]	CD34 [x10^6]	CD3 [x10^7]	PBMC	LC	PBMC	LC	PBMC	LC	PBMC	LC	PBMC	LC	(day)
No. 1	2.7	4.0	0.9	26.3	0.0	7.7	0.0	0.0	0.0	n.d.	n.d.	n.d.	n.d.	+70
No. 2	6.4	13.7	3.7	41.0	0.0	36.4	1.9	[b]		[b]		[b]		died d + 60
No. 3	3.7	8.2	2.0	31.0	0.0	67.4	6.3	100.0	16.5	100.0	55.4	100.0	88.6	no
No. 4	1.9	3.6	1.8	17.8	0.0	64.1	41.9	100.0	88.5	100.0	90.0	100.0	95.6	no
No. 5	11.8	10.3	7.9	31.7	2.0[a]	49.7	16.3	63.9	13.9	n.d.	n.d.	80.1	81.4	no
No. 6	6.2	18.2	3.4	58.1	0.0	39.9	0.0	41.1	12.1	7.7	17.0	0.0	35.9	+391
No. 7	7.6	6.7	3.5	25.9	0.0	21.1	2.3	92.3	3.8	25.4	6.2	17.5	22.7	no
No. 8	2.2	2.6	1.1	14.7	7.2[a]	3.1	7.2	5.0	5.1	0.0	7.9	0.0	5.0	+70
No. 9	3.1	3.0	1.8	14.0	0.0	10.5	0.0	0.0	0.0	0.0	0.0	n.d.	n.d.	+91
Median	3.7	6.7	2.0	26.3	0.0	36.4	2.3	52.5	8.6	16.6	12.5	48.8	58.7	

n.d. not determined

[a]LC chimerism test results for these dogs were already 3 % (No. 5) and 7 % (No. 8) before transplantation despite repeated testing. Therefore, d + 28 chimerism might be considered as not present

[b]died day +60

Discussion

The aim of this study was to characterize the development of LC donor chimerism in the skin after NM-HSCT. For this purpose skin biopsies were taken from 9 transplanted dogs before and at different times after NM-HSCT.

Studies describing the kinetic of LC chimerism after myeloablative or reduced-intensity conditioning were conducted previously [12, 13], but data analysing LC chimerism following NM-HSCT still remain rare.

The herein gained results showed a moderate reduction of LC counts following NM-conditioning. The cell number decreased from day 0 to +28 by half (1.5 × 10^4/100 mm^2) and recovered to the initial value at day +56. In myeloablative regimens a LC nadir of 0.2 × 10^4/100 mm^2 during the first month was observed and the LC count increased to its normal level within 4-12 months after HSCT [21, 22]. These results demonstrated a considerably lower decrease and a faster recovery of LC numbers after NM-HSCT when compared to the kinetics seen in myeloablative regimens.

The donor LC chimerism following NM-HSCT increased slowly. In none of the examined dogs donor LC were detectable until day +56. Even at day +105 the present LC were mainly of host origin and the development of LC chimerism was not finished within 1 year after HSCT. In contrast, data from myeloablative studies certainly had shown a rapid replacement of host LC by donor derived LC as early as day +56 after HSCT [13]. The retardation in donor LC engraftment in our NM-HSCT study was even more pronounced than the delay previously reported after reduced-intensity conditioning, where by day +100 the majority of LC were donor in origin [12]. Previous studies demonstrated that the recruitment of circulating LC precursors does not only depend on proinflammatory chemokines as CCL20, but also on available LC sites in the epidermis [11, 23]. We assume that the availability of LC sites in the epidermis was reduced due to a less efficient depletion of host LC by NM-conditioning. Therefore, the recruitment of donor LC precursor could be hampered, beeing the reason for a delayed donor LC engraftment after NM-HSCT compared to myeloablative regimens.

In addition, a small fraction of LC is able to perform in situ proliferation [23–25]. This self-reproducing capacity may explain why the reduction of LC number by half was not followed by a 50 % LC donor chimerism after reaching initial cell counts in our study.

We also analysed the development of donor chimerism in LC comparatively to the ratio seen in granulocytes and PBMC. The significantly delayed donor LC engraftment in our dogs is in accordance with the reduced LC chimerism compared to DC chimerism in peripheral blood or the bone marrow as described in a current NM-HSCT study [26]. Dog No. 6 which experienced late graft rejection even displayed a continuous increase of LC donor chimerism, whereas chimerism in peripheral blood was not detectable any longer. This observation is potentially caused by the ability of LC to proliferate in the epidermis [23–25]. Furthermore, dogs showing a 100 % donor chimerism in granulocytes and PBMC also reached the highest LC donor chimerism. Correlation analysis confirmed a strong relationship between LC and PBMC chimerism in our study. In contrast, in previous publications no correlation between dendritic cell chimerism in the blood and in the skin has been described [11, 12].

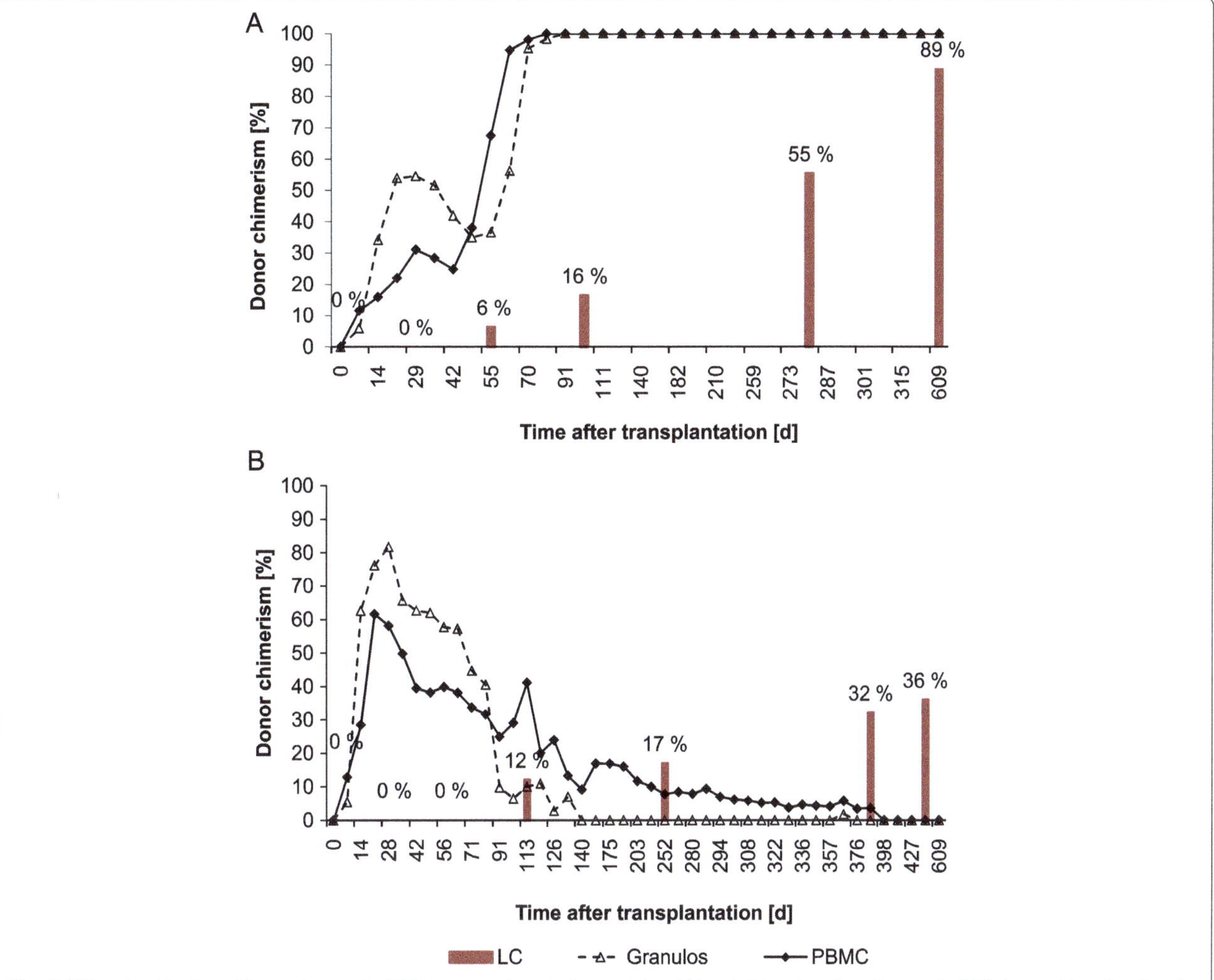

Fig. 3 Chimerism kinetics of Langerhans cells (LC) in comparison to the peripheral blood chimerism. Development of LC donor chimerism (bars) compared with donor chimerism of PBMC (solid line) and granulocytes (dotted line) after 2 Gy nonmyeloablative HSCT in two dogs. **a** Dog No. 3 with full donor chimerism in peripheral blood. Continuously increasing LC donor chimerism starting at day +56 after HSCT at a time when the dog experienced strong engraftment in the peripheral blood. Donor chimerism of LC developed delayed compared to donor chimerism in the peripheral blood and did not achieve the peripheral blood levels during the observation period **b** Dog No 6 with initial engraftment and subsequent late graft rejection. Despite high initial donor chimerism levels in the peripheral blood of 82 % (granulocytes d +28) and 62 % (PBMC d +21) first LC donor chimerism was not detected before day +112 probably as a consequence of decreasing peripheral blood chimerism levels starting 4 weeks after HSCT. Interestingly, although donor chimerism values of the peripheral blood continuously declined and the graft was eventually rejected at day +391 a continuously increasing LC donor chimerism was observed also beyond the date of graft rejection

One dog in this study suffered from acute GVHD after transplantation. The GVHD occurred at day +70 and the dog rapidly developed a high LC donor chimerism until day +105. Whether the earlier onset of donor LC chimerism has triggered GVHD, or whether the development of acute GVHD may have facilitated the rapid replacement of host LC with donor derived LC cannot be concluded from this single case.

Conclusions

Our study indicates that LC chimerism kinetics are delayed following NM-HSCT compared to chimerism development in the peripheral blood. Highest donor LC engraftment rates were observed in dogs with full donor peripheral blood chimerism and the LC chimerism correlates with the chimerism in PBMC. The kinetic of LC chimerism after NM-HSCT seems to be delayed in comparison to published data on the development of LC chimerism after myeloablative and reduced-intensity conditioning as well. Recipient LC are present in the skin even 1 year after NM-HSCT. Whether this difference in the kinetic of LC chimerism might be responsible for the delayed onset of acute skin GVHD following NM-HSCT remains to be investigated in future studies.

Competing interests

The authors declare that they have no competing interests.

Authors' contributions

CJ, MF, SL have made substantial contributions to conception and design of the study. SP, SL, AK, GK, AS, IL, and LJ have been involved in acquisition, analyses and interpretation of data. SP, CJ, HME, CR, and SL have been involved in drafting the manuscript as well as revising it critically for important intellectual content. All authors read and approved the final manuscript.

Acknowledgement

The authors thank the technicians of the shared animal facility for their excellent and dedicated care of the animals. This work was supported by the German Research Council (Deutsche Forschungsgemeinschaft) grants JU 417/2-2 and SFB Transregio 37, SP A2.

Author details

[1]Department of Hematology, Oncology, Palliative Medicine, Division of Medicine, University of Rostock, Ernst-Heydemann-Str. 6, 18057 Rostock, Germany. [2]Institute of Legal Medicine, Division of Medicine, University of Rostock, St.-Georg-Str. 108, 18055 Rostock, Germany. [3]Electron Microscopic Centre, Division of Medicine, University of Rostock, Strempelstr. 14, 18057 Rostock, Germany.

References

1. Slavin S, Nagler A, Naparstek E, Kapelushnik Y, Aker M, Cividalli G, et al. Nonmyeloablative stem cell transplantation and cell therapy as an alternative to conventional bone marrow transplantation with lethal cytoreduction for the treatment of malignant and nonmalignant hematologic diseases. Blood. 1998;91:756–63.
2. McSweeney PA, Niederwieser D, Shizuru JA, Sandmaier BM, Molina AJ, Maloney DG, et al. Hematopoietic cell transplantation in older patients with hematologic malignancies: replacing high-dose cytotoxic therapy with graft-versus-tumor effects. Blood. 2001;97:3390–400.
3. Diaconescu R, Storb R. Allogeneic hematopoietic cell transplantation: from experimental biology to clinical care. J Cancer Res Clin Oncol. 2005;131:1–13.
4. Khouri IF, Keating M, Körbling M, Przepiorka D, Anderlini P, O'Brien S, et al. Transplant-lite: induction of graft-versus-malignancy using fludarabine-based nonablative chemotherapy and allogeneic blood progenitor-cell transplantation as treatment for lymphoid malignancies. J Clin Oncol. 1998; 16:2817–24.
5. Sung AD, Chao NJ. Concise review: acute graft-versus-host disease: immunobiology, prevention, and treatment. Stem Cells Transl Med. 2013;2:25–32.
6. Mielcarek M, Martin PJ, Leisenring W, Flowers ME, Maloney DG, Sandmaier BM, et al. Graft-versus-host disease after nonmyeloablative versus conventional hematopoietic stem cell transplantation. Blood. 2003;102:756–62.
7. Banchereau J, Briere F, Caux C, Davoust J, Lebecque S, Liu YJ, et al. Immunobiology of dendritic cells. Annu Rev Immunol. 2000;18:767–811.
8. Stingl G, Tamaki K, Katz SI. Origin and function of epidermal Langerhans cells. Immunol Rev. 1980;53:149–74.
9. Romani N, Clausen BE, Stoitzner P. Langerhans cells and more: langerin-expressing dendritic cell subsets in the skin. Immunol Rev. 2010;234:120–41.
10. Romani N, Brunner PM, Stingl G. Changing views of the role of Langerhans cells. J Invest Dermatol. 2012;132:872–81.
11. Merad M, Hoffmann P, Ranheim E, Slaymaker S, Manz MG, Lira SA, et al. Depletion of host Langerhans cells before transplantation of donor alloreactive T cells prevents skin graft-versus-host disease. Nat Med. 2004;10:510–17.
12. Collin MP, Hart DNJ, Jackson GH, Cook G, Cavet J, Mackinnon S, et al. The fate of human Langerhans cells in hematopoietic stem cell transplantation. J Exp Med. 2006;203:27–33.
13. Auffermann-Gretzinger S, Eger L, Bornhäuser M, Schäkel K, Oelschlaegel U, Schaich M, et al. Fast appearance of donor dendritic cells in human skin: dynamics of skin and blood dendritic cells after allogeneic hematopoietic cell transplantation. Transplantation. 2006;81:866–73.
14. Storb R, Yu C, Wagner JL, Deeg HJ, Nash RA, Kiem HP, et al. Stable mixed hematopoietic chimerism in DLA-identical littermate dogs given sublethal total body irradiation before and pharmacological immunosuppression after marrow transplantation. Blood. 1997;89:3048–54.
15. Mack GS. Cancer researchers usher in dog days of medicine. Nat Med. 2005; 11:1018.
16. Baron F, Sandmaier BM. Chimerism and outcomes after allogeneic hematopoietic cell transplantation following nonmyeloablative conditioning. Leukemia. 2006;20: 1690–700.
17. Burnett RC, Francisco LV, DeRose SA, Storb R, Ostrander EA. Identification and characterization of a highly polymorphic microsatellite marker within the canine MHC Class I region. Mamm Genome. 1995;6:684–85.
18. Wagner JL, Burnett RC, DeRose SA, Francisco LV, Storb R, Ostrander EA. Histocompatibility testing of dog families with highly microsatellite markers. Transplantation. 1996;62:876–77.
19. Junghanss C, Rathsack S, Wacke R, Weirich V, Vogel H, Drewelow B, et al. Everolimus in combination with cyclosporin a as pre- and posttransplantation immunosuppressive therapy in nonmyeloablative allogeneic hematopoietic stem cell transplantation. Biol Blood Marrow Transplant. 2012;18:1061–68.
20. Hilgendorf I, Weirich V, Zeng L, Koppitz E, Wegener R, Freund, et al. Canine haematopoietic chimerism analyses by semiquantitative fluorescence detection of variable number of tandem repeat polymorphism. Vet Res Commun. 2005;29:103–10.
21. Volc-Platzer B, Rappersberger K, Mosberger I, Hinterberger W, Emminger-Schmidmeier W, Radaszkiewicz T, et al. Sequential immunohistologic analysis of the skin following allogeneic bone marrow transplantation. J Invest Dermatol. 1988;91:162–68.
22. Perreault C, Pelletier M, Landry D, Gyger M. Study of Langerhans cells after allogeneic bone marrow transplantation. Blood. 1984;63:807–11.
23. Merad M, Manz MG, Karsunky H, Wagers A, Peters W, Charo I, et al. Langerhans cells renew in the skin throughout life under steady-state conditions. Nat Immunol. 2002;3:1135–41.
24. Kanitakis J, Morelon E, Petruzzo P, Badet L, Dubernard J-M. Self-renewal capacity of human epidermal Langerhans cells: observations made on a composite tissue allograft. Exp Dermatol. 2011;20:145–6.
25. Czernielewski JM, Demarchez M. Further evidence for the self-reproducing capacity of Langerhans cells in human skin. J Invest Dermatol. 1987;88:17–20.
26. Mielcarek M, Kirkorian AY, Hackman RC, Price J, Storer BE, Wood BL, et al. Langerhans cell homeostasis and turnover after nonmyeloablative and myeloablative allogeneic hematopoietic cell transplantation. Transplantation. 2014;98:563–8.

11

Effect of anti-tuberculosis drugs on hematological profiles of tuberculosis patients attending at University of Gondar Hospital, Northwest Ethiopia

Eyuel Kassa[1], Bamlaku Enawgaw[1], Aschalew Gelaw[2] and Baye Gelaw[2*]

Abstract

Background: Tuberculosis (TB) treatment may present significant hematological disorder and some anti-TB drugs also have serious side effects. Although many other diseases may be reflected by the blood and its constituents, the abnormalities of red cells, white cells, platelets, and clotting factors are considered to be primary hematologic disorder as a result of tuberculosis treatment. The aim of this study was to determine hematological profiles of TB patients before and after intensive phase treatment.

Objective: The aim of this study was to determine hematological profiles of TB patients before and after intensive phase treatment.

Methods: Smear positive new TB patients were recruited successively and socio-demographic characteristics were collected using pre-tested questionnaire. About 5 ml of venous blood was collected from each patient and the hematological profiles were determined using Mindry BC 3000 plus automated hematology analyzer.

Result: The hematological profiles of TB patients showed statistically significant difference in hematocrit (38.5 % versus 35.7 %), hemoglobin (12.7 g/lversus11.8 g/l) and platelet (268×10^3/μlversus239×10^3/μl) values of patients before initiation of treatment and after completion of the intensive phase of tuberculosis treatment, respectively ($P < 0.05$). The red cell distribution width (RDW) of treatment naïve TB patients was by far lower (17.6 ± 7.09 %) than the corresponding RDW (31.9 ± 5.19 %) of intensive phase treatment completed patients. Among TB patients that had high platelet distribution width (PDW) ($n = 11$) before initiation of TB treatment, 10 demonstrated lower PDW values after completion of the intensive phase. There was no significant difference on total white blood cell count among TB patients before and after completion of the 2 month treatment.

Conclusion: The levels of hemoglobin, hematocrit and platelet count of the TB patients were significantly lowered after completion of the intensive phase of TB treatment. Significant variation of the RDW and PDW were also observed among treatment naïve and treatment completed patients. Hematological abnormalities resulted from TB treatment should be assessed continuously throughout the course of tuberculosis therapy.

Keywords: Tuberculosis, Haematological profile, Intensive phase, Anti-TB drugs

* Correspondence: tedybayegelaw@gmail.com
[2]Department of Medical Microbiology, School of Biomedical and Laboratory Sciences, College of Medicine and Health Sciences, University of Gondar, Gondar, Ethiopia
Full list of author information is available at the end of the article

Background

Tuberculosis (TB) is a contagious disease that can affect almost any tissue and organs of the human body but mainly cause infection of the lungs [1]. Tuberculosis is a major public health problem throughout the world. About a third of the world's population is estimated to be infected with tubercle bacilli and hence at risk of developing active TB disease. The burden of TB is highest in Africa, Asia, India and China together accounting for almost 40 % of the world's TB cases [2]. About 2.4 million new TB cases and 540,000 TB-related deaths occur in sub-Saharan Africa annually [3]. Ethiopia is among the countries most heavily affected by TB [4]. The annual TB incidence of Ethiopia is estimated to be 341/100,000. Tuberculosis mortality rate is 73/100,000 and the prevalence of all forms of TB is estimated to be 546/100,000 [5].

TB is a curable disease although drug resistance is one of the major challenges in the treatment, prevention and control of the disease. However, the use of anti-TB drugs is not free from side effects. Allergic reactions, fever, rash, vasculitis, nausea, vomiting, hepatotoxicity, hepatocellular inflammation, peripheral neuropathy and others are some of the common side effects associated with TB treatment [6]. In addition, a wide range of hematological abnormalities has been reported as a result of administration of anti-TB drugs. The major hematological disorder due to anti-TB drug is aplastic anemia. Aplastic anemia is a hypo- regenerative bone marrow disorder characterized by a reduction in the amount of haemopoitic bone marrow and pancytopenia. It has been reported that pancytopenia due to aplastic anemia of moderate severity was observed in a patient while receiving anti-tuberculosis therapy, probably caused by an idiosyncratic reaction to streptomycin. Although the total leukocyte and platelet counts could be depressed after cessations of drugs, physicians rarely suspect anti-tuberculosis induced hematological complications which may have fatal consequences [7].

Hematological disorders arise through a variety of mechanisms and etiologies. Drug-induced hematological disorders can span almost the entire spectrum of hematology, affecting red cells, white cells, platelets, and the coagulation system. The wide spectrum of drug-induced hematologic syndromes is mediated by a variety of mechanisms, including immune effects, interactions with enzymatic pathways, and direct inhibition of hematopoiesis. Drug-induced syndromes include hemolytic anemia, red cell aplasia, sideroblastic anemia, megaloblastic anemia, polycythemia, aplastic anemia, leukocytosis and others. There are four possible relationships of tuberculosis to hematologic disease. These are the hematologic disease predisposes to tuberculosis reactivation. Drugs may cause idiosyncratic reactions, malabsorption, interference with iron metabolism, and hemolysis in patients with red blood cell enzyme deficiencies. Idiosyncratic reactions manifested by depression of any or all of the three cellular blood elements (white cells, red cells and platelets) together with the coagulation system may be caused by any of the anti-tuberculosis drugs [8, 9].

The magnitude of drug induced hematological abnormalities had been investigated in different parts of the world. For example, leucopenia as a result of rifampicin and isoniazid therapy was reported in Japan [10]. Anti-TB drug induced normocytic normochromic anemia was the most common abnormality observed in Malaysia [11] and a 74 % prevalence of anemia together with 26 % Leukocytosis, 24 % Thrombocytosis was reported in India [12]. In a study conducted in South Africa, a 15 % leucopenia, 23 % thrombocytopenia and 87 % lymphopenia was reported as a result of anti-TB drug treatment [13]. By another study conducted in Nigeria, anti-TB drug induced hematological abnormality were reported 93.6, 22.3, 45.2 and 4.8 % for anemia, leukocytosis, neutrophilia, and lymphopaenia, respectively [14]. Moreover, in Tanzania an 86 % anti-TB drug induced anemia was reported [15].

Different reports showed that altered hematopoiesis occurs in TB patients. Hematological changes associated with tuberculosis treatments have been investigated in many parts of the world. However, to the best of our knowledge, there is no comprehensive study assessed the hematological abnormalities among TB patients in Ethiopia in general and in Gondar in particular. Hence, this study was designed to determine the effect of anti-TB drugs on hematological profile among TB patients. In the present study, hematological findings amongTB patients before initiation and after completion of the intensive phase of tuberculosis treatment were assessed.

Methods

Study design, area and setting

A longitudinal prospective study was conducted from February to June 2014 at the University of Gondar (UoG) hospital, Northwest Ethiopia. The hospital is found in Gondar town. Gondar town is located in the North Gondar Zone of the Amhara Region, North of Lake Tana, Northwestern Ethiopia, and 748 km far from Addis Ababa. The town has a latitude and longitude of 12°36′N 37°28′E with an elevation of 2133 m above sea level. Based on figures from the Central Statistical Agency in 2008, Gondar has an estimated total population of 231,977. University of Gondar hospital is a referral hospital for Northwestern Ethiopia with more than 400 beds serving a population of about 5 million. The Hospital is one of the biggest tertiary level referral and teaching hospitals in the region. A large number of people from the surrounding zones and nearby regions visit the hospital both for inpatient and as an outpatient treatment.

Populations

The source population was all TB suspected patients (both pulmonary and extra pulmonary) attending for health service at the University of Gondar Hospital. The study population were smear positive pulmonary tuberculosis patients and all confirmed extra-pulmonary TB patients who took all the intensive phase of treatment at the Directly Observed Treatment Short course (DOTS) clinic of University of Gondar hospital during the study period. In this study, TB patient less than 5 years of age and greater than 65 years of age, retreatment cases, patient with known organ impairment, malignant cases (cancer and chronic patients) and HIV patients were excluded from the study.

Sample size determination and sampling technique

Time delimited consecutive sampling technique was employed to recruit the study subjects. All newly diagnosed TB patients who were confirmed for tuberculosis infection and seeking for anti-TB treatment at the University of Gondar Teaching Hospital DOTS clinic during the study period were included. By using the inclusion and exclusion criteria's set for the study, a total of 168 new TB patients were recruited and involved in this study.

Socio-demographic data

Socio-demographic characteristics such as age, sex, marital status, residence and clinical information such as WHO clinical stage, use of myelo-suppressive drugs, loss of appetite, weight loss, night sweats and fever were gathered using pre-tested and structured questionnaire. A trained clinical nurse and laboratory technologist working at the DOTS clinic of the University of Gondar hospital collected the socio-demographic characteristics of the TB patients.

Sputum sample collection and microscopy

Sputum samples were collected using dry, clean, leak proof, translucent and screw-capped plastic containers with a capacity of 30 ml. Smears were prepared and air dried then stained with Ziehl-Neelsen (ZN) stain. Briefly, smears were genteelly heat fixed and each smear was flooded with carbolfuchsin solution. On each preparation, heat was applied until steaming and allowed to stand for 5 min. After washing with tap water, smear was decolorized with acid alcohol for 1 min and washed with tap water and counter stained with methylene blue for 30 s, washed and air dried. Slides were examined under 100× oil immersion objective with bright field illumination. Microscopy results were recorded following the WHO reporting methods as negative, actual number of acid-fast bacilli (AFB), 1+, 2+ and 3 + .

Blood sample collection and determination of hematological parameters

About 5 ml of venous blood was collected aseptically by using EDTA tube from each of the selected study subjects. following collection, the EDTA tube was labeled with code number. The blood sample was collected from each study subject before initiation of anti-TB drugs and after completion of the 2 month intensive phase treatment. Hematologic profiles such as Red blood cell count, hemoglobin level, hematocrit (HCT), Red blood cell indices such as mean corpuscular volume (MCV), mean corpuscular haemoglobin (MCH), mean corpuscular haemoglobin concentration (MCHC), Red cell distribution width (RDW), total white blood cell count (WBC), WBC differential count, Platelet count, Mean Platelet Volume (MPV) and platelet cell distribution width (PDW) were determined using Mindray automated hematology analyzer following the manufacturers instruction and the Standard Operational Procedures (SOP) of the University of Gondar hospital laboratory.

Quality control

The reliability of the study findings were guaranteed by implementing quality control (QC) measures throughout the whole process of the laboratory work. All materials, equipment and procedures were adequately controlled. Blood samples were collected free of hemolysis, clot, with sufficient quantity (5 ml) and correctly labeled with patients identification number. The performance of the hematology analyzer was check by running normal, low and high blood controls. During a condition where flags were found with automation hematological parameters, manual differential count was performed. Sputum samples with an AFB score of 1+ ($n = 10$) was used to assess the reliability of microscopic examinations. These samples were stained by Ziehl-Neelsen stain and examined by two laboratory technologists blinded from each other. The coefficient of variation (CV) was found 0.016 which shows that the result of the two laboratory technologists was 99.984 % consistent. The questionnaire was prepared in English, translated to local Amharic language and then translated back to English to check for consistency. Data on Socio-demographic and TB related medical history were collected by trained nurses under the supervision of the investigators.

Data analysis

Data were checked, sorted, categorized and coded manually then transferred to SPSS version 20 statistical packages for analysis. Frequencies and cross tabulations were used to summarize descriptive statistics. Paired t test was used in the analysis to compare the hematologic values before initiation and after completion of the intensive phase of tuberculosis treatment. A P values less than 0.05 were considered statistically significant.

Ethical consideration

Ethical approval was obtained from an ethical review committee organized by the School of Biomedical and Laboratory Sciences which was mandated by the College of Medicine and health Sciences, University of Gondar. A permission and support letter was also obtained from University of Gondar hospital and both verbal and written consent was obtained from each participant. All the consent procedures were approved by the ethical approval committee of the School of Biomedical and Laboratory Sciences. In the case of children, both verbal and written consent were taken from the guardian that was also approved by the ethical review committee. The purpose and importance of the study was explained to each study participants. To ensure confidentiality of participants information, anonymous typing was applied where by the name of the participant and any identifier of participants were not written on the questionnaire, and during the interview to keep the privacy, they were interviewed alone. The laboratory findings of each study participant were communicated with the responsible clinician assigned at TB clinic. Above all the data was collected after full written consent was obtained from each study participates.

Results

Characteristics of the study participants

A total of 168 HIV negative new TB patients were included in this study. Ninety six (56.5 %) of the TB patients were males and the other 73 (43.5 %) were females. The mean age of the study participants was 34.8 ± 15.3 years ranging from 5 to 65 years. Sixty-two (36.9 %) TB patient were within the age group 5–25, 62 (36.9 %) within the age group 26–44 and the other 44 (26.2 %) within 45–65 years of age. Forty-seven percent ($n = 79$) were urban dwellers and the other 53 % ($n = 89$) were living in rural areas. The clinical and laboratory data of the TB patients showed that 87 (51.8 %) and 81 (48.2 %) were pulmonary and extra pulmonary cases.

Association between hematological parameters with the age and sex of the TB patients before and after completion of the intensive phase treatment

Tuberculosis confirmed patients were investigated to assess their hematological profile prior initiation of anti-TB treatment and after completion of the intensive phase treatment. The hematological profiles assessed were red blood cell count, hemoglobin concentration, hematocrit, red cell indices, total white blood cell count, white blood cell differential count, red blood cell distribution width, platelet distribution width, platelet count and mixed cells (eosinophile, monocyte and basophile) count. Analysis of the demographic characteristics of the TB patients such as age and sex versus hematological parameters demonstrated that there was significant difference on Hgb and Hct concentrations ($P < 0.001$) before initiation and after completitions of the intensive phase treatment. In addition, a significant difference on RBC among patients with the age group 45–65 years was observed ($P = 0.030$). The RDW-CV parameter of female patients and the PLT count of male patients were also significantly different ($P = 0.002$ and 0.031 respectively) (Table 1). However, there was no significant difference in WBC parameters and PDW versus the age and sex of the TB patients.

Assessment of anemia

The magnitude of anemia among TB patients before initiation and after completion of the intensive phase of treatment was assessed using red blood cell count (RBC), hemoglobin (Hgb) and hematocrit (Hct) values. The average RBC of the TB patients before initiation of anti-TB treatment was relatively similar to that of RBC after completion of the intensive phase of tuberculosis treatment ($4.25 \times 10^3 \pm 0.83$ versus $4.42 \times 10^3 \pm 0.824$, respectively) (Table 2). Many of the TB patients that had normal RBC before initiation of tuberculosis treatment ($n = 72$) demonstrated also normal RBC after completion of the intensive phase ($n = 69$) of treatment. However, 54 % of the TB patients had lower RBC before initiation and after completion of the intensive phase of treatment. Nevertheless, data showed no statistically significant difference on the RBC of TB patients before initiation and after completion of the intensive phase of tuberculosis treatment. The average Hgb concentration of the TB patients before initiation of tuberculosis treatment was slightly higher (12.7 ± 2.09 g/dl) than the corresponding Hgb concentration determined after completion of the intensive phase of treatment (11.8 ± 1.68 g/dl). Similarly, the average packed cell volume (Hct) was also relatively higher before initiation of treatment (38.5 ± 2.42 %) than the corresponding concentration after completion of the 2 month treatment (35.7 ± 2.31 %). In this study, 55 % of the TB patients ($n = 92$) had low Hgb concentration and the Hct values of 86 TB patients (51 %) was found low before initiation of anti-tuberculosis treatment. The proportion of TB patients with low Hgb and Hct concentration was by far increased (72 %) after completion of the intensive phase of TB treatment. Among the TB patients that had higher Hct concentration ($n = 13$) before initiation of anti-TB treatment, only 4 resulted similarly higher concentration. On the other hand, among 69 and 76 patients that had normal Hct and Hgb concentration

Table 1 Hematological parameters that demonstrated significant difference based on the age and sex of TB patients before initiation of anti-TB drugs compared with after completion of the intensive phase of treatment

			Before treatment	After treatment	*P*-value
RBC × 10^6/ µl	Sex	Male	4.27 ± 0.92	4.43 ± 0.92	0.235
		Female	4.24 ± 0.72	4.42 ± 0.68	0.143
	Age	5 – 25	4.26 ± 0.77	4.42 ± 0.89	0.320
		26 – 44	4.37 ± 0.75	4.33 ± 0.68	0.747
		45 – 65	4.09 ± 1.01	4.58 ± 0.92	0.030*
Hgb (g/dl)	Sex	Male	12.7 ± 2.1	11.8 ± 1.5	0.000*
		Female	12.8 ± 2.1	11.8 ± 1.9	0.000*
	Age	5 – 25	12.9 ± 2	11.8 ± 1.8	0.000*
		26 – 44	12.9 ± 1.8	12 ± 1.4	0.001*
		45 – 65	12.4 ± 2.5	11.5 ± 1.8	0.000*
HCT (%)	Sex	Male	38.6 ± 6	35.8 ± 4.4	0.000*
		Female	38.9 ± 5.5	35.7 ± 5.4	0.000*
	Age	5 – 25	39.1 ± 5.7	35.7 ± 5.5	0.000*
		26 – 44	38.9 ± 4.9	36.6 ± 4	0.001*
		45 – 65	37.9 ± 6.8	34.7 ± 5	0.000*
MCV (fl)	Sex	Male	88.4 ± 6.9	89.4 ± 9.1	0.036*
		Female	89.4 ± 6.7	90.9 ± 5.1	0.143
	Age	5 – 25	89.4 ± 7.3	90.2 ± 5.1	0.486
		26 – 44	88.3 ± 5.8	91.2 ± 5.8	0.013*
		45 – 65	88.7 ± 7.6	90.4 ± 5.2	0.241
MCH (pg)	Sex	Male	28.9 ± 3.3	29.6 ± 2.3	0.143
		Female	29.2 ± 2.6	30.1 ± 2	0.040*
	Age	5 – 25	29.3 ± 3	29.7 ± 2.1	0.427
		26 – 44	29.1 ± 3.1	29.7 ± 2.5	0.253
		45 – 65	28.5 ± 3	30 ± 2	0.012*
MCHC (%)	Sex	Male	32.7 ± 2	32.7 ± 1.3	0.878
		Female	32.6 ± 1.4	33.1 ± 1.1	0.049*
	Age	5 – 25	32.6 ± 1.6	32.9 ± 1.3	0.357
		26 – 44	33 ± 1.9	32.7 ± 1.3	0.390
		45 – 65	32.2 ± 1.6	33.1 ± 1	0.003*
RDW CV (%)	Sex	Male	14.4 ± 1.4	14.2 ± 1.2	0.311
		Female	14.5 ± 1.7	13.9 ± 1.2	0.02*
	Age	5 – 25	14.4 ± 1.4	14.1 ± 1.3	0.143
		26 – 44	14.3 ± 1.4	14.1 ± 1.2	0.477
		45 – 65	14.6 ± 1.8	14 ± 1.1	0.059
PLT × 10^3/µl	Sex	Male	267 ± 106	232 ± 109	0.031*
		Female	270 ± 101	250 ± 86	0.169
	Age	5 – 25	258 ± 105	250 ± 116	0.697
		26 – 44	274 ± 101	246 ± 72	0.085
		45 – 65	275 ± 105	216 ± 108	0.006*

* = significant association

Table 2 Hematological profiles of tuberculosis patients before and after initiation of anti-TB treatment at University of Gondar Teaching hospital, 2014

Variable	Before treatmentof TB Mean (SD)	After treatmentof TB Mean (SD)	P-Value
RBC/µl	4.25×10^6 (0.83)	4.42×10^6 (0.824)	0.072
WBC/ µl	7.5×10^3 (3.76)	7.08×10^3 (3.27)	0.224
Hgb (g/dl)	12.7 (2.09)	11.8 (1.68)	0.000*
HCT (%)	38.5 (2.42)	35.7 (2.31)	0.000*
MCV (fl)	88.8 (6.8)	89.7 (8.4)	0.268
MCH (Pg)	30.13 (5.0)	29.03 (3.0)	0.018*
MCHC (g/dl)	30.13 (2.91)	29.43 (7.1)	0.000*
RDW-CV	17.6 (7.09)	31.9 (5.19)	0.000*
PLT/ µl	268×10^3 (103.2)	239.93 (99.8)	0.01*
PDW	17.01 (4.79)	15.7 (0.61)	0.001*
Lymphocyte	1.96×10^3 (0.94)	2.08×10^3 (1.36)	0.375
Mixed cell	0.74×10^3 (0.422)	0.69×10^3 (0.425)	0.272
Neutrophil	4.37×10^3 (2.42)	4.08×10^3 (2.31)	0.230

RBC red blood cell, *WBC* White blood cell, *HCT* Haematocrit, *HGB* Haemoglobin, *MCV* mean corpuscular volume, *MCH* mean haemoglobin, *MCHC* mean haemoglobin concentration, *RDW-CV* red cell distribution width, *PLT* platelet, *PDW* Platelet distribution width, *fl* femto litter (10^{-15}L), *pg* pico-gram (10^{-12}g), * significant association

before initiation of anti-TB treatment, only 42 and 47 demonstrated normal concentrations respectively after completion of the intensive phase treatment (Table 3). Moreover, data showed a significant decreased level of Hgb concentration and Hct value after completion of the 2 month tuberculosis treatment compared to the pre-treatment level ($P = 0.00$).

Leukocytosis versus leukopenia

The average total WBC of TB patients before treatment ($7.5 \times 10^3 \pm 3.76$) was slightly lower than the corresponding average WBC after completion of the 2 month treatment ($7.08 \times 10^3 \pm 3.27$). The total WBC of 24 TB patients (14.3 %) enumerated before initiation of TB treatment was low but that of 115 (68.5 %) and 29 (17.3) patients were normal and high, respectively. The proportion of tuberculosis patients with low WBC was slightly raised 18.5 % ($n = 31$) when examined after completion of the intensive phase of treatment. However, there was no statistically significant difference on total WBC among TB patients before initiation and after completion of the 2 month tuberculosis treatment. The lymphocyte, neutrophil and mixed cell (eosinophil, monocyte and basophil) differential WBC count of the TB patients showed no statistically significant difference among TB patients before and after initiation of tuberculosis treatment. However, the proportion of TB patients with high neutrophil count was raised from 7.7 % ($n = 13$) of treatment naïve phase to 14.3 % ($n = 24$) after completion of the 2 month tuberculosis treatment.

Association of tuberculosis treatment with platelet count

The mean thrombocyte count among TB patients before administration of anti-TB drugs was $268 \times 10^3 \pm 103.2$. The corresponding platelet counts among TB patients after completion of the 2 month treatment was slightly lower ($239 \times 10^3 \pm 99.8$). However, data showed no statistically significant difference on platelet count among TB patients before initiation and after completion of the intensive phase tuberculosis treatment. The proportion of TB patients with low platelet count was slightly increased after completion of tuberculosis treatment ($n = 25$; 14.9 %) compared to the corresponding platelet count among tuberculosis treatment naïve patients ($n = 22$; 13.1 %). On the other hand, significantly reduced proportion of TB patients with high platelet count was observed (8.9 %; $n = 15$) after completion of the intensive phase of TB treatment compared to the proportion of TB patients with high platelet count (19.6 %; $n = 33$) among treatment naïve TB patients. Moreover, data showed significant difference in the proportion of TB patients with both low and high platelet count after completion of the 2 month treatment compared with treatment naïve patients ($P = 0.01$).

Red blood cell indices during tuberculosis treatment

The average MCV of the TB patients before initiation of tuberculosis treatment and after completion of the 2 month treatment was nearly similar (88.8 ± 6.8 versus 89.7 ± 8.4, respectively). A slightly reduced MCH (29.03 ± 3.0) was observed after completion of the intensive phase tuberculosis treatment compared with the average MCH before initiation of treatment (30.13 ± 5.0).

Table 3 The proportion of TB patients with low, normal and high hematological profile before initiation and after completion of the intensive phase tuberculosis treatment at University of Gondar hospital, 2014

Parameters	Category	Before TB treatment	After TB treatment	Reference Intervals	*P*-Value
RBC	Low	91 (54.2)	92 (54.8)		0.92
	Normal	72 (42.9)	69 (41.1)	$M = 4.5\text{-}6.2 \times 10^6/\mu l$ $F = 4.0\text{-}5.5 \times 10^6/\mu l$	
	High	5 (3)	7 (4.2)		
WBC	Low	24 (14.3)	31 (18.5)		0.262
	Normal	115 (68.5)	113 (67.3)	$4.0 - 10.0 \times 10^3/\mu l$	
	High	29 (17.3)	24 (14.3)		
HCT	Low	86 (51.2)	122 (72.6)		0.000*
	Normal	69 (41.1)	42 (25.0)	M = 40 -52 % F =36 – 47 %	
	High	13 (7.7)	4 (2.4)		
HGB	Low	92 (54.8)	121 (72)		0.000*
	Normal	76 (45.2)	47 (28)	M = 13 – 18 g/dl F = 12–16 g/dl	
	High	0 (0)	0 (0)		
MCV	Low	13 (7.7)	10 (6)		0.589
	normal	129 (76.8)	130 (77.4)	80 – 100 fl	
	high	26 (15.5)	28 (16.7)		
MCH	low	37 (22)	18 (10.7)		0.000*
	Normal	96 (57.1)	105 (62.5)	27 – 32 pg	
	High	35 (20.8)	45 (26.8)		
MCHC	low	75 (44.6)	163 (98.2)		0.000*
	normal	90 (53.6)	3 (1.8)	31.5 – 36 g/dl	
RDW_CV	Normal	118 (70.2)	9 (5.4)	11.5 - 14.5 %	0.000*
	high	50 (29.8)	159 (94.6)		
PLT	low	22 (13.1)	25 (14.9)		0.01*
	normal	113 (67.3)	128 (76.2)	$150 - 450 \times 10^3/\mu l$	
	High	33 (19.6)	15 (8.9)		
PDW	Normal	157 (93.5)	167 (99.4)	10 -17 %	0.000*
	high	11 (6.5)	1 (0.6)		
Lymphocyte	low	4 (2.4)	6 (3.6)		1.000
	Normal	160 (95.2)	156 (92.9)	$1.5 - 4.5 \times 10^3/\mu l$	
	high	4 (2.4)	6 (3.6)		
Mixed cell	Normal	160 (95.2)	165 (98.2)	$0.26 - 1.3 \times 10^3/\mu l$	0.960
	high	8 (4.8)	3 (1.8)		
Neutrophil	Low	13 (7.7)	24 (14.3)		0.233
	Normal	136 (81)	124 (73.8)	$2.0 - 7.0 \times 10^3/\mu l$	
	High	19 (11.3)	20 (11.9)		

* = significant association. Hematological parameter values less than and greater than the reference intervals are categorized as low and high respectively

Similarly, the MCHC was also slightly reduced after completion of the 2 month treatment compared with before initiation of treatment (29.43 ± 7.1 versus 30.13 ± 2.91, respectively). The difference in MCH and MCHC among TB treatment naïve and TB patients completed the intensive phase was found statistically significant ($P \le 0.018$). In this study, 7.7 % ($n = 13$) of the TB patients had low MCV before initiation of anti-TB treatment. The proportion of TB patients with low MCV was slightly reduced (6 %; $n = 10$) after completion of the intensive phase treatment. The majority of the TB patients (57.1 %; $n = 96$) had normal MCH before initiation of treatment and the proportion of TB patients with normal MCH risen to 108 (62.5 %) after completion of the intensive phase treatment. Forty-five percent ($n = 75$) of the TB patients had low MCHC before initiation of treatment. The proportion of TB patients that had low MCHC was significantly raised (98.2 %; $n = 163$) after completion of the intensive phase treatment. The proportion of TB patients with normal MCHC before initiation of TB treatment was 53.6 % ($n = 90$). However, only 1.8 % ($n = 3$) of the TB patients that had normal MCHC before initiation of tuberculosis treatment had also normal MCHC after completion of the intensive phase treatment.

Red blood cell and Platelet distribution width during tuberculosis treatment

The mean red blood cell distribution width (RDW) among treatment naïve TB patients (17.6 ± 7.09 %) was by far lower than the corresponding RDW (31.9 ± 5.19 fl) of TB patients determined after completion of the intensive phase of treatment. This difference was also statistically significant ($P = 0.00$). Contrary to RDW, the mean platelet distribution width (PDW) among treatment naïve TB patients (17.01 ± 4.79 %) was higher than that of TB patients completed the intensive phase of treatment (15.7 ± 0.61 %). Moreover, data also showed statistically significant difference on PDW among treatment naïve TB patients compared with TB patients completed the intensive phase of treatment ($P = 0.00$) (Table 2).

In this study, 70.2 % ($n = 118$) of TB patients had normal RDW before initiation of anti-TB treatment. However, the proportion of TB patients that had normal RDW was by far reduced to 5.4 % ($n = 9$) after completion of the intensive phase treatment. On the other hand, the proportion of TB patients with high RDW which was 29.8 % ($n = 50$) was raised to 94.6 % ($n = 159$) after completion of the intensive phase of tuberculosis treatment. Moreover, data showed statistically significant difference on the proportion of TB patients with high/low RDW before initiation and after completion of the intensive phase of tuberculosis treatment ($P = 0.00$) (Table 3).

The proportion of TB patients that had normal PDW (93.5 %; $n = 157$) before initiation of treatment was relatively similar to the corresponding proportion of TB patients that had normal PDW (99.4 %; $n = 167$) after completion of the 2 month treatment. Eleven TB patients (6.5 %) had high PDW before initiation of tuberculosis treatment but only 1 patient showed high PDW after completion of the intensive phase of treatment and the difference was statistically significant ($P = 0.00$).

Discussion

Tuberculosis exerts incredible varieties of hematologic effects and hematologic abnormality is a common finding among TB patients. These abnormalities involves both cell lines and plasma components. Anti-tuberculosis therapy has its own spectrum of hematologic toxicity and blood cell abnormalities [16]. The current study compared the hematologic profile of HIV negative TB patients before initiation of treatment and after completion of the intensive phase of tuberculosis treatment.

In the current study, the average RBC of the TB patients before initiation of anti-TB treatment was relatively similar to that of RBC after completion of the intensive phase of tuberculosis treatment. The average RBC of the TB patients were $4.25 \times 10^6 \pm 0.83$ versus $4.42 \times 10^6 \pm 0.824$ before treatment and after completion of the intensive phase treatment, respectively, which is nearly similar to the lower limits of the reference values for male and female adults (4.7 and 4.2 million cells per microliter (cells/μL), respectively). Previously Tsegay et al. [17] reported reference range of erythrocyte counts, 5.1×10^{12}/l (males) and 4.5×10^{12}/l (females) for healthy adult Ethiopians.

The hemoglobin concentration and packed cell volume were slightly higher among treatment naïve TB patients compared with those received anti-TB treatment for 2 months. However, the proportion of TB patients with low hemoglobin and hematocrit concentration was significantly increased (72 %) after completion of the intensive phase of TB treatment. All chronic infections including TB can cause anemia [18]. Various pathogenesis have been suggested in TB-associated anemia, but most studies have been shown suppression of erythropoiesis by inflammatory mediators as a cause of anemia [19]. Nutritional deficiency and malabsorption syndrome can deepen the severity of anemia [20]. The possible mechanisms for the development of anemia during tuberculosis infection may be due to nutritional insufficiency, impaired iron utilization, mala-absorption, bone marrow granuloma and shortened duration of RBC survival [21]. Weiss [18], Means [22] and Nemeth et al. [23] explain the mechanism behind the occurrence of anemia in pulmonary tuberculosis patients saying that the invasion of bacteria leads to activation of T-lymphocyte and macrophages, which induce the production of the cytokines like interferon gamma (IFN-γ), tumor necrosis factor alpha (TNF-α), Interlukin-1 (IL-1) and interlukin-6 (IL-6) which with their products will cause diversion of iron into iron stores in the reticulo-endothelial system resulting in decreased iron concentrations in the plasma thus limiting its availability to red cells for hemoglobin synthesis, inhibition of erythroid progenitor cell proliferation and in appropriate production and activity of erythropoietin which may lead to anemia and suboptimal response of the bone marrow to anemia, respectively. The high proportion of TB patients with reduced hemoglobin and hematocrit concentration after completion of the intensive phase of tuberculosis treatment may suggest drug induced anemia among TB patients. Drugs can induce variety of hematological disorders affecting RBCs, WBCs and plateltes. Drug induced syndromes includes hemolytic anemia, methemoglobinemia, red cell aplasia, sideroblastic anemia, megaloblastic anemia, polycythemia and aplastic anemia [8].

The total WBC count of TB patients before initiation of anti-TB drugs was relatively similar to that of total WBC count after completion of the intensive phase of treatment. However, the proportion of TB patients with low total WBC count was raised from 14.3 % before initiation of treatment to 18.5 % after completion of the intensive phase treatment. On the other hand, the proportion of TB Patients with high neutrophil differential count was increased from 7.7 % before treatment to 14.3 % after completion of the intensive phase of treatment. Nevertheless, there was no leukocytosis neither before initiation of treatment nor after completion of the 2 month treatment. In a study designed to assess the hematological abnormalities of TB patients, Singh et al. [24] reported a 25 % leukopenia and a 22 % neutropenia among TB patients. Drug induced neutropenia was also reported in association with various analgesics, psychotropic's, anti-convulsions, anti-thyroid drugs, antihistaminics, anti-rheumatics, gastro-intestinal drugs, antimicrobials and cardiovascular drugs [25].

The result of the current study showed that platelet count was another important hematological profile that showed significant difference when the count before initiation of tuberculosis treatment was compared to that of platelet count after completion of the 2 month tuberculosis treatment ($P = 0.010$). Almost half of the TB patients that had high platelet count before treatment showed decreased platelet count after completion of the intensive phase. This finding is supported by a report from India and was suggested that decrease in platelet count could possibly be due to the effect of anti-TB drugs and immune destruction of platelets [26]. Classical causes of drug-induced thrombocytopenia are the quinine and quinine-like drugs [27]. The thrombocytopenia induced by these drugs is caused by antibody that is nonreactive in the absence of drug, but binds to epitopes on platelet membrane, glycoproteins IIb/IIIa or Ib/IX, when the sensitizing drug is present. Vancomycin can also be associated with marked thrombocytopenia and demonstrable drug-dependent antibodies in the serum [28]. Other drugs associated with thrombocytopenia include antimicrobials (sulfanomides, rifampin, linezolid), anti-inflammatory drugs, anti-neoplastics, anti-depressants, benzodiazepines, anti-convulsants (carbamazepine, phenytoin, valproic acid) as well as cardiac and anti-hypertensive drugs [29, 30].

In the current study, the MCV values before and after treatments were not significantly changed. However, the differences in the MCH and MCHC values were significantly different when the values were compared before and after completion of the intensive phase of TB treatment. Previous reports showed that the red cell indices in the untreated male pulmonary TB patients showed lower values as compared to normal males. In addition, it was also found that the MCH and MCHC among male pulmonary TB patients were significantly lower when compared with normal males [31, 32]. Different study reports showed that after anti-tuberculosis treatment with streptomycin, rifampicin and isoniazid, the RBC indices were affected and reached closer to normal values. Moreover, RBC morphology in pulmonary TB patients was found to be mainly normocytic normochromic type and during medication, the blood film showed normochromic pictures [31, 33, 34] which suggests the effects of tuberculosis treatment on the restoration of RBC morphology.

The mean RDW of TB patients determined after completion of the intensive phase of treatment (31.9 ± 5.19 %) was significantly different from the corresponding RDW of treatment naïve TB patients (17.6 ± 7.09 %). Opposite to the RDW, the PDW among treatment naïve TB patients (17.01 ± 4.79 %) was higher than the PDW of TB patients measured after completing the intensive phase of treatment (15.7 ± 0.61 %). Moreover, TB patients that had high PDW before treatment ($n = 10$) showed reduced PDW after completion of the 2 month anti-TB treatment. Red cell distribution width and PDW measure the variation of RBC and platelete volume. The normal reference range of RDW-CV in adult humans was reported 11.5 to 14.5 % [35] while that of PDW 9–16.56 % for men and 8–13.3 % for women [36]. Nowadays, RDW is used to diagnose anemia. Domingo et al. [37] reported greater decrease in hemoglobin concentration in patients with higher values for RDW. Red cell distribution width is often used to differentiate anemia of mixed causes from anemia of a single cause. There are reports that documented deficiency of vitamin B12, or folate produce macrocytic anemia (large cell anemia) in which the RDW is elevated in roughly two-thirds of all cases [38]. However, varied size distribution of RBC is the hallmark of iron deficiency anemia, and as such shows increased RDW in virtually all cases [39]. Long term exposure to anti-tuberculosis medication increases the risk of adverse drug reactions and toxicity. Isoniazid and rifampicin may directly cause hemolytic anemia, as can pyrazinamide cause sidroblastic anemia [40]. Others have suggested that anemia is seen as part of the clinical manifestation of tuberculosis and as a consequence of a chronic disease. In general, tuberculosis patients have a higher predisposition to develop gastro-intestinal absorption problems, consequently leading to anemia [20] and elevated RDW is associated with anemia. At a condition when there is microcytic RBCs produced prior to treatment and normocytic RBCs produced after completion of treatment in the circulation leads to high size variation (increase RDW value). Lee et al. [20] showed that anemia is a common hematological abnormality in patients and Baynes et al. [19] states that RDW values in chronic inflammatory disorder like tuberculosis similar with the RDW values occurring in iron-deficiency anemia which is in line with the current study.

Platelet distribution width directly measures the variability in platelet size and has been used to differentiate disorders of platelets such as essential thrombocythemia from reactive thrombocytosis [41]. In the present study, PDW of TB patients was significantly reduced after taking anti-TB drugs for 2 months. Previously, Tozkoparan et al. [42] reported that there were significantly higher PDW values (40 ± 23.5) among TB patients which decreased significantly with anti-tuberculosis therapy. Thrombocytopenia is a serious side effect that potentially caused by anti-TB drugs which occurs mostly due to rifampicin (RIF) [43]. The main mechanisms of thrombocytopenia are decreased production or increased destruction of platelets. The drug binds non-covalently to membrane glycol-proteins to produce compound epitopes or induce conformational changes which antibodies are specific. In addition, RIF-dependant antibodies attach to thrombocytes and cause increased destruction [44]. However, the exact mechanism of INH-induced thrombocythemia is not known.

The result of this study showed that the Hgb concentration, HCT, PLT and PDW values were reduced after completion of the intensive phase of tuberculosis treatment. This is due to the fact that iron is critical for *Mycobacterium tuberculosis* growth in macrophages in turn causes iron deficiency anemia. After the intensive phase treatment, there will be sufficient iron in the body and starts production of normal erythrocytes. This study finding is supported by Tozkoparan et al. [42] that indicates significantly lower PDW values with anti-tuberculosis therapy. Also another study by Sahin et al. [45] indicates that reactive thrombocytosis and PDW develop frequently in PTB and there is a relation with acute phase reactants, which is the inflammatory response and decreased after treatment.

Conclusion

The levels of hemoglobin, hematocrit and platelet count of the TB patients were significantly lowered after completion of the intensive phase of TB treatment compared with the corresponding values before initiation of anti-TB treatment. The RDW and PDW also showed significant variation before initiation and after completion of the 2 month tuberculosis treatment. The varied hematological abnormalities observed in TB patients after intensive phase tuberculosis therapy suggests the need for continuous monitoring and evaluation of TB patients for adverse hematological abnormalities during tuberculosis treatment. Anemia was found to be one of the most common hematological abnormalities among patients taking anti-tuberculosis treatment. Thus anemia and thrombocytopenia should be regularly checked during tuberculosis treatment.

Limitation of the study

The limitation of this study was the relatively small sample size which is the result of the nature of the study as longitudinal study are time consuming and costly. We were also unable to determine the effect of anti-TB drugs after completion of the 6 month treatment.

Competing interest

The authors declare that they have no competing interests.

Author's contribution

This work was accomplished in collaboration between all authors. Author EK designed the study, wrote the proposal and collected laboratory data. Author BG commented the protocol, analyzed the data and prepared the manuscript for publication. Author BE managed the literature search and involved in data analysis. Author AG participated in data analysis, literature search and laboratory investigation. All authors read and approved the final manuscript.

Acknowledgements

We would like to thank the school of Biomedical and laboratory Sciences, University of Gondar for financial support. Our special thanks also go to all patients involved in this study.

Author details

[1]Department of Hematology and Immunohematology, School of Biomedical and Laboratory Sciences, College of Medicine and Health Sciences (CMHS), University of Gondar (UOG), Gondar, Ethiopia. [2]Department of Medical Microbiology, School of Biomedical and Laboratory Sciences, College of Medicine and Health Sciences, University of Gondar, Gondar, Ethiopia.

References

1. World Health Organization. Global tuberculosis control: WHO report 2010. Geneva, Switzerland: WHO; 2010.
2. Federal Ministry of Health Ethiopia. Tuberculosis, leprosy and TB/HIV prevention and control programme manual. 4th ed. Addis Ababa: MOH; 2008.
3. World Health Organization. WHO declares TB an emergency in Africa. Call for urgent and extraordinary actions to halt a worsening epidemic. Geneva, Switzerland: WHO; 2005.
4. World Health Organization. Global tuberculosis control: surveillance, planning, financing. WHO report 2008; No. 393. Geneva, Switzerland: WHO; 2008.
5. World Health Organization. Global tuberculosis control: surveillance, planning, financing. WHO report 2007. Geneva, Switzerland: WHO; 2007.
6. Loulergue P, Mir O, Dhote R. Pure red blood cell aplasia and isoniazid use. Emerg Infect Dis. 2007;13(9):1427.
7. Agarwal AK, Chugh IM, Panjabi C, Dewan S, Shah A. Asymptomatic aplastic anaemia in a patient receiving anti-tuberculosis treatment. Indian J Tuberc. 2001;48(2):97–100.

8. Mintzer DM, Billet SN, Chmielewski L. Drug-induced hematologic syndromes. Adv. Hematol. 2009;2009:495863. doi:10.1155/2009/495863.
9. Whitfield CL. Hematologic abnormalities in tuberculous patients. Arch Intern Med. 1970;126(4):698.
10. Nagayama N, Shishido Y, Masuda K, Baba M, Tamura A, Nagai H, et al. Leukopenia due to anti-tuberculous chemotherapy including rifampicin and isoniazid. Kekkaku: [Tuberculosis]. 2004;79(5):341–8.
11. Muzaffar TM, Shaifuzain AR, Imran Y, Haslina MN. Hematological changes in tuberculous spondylitis patients at the Hospital Universiti Sains Malaysia. Southeast Asian J Trop Med Public Health. 2008;39(4):686–9.
12. Yaranal PJ, Umashankar T, Harish SG. Hematological profile in pulmonary tuberculosis. Int J Health Rehabil Sci. 2013;2(1):50–5.
13. Maartens G, Willcox PA, Benatar SR. Miliary tuberculosis: rapid diagnosis, hematologic abnormalities, and outcome in 109 treated adults. Am J Med. 1990;89(3):291–6.
14. Olaniyi J, Aken'Ova Y. Haematological profile of patients with pulmonary tuberculosis in Ibadan, Nigeria. Afr J Med Med Sci. 2003;32(3):239–42.
15. Koju D, Rao B, Shrestha B, Shakya R, Makaju R. Occurrence of side effects from anti-tuberculosis drugs in urban Nepalese population under DOTS treatment. Kathmandu University J Sci Eng Technol. 2005;1(1):1–2.
16. Oyer RA, Schlossberg D. Hematologic changes in tuberculosis. In: Schlossberg D, editor. Tuberculosis & Nontuberculous Mycobacterial infections. 5th ed. New Delhi: Tata McGraw-Hill; 2007. pp. 357–64.
17. Tsegaye A, Messele T, Tilahun T, Hailu E, Sahlu T, Doorly R, et al. Immunohematological reference ranges for adult Ethiopians. Clin Diagn Lab Immunol. 1999;6(3):410–4.
18. Weiss G. Pathogenesis and treatment of anaemia of chronic disease. Blood Rev. 2002;16(2):87–96.
19. Baynes R, Flax H, Bothwell T, Bezwoda W, Atkinson P, Mendelow B. Red blood cell distribution width in the anemia secondary to tuberculosis. Am J Clin Pathol. 1986;85(2):226–9.
20. Lee SW, Kang Y, Yoon YS, Um S-W, Lee SM, Yoo C-G, et al. The prevalence and evolution of anemia associated with tuberculosis. J Korean Med Sci. 2006;21(6):1028–32.
21. Berkowitz FE. Hemolysis and infection: categories and mechanisms of their interrelationship. Review of Infectious Diseases. 1991;13(6):1151–62.
22. Means Jr RT. Recent developments in the anemia of chronic disease. Curr Hematol Rep. 2003;2(2):116–21.
23. Nemeth E, Rivera S, Gabayan V, Keller C, Taudorf S, Pedersen BK, et al. IL-6 mediates hypoferremia of inflammation by inducing the synthesis of the iron regulatory hormone hepcidin. J Clin Investig. 2004;113(9):1271.
24. Singh K, Ahulwalia G, Sharma S, Saxena R, Chaudhary V, Anant M. Significance of haematological manifestations in patients with tuberculosis. J Assoc Physicians India. 2001;49(788):790–4.
25. Bhatt V, Saleem A. Drug-induced neutropenia–pathophysiology, clinical features, and management. Ann Clin Lab Sci. 2004;34(2):131–7.
26. Nagu TJ, Spiegelman D, Hertzmark E, Aboud S, Makani J, Matee MI, et al. Anemia at the initiation of tuberculosis therapy is associated with delayed sputum conversion among pulmonary tuberculosis patients in Dar-es-Salaam, Tanzania. PLoS One. 2014;9(3), e91229.
27. Bougie DW, Wilker PR, Aster RH. Patients with quinine-induced immune thrombocytopenia have both drug-dependent and drug-specific antibodies. Blood. 2006;108(3):922–7.
28. Von Drygalski A, Curtis BR, Bougie DW, McFarland JG, Ahl S, Limbu I, et al. Vancomycin-induced immune thrombocytopenia. N Engl J Med. 2007; 356(9):904–10.
29. Aster RH, Bougie DW. Drug-induced immune thrombocytopenia. N Engl J Med. 2007;357(6):580–7.
30. Visentin GP, Liu CY. Drug-induced thrombocytopenia. Hematol Oncol Clin North Am. 2007;21(4):685–96.
31. Baynes R, Flax H, Bothwell T, Bezwoda W, MacPhail A, Atkinson P, et al. Haematological and iron-related measurements in active pulmonary tuberculosis. Scand J Haematol. 1986;36(3):280–7.
32. Morris CD, Bird AR, Nell H. The haematological and biochemical changes in severe pulmonary tuberculosis. QJM. 1989;73(3):1151–9.
33. Lombard E, Mansvelt E. Haematological changes associated with miliary tuberculosis of the bone marrow. Tuber Lung Dis. 1993;74(2):131–5.
34. Dosumu E. Pattern of some haematological indices in newly diagnosed pulmonary tuberculosis cases in Iwo, Nigeria: diagnostic and therapeutic implications. Niger J Med. 2000;10(1):18–20.
35. Vajpayee N, Graham S, Bem S. Basic examination of blood and bone marrow. In: McPherson RA, Pincus MR, editors. Henry's clinical diagnosis and management by laboratory methods. 22nd ed. Philadelphia, PA: Elsevier/ Saunders; 2011. p. 30.
36. Subhashree A, Parameaswari P, Shanthi B, Revathy C, Parijatham B. The reference intervals for the haematological parameters in healthy adult population of chennai, southern India. J Clin Diagn Res. 2012;6(10):1675–80.
37. Pascual-Figal DA, Bonaque JC, Manzano-Fernández S, Fernández A, Garrido IP, Pastor-Perez F, et al. Red blood cell distribution width predicts new-onset anemia in heart failure patients. Int J Cardiol. 2012;160(3):196–200.
38. Bessman J, Gilmer Jr P, Gardner FH. Improved classification of anemias by MCV and RDW. Am J Clin Pathol. 1983;80(3):322–6.
39. Abdelrahman EG, Gasim GI, Musa IR, Elbashir LM, Adam I. Red blood cell distribution width and iron deficiency anemia among pregnant Sudanese women. Diagn Pathol. 2012;7(168):1596–7.
40. Rieder HL. Intervention for tuberculosis control and elimination. Paris, International Union Against Tuberculosis and Lung Disease, 2002:pp.554. https://books.google.com.et/books?isbn=1444113542.
41. Osselaer J-C, Jamart J, Scheiff J-M. Platelet distribution width for differential diagnosis of thrombocytosis. Clin Chem. 1997;43(6):1072–6.
42. Tozkoparan E, Deniz O, Ucar E, Bilgic H, Ekiz K. Changes in platelet count and indices in pulmonary tuberculosis. Clin Chem Lab Med. 2007;45(8): 1009–13.
43. Yakar F, Yildiz N, Yakar A, Kılıçaslan Z. Isoniazid-and rifampicin-induced thrombocytopenia. Multidiscip Respir Med. 2013;8(1):13.
44. George JN, Raskob GE, Shah SR, Rizvi MA, Hamilton SA, Osborne S, et al. Drug-induced thrombocytopenia: a systematic review of published case reports. Ann Intern Med. 1998;129(11):886–90.
45. Sahin F, Yazar E, Yıldız P. Prominent features of platelet count, plateletcrit, mean platelet volume and platelet distribution width in pulmonary tuberculosis. Multidiscip Respir Med. 2012;7(1):38.

12

Diagnostic utility of zinc protoporphyrin to detect iron deficiency in Kenyan preschool children: a community-based survey

Emily M. Teshome[1,2*], Andrew M. Prentice[1,2], Ayşe Y. Demir[3], Pauline E.A. Andang'o[4] and Hans Verhoef[1,2,5]

Abstract

Background: Zinc protoporphyrin (ZPP) has been used to screen and manage iron deficiency in individual children, but it has also been recommended to assess population iron status. The diagnostic utility of ZPP used in combination with haemoglobin concentration has not been evaluated in pre-school children. We aimed to a) identify factors associated with ZPP in children aged 12–36 months; b) assess the diagnostic performance and utility of ZPP, either alone or in combination with haemoglobin, to detect iron deficiency.

Methods: We used baseline data from 338 Kenyan children enrolled in a community-based randomised trial. To identify factors related to ZZP measured in whole blood or erythrocytes, we used bivariate and multiple linear regression analysis. To assess diagnostic performance, we excluded children with elevated plasma concentrations of C-reactive protein or α_1-acid glycoprotein, and with *Plasmodium* infection, and we analysed receiver operating characteristics (ROC) curves, with iron deficiency defined as plasma ferritin concentration < 12 μg/L. We also developed models to assess the diagnostic utility of ZPP and haemoglobin concentration when used to screen for iron deficiency.

Results: Whole blood ZPP and erythrocyte ZPP were independently associated with haemoglobin concentration, *Plasmodium* infection and plasma concentrations of soluble transferrin receptor, ferritin, and C-reactive protein. In children without inflammation or *Plasmodium* infection, the prevalence of true iron deficiency was 32.1%, compared to prevalence of 97.5% and 95.1% when assessed by whole blood ZPP and erythrocyte ZPP with conventional cut-off points (70 μmol/mol and 40 μmol/mol haem, respectively). Addition of whole blood ZPP or erythrocyte ZPP to haemoglobin concentration increased the area-under-the-ROC-curve (84.0%, $p = 0.003$, and 84.2%, $p = 0.001$, respectively, versus 62.7%). A diagnostic rule (0.038689 [haemoglobin concentration, g/L] + 0.00694 [whole blood ZPP, μmol/mol haem] >5.93120) correctly ruled out iron deficiency in 37.4%–53.7% of children screened, depending on the true prevalence, with both specificity and negative predictive value ≥90%.

Conclusions: In young children, whole blood ZPP and erythrocyte ZPP have added diagnostic value in detecting iron deficiency compared to haemoglobin concentration alone. A single diagnostic score based on haemoglobin concentration and whole blood ZPP can rule out iron deficiency in a substantial proportion of children screened.

Keywords: Erythrocyte protoporphyrin, Inflammation, Iron deficiency, Kenya, Malaria, *Plasmodium*, Child, Preschool, Zinc protoporphyrin

* Correspondence:
Emily.teshome@lshtm.ac.uk; emily_mwadimew@yahoo.com
[1]MRCG Keneba at MRC Unit The Gambia, PO Box 273, Banjul, The Gambia
[2]MRC International Nutrition Group, Faculty of Epidemiology and Population Heath, London School of Hygiene and Tropical Medicine, Keppel Street, London WC1E7HT, UK
Full list of author information is available at the end of the article

Background

Zinc protoporphyrin (ZPP) is formed in erythrocytes when the iron supply for erythropoiesis is less than required, or when iron utilization is impaired. In such conditions of iron-deficient erythropoiesis, protoporphyrin IX, the immediate precursor of haem, incorporates an atom of zinc rather than iron, resulting in the formation of ZPP instead of haem. Thus, depleted iron stores or a decrease in circulating iron in the bone marrow lead to elevated ZPP concentrations in whole blood or erythrocytes [1, 2].

ZPP can be determined rapidly and at low assay cost by haematofluorometer. It has been used to screen and manage iron deficiency in individual children, but it has also been a recommended marker to assess population iron status in cross-sectional studies, together with haemoglobin concentration [1, 3].

One possible application concerns the use of a single score that captures the diagnostic information of both whole blood ZPP and haemoglobin concentration in a screen-and-treat approach to manage iron deficiency in preschool children. Such diagnostic utility has not been assessed in pre-school children. We found earlier, however, that both whole blood ZPP and erythrocyte ZPP have little diagnostic utility as a screening marker to manage iron deficiency in pregnant women, whether used as single tests or combined with haemoglobin concentration [4].

The present study aimed to identify factors associated with ZPP measured in whole blood or erythrocytes from preschool children. We also assessed the diagnostic performance and utility of ZPP, either alone or in combination with haemoglobin concentration, in detecting iron deficiency defined as plasma ferritin concentration < 12 μg/L in children without inflammation or *Plasmodium* infection.

Methods

Study setting and population

The present study made use of samples that were collected at baseline in a randomised placebo-controlled trial to show non-inferiority of home fortification with 3 mg iron as NaFeEDTA compared with 12.5 mg iron as encapsulated ferrous fumarate. The main results of this trial will be reported elsewhere [5]. The study was conducted in children aged 12–36 months from January–December 2014 in Kisumu-West District, Kenya, an area that is located at around 1350 m above sea level. To recruit the children, community health workers compiled a list of parents with children within the eligible age range in a predefined study area and invited parents to bring all of them for screening to the research clinic, where parents were asked to sign an informed consent form.

Collection of data and samples

We determined weight and height using Salter Scale (UNICEF, catalogue 0145555, Copenhagen, Denmark) and height/recumbent length boards (UNICEF, catalogue 0114500, Copenhagen, Denmark) within 100 g and 1 mm, respectively. Phlebotomists collected 4 mL venous blood in tubes containing Li-heparin. An aliquot of blood was centrifuged, plasma was transferred to a microtube, centrifuged, and stored immediately in liquid nitrogen (−196 °C). The erythrocyte sediment was washed and centrifuged three times with isotonic phosphate-buffered saline. We assessed haemoglobin concentration (HemoCue 301, Ängelholm, Sweden) in duplicate, and zinc protoporphyrin: haem ratio (AVIV haematofluorometer, model 206D, Lakewood NJ, USA) in whole blood and in erythrocytes, each in triplicate. For quality control of the haematofluorometer, we used erythrocyte controls for low, medium and high ZPP values from the manufacturer (Aviv) and as per manufacturer's instructions. Measurements were within the acceptable range throughout the study.

ZPP in washed erythrocytes is considered a more valid measure of iron-deficient erythropoiesis when compared to ZPP in whole blood because the washing process removes substances dissolved in plasma such as bilirubin and riboflavin that can fluoresce at a wavelength similar to that of ZPP.

We used two rapid diagnostic tests to detect *Plasmodium* antigenaemia. CareStart G0151 (AccessBio, USA; http://www.accessbio.net/) can detect lactate hydrogenase (pLDH) produced by either *P. falciparum* or *Plasmodium* species other than *P. falciparum* (i.e. *P. ovale, P. malariae* or *P. vivax*). CareStart G0171 can detect histidine-rich protein-2 (HRP2), which is produced exclusively by *P. falciparum*.

Plasma iron indicators (concentrations of ferritin and soluble transferrin receptor), inflammation indicators (concentrations of C-reactive protein and α-1-acid glycoprotein) and other nutritional markers (concentrations of albumin and vitamin B_{12}) were measured on an Abbott Architect C16000 and i2000 SR analyser at Meander Medical Centre, Amersfoort, The Netherlands, with reagents from and as per instructions of the manufacturer.

Eligibility criteria

After data and blood samples were collected but before randomisation to intervention, children were given pre-medication (3-day courses of dihydroartemisinin-piperaquine and albendazole; a single dose of praziquantel). Children were eligible for enrolment in the trial and the present study if: aged 12–36 months, resident in the study area; parental consent form signed by both parents; not acutely sick or febrile (axillary temperature ≥ 37.5 °C) at the time of recruitment; absence of reported or suspected major systemic disorder (e.g. HIV infection, sickle cell disease); no use of antiretroviral drugs against HIV, rifampicin, carbamazepine, phenytoin or phenobarbital and no twin sibling. Children were excluded if: haemoglobin concentration < 70 g/L (for ethical reasons, because the trial had a placebo arm); severely wasted (weight-for-height z-score < −3 SD); known allergy to dihydro artemisinin-piperaquine, benzimidazole or praziquantel; parent-reported history of using antihelminthic drugs in the 1-month period before the screening date; not at risk of malaria (e.g. children who received chemoprophylaxis against malaria because of HIV infection or sickle cell disease); they received their first dose of dihydroartemisinin-piperaquine at the research clinic and did not complete the prescribed second and third doses at home.

Sample size determination

We included all children enrolled in the trial in the present study. Our sample size calculations were based on our primary aim to show non-inferiority of the haemoglobin concentration response to home fortification with 3 mg iron as NaFeEDTA compared with 12.5 mg iron as ferrous fumarate intention. Because this aim is irrelevant to the present study, these calculations are not reported here, although they are available elsewhere [5].

Statistical analysis

Definitions

Anthropometric indices were calculated by comparing measurements with the standards WHO Growth Standards [6]. For whole blood and erythrocyte ZPP, we used a cut-off value of 70 μmol/mol haem (2.7 μg/g haemoglobin), corresponding to the 95% upper limit of the reference values for women and children participating in the US National Health and Nutrition Examination Survey (NHANES) II, from which individuals with anaemia, low transferrin saturation and elevated blood lead concentrations had been excluded [1–3]. For erythrocyte ZPP, we also used a cut-off point of 40 μmol/mol haem, which is based on several small studies comparing iron-deficient and iron-replete individuals [7].

We defined iron deficiency as the absence or near-absence of storage iron, indicated by plasma ferritin concentration < 12 μg/L [8]. Because this definition is recommended by WHO to measure population iron status except where inflammation is prevalent [2], we considered it to be valid only in children without inflammation, *Plasmodium* infection, or HIV infection. In addition, we used the following definitions: anaemia: haemoglobin concentration < 108 g/L (i.e. 110 g/L reference range for children aged 6–59 months, at sea level, minus 2 g/L adjustment for an altitude at 1000–1500 m above sea level) [9]; inflammation: plasma concentrations of C-reactive protein concentration > 5 mg/L [10] and/or α_1-acid glycoprotein concentration > 1 g/L [11]; being stunted or wasted: height-for-age or weight-for-height z-score < −2 SD; [6] *P. falciparum* infection: presence in blood of HRP2 or *P. falciparum*-specific pLDH; any *Plasmodium* infection: presence of HRP2 or pLDH specific to either *P. falciparum* or human *Plasmodium* species other than *P. falciparum*; low vitamin B_{12} status: plasma vitamin B_{12} concentration < 150 pmol/L.

Description of the study population

We calculated prevalence values for binary variables, means with corresponding SDs for variables with an approximately normal distribution, and quartiles for continuous variables that were not normally distributed. Because some of the plasma markers used (ferritin, albumin, vitamin B_{12}) can act as acute phase reactants we also described these characteristics in children without inflammation or *Plasmodium* infection.

Factors associated with ZPP

We explored associations between ZPP and personal characteristics (age, sex), inflammation markers, iron markers, *Plasmodium* infection and other plasma markers (albumin and vitamin B_{12} concentrations). Groups were compared assuming t-distributions of ZPP values that were normalised by log-transformation. Exponentiation of results yielded group differences that were expressed as relative differences.

We inspected scatterplots and used simple linear regression analysis to assess associations between ZPP (log-transformed) and explanatory variables with continuous outcomes. Some explanatory factors were untransformed, with the implicit assumption that ZPP values can increase or decrease exponentially with an absolute increment in the explanatory variable; in other cases, log-transformation of the explanatory factor yielded a better model fit, indicating that ZPP values and explanatory variables change at rates that are proportional to their current values. In such cases, variation in the independent variable was expressed as geometric standard deviation, i.e. a dimensionless, multiplicative factor such that dividing or multiplication of the geometric mean by this ratio indicates a variation that is equivalent to subtraction or addition of one standard deviation on a log-transformed scale [12].

We subsequently used multiple linear regression analyses to identify factors that were independently associated with ZPP. Given a linear association between continuous variables, dichotomisation generally results in loss of statistical precision [13]. Thus we preferred to use continuous variables that were shown to be linearly associated with ZPP in the bivariate analyses. Our analysis started with a full model that included haemoglobin concentration, *Plasmodium* infection, and plasma concentrations of ferritin, soluble transferrin receptor, C-reactive protein, α_1-acid glycoprotein, albumin, vitamin B_{12}, sex (binary) and age class (binary). All plasma markers except albumin and vitamin B_{12} were log-transformed. Factors were manually eliminated using a backward elimination process with a removal criterion of $p > 0.05$.

Diagnostic performance of ZPP to detect iron deficiency

This part of the analysis was restricted to children without inflammation (i.e. plasma concentrations of C-reactive protein <5 mg/L and/or α_1-acid glycoprotein <1 g/L) and without *Plasmodium* infection. We used logistic discriminant analysis to model the probability of iron deficiency as a function of continuous explanatory variables, either alone or combined.

We used the pROC package [14] within R vs. 3.2.0 (www.r-project.org) to produce and analyse receiver operating characteristics (ROC) curves, with comparison of areas-under-the-curve (AUCs) by DeLong's test for paired curves. Partial AUCs were computed with a correction to achieve a maximal value of 1.0 and a non-discriminant value of 0.5, whatever the range of specificity or sensitivity values. Confidence intervals of estimates for partial areas-under-the-curve (pAUCs) were computed by stratified bootstrapping with 10,000 replicates.

Diagnostic utility of ZPP to estimate prevalence of iron deficiency

First, we assessed the diagnostic performance of ZPP to estimate the prevalence of iron deficiency, using two commonly used cut-off points for ZPP, namely whole blood ZPP >70 µmol/mol haem and erythrocyte ZPP >40 µmol/mol haem (see preceding paragraphs). We used Wilson's method to calculate confidence intervals around proportions [15, 16]; for sensitivity and specificity, and for the pair of predictive values, we calculated 97.5% univariate CIs. The cross-product of these univariate CIs, considered together, form a joint 95% confidence region for both population parameters [17].

Second, as an example, we used our data to explore the utility of using the combination of haemoglobin concentration and ZPP to screen for iron deficiency (Additional file 1), with cut-points chosen to ensure a high sensitivity so that most cases are detected, at the cost of false positives that could be eliminated by further diagnostic tests. Children can be excluded from further testing if negative test results correctly identify children without iron deficiency in the vast majority of cases. Such a strategy may be desirable in community-based surveys with relatively low prevalence of iron deficiency, but also in medical practice with higher prevalence values (because of self-selection). Thus we estimated the proportion of children who could be eliminated from further testing in settings with a prevalence range for iron deficiency of 0%–50%, which probably covers the vast majority of community settings, with arbitrarily selected sensitivity values and negative predictive values of >90%. Because of its ease of measurement, we limited this assessment with ZPP being measured in whole blood.

Results

We enrolled 338 children into the study.

Description of the study population

The prevalence of iron deficiency, measured in children without inflammation or *Plasmodium* infection, was 32.1%; when measured in all children (Table 1), this value was 17.1%. Whole blood ZPP > 70 µmol/mol haem occurred in 97.9% and erythrocyte ZPP > 40 µmol/mol occurred in 96.7% of children. The prevalence of anaemia was 55.6%, but there were virtually no children with low vitamin B_{12} status. Inflammation, assessed by plasma concentrations of C-reactive protein and α_1-acid glycoprotein, occurred in 66.9% of children, and was mostly mild. Of 226 children with inflammation, 98 (43.4%) had elevated concentrations of α_1-acid glycoprotein with normal C-reactive protein concentrations, 11 (4.9%) had elevated C-reactive protein concentrations with normal concentrations of α_1-acid glycoprotein, and 117 (51.8%) had elevated concentrations of both markers. Of children who carried *Plasmodium* parasites (36.4% = 123/338), only 1 was infected with *Plasmodium* species other than *P. falciparum*.

Factors associated with ZPP: Crude analysis

In bivariate analysis, both whole blood and erythrocyte ZPP were strongly elevated in iron deficiency, anaemia and *Plasmodium* infection; they declined with increasing haemoglobin and plasma ferritin concentrations; and they increased with plasma transferrin receptor concentration (Table 2). Whole blood ZPP was also associated with increased plasma concentrations of α_1-acid glycoprotein and C-reactive protein concentration; a higher prevalence of inflammation as defined by α_1-acid glycoprotein >1 g/L; decreased plasma albumin concentration, and increased plasma vitamin B_{12} concentration. Although erythrocyte ZPP was reduced in children aged 24–36 months and, seemed higher in boys than in girls, there was no evidence that it was associated with inflammation, however defined, or with either of the

Table 1 Characteristics of the study population

	All children		Children without inflammation or *Plasmodium* infection	
n	338		84	
Age				
12–23.99 months	53.6%	(181)	54.8%	(46)
24–36 months	46.4%	(157)	45.2%	(38)
Sex, male	55.0%	(186)	47.6%	(40)
Height-for-age z-score, SD	−1.33	(1.4)	−0.91	(1.5)
Stunted (height-for-age z-score < −2 SD)	30.2%	(102)	14.3%	(12)
Weight-for-height z-score, SD	−0.14	(1.0)	−0.15	(0.97)
Wasted (weight-for-age z-score < −2 SD)	3.0%	(10)	2.4%	(2)
Whole blood ZPP, μmol/mol haem	181	[124–282]	131	[98–239]
Whole blood ZPP > 70 μmol/mol haem	97.9%	(331)	97.6%	(82)
Erythrocyte ZPP, μmol/mol haem	142	[86–246]	117	[69–215]
Erythrocyte ZPP > 70 μmol/mol haem	83.1%	(281)	72.6%	(61)
Erythrocyte ZPP > 40 μmol/mol haem	96.7%	(327)	95.2%	(80)
Haemoglobin concentration, g/L	105.0	(13.2)	111.7	(10.0)
Anaemia (haemoglobin concentration < 108 g/L)	55.6%	(188)	34.5%	(29)
Plasma ferritin concentration, μg/L	35.3	[17.1–67.2][a]	17.3	[10.3–28.8][b]
Iron status[c]				
Deficient	17.1%	(57/333)	32.1%	(27/81)
Replete	23.1%	(77/333)	64.3%	(54/81)
Uncertain	59.8%	(199/333)	Not applicable	
Plasma sTfR concentration, mg/L	2.43	[1.84–3.30]	2.11	[1.50–2.94]
Plasma albumin concentration, g/L	34.8	(3.9)	37.4	(2.2)
Plasma vitamin B_{12} concentration, pmol/L	400	[307–559][d]	356	[283–452][e]
Plasma vitamin B_{12} concentration < 150 pmol/L	1.2%	(4/332)	1.2%	(1/80)
Plasma CRP concentration, mg/L	2.9	[0.8–9.2]	Not applicable	
Plasma AGP concentration, g/L	1.16	[0.9–1.55]	Not applicable	
Inflammation				
Plasma CRP concentration > 5 mg/L	37.9%	(128)	Not applicable	
Plasma AGP concentration > 1.0 g/L	63.6%	(215)	Not applicable	
Plasma CRP concentration > 5 mg/L, or plasma AGP concentration > 1.0 g/L	66.9%	(226)	Not applicable	
Plasmodium infection				
P. falciparum	36.1%	(122)	Not applicable	
Plasmodium spp. other than *P. falciparum*	0.3%	(1)	Not applicable	
Missing	0.9%	(3)	Not applicable	

Values indicate mean (SD), median [25th and 75th percentile] or % (*n*)
AGP α_1-acid glycoprotein, *CRP* C-reactive protein, *sTfR* soluble transferrin receptor, *ZPP* zinc protoporphyrin
Missing values, due to insufficient plasma volumes for analysis, resulted in [a]*n* = 333, [b]*n* = 81; [c]*Deficient:* plasma ferritin concentration < 12 μg/L, regardless of the presence or absence of inflammation; *replete:* plasma ferritin concentration ≥ 12 μg/L, in the absence of inflammation; *uncertain:* plasma ferritin concentration ≥ 12 μg/L, in the presence of inflammation defined as plasma concentrations of CRP > 5 mg/L or AGP > 1.0 g/L. Missing values, due to insufficient plasma volumes for analysis, resulted in [d]*n* = 332 and [e]*n* = 80

two plasma inflammation markers. We found no evidence that ZPP, whether measured in whole blood or erythrocytes, was associated with z-scores for height-for-age or weight-for-height, or with being stunted or wasted.

Factors associated with ZPP: Multiple linear regression analysis

In multivariate analysis, there was no evidence that ZPP, whether measured in whole blood or erythrocytes, was associated with plasma concentrations of α_1-acid

Table 2 Factors associated with ZPP-haem ratio measured in whole blood or erythrocytes, crude analysis[a]

Factor	Number	Whole blood ZPP-haem ratio			Erythrocyte ZPP-haem ratio		
		Geometric mean	Δ[b]	(95% CI)	Geometric mean	Δ[b]	(95% CI)
Age							
12–23.99 months	162	199	Ref		163	Ref	
24–36 months	176	178	−10.8%	(−21.2% to 0.9%)	134	−18.1%	(−4.3% to −29.9%)
Sex							
Girls	152	179	Ref		135	Ref	
Boys	186	195	9.4%	(−3.4% to 23.8%)	158	16.4%	(−0.5% to 36.1%)
Inflammation (CRP concentration > 5 mg/L)							
No	210	180	Ref		144	Ref	
Yes	128	201	11.4%	(−1.9% to 26.5%)	153	6.6%	(−9.3% to 25.4%)
Inflammation (AGP concentration > 1 g/L)							
No	123	166	Ref		136	Ref	
Yes	215	201	21.4%	(7.0% to 37.9%)	154	13.3%	(−3.7% to 33.3%)
Inflammation (CRP concentration > 5 mg/L or AGP concentration > 1 g/L)							
No	112	166	Ref		137	Ref	
Yes	226	199	20.0%	(5.4% to 36.7%)	153	11.4%	(−5.6% to 31.6%)
Iron deficiency (ferritin concentration < 12 μg/L)							
No	276	173	Ref		132	Ref	
Yes	57	278	60.4%	(36.9% to 87.8%)	255	93.6%	(58.8% to 136.0%)
Anaemia							
No	150	135	Ref		103	Ref	
Yes	188	244	81.4%	(63.3% to 101.4%)	195	89.1%	(64.3% to 117.5%)
Plasmodium infection, any species							
No	212	167	Ref		131	Ref	
Yes	123	230	37.5%	(21.5% to 55.6%)	180	38.1%	(18.6% to 60.8%)
Plasma ferritin concentration, 5.11-fold change[d, e]			−16.7%	(−24.6% to −7.9%)		−18.1%	(−24.1% to −11.6%)
Plasma sTfR concentration, 1.43-fold change[d]			38.3%	(34.0% to 42.7.0%)		66.8%	(57.7% to 76.4%)
Plasma CRP concentration, 2.72-fold change[d]			3.5%	(0.8% to 6.2%)		6.8%	(−1.2% to 15.5%)
Plasma AGP concentration, 1.60-fold change[d]			23.7%	(10.0% to 39.1%)		7.1%	(−1.0% to 15.8%)
Haemoglobin concentration, change by 13.2 g/L[f, g]			29.8%	(−33.1% to −26.2%)		−31.5%	(−35.9% to −26.7%)
Plasma albumin concentration, change by 3.9 g/L[f]			−7.0%	(−12.5% to −1.1%)		−1.4%	(−8.9% to 6.7%)
Plasma vitamin B_{12} concentration, change by 213 pmol/L[f]			7.0%	(0.6% to 13.9%)		6.1%	(−2.0% to 14.8%)

AGP α_1-acid glycoprotein, *CRP* C-reactive protein, *GSD* geometric standard deviation, *Ref* reference, *SD* standard deviation, *sTfR* soluble transferrin receptor, *ZPP* zinc protoporphyrin

[a]ZPP values were normalised by log-transformation; exponentiation of results yielded associations being expressed as relative differences; [b]Difference; [c]Based on HRP2- and pLDH-based dipstick test results; [d]Corresponding to 1 geometric standard deviation; [e]For example, a 5.11-fold increase in plasma ferritin concentration, which corresponds to a variation that is equivalent to addition of 1 SD on a log-transformed scale, is associated with a reduction in the whole blood ZPP-haem ratio by 16.7%; [f]Corresponding to 1 SD; [g]For example, an increase in haemoglobin concentration by 13.2 g/L, which corresponds to an increase by 1 SD, is associated with a reduction in the whole blood ZPP-haem ratio by 29.8%

glycoprotein and vitamin B_{12}, or with sex or age class. Thus, these factors were eliminated from the models shown in Table 3.

Whole blood ZPP was independently associated with decreased concentrations of haemoglobin and ferritin and with increased plasma concentrations of transferrin

Table 3 Factors associated with ZPP-haem ratio measured in whole blood or erythrocytes, multiple linear regression analysis[a]

	Whole blood ZPP-haem ratio (model 1)		Whole blood ZPP-haem ratio (model 2)		Erythrocyte ZPP-haem ratio	
	Δ[b]	(95% CI)	Δ[b]	(95% CI)	Δ[b]	(95% CI)
Plasma ferritin concentration, 5.11-fold change[c]	−10.1%	(−14.3% to −5.6%)	−9.6%	(−14.0% to −4.9%)	−15.5%	(−21.1% to −9.5%)
Plasma sTfR concentration, 1.43-fold change[c]	34.8%	(28.3% to 41.7%)	34.9%	(28.3% to 41.8%)	45.3%	(35.7% to 55.6%)
Plasma CRP concentration, 2.72-fold change[c]	5.0%	(0.1% to 10.0%)	5.4%	(0.4% to 10.5%)	9.8%	(2.8% to 17.2%)
Haemoglobin concentration, change by 13.2 g/L[d]	−13.9%	(−18.3% to −9.4%)	−14.9%	(−19.4% to −10.1%)	−14.5%	(−20.7% to −7.9%)
Plasmodium infection, any species[e]	17.3%	(7.8% to 27.7%)	16.8%	(7.4% to 27.2%)	93.3%	(23.8% to 202.0%)
Plasma albumin concentration, change by 3.9 g/L[d]	—	(eliminated)	3.0%	(−1.7% to 8.0%)	2.2%	(0.5% to 4.0%)

CRP C-reactive protein, *sTfR* soluble transferrin receptor, *ZPP* zinc protoporphyrin
[a]ZPP values were normalised by log-transformation; exponentiation of results yielded associations being expressed as relative differences. Plasma concentrations of α_1-acid glycoprotein (log-transformed), vitamin B_{12} (log-transformed), sex (binary) and age class (binary) were eliminated from all models through a manual stepwise backward elimination process with an removal criterion of $p > 0.05$; [b]Difference; [c]Corresponding to 1 geometric standard deviation; [d]Corresponding to 1 SD; [e]Based on HRP2- and pLDH-based dipstick test results

receptor and C-reactive protein (Table 3). Of all biochemical markers, plasma transferrin receptor concentration showed the strongest association with whole blood and erythrocyte ZPP. Similar results were found with erythrocyte ZPP as dependent variable. *Plasmodium* infection was associated with elevated whole blood ZPP, and an even more pronounced elevation in erythrocyte ZPP values. There was a mild association between plasma albumin concentration and erythrocyte ZPP, but retention of this factor in the model for whole blood ZPP did not appreciably change the magnitude of the association for other factors.

Diagnostic performance of ZPP to detect iron deficiency

ROC curve analysis showed that whole blood and erythrocyte ZPP had similar diagnostic performance (AUC values: 79.1% and 81.2%, respectively; $p = 0.36$) in detecting iron deficiency, but either marker performed better than haemoglobin concentration (AUC: 62.7%) (Fig. 1a; Table in Fig. 1). The diagnostic accuracy was further improved by combining either whole blood or erythrocyte ZPP with haemoglobin (Fig. 1b, p=0.003; and Fig. 1c, p=0.001, respectively).

Overall, there was no evidence that the diagnostic accuracy differed between the combination of haemoglobin concentration with erythrocyte ZPP and the combination of haemoglobin concentration with whole blood ZPP (AUCs: 84.2% versus 84.0%; $p = 0.91$). The ROCs for these markers crossed (Fig. 1d) at a sensitivity of 81.5%, corresponding to $0.07195[Hb] + 0.01449[ZZP_{whole}] = 10.39334$ (where Hb and ZPP_{whole} indicate haemoglobin concentration in g/L and whole blood ZPP:haem ratio in μmol/mol, respectively; in this equation, parameter estimates are shown with 5 decimals to avoid misclassification due to multiplication of rounding errors). At all sensitivity values above this cut-off (Fig. 1d, red rectangle), the diagnostic accuracy of the combination of erythrocyte ZPP with haemoglobin concentration was superior to the combination of whole blood ZPP with haemoglobin concentration (corrected pAUCs: 76.3% versus 70.4%, $p = 0.04$).

Diagnostic utility of ZPP

When whole blood ZPP was considered without additional markers to detect iron deficiency, a conventional threshold of 70 μmol/mol haem resulted in the following estimates (Table 4): sensitivity: 100%; specificity: 3.7%, positive predictive value: 34.2%; prevalence: 97.5% (as compared to a 'true' prevalence of 32.1%; Table 1). Corresponding values for an erythrocyte ZPP threshold of 40 μmol/mol haem were: 100%, 7.4%, 35.1% and 95.1%.

Within a prevalence range of iron deficiency of <14.1%, a diagnostic rule of haemoglobin concentration > 122 g/L would rule out iron deficiency in 14.1%–14.8% of children tested, depending on the actual prevalence, with both sensitivity and negative predictive value >90% (Fig. 2). Similarly, within a prevalence range of iron deficiency of <28.6%, whole blood ZPP > 99 μmol/mol haem would rule out iron deficiency in 28.6%–36% of children tested; and within a prevalence range of 37.4%, $0.038689\ [Hb] + 0.00694\ [\text{whole blood ZPP}] > 5.93120$ would rule out iron deficiency in 37.4%–53.7% of children. At all prevalence values exceeding these ranges, these diagnostic tests would not be able to rule out children with the predefined diagnostic criteria (i.e. both sensitivity and negative predictive value should be 90%), and all children would need to undergo further diagnostic work-up using more advanced tests.

Discussion

In our population, virtually all children had whole blood ZPP values exceeding conventional cut-off points of 70 μmol/mol haem, resulting in very low specificity and gross overestimates of the 'true' prevalence of iron deficiency of 32.1%, whether assessed in the overall

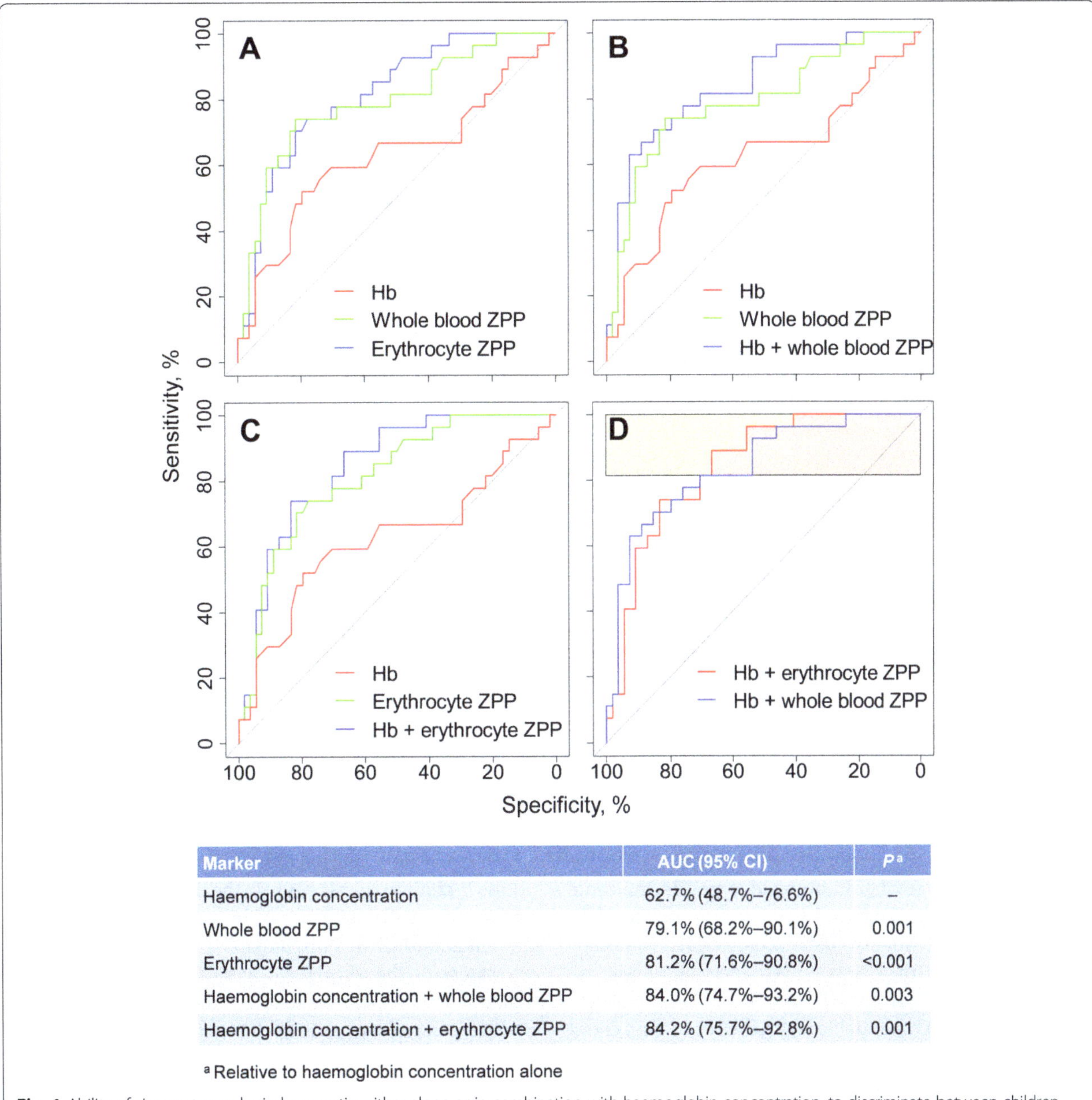

Marker	AUC (95% CI)	P^a
Haemoglobin concentration	62.7% (48.7%–76.6%)	–
Whole blood ZPP	79.1% (68.2%–90.1%)	0.001
Erythrocyte ZPP	81.2% (71.6%–90.8%)	<0.001
Haemoglobin concentration + whole blood ZPP	84.0% (74.7%–93.2%)	0.003
Haemoglobin concentration + erythrocyte ZPP	84.2% (75.7%–92.8%)	0.001

[a] Relative to haemoglobin concentration alone

Fig. 1 Ability of zinc protoporphyrin-haem ratio, either alone or in combination with haemoglobin concentration, to discriminate between children with and without iron deficiency. Panel **a**: Receiver operating characteristics (ROC) curves for various blood markers, used alone, to discriminate between iron-deficient and iron-replete children. Panel **b**: As in Panel **a**, with haemoglobin concentration and whole blood ZPP, alone and in combination. Panel **c**: As in Panel **a**, with haemoglobin concentration and erythrocyte ZPP, alone and in combination. Panel **d**: As in Panel **a**, with combined haemoglobin concentration and whole blood ZPP, versus combined haemoglobin concentration and erythrocyte ZPP. Hb: haemoglobin concentration. Grey diagonal lines in ROC curves indicate a 'worst' possible test, which has no discriminatory value and an area-under-the-curve (AUC) of 0.5. An ideal marker would have a curve that runs from the lower-left via the upper-left to the upper-right corner, yielding an AUC of 1.0

population or when restricted to those without inflammation and without *Plasmodium* infection. A similar problem was noted with erythrocyte ZPP > 40 μmol/mol haem. Both whole blood ZPP and erythrocyte ZPP were independently associated with *Plasmodium* infection and plasma C-reactive protein concentration. ZPP, whether measured in whole blood or erythrocytes, yielded higher diagnostic accuracy in detecting iron deficiency than haemoglobin concentration alone, and also improved this diagnostic accuracy when used in combination with haemoglobin concentration. When applied in a screen-and-treat strategy to control iron deficiency in paediatric populations with a prevalence of iron deficiency of <37.4% (which covers most settings in developing countries), our data suggest that a diagnostic rule of 0.038689 [Hb] + 0.00694 [whole blood ZPP] > 5.93120

Table 4 Diagnostic performance of zinc protoporphyrin-haem ratio, with dichotomised test results, to detect iron deficiency

	n/n	Estimate	(CI)
Whole blood ZPP > 70 µmol/mol haem			
Sensitivity	27/27	100.0%	(84.4%–100.0%)[a]
Specificity	2/54	3.7%	(0.9%–14.4%)[a]
Positive predictive value	27/79	34.2%	(23.5%–46.7%)[a]
Negative predictive value	2/2	100.0%	(28.6%–100.0%)[a]
Prevalence	79/81	97.5%	(91.4%–99.3%)[b]
Erythrocyte ZPP > 40 µmol/mol haem			
Sensitivity	27/27	100.0%	(84.4%–100.0%)[a]
Specificity	4/50	7.4%	(2.6%–19.5%)[a]
Positive predictive value	27/77	35.1%	(24.2%–47.8%)[a]
Negative predictive value	4/4	100.0%	(44.4%–100.0%)[a]
Prevalence	77/81	95.1%	(88.0%–98.1%)[b]

[a]97.5% CI; [b]95% CI

can correctly identify 90% of children with iron deficiency, and correctly rule out iron deficiency in 37.4%–53.7% of children who are tested, depending on the true prevalence.

Lead poisoning can cause elevated ZPP values, but lead exposure is presumably low in rural African children. Thus, the high ZPP values found in this study population may have been due to a combination of factors causing an inadequate supply of iron to erythroblasts (iron deficiency, inflammation) and increased erythropoiesis (haemolysis due to *Plasmodium* infection and possibly selected hereditary disorders such as glucose-6-phosphate dehydrogenase deficiency, sickle cell and α^+-thalassaemia). In a previous trial in the same area as the present study, α^+-thalassaemia occurred in 48.8% of pregnant women (heterozygotes: 41.3%; homozygotes: 7.5%), but there was no evidence that it was associated with ZPP [4]. In a nearby area, the prevalence of sickle cell trait and sickle cell disease in preschool children was 17.1% and 1.6%, respectively; genotypes indicating G6PD deficiency occurred in 8.2% of males and 6.8% of children overall, whilst the prevalence of haptoglobin 2–2 genotype was 20.4% [17, 18] A study in Gambian children aged 2–6 years, however, failed to find an association between haptoglobin genotype and ZPP [19].

We found a particularly strong relationship between ZPP, whether measured in whole blood or erythrocytes, and plasma transferrin receptor concentration. This is not surprising because both are markers for iron-deficient erythropoiesis. Consistent with our data, ZPP is known to be increased in iron deficiency, inflammation and other causes of an inadequate iron supply to erythroblasts. The increase in whole blood ZPP that was associated with *Plasmodium* infection may be due in part to the formation of bilirubin and other haemoglobin breakdown products in plasma that result from haemolysis and that fluoresce in the same wavelength range as protoporphyrins. *Plasmodium* infection was also associated with an even larger increase in erythrocyte ZPP, independently of inflammation. This was unexpected because erythrocytes lack plasma constituents, which are removed by washing. A possible explanation is that haemolysis-induced increase in erythropoietin activity under influence of *Plasmodium* infection drives up the demand for iron in the erythron. We have not been able to find previous reports of an association between erythrocyte ZPP and plasma albumin concentration, which could be a spurious finding.

One limitation of our study is the difficulty of measuring iron status in the presence of inflammation. Throughout the remainder of this discussion, it should be noted that we assessed the diagnostic performance and ZPP in children without inflammation and without *Plasmodium* infection, because plasma ferritin concentration can be elevated in the presence of infection-induced inflammation independently of iron status. We used this approach in favour of other biomarkers and approaches that have been proposed.

In one method [20, 21], fixed correction factors for serum ferritin concentrations are computed based on geometric mean values in groups that are defined by cross-classification of individuals by two inflammation markers (serum concentrations of C-reactive protein >5 g/L and α_1-acid glycoprotein >1.0 g/L). The resulting ratios in geometric mean values are used to adjust individual values, and deficiency is determined on the basis of these adjusted values. This method has the disadvantages, however, that it is not validated using a reference standard, its validity depends on untested and perhaps invalid assumptions, and it does not take into account likely between-person variability in the response of

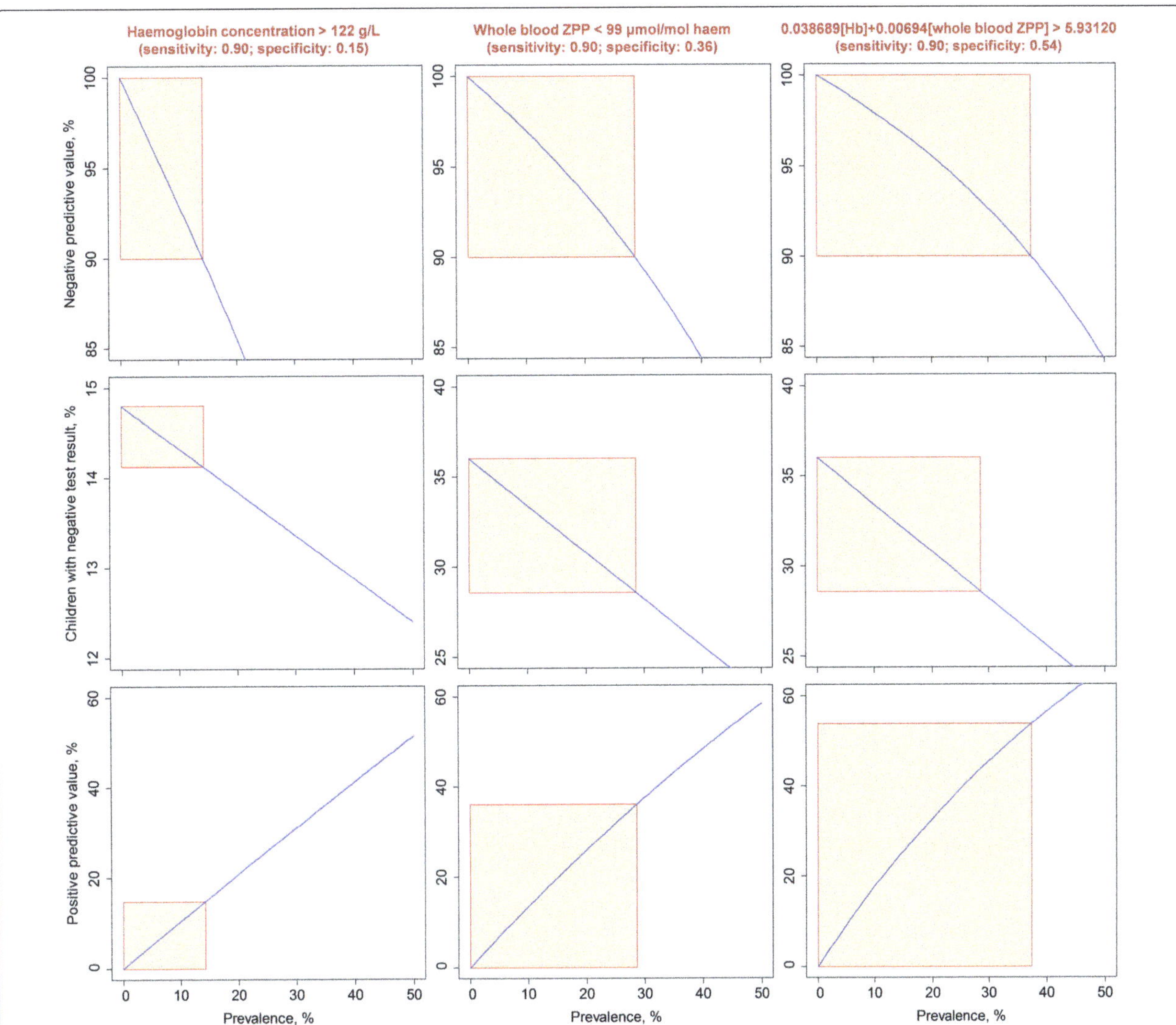

Fig. 2 Application of a diagnostic strategy to rule out iron deficiency. [Hb]: haemoglobin concentration, expressed in g/L; [whole blood ZPP]: whole blood ZPP content, expressed in µmol/mol haem. The diagnostic strategy in a screen-and-treat survey is based on two criteria: a) the probability of correctly diagnosing iron deficiency should exceed 90%; and b) iron deficiency can be ruled out if the probability of a negative test result being correct (negative predictive value) exceeds 90%. To meet the first requirement, a cut-off point for each diagnostic test result (top) is selected to yield a sensitivity of 90%; the corresponding specificity value is obtained from the ROC curves (Fig. 1). For haemoglobin concentration and whole blood ZPP, the cut-off points were 122 g/L and 99 µmol/mol haem; the corresponding specificity values were 14.8% and 36.0%, respectively. When these markers were combined in a single diagnostic rule, 0.038689 [Hb] + 0.00694 [whole blood ZPP] > 5.93120 had a specificity of 53.7%. The negative predictive value (top panels, *blue* lines) depends on sensitivity and specificity values thus fixed, and the prevalence of iron deficiency. The second diagnostic criterion, i.e. the negative predictive value should exceed 90%, applies only within a limited prevalence range (top panels, red rectangle); at prevalence values exceeding this range, the negative predictive value will be below 90% and iron deficiency cannot be ruled out with diagnostic test applied (top). The percentage of children with a negative test result declines linearly with the prevalence of iron deficiency (middle panels, blue lines). The percentage of children for whom iron deficiency can be ruled out (middle panels, Y-intercepts of red rectangles) depends on the prevalence range in which the negative predictive value exceeds 90% (top panels, red rectangles). With fixed sensitivity and specificity values, the positive predictive value (bottom panels, blue lines) increase monotonically with the prevalence of iron deficiency. Within the prevalence range in which the negative predictive value exceeds 90% (top panels, *red* rectangles), the highest positive predictive value is 54% (for combined use of haemoglobin concentration and whole blood ZPP), indicating that additional tests (i.e. other than haemoglobin concentration and whole blood ZPP) are required to accurately determine iron status. For example, haemoglobin concentration > 122 g/L (left panels) has 90% sensitivity of detecting iron deficiency; at a true prevalence of iron deficiency <14.1%, a negative test result obtained with this decision rules out iron deficiency with a probability of 90% (upper left panel, red rectangle). Depending on the true prevalence of iron deficiency, such a cut-off for haemoglobin concentration would result in iron deficiency being ruled out in 14.1%–14.8% of children who are tested (middle left panel, red rectangle). Similarly, within a prevalence range < 28.6%, whole blood ZPP > 99 µmol/mol haem rules out iron deficiency in 28.6%–36% of children tested. Within a prevalence range of <37.4%, 0.038689 [Hb] + 0.00694 [whole blood ZPP] > 5.93120 rules out iron deficiency in 37.4%–53.7% of children

ferritin concentration to inflammation. Another limitation is the possibility that plasma ferritin concentration is possibly elevated at levels of inflammatory markers within the normal range (serum C-reactive protein concentration < 5 mg/L or plasma α_1-acid glycoprotein concentration < 1.0 g/L). This limitation also applies, of course, to the restriction method used in the analysis of the present paper.

Recently, it has been proposed to adjust values using regression analysis [12]. Although this approach offers several theoretical advantages, its validity remains to be investigated by comparison with a reference standard. The ratio of concentrations of soluble transferrin receptor/log ferritin has been suggested as a marker of body iron content but its use to detect iron deficiency remains problematic for reasons discussed elsewhere [4].

Our results clearly show that, in the absence of inflammation or *Plasmodium* infection, ZPP has added diagnostic value in detecting iron deficiency over haemoglobin concentration alone. This added value applied both to ZPP measured in whole blood or erythrocytes. By contrast, we found that the diagnostic performance of haemoglobin concentration in detecting iron deficiency was similar in pregnant women (AUC: 61%, [4]) as in children (AUC: 63%, present study); in pregnant women, however, replacement of haemoglobin concentration by ZPP, or addition by ZPP to haemoglobin concentration, whether measured in whole blood or in erythrocytes, had little diagnostic value [4].

When combined with haemoglobin concentration, whole blood ZPP or erythrocyte ZPP yielded AUC values for the ROC curves of approximately 84%. Whether this accuracy is satisfactory depends on the purpose of testing. Conventional cut-off points for whole blood ZPP and erythrocyte ZPP are clearly inappropriate and produce gross overestimates of prevalence and a very low positive predictive value (Table 5 in this paper; see also [4]) due to their low specificity. Mwangi et al. 2014 [4], reported how cut-off points can be manipulated to minimize bias in the estimation of population prevalence. In the present paper, we have shown how cut-off points for haemoglobin and whole blood ZPP, either alone or in combination, can be calibrated in a screen-and-treat strategy to identify individuals with iron deficiency at community level. Screening generally requires the selection of a cut-off point to ensure a high sensitivity for the test or combination of tests to be employed. Such high sensitivity ensures that most cases are detected, at the cost of false positives that can be eliminated by further diagnostic tests. Although the accuracy of this approach is insufficient to give a final diagnosis in all individuals, the combination of haemoglobin concentration and whole blood ZPP can constitute a rapid and convenient method to rule out iron deficiency in a substantial proportion of children screened. Although we considered the example of screening at community level, a similar strategy can be employed in clinical practice to identify children who may need referral to higher levels of care for further testing. When $0.07195[Hb] + 0.01449[ZZP_{whole}] < 10.39334$, the diagnostic accuracy may be improved by using a combination of erythrocyte ZPP with haemoglobin concentration, but the improved diagnostic accuracy thus achieved must be weighed against the procedure of washing red cells, which may be cumbersome in practice.

One problem that has not been solved in our study is the difficulty in detecting iron deficiency in the presence of inflammation. The associations found between ZPP and *Plasmodium* infection and between ZPP and C-reactive protein, underscore the importance of this issue. Further research is required to extend and validate our approach with appropriately selected reference standard for iron deficiency in a population that included individuals with inflammation and infections. Because point-of-care tests are rapidly developing, with quantitative tests already being commercially available for plasma concentrations of ferritin and C-reactive protein, and for various infections, this is likely to be a fruitful area of future research.

Conclusion

In Kenyan preschool children, ZPP, whether measured in whole blood or in erythrocytes, has added diagnostic value in detecting iron deficiency over haemoglobin concentration alone. When used in a screen-and-treat approach, combination of haemoglobin concentration and whole blood ZPP in a single diagnostic score can be used as a rapid and convenient testing method to rule out iron deficiency in a substantial proportion of children screened.

Abbreviations

AGP: α_1-acid glycoprotein; AUC: Area-under-the-curve; CRP: C-reactive protein; EP: Erythrocyte protoporphyrin; FEP: Free erythrocyte protoporphyrin; Hb: haemoglobin concentration; HRP2: Histidine-rich protein-2; IPT: Intermittent preventive treatment; pLDH: *Plasmodium* lactate dehydrogenase; ROC: Receiver operating characteristics; WHO: World Health Organization; ZPP: Zinc protoporphyrin

Acknowledgements

This work was supported by DSM Sight and Life and MRC for personal grant to ET. We thank local authorities, field staff, community workers, research assistants, and students involved in the study.

Funding
The study was funded by Sight and Life, a non-profit organisation established by Royal DSM Chemicals, Heerlen, The Netherlands, and International Nutrition Group of the Medical Research Council, UK. Micronutrients other than iron were included in the supplements at the request of Sight and Life; the funder had no further role in study design, data collection and analysis, preparation of the manuscript or decision to publish.

Authors' contributions
ET assisted in the study design and coordinated field work. PEAA supervised field work. AYD supervised biochemical analyses. HV conceived, designed, and supervised all aspects of the study. ET and HV conducted statistical analyses and prepared the first draft manuscript. All authors read and approved the final manuscript.

Competing interests
The authors declare that they have no competing interests.

Author details
[1]MRCG Keneba at MRC Unit The Gambia, PO Box 273, Banjul, The Gambia. [2]MRC International Nutrition Group, Faculty of Epidemiology and Population Heath, London School of Hygiene and Tropical Medicine, Keppel Street, London WC1E7HT, UK. [3]Meander Medical Centre, Laboratory for Clinical Chemistry, Maatweg 3, 3813 TZ, Amersfoort, Netherlands. [4]School of Public Health and Community Development, Maseno University, Private Bag, Maseno, Kenya. [5]Division of Human Nutrition and Cell Biology and Immunology Group, Wageningen University, P.O. Box 17, 6700 AA Wageningen, The Netherlands.

References
1. Erythrocyte protoporphyrin testing; approved guideline. NCCLS document C42-A. National Committee for Clinical Laboratory Standards: Wayne, PA; 1996.
2. Assessing the iron status of populations, 2nd ed. Report of a joint World Health Organization/Centers for Disease Control and Prevention technical consultation on the assessment of iron status at the population level (Geneva, Switzerland: 6–8 April 2004). Geneva, Switzerland: World Health Organization; 2007.
3. UN Children's Fund/UN University/World Health Organization: Iron deficiency anaemia: assessment, prevention, and control. a guide for programme managers. Document reference WHO/NHD/01.3. Geneva, Switzerland: World Health Organization; 2001.
4. Mwangi MN, Maskey S, Andango PE, Shinali NK, Roth JM, Trijsburg L, et al. Diagnostic utility of zinc protoporphyrin to detect iron deficiency in Kenyan pregnant women. BMC Med. 2014;12:229.
5. Teshome EM, Andang o PEA, Osoti V, Terwel SR, Otieno W, Demir AY, Prentice AM, Verhoef H. Daily home fortification with iron as ferrous fumarate versus NaFeEDTA: a randomised, placebo-controlled, non-inferiority trial in Kenyan children. BMC Med. 2017; [in press]
6. WHO Multicentre Growth Reference Study Group. WHO child growth standards: length/height-for-age, weight-for-age, weight-for-length, weight-for-height and body mass index-for-age: methods and development. Geneva: World Health Organization; 2006.
7. Hastka J, Lasserre J, Schwarzbeck A, Strauch M, Hehlmann R. Washing erythrocytes to remove interferents in measurements of zinc protoporphyrin by front-face hematofluorometry. Clin Chem. 1992;38(11):2184–9.
8. Hastka J, Lasserre J, Schwarzbeck A, Hehlmann R. Central role of zinc protoporphyrin in staging iron deficiency. Clin Chem. 1994;40(5):768–73.
9. Serum ferritin concentrations for the assessment of iron status and iron deficiency in populations. Document reference WHO/NMH/NHD/MNM/11.2. Geneva, Switzerland: World Health Organization; 2011.
10. Haemoglobin concentrations for the diagnosis of anaemia and assessment of severity. Document reference WHO/NMH/NHD/MNM/11.1. Geneva, Switzerland: World Health Organization; 2011.
11. Abraham K, Muller C, Gruters A, Wahn U, Schweigert FJ. Minimal inflammation, acute phase response and avoidance of misclassification of vitamin a and iron status in infants—importance of a high-sensitivity C-reactive protein (CRP) assay. Int J Vitam Nutr Res. 2003;73(6):423–30.
12. Suchdev PS, Namaste SML, Aaron GJ, Raiten DJ, Brown KH, Flores-Ayala R. On behalf of the BRINDA working group. Overview of the biomarkers reflecting inflammation and nutritional determinants of anemia (BRINDA) project. Adv Nutr. 2016;7(2):349–56.
13. Bland JM, Altman DG. Measurement error proportional to the mean. BMJ. 1996;313(7049):106.
14. Royston P, Altman DG, Sauerbrei W. Dichotomizing continuous predictors in multiple regression: a bad idea. Stat Med. 2006;25(1):127–41.
15. Robin X, Turck N, Hainard A, Tiberti N, Lisacek F, Sanchez J-C, Müller M. pROC: an open-source package for R and S+ to analyze and compare ROC curves. BMC Bioinformatics. 2011;12:77.
16. Altman DG, Machin D, Bryant TN, Gardner MJ (eds.). Statistics with confidence, 2nd ed. London, BMJ Books; 2000. (including CIA software).
17. Suchdev PS, Ruth LJ, Earley M, Macharia A, Williams TN. The burden and consequences of inherited blood disorders among young children in western Kenya. Matern Child Nutr. 2014;10(1):135–44.
18. Tsang BL, Sullivan KM, Ruth LJ, Williams TN, Suchdev PS. Nutritional status of young children with inherited blood disorders in western Kenya. Am J Trop Med Hyg. 2014;90(5):955–62.
19. Atkinson SH, Rockett K, Sirugo G, Bejon PA, Fulford A, O'Connell MA, Bailey R, Kwiatkowski DP, Prentice AM. Seasonal childhood anaemia in West Africa is associated with the haptoglobin 2-2 genotype. PLoS Med. 2006;3(5):e172.
20. Altman DG. Why we need confidence intervals. World J Surg. 2005;29:554–6.
21. Pepe MS. The statistical evaluation of medical tests for classification and prediction. Oxford: Oxford University Press; 2003.

Characteristics of chronic lymphocytic leukemia in Senegal

Abibatou Sall[1*], Awa Oumar Touré[1], Fatimata Bintou Sall[1], Moussa Ndour[1], Seynabou Fall[2], Abdoulaye Sène[1], Blaise Félix Faye[1], Moussa Seck[1], Macoura Gadji[1], Tandakha Ndiaye Dièye[1], Claire Mathiot[3], Sophie Reynaud[4], Saliou Diop[1] and Martine Raphaël[5]

Abstract

Background: Chronic lymphocytic leukemia (CLL) is a mature B-cell neoplasm characterized by the expansion of CD5-positive lymphocytes in peripheral blood. While CLL is the most common type of leukemia in Western populations, the disease is rare in Africans. Hence, clinical and laboratory data and studies of CLL in Sub Saharan populations have been limited. The aims of this study were to analyze the characteristics of senegalese patients with CLL at the time of the diagnosis and to identify the correlation between clinical characteristics (Binet stage) with age, gender, laboratory parameters and chromosomal abnormalities.

Methods: In this study, we investigated the clinical and laboratory characteristics of CLL in Senegal. A total of 40 patients who had been diagnosed with CLL during the period from July 2011 to April 2015 in Senegal were evaluated. Cytology and immunophenotype were performed in all patients to confirm the diagnosis. The prognosis factors such as Binet staging, CD38 and cytogenetic abnormalities were studied. The statistical analysis was performed using STATA version 13 (Stata college station Texas). Each patient signed a free and informed consent form before participating in the study.

Results: The mean age was 61 years ranged from 48 to 85. There were 31 males and only 9 females (sex ratio M : F = 3,44). At diagnosic, 82.5 % of the patients were classified as having advanced Binet stages B or C. The prognosis marker CD38 was positive in 28 patients. Cytogenetic abnormalities studied by FISH were performed in 25 patients, among them, 68 % (17 cases) had at least one cytogenetic abnormality and 28 % had 2 simultaneous cytogenetic abnormalities.

Conclusion: Africans may present with CLL at a younger age and our data suggest that CLL in Senegal may be more aggressive than in Western populations.

Keywords: Chronic lymphocytic leukemia, Clinic, Cytology, Immunophenotype, Cytogenetic abnormalities

Background

Chronic lymphocytic leukemia (CLL) is the most frequent form of leukemia in Western countries [1, 2]. The median age at diagnosis ranges between 67 and 72 years and males are more likely to develop the disease than females [3, 4]. CLL is characterized by clonal proliferation and accumulation of mature, typically CD5-positive B-cells within the blood, bone marrow, lymph nodes, and spleen [5]. It is a heterogeneous disease which can present as an aggressive and life threatening leukemia or as an indolent form that will not require treatment over decades. Rai et al. (1975) [6] and Binet et al. (1981) [7] staging systems are the standard clinical staging to estimate prognosis of patients. However, both systems fail to indicate the higher risk of progression among patients in early stages of the disease. These clinical staging systems were complemented by prognostic markers based on : serum prognostic factors, immunoglobulin heavy chain variable region (*IGHV*) mutation status, some cytogenetic abnormalities, cell membrane expression of CD38, and intracellular expression of zeta-associated protein-70 (ZAP- 70) [5, 8, 9].

As CLL is a rare disease in Africa [10, 11], clinical and laboratory data and studies in Sub Saharan populations

* Correspondence: sallabibatou@gmail.com
[1]Hematology, Cheikh Anta Diop University, Dakar, Senegal
Full list of author information is available at the end of the article

have been limited. In this first study of CLL in Senegal, we have investigated the clinico-biological characteristics of the disease at time of diagnosis.

The first objective of this current study was to analyze the characteristics of senegalese patients with CLL at the time of the diagnosis. The second objective was to identify the correlation between clinical characteristics (Binet stage) with age, gender, laboratory parameters and chromosomal abnormalities.

Methods

Patients

In a prospective study, a total of 40 patients diagnosed with CLL between July 2011 to April 2015, in different hospitals in Senegal were evaluated. The diagnosis was based on morphological and immunophenotypical findings according the World Health Organization (WHO) classification (2008) [12]. The patients were not treated at diagnosis and clinical characteristics including age, gender, symptoms and clinical features were provided by referring physicians. All of the patients were classified using the Binet staging system as one of the three groups (A, B or C). The Binet staging system [7] is based on the number of involved areas, as defined by the presence of enlarged lymph nodes of greater than 1 cm in diameter or organomegaly, and on whether there is anemia or thrombocytopenia. Binet stages are defined as follows:

- Stage A : Hemoglobin (Hb) more than 10 g/dL and platelets above 100 x 10^9/L and to two of the superfical lymph nodes involved.
- Stage B : Hb above 10 g/dl and platelets above 100 x 10^9/L and organomegaly greater than that defined for Stage A (i.e., three or more areas of nodal or organ enlargement).
- Stage C : All patients who have Hb of less than 10 g/dL and/or a platelet count of less than 100 x 10^9/L, irrespective of organomegaly.

Peripheral Blood cells Counts

The peripheral blood cells counts were performed on the Symex XT2000i ™ (Sysmex Diagnostics, Japan) and a blood smear stained by May Grunwald Giemsa was obtained for all patients.

Immunophenotypical analysis

In each patient, immunophenotype of leukemic cells was performed by flow cytometry, using the FacsCalibur™ flow cytometer (Becton Dickinson, CA, USA). Different panels of antibodies were used to assess the immunophenotype CLL scoring system proposed by Matutes et al. [13]. These monoclonal antibodies were : CD45-APC/CD19-PerCP/kappa-FITC/lambda-PE/CD5-PE/FMC7-FITC/CD22-FITC/CD23-PE/CD10-FITC/CD38-PE/CD11c-PE/CD25-FITC/CD103-FITC. Data were acquired and analyzed with the BD CellQuest Pro software (Becton Dickinson).

Fluorescence in situ hybridization

Cytogenetic abnormalities were determined by Fluorescence in situ hybridization (FISH) on peripheral blood using Vysis probes (Abbott) according to the manufacturer recommandations. The following abnormalities : del13q14 (D13S319 probe), del 11q22 (ATM probe), del17p13 (TP53 probe) and trisomy 12 (CEP 12 DNA Probe) were tested.

Ethical considerations

The study was approved by the « Research Ethics Committee » of Cheikh Anta Diop University and each patient signed a free and informed consent form before participating. A written consent for publication of personal information, such as that contained in table, was obtained from all participants. Written consent to publish the images contained in Fig. 1 was also obtained from the relevant participant.

Statistical analysis

Data were collected using Microsoft Excel Spreadsheet and then transferred to Stata for data management and statistical analysis. Continuous variables were described as mean with standard deviation or as median with inter quartile range if the variable was not normally distributed. Qualitative variables were described as proportion. For the bivariate analysis, difference between means was tested using the student *t*-test or the Mann–Whitney non-parametric depending on the normality assumption. Association between categorical variables was performed using the Pearson chi-square test or the Fisher exact test. The estimations were done within a 95 % confidence level and the entire statistical tests were significant when the p value was below the threshold level of 0.05. The statistical analysis was performed using STATA version 13 (Stata college station Texas).

Results

Of the 40 patients studied, 31 were males and only 9 females (sex ratio M : F = 3,44). The mean age was 61 years ranged from 48 to 85. Table 1 shows the age and sex distribution of the CLL patients in this study. CLL occurred frequently between 55–70 years (55 % of patients). Just over one quarter of patients was under 50 years old.

The most frequently found symptoms were related to tumor syndrome; it was mainly discomfort, pain or mass abodominal observed in 80 % of cases. Signs of impaired general condition: weight loss, asthenia or anorexia were

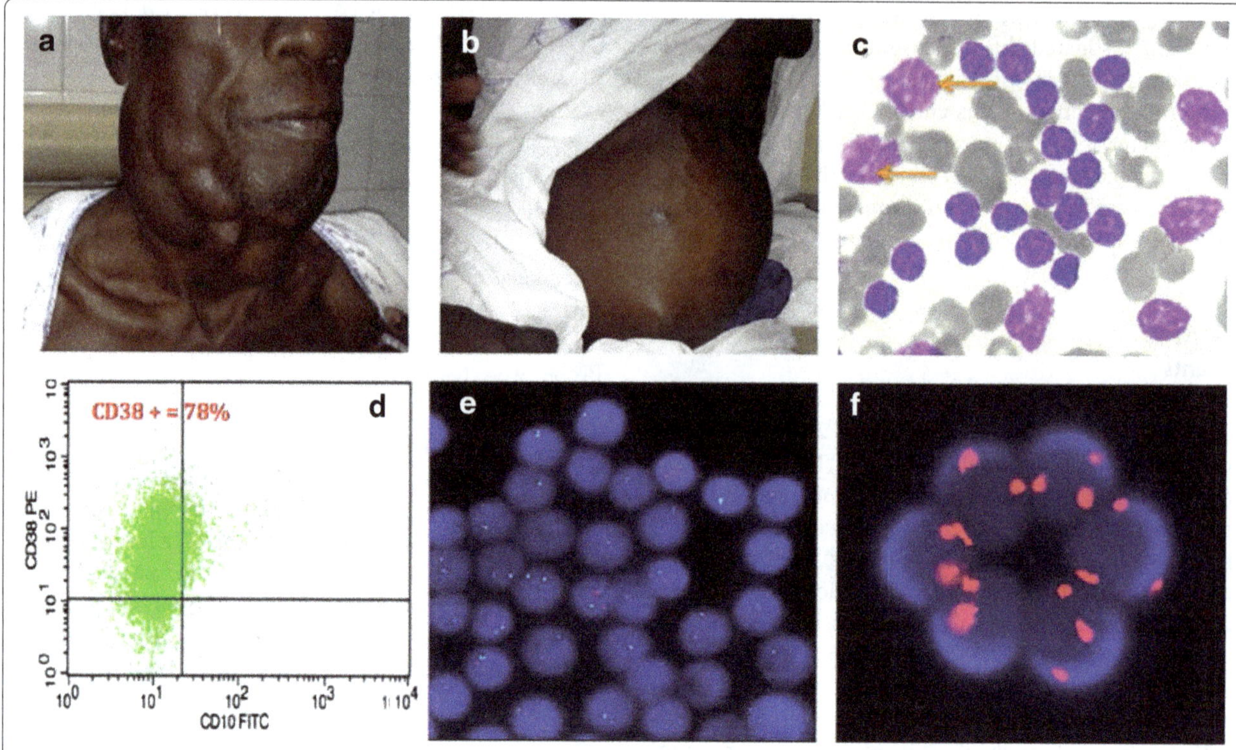

Fig. 1 **a** Bulky cervical lymph nodes. **b** Huge splenomegaly with splenic abcess. **c** Peripheral blood smear, typical small lymphocytes,with hypermature clumped chromatin and scanty cytoplasm. Presence of smudge cells (arrows). **d** Immunophenotype with CD38 positivity. **e** FISH, bi allelic deletion of 13q. **f** trisomy 12 (FISH)

found respectively in 52.5- 65 -30 % of cases. There was only one patient with a bleeding symptoms (Table 2).

Clinically, tumor syndrome was evident in most patients. The enlarged lymph nodes were present in 72 % of patients (Fig. 1a) and 26 patients had a palpable spleen of which 40 % had at least one splenomegaly according to Hackett type III (Fig. 1b).

The average lymphocytosis was very high : 186.68x10^9/L, ranges between : 5.03 to 869x10^9/L. The blood smears showed mature lymphocytes with clumped chromatin and scanty cytoplasm (Fig. 1c). Prolymphocytes, counted in all cases, were present in only 9 cases and the percentage was below 15 %. Smudge cells (Fig. 1c, arrows) were observed in almost all peripheral blood smears except in 3 cases.

Table 1 Age and sex distribution

Variables	Number	Proportion (%)
Age groups (years)		
<55	11	27.5
55–70	22	55
>70	7	17.5
Sex		
Male	31	77.5
Female	9	22.5

The mean hemoglobin level was 9.5 g/dl (Ranges: 3.9 to 15.2), 55 % of patients had an hemoglobin less than 10 g/dl. Thrombocytopenia was observed in 21 patients. The platelets count was below 50x10^9/L in 6 patients (patients : 3, 15, 18, 23, 32, 40. Table 3) and the mean platelets levels was 149.07x10^9/L (Ranges: 21- 452x10^9/L) (Table 3).

At diagnosis, 82.5 % of patients dysplayed an advanced Binet clinical stage : 22.5 % were stage B and 62.5 % were stage C. Only 7 patients were in stage A.

The Matutes scoring was 4 or 5 in almost all patients confirming the CLL diagnosis. Three patients had an atypical CLL with a score at 3/5.

The prognosis marker CD38 was positive (Fig. 1d) in 28 patients of the series, including 4 patients in stage A (Table 4).

Cytogenetic abnormalities studied by FISH were performed in 25 patients, among them, 68 % (17 cases) had at least one cytogenetic abnormality and 28 % had 2 simultaneous cytogenetic abnormalities.

The 13q deletion was found in 44 % of cases (11/25) and 3 patients (patients 6, 15, 23. Table 3) had a biallelic deletion (Fig. 1e). Seven patients had trisomy 12 (Fig. 1f) while 11q and 17p deletions were found in 3 cases each.

Table 2 Clinical features in our patients

Clinical features	Number (l = 40)	Proportion (%)
Symptoms		
Weight loss	21	52.5
Abdominal pain/discomfort	19	47.5
Abdominal mass	13	32.5
Weakness	26	65
Cervical, axillary or inguinal mass	19	47.5
Anorexia	12	30
Fever	07	17.5
Nght swaet	03	7.5
Bleeding	01	2.5
Signs		
Anaemia- Pallor	25	62.5
Lymphadenopathy (cervical, axillary, inguinal)	36	72
No lymphadenopathy	04	10
Splenomegaly		
- moderate (I, II Hackett)	11	27.5
- gross splenomegaly (III, IV,V Hackett)	16	40
Spleen no palpable	13	32.5
Hepatomegaly	06	15
Respiratory tract infection	04	10

Note that patients with bi allelic deletion of 13q or 17p deletion were in stage C (Table 3). Twenty four percent of patients on Stage A or B had at least one cytogenetic abnormality versus 66.7 % in stage C. However this difference was not statistically significant (p value = 0.23 Table 4). The deletion of the long arm of the chromosome 11 were observed in 8.3 % of patients with stage A or B and in 15, 4 % of patients classified in the advanced stage (stage C). The statistical test shows that this difference was not significant (p = 0.58). In addition, the deletion of the short arm of the chromosome 17 was not observed in any patient on stage A or B, whereas this abnormality was detected in 24 % of patients on stage C (Table 4).

The number of lymphocytes count was significantly greater in patients with stage C than in those in the group with stages A or B (p = 0.005). The average number of lymphocytes was 269.5 x 10^9/L in the advanced stage group compared to 61.5 x 10^9/L in patients classified in stage A or B.

Discussion

Chronic lymphocytic leukaemia (CLL) is the most common form of leukaemia in Western countries [1, 2] while it is extremely rare in Africa [10, 11]. In 3 years, only 40 patients with CLL were identified in several centers of Senegal with an average age of 61 years (Ranges : 48–85 years). This average age is comparable to Nigerian [10, 11] and Ethiopian [14] studies which found respectively a mean age of 60, 56 and 55 years.

However, this average age at diagnosis is somewhat higher in Western Countries : American (72 years) [5], English (74 years) [15] or French (72 years) [16]. There is at least 10 years between the age of onset of CLL in African compared to Westerners. We speculate that Africans present with CLL at a younger age than Western patients.

These data may support the idea that environmental factors, remaining to be identified, may be involved. It has been postulated that CLL occurring in younger adults in Africa is a consequence of recurrent malaria and other infections, resulting in a polyclonal B-cell proliferation which in an extreme form is hyper reactive malarial splenomegaly [17].

Male dominance has been reported in the most published series [5, 10, 15, 16]. In ours, male dominance was evident with a ratio M/F = 3.44. A different evolution according to gender was however raised and proved [3, 18, 19]. Catovsky et al. [4] demonstrates that CLL runs a more benign clinical course in women than in men. Women were more likely to have Binet stage A than B or C; their overall survival rates at 10 years were better than for men and they had a better overall response to treatment. No good hypothesis have been advanced to explain the observed trend for a better outcome in women. However, the implications of gender differences in the pathogenesis of CLL and its treatment require further studies. Among our 40 cases, 9 were women (4 in stage A or B and 5 in stage C). We have not however found significant differences between men and women compared to Binet stages (p = 0.75).

CD38 is a well-known lymphocyte differentiation antigen with proposed receptor and adhesion molecule functions. In mature circulating B cells, CD38 ligation induced proliferation by promoting the expression of CD25, MHC-II, and certain cytokines [20, 21].

The prognosis role of CD38 in CLL was first proposed on the basis of an immunophenotypical study of CLL cases with known IGHV sequences. CD38 predicted shorter overall survival rates when expressed on 30 % or more CLL cells [22]. Since this report in 1999, CD38 expression has been well established as an independent prognostic factor in CLL by numerous reports, but with various cut-off levels. While Del Poeta et al. [23] and Hamblin et al. [24] proposed 30 % as the best cut-off, others proposed 20 % [25] or even 7 % [26]. Further cooperative studies are still necessary to define a common cut-off level. We use the cut-off of 30 % in our patients. The CD38 were express in 70 % of patients from the series; 12 of them were stage A or B and 16 patients in stage C in the Binet system. We did not find significant difference between the expression of CD38 and the different stages of Binet (p = 0.75).

Table 3 Characteristics of 40 CLL patients

Patients N°	Age/ Sex	Lymphocytesx10^9/ L	Haemoglobin g/dl	Platelests x10^9/L	Binet Stage	CD38 expression*	Deletion of 13q ($n = 11/25$)	Deletion of 11q ($n = 3/25$)	Trisomy 12 ($n = 7/25$)	Deletion of 17p ($n = 3/25$)
1	63/F	33.4	13.3	279	A	+	-	-	-	-
2	50/F	268.8	8.4	140	C	+	-	-	Yes	-
3	65/M	52.248	12.4	24	B	+	Yes	-	-	-
4	53/M	831.14	5.2	69	C	+	Yes	Yes	-	-
5	54/M	225.5	7.5	137	C	Negative	Yes	-	-	-
6	69/M	179.5	4.4	81	C	+	Yes (biallelic)	-	-	-
7	80/M	49	11.2	200	A	Negative	-	-	-	-
8	63/M	230	9.3	206	C	+	-	-	Yes	Yes
9	50/M	58	8.8	66	C	+	-	Yes	-	-
10	51/M	88.55	9.5	97	C	+	-	-	-	-
11	63/M	145.78	9.7	203	C	Negative	Yes	-	-	Yes
12	59/M	42.6	10.3	126	B	+	yes	-	Yes	-
13	67/M	5.8	15.2	220	A	+	-	-	-	-
14	67/F	6.4	11.6	332	A	+	Yes	-	-	-
15	70/M	491.4	6	31	C	+	Yes (biallelic)	-	Yes	-
16	57/F	12.8	13	229	A	+	-	-	-	-
17	80/F	93.34	13.2	157	B	+	Yes	-	Yes	-
18	60/M	82.3	7.9	28	C	Negative	-	-	Yes	-
19	85/M	397	8.9	108	C	+	-	-	-	Yes
20	54/M	87.8	10.7	239	A	Negative	-	-	-	-
21	60/M	16.38	12.6	276	B	+	-	-	-	-
22	63/M	789.2	8	262	C	Negative	-	-	-	-
23	54/M	51.76	4.9	44	C	+	Yes (biallelic)	-	-	-
24	67/M	201.5	10.3	263	B	+	-	-	yes	-
25	60/M	171	12	203	B	+	yes	yes	-	-
26	72/M	15	6.5	115	C	Negative				
27	58/M	7.1	12.1	146	A	Negative				
28	73/M	241	7.6	242	C	+				
29	74/M	12.7	10.9	157	B	Negative				
30	63/M	734	8.8	151	C	Negative				
31	68/M	5.03	12.1	64	C	+				
32	48/M	165.33	6.7	34	C	Negative				
33	60/M	85.5	11	152	B	+				
34	52/M	156.3	11.2	452	B	+				
35	48/F	365.8	9.7	76	C	+				
36	78/F	198	7.4	115	C	+				
37	54/F	27	9.8	88	C	+				
38	59/M	131	12.8	76	C	Negative				
39	64/F	869	9	54	C	+				
40	55/M	114.41	3.9	21	C	+				
Mean	186.68	9.5	149.07							

CD38 expression : positive if >30 %

Table 4 Correlation between clinical stage and laboratory findings

Characteristics	Clinical staging system according to Binet and al.		
	Either stage A or B	Stage C	*P value**
	N (%)	N (%)	
Age (years) $n = 40$			
<55	2 (12.5)	9(37.5)	0.1
55-70	11 (68.7)	11(45.8)	
<70	3 (18.75)	4 (16.67)	
Sex ($n = 40$)			
Male	12 (75)	19 (20)	0.75
Female	4 (25)	5 (80)	
Average lymphocytes x10^9/L ($n = 40$)	61.5	269.5	0.005*
At least one cytogenetic abnormality ($n = 25$)			
Yes	06 (24)	11 (44)	0.097
No	06 (24)	02 (08)	
Deletion 13q			
Yes	05 (42)	06 (46.15)	0.82
No	07 (58)	07 (53.85)	
Deletion 11q			
Yes	1 (8.3)	2(15.4)	0.58
No	11 (91.7)	11(84.6)	
Trisomy 12			
Yes	03 (25)	04 (31)	0.74
No	9 (75)	9 (71)	
Deletion 17p			
Yes	00 (00)	03 (24)	0.07
No	12 (100)	10 (76)	
CD38 expression ($n = 40$)			
Positive	12 (75)	16 (67)	0.75
Negative	04 (25)	08 (33)	

The others evaluated prognostic factors were cytogenetic abnormalities perfomed by FISH. The 13q deletion was found in 11 patients (44 %), 6 of them were in stage C. Deletions on the long arm of chromosome 13, specifically involving band 13q14 (del (13q14)) represent the single most frequently observed cytogenetic aberration in CLL, occurring in approx. 55 % of all cases [5]. An isolated del 13q14 is typically characterized by a benign course of the disease. Three of our patients had a biallelic deletion of 13q and they were all in Binet stage C. Nevertheless it has been demonstrated that, there was no difference in the baseline characteristics between patients with CLL who had monoallelic or biallelic deletion of 13q. In addition, there was no significant difference in endpoints, including time to treatment [27]. Interestingly, it has been shown that the size of the 13q deletion is associated with outcome, since patients with CLL with larger aberrations have a shorter time to treatment and overall survival, indicating that several genes included in the deletion have an effect on the disease course [28, 29].

Trisomy 12 is detected in 11–16 % of patients at diagnosis [9] and is associated with an intermediate prognosis [9, 30, 31]. Seven of our patients had trisomy 12 (28 %) including 4 stage C Binet ($p = 0.74$). The genes involved in the pathogenesis of CLL carrying a trisomy 12 are largely unknown. Furthermore, the prognostic relevance of trisomy 12 remains a matter of debate [32].

The deletions of 11q22-q23 and 17p13 are known to be associated with poor prognosis in CLL [5, 9, 31, 32]. The deletion of 11q is most often monoallelic and carried by 10–17 % of patients with CLL [9, 30]. The minimal deleted region is known to encode several tumor suppressor genes including *ATM* which plays an important role in cell cycle regulation. The deletion of 17p is detected at a frequency of 3–7 % at diagnosis [9, 30]. The 17p deletion often involves the entire p-arm, but some losses are focused to the 17p13.1 region, which encodes the *TP53* gene among several other genes. This gene is a key regulator of the cell cycle. The 11q deletion was found in 2 patients in stage C and 1 B stage while the 3 patients with 17p deletion were all in stage C. No significance was found between these poor prognosis deletions and Binet clinical stages (Table 4). This could be explained by the small size of our series as Lai et al. [33] obtained significant differences in the distribution of p53 deletion according to Binet classification system (P = 0.008).

The number of lymphocytes count was significantly greater in patients with stage C than in those in the group with stages A or B (p = 0.005). A high lymphocytosis could be associated to poor prognosis in African with CLL. However Shvidel et al. [34] demonstrated that although CLL patients presenting with hyperleukocytosis at diagnosis generally have an aggressive clinical course, this is not an independent predictor of survival in CLL. In any case, further studies are needed to better define the role of lymphocytosis in prognostic factors for CLL.

Conclusion

This study helps to define the characteristics of CLL in sub-Saharan Africa. The patient type would be aged 60 years with a major tumor syndrome, higher lymphocytosis to 150 x 10^9/L, stage C according to Binet clinical stage, positivity of CD38 and at least one cytogenetic abnormality at biological level.

CLL is certainly much less common in Africa than in Western countries but African patients seem to have a worse prognosis compared to Westerners. We assess time to treatment and the time of overall survival at 5 years to better answer this question.

Abbreviations

CLL: Chronic lymphocytic leukemia; FISH: Fluorescence in situ hybridization; IGVH: Immunoglobulin heavy chain variable region; Zap 70: Zeta-associated protein 70; WHO: World Health Organization; Hb: Hemoglobin; MCH II: Major histocompatibility complex class II.

Competing interest

The authors declare that they have no competing interest.

Authors' contributions

SF, BFF, MS, SD provided clinical data. AS, FBS, AOT and AS participated on cytologic studies. AS, MN, CM, TND carried out the immunophenotypic analysis. AS, MG, SR participated on cytogenetic studies. AS, AOT and MR made substantial contributions to conception and design as well as to analysis and interpretation of data. All authors read and approved the final manuscript.

Acknowledgements

We thank INCa (Institut National du Cancer) and AMCC (Alliance mondiale contre le Cancer) for their support.

Financial disclosures

The authors have no financial relationships relevant to this article to disclose.

Author details

[1]Hematology, Cheikh Anta Diop University, Dakar, Senegal. [2]Hematology, Aristide Le Dantec Hospital, Dakar, Senegal. [3]Curie Institute, Paris, France. [4]Hematology, University Hospital, Nice, France. [5]University Paris XI, Paris, France.

References

1. National Cancer Institute: Surveillance, Epidemiology, and End Results: Populations (1969–2010). http://seer.cancer.gov.
2. Sant M, Allemani C, Tereanu C, De Angelis R, Capocaccia R, Visser O, et al. Incidence of hematologic malignancies in Europe by morphologic subtype: results of the HAEMACARE project. Blood. 2010;116(19):3724–34.
3. Molica S. Sex differences in incidence and outcome of chronic lymphocytic leukemia patients. Leuk Lymphoma. 2006;47:1477–80.
4. Catovsky D, Wade R, Else M. The clinical significance of patients' sex in chronic lymphocytic leukemia. Haematologica. 2014;99(6):1088–94.
5. Hallek M. Chronic lymphocytic leukemia: 2015 Update on diagnosis, risk stratification, and treatment. Am J Hematol. 2015;90(5):446–60.
6. Rai KR, Sawitsky A, Cronkite EP, et al. Clinical staging of chronic lymphocytic leukemia. Blood. 1975;46:219–34.
7. Binet JL, Auquier A, Dighiero G, et al. A new prognostic classification of chronic lymphocytic leukemia derived from a multivariate survival analysis. Cancer. 1981;48:198–204.
8. Cramer P, Hallek M. Prognostic factors in chronic lymphocytic leukemia. « what do we need to know? ». Nat Rev Clin Oncol. 2011;8:38–47.
9. Rosenquist R, Cortese D, Bhoi S, Mansouri L, Gunnarsson R. Prognostic markers and their clinical applicability in chronic lymphocytic leukemia: where do we stand? Leuk Lymphoma. 2013;54(11):2351–64.
10. Salawu L, Bolarinwa RA, Durosinmi MA. Chronic lymphocytic leukaemia: a-twenty-years experience and problems in Ile-Ife, South-Western Nigeria. Afr Health Sci. 2010;10(2):187–92.
11. Omoti CE, Awodu OA, Bazuaye GN. Chronic lymphoid leukaemia: clinico-haematological correlation and outcome in a single institution in Niger Delta region of Nigeria. Int J Lab Hematol. 2007;29(6):426–32.
12. Müller-Hermelink HK, Montserrat E, Catovsky D, et al. Chronic lymphocytic leukemia/small lymphocytic lymphoma. In: Swerdlow SH, Campo E, Harris NL et al. editors. World Health Organization Classification of Tumours of Haematopoietic and Lymphoid Tissues. Lyon: IARC 4th Edition; 2008. pp 180–182.
13. Matutes E, Owusu-Ankomah K, Morilla R, et al. The immunological profile of B-cell disorders and proposal of a scoring system for the diagnosis of CLL. Leukemia. 1994;8:1640–5.
14. Shamebo M, Gebremedhin A. Chronic lymphocytic leukaemia in Ethiopians. East Afr Med J. 1996;73(10):643–6.
15. Pfeil AM, Imfeld P, Pettengell R, Jick SS, Szucs TD, Meier CR, Schwenkglenks M. Trends in incidence and medical resource utilisation in patients with chronic lymphocytic leukaemia: insights from the UK Clinical Practice Research Datalink (CPRD). Ann Hematol. 2015;94(3):421–9.
16. Projections de l'incidence et de la mortalité par cancer en France en 2011. Cancers/Surveillance épidémiologique des cancers/Projections Estimations de l'incidence et de la mortalité en France en 2011.
17. Fleming AF, Terunuma H, Tembo C, et al. Leukaemias in Zambia. Leukaemia. 1999;13:1292–3.
18. Molica S, Mauro FR, Callea V, Gentile M, Giannarelli D, Lopez M, et al. GIMEMA CLL Study Group. A gender-based score system predicts the clinical outcome of patients with early B-cell chronic lympho- cytic leukemia. Leuk Lymphoma. 2005;46(4):553–60.
19. Chen C, Puvvada S. Prognostic Factors for Chronic Lymphocytic Leukemia. Curr Hematol Malig Rep. 2016;11(1):37–42.
20. Malavasi F, Deaglio S, Funaro A, Ferrero E, Horenstein AL, Ortolan E, et al. Evolution and function of the ADP ribosyl cyclase/CD38 gene family in physiology and pathology. Physiol Rev. 2008;88(3):841–86.
21. Funaro A, Morra M, Calosso L, Zini MG, Ausiello CM. Malavasi F Role of the human CD38 molecule in B cell activation and proliferation. Tissue Antigens. 1997;49(1):7–15.
22. Damle RN, Wasil T, Fais F, Ghiotto F, Valetto A, Allen SL, Buchbinder A, Budman D, Dittmar K, Kolitz J, Lichtman SM, Schulman P, Vinciguerra VP, Rai KR, Ferrarini M, Chiorazzi N. Ig V gene mutation status and CD38 expression as novel prognostic indicators in chronic lymphocytic leukemia. Blood. 1999;94(6):1840–47.
23. Del Poeta G, Maurillo L, Venditti A, Buccisano F, Epiceno AM, Capelli G, Tamburini A, Suppo G, Battaglia A, Del Principe MI, Del Moro B, Masi M, Amadori S. Clinical significance of CD38 expression in chronic lymphocytic leukemia. Blood. 2001;98(9):2633–39.

24. Hamblin TJ, Orchard JA, Ibbotson RE, Davis Z, Thomas PW, Stevenson FK, Oscier DG. CD38 expression and immunoglobulin variable region mutations are independent prognostic variables in chronic lymphocytic leukemia, but CD38 expression may vary during the course of the disease. Blood. 2002; 99(3):1023–9.
25. Durig J, Naschar M, Schmucker U, Renzing-Kohler K, Holter T, Huttmann A, Duhrsen U. CD38 expression is an important prognostic marker in chronic lymphocytic leukaemia. Leuk Off J Leuk Soc Am Leuk Res Fund UK. 2002; 16(1):30–5.
26. Thornton PD, Fernandez C, Giustolisi GM, Morilla R, Atkinson S, A'Hern RP, Matutes E, Catovsky D. CD38 expression as a prognostic indicator in chronic lymphocytic leukaemia. Hematol J: Off J Eur Haematol Assoc/EHA. 2004; 5(2):145–51.
27. Garg R, Wierda W, Ferrajoli A, Abruzzo L, Pierce S, Lerner S, Keating M, O'Brien S. The prognostic difference of monoallelic versus biallelic deletion of 13q in chronic lymphocytic leukemia. Cancer. 2012;118(14):3531–7.
28. Ouillette P, Erba H, Kujawski L, et al. Integrated genomic profiling of chronic lymphocytic leukemia identifies subtypes of deletion 13q14. Cancer Res. 2008;68:1012–21.
29. Parker H, Rose-Zerilli MJ, Parker A, et al. 13q deletion anatomy and disease progression in patients with chronic lymphocytic leukemia. Leukemia. 2011; 25:489–97.
30. Gunnarsson R, Mansouri L, Isaksson A, et al. Array-based genomic screening at diagnosis and during follow-up in chronic lymphocytic leukemia. Haematologica. 2011;96:1161–9.
31. Smolewski P, Witkowska M, Korycka-Wołowiec A. New insights into biology, prognostic factors, and current therapeutic strategies in chronic lymphocytic leukemia. ISRN Oncol 2013: 740615. 740615. doi: 10.1155/2013/740615.
32. Hallek M. Chronic lymphocytic leukemia: 2013 update on diagnosis, risk stratification and treatment. Am J Hematol. 2013;88(9):803–16.
33. Lai YY, Huang XJ. Cytogenetic characteristics of B cell chronic lymphocytic leukemia in 275 Chinese patients by fluorescence in situ hybridization: a multicenter study. Chin Med J. 2011;124(16):2417–22.
34. Shvidel L, Bairey O, Tadmor T, Braester A, Ruchlemer R, Fineman R, Joffe E, Berrebi A, Polliack A. Absolute lymphocyte count with extreme hyperleukocytosis does not have a prognostic impact in chronic lymphocytic leukemia. Anticancer Res. 2015;35(5):2861–6.

14

Hospitalization for pulmonary embolism associated with antecedent testosterone or estrogen therapy in patients found to have familial and acquired thrombophilia

Marloe Prince[*†], Charles J. Glueck[†], Parth Shah[†], Ashwin Kumar[†], Michael Goldenberg[†], Matan Rothschild[†], Nasim Motayar[†], Vybhav Jetty[†], Kevin Lee[†] and Ping Wang[†]

Abstract

Background: In patients hospitalized over a 4 year period for pulmonary embolism (PE), we assessed relationships of testosterone (TT) and estrogen therapy (ET) anteceding PE in patients found to have familial-acquired thrombophilia.

Methods: From 2011 through 2014, 347 patients were hospitalized in Cincinnati Mercy Hospitals with PE. Retrospective chart review was used to identify patients receiving TT or ET before PE; coagulation studies were done prospectively if necessary.

Results: Preceding hospitalization for PE, 8 of 154 men (5 %) used TT, and 24 of 193 women (12 %) used ET. The median number of months from the initiation of TT or ET to development of PE was 7 months in men and 18 months in women. Of the 6 men having coagulation measures, all had ≥ 1 thrombophilia, and of the 18 women having measures of coagulation, 16 had ≥ 1 thrombophilia. The sensitivity of a previous history of thrombosis to predict PE was low, 25 % (2/8 men), 4 % (1/24 women).

Conclusions: Of 154 men hospitalized for PE, 8 (5 %) used TT, and of 193 women, 24 (12 %) used ET. Our data suggests that PE is an important complication of TT in men and ET in women, in part reflecting an interaction between familial and acquired thrombophilia and exogenous hormone use.

Keywords: Thrombophilia, Testosterone, Estrogen, Pulmonary embolus

Background

When testosterone therapy (TT) is given to men or women with underlying familial or acquired thrombophilia, venous thromboembolism (VTE), deep venous thrombosis (DVT), pulmonary emboli (PE), ocular thrombosis, and osteonecrosis may occur [1–8]. In 67 recently reported cases of VTE, Glueck et al. [8] compared thrombophilia in 67 cases (59 men and 8 women) with thrombotic events after starting testosterone therapy versus 111 patient controls having unprovoked venous thrombotic events without TT. In the 67 patients, thrombosis (47 deep venous thrombosis-pulmonary embolism, 16 osteonecrosis, and 4 ocular thrombosis) occurred 6 months (median) after starting TT. Cases differed from controls for factor V Leiden heterozygosity (16 of the 67 [24 %] vs 13 [12 %] of the 111, P = .038) and for lupus anticoagulant (9 [14 %] of the 64 vs 4 [4 %] of the 106, P = .019). After a first thrombotic event and continuing TT, 11 cases had a second thrombotic event, despite adequate anticoagulation, 6 of whom, still anticoagulated, had a third thrombosis. Screening for thrombophilia before starting TT should identify men and women at high risk for thrombotic events with an adverse risk-benefit ratio for TT. Glueck et al. [8] concluded that when TT is given to patients with familial and acquired thrombophilia, thrombosis may occur and recur in thrombophilic men despite anticoagulation.

* Correspondence: Marloe.prince@gmail.com
[†]Equal contributors
From the Internal Medicine Residency Program, Cholesterol, Metabolism, and Thrombosis Center of the Jewish Hospital of Cincinnati, 2135 Dana Avenue, Suite 430, Cincinnati, OH 45207, USA

About 10 % of patients with symptomatic DVTs develop severe post thrombotic syndrome within 5 years [9]. Despite adequate treatment, up to 25 % of patients with symptomatic DVT-PE have recurrent VTE within 5 years [10]. Moreover, 25 % of patients with VTE do not survive the first year after diagnosis [11].

In 596 men hospitalized for DVT-PE, we previously reported that 7 (1.2 %) had taken TT before and at time of their admission [3]. Of these 7 men, all 5 who had evaluation of thrombophilia-hypofibrinolysis were found to have previously undiagnosed procoagulants. Separately, we studied 147 men hospitalized for DVT-PE, finding 2 (1.4 %) with antecedent TT use [5]. Both men had previously undiagnosed thrombophilia [5]. Parallel to the TT-VTE relationship in men, estrogen-progestin birth control pills (BCP) and hormone replacement therapy (HRT) in women are associated with VTE [12–14], and the issue of screening for thrombophilia before prescription of BCP or HRT is contentious because of cost-effectiveness issues [15].

In 347 patients (154 men, 193 women) hospitalized over a 4-year period for pulmonary embolism, we investigated testosterone and estrogen therapy (ET) use anteceding PE, and studies of procoagulants in TT and ET users.

Methods

Patients

Ethics, consent

The study was carried out following a protocol approved by the Jewish Hospital Institutional Review Board, with signed informed consent. No identifiable clinical data is presented.

From 2011 through 2014, using review of electronic medical records, 347 patients were hospitalized in Cincinnati Mercy Hospitals with PE. Only patients hospitalized for PE were studied. Retrospective chart review was used to document TT or ET use anteceding PE. We prospectively performed coagulation studies in those patients who used TT or ET, not having previous evaluation of thrombophilia-hypofibrinolysis.

Retrospectively, we reviewed coagulation data obtained at hospitalization for PE from electronic medical records in two other groups of patients not exposed to TT or ET, 78 with cancer associated with PE (17 had coagulation data), and 237 free of cancer (116 had coagulation data).

Studies of thrombophilia and hypofibrinolysis

PCR measures of the Factor V Leiden, prothrombin, MTHFR mutations and serologic measures of activated protein C resistance [16, 17], antigenic proteins antithrombin III, C, total S, free S, homocysteine, factors VIII and XI [18, 19], the lupus anticoagulant, and anticardiolipin antibodies were carried out using established methods [20–22].

PCR measures of the 4G/5G mutation in the plasminogen activator inhibitor (Serpine1) gene [8, 23–25] were carried out using established methods [20–22]. Serologic studies of plasminogen activator inhibitor activity were not done.

Statistical methods

Within gender, users and non-users of ET/TT were compared by Fisher's exact test and by Wilcoxon tests. Thrombophilia in the 24 hormone users (6 men on TT, 18 women on ET) was compared to 116 cases (62 men, 54 women) with PE, not receiving TT or ET and free of cancer, and to 17 cases (9 men, 8 women) with cancer, not receiving TT or ET by Fisher's exact test.

Results

Preceding hospitalization for PE, of the 154 men and 193 women, 8 men (5 % of men) used TT, 24 women (12 % of women) used ET (16 estrogen-progestin birth control pills [BCP], 6 hormone replacement therapy [HRT], 2 progesterone), Fig. 1, Table 1. From the initiation of TT or ET to development of PE, the median time was 7 months in men and 18 months in women.

Median age in the 8 men was 56, marginally (p = .068) younger than in the 146 men not on TT (65). Median age in the 24 women with PE on ET was 38, younger than 169 women not taking ET (69, p < .0001), Table 1. Women taking ET with subsequent PE were less likely

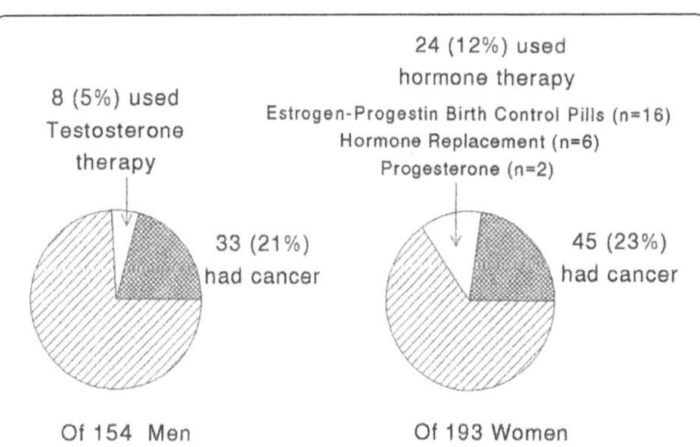

Fig. 1 Percent of 154 men admitted with pulmonary embolism (PE) who used testosterone therapy before PE, and the percent who had cancer associated with PE. Percent of 193 women admitted with pulmonary embolism (PE) who used estrogen-progestin birth control pills (n = 16), estrogen-progestin hormone replacement therapy (n = 6) or progesterone (n = 2) before PE, and percent who had cancer associated with PE

Table 1 Demographics in 347 pulmonary embolism patients (193 women, 154 men), by gender and by hormone use

Women			
	Hormone user, n = 24 (12 %)	Non user, n = 169 (88 %)	all women n = 193 (100 %)
Age (year)	42 ± 13, median 38****	66 ± 17, median 69	63 ± 18, median 65
Smoking	7/24 (29 %)*	96/169 (57 %)	103/193 (53 %)
Hormone	BC pill 16 (67 %) Estrogen 6 (25 %) Progesterone 2 (8 %)		
Cancer	0/24 (0 %)**	45/169 (27 %)	45/193 (23 %)
DM	2/24 (8 %)	42/169 (25 %)	44/193 (23 %)
Death	0/24 (0 %)	3/169 (2 %)	3/193 (2 %)
Thrombosis history	1/24 (4 %)*	40/168 (24 %), 1 missing	41/193 (21 %)
Men			
	Hormone user, n = 8 (5 %)	Non user n = 146 (95 %)	All men n = 154 (100 %)
Age (year)	48 ± 23, median 56	63 ± 17, median 65	62 ± 17, median 64
Smoking	5/8 (63 %)	103/146 (71 %)	108/154 (70 %)
Hormone	Testosterone		
Cancer	0/8 (0 %)	33/146 (23 %)	33/154 (21 %)
DM	2/8 (25 %)	31/146 (21 %)	33/154 (21 %)
Death	0/8 (0 %)	2/146 (1 %)	2/154 (1 %)
Thrombosis history	2/8 (25 %)	31/146 (21 %)	33/154 (21 %)

* $p < .05$, ** $p < .01$, comparing hormone user vs non user in each gender by Fisher's exact test
**** $p < .0001$, comparing hormone user vs non user in each gender by Wilcoxon test

than women not taking ET to have cancer, and were less likely to have a previous thrombosis history (4 % vs 24 %, $p < .05$), Table 1.

Of the 8 men using TT before their PE, 6 used TT gels, 50 mg/day, and 2 had intra muscular TT 50 mg/week. Of these 8 men, 5 (63 %) smoked, 2 had a previous history of thrombotic events, and 2 had type 2 diabetes, Table 1.

Coagulation evaluations were done in 6 of the 8 men with TT anteceding PE, Table 2. All 6 had ≥ 1 thrombophilia or hypofibrinolysis: 1 heterozygous for the G20210A prothrombin gene mutation, 1 homozygous for the 4G4G PAI-1 gene mutation, 1 with high factor VIII, 1 with high ACLA IgG, 3 with high homocysteine (1 of whom had MTHFR C677T homozygosity), 2 with low protein C, 2 with low protein S, and 2 with low free protein S, Table 2. Two of 8 men had Klinefelters syndrome.

Of the 24 women taking ET before PE, 2 were diabetic, 1 had a previous history of thrombosis and 7 (29 %) smoked, Table 1.

Of the 24 women, 18 had measures of coagulation, and 16 (89 %) had ≥ 1 thrombophilia (Table 3). Four women were V Leiden heterozygotes, 1 prothrombin

Table 2 Abnormal measures of thrombophilia and hypofibrinolysis in 8 men who using testosterone therapy before pulmonary embolism (6 men had coagulation measures)

	PTG	MTHFR	PAIG	Homocysteine	Factor VIII	ACLA IgG	Pro C	PRO S	Free S
Abnormal range	TC/TT	TT	4G4G	Dated cut point[a]	> 150 %	Dated cut point[b]	< 73 %	< 63 %	< 66 %
ID# 1				12.0			61		
2	TC					18.0			57
4								64	
5			4G4G		223		47	49	43
6		TT		17.3					
7				11.0					

[a]dated cut point for Homocysteine high: ≥ 15 (11/15/08-12/2/14); ≥ 10.4 (after 12/3/14)
[b]dated cut point for IgG high: ≥ 23 GPL (before 10/31/12); ≥ 15 (after 11/1/12)

Table 3 Abnormal measures of thrombophilia and hypofibrinolysis in 24 women who used hormone replacement therapy on estrogen-progestin oral contraceptives before pulmonary embolism (18 women had coagulation measures)

	FactorV	PTG	Factor VIII	FactorXI	ACLAIgG	ACLAIgM	Lupus anticoagulant	Pro S	Free S	Anti III
Abnormal range	TC/TT	TC/TT	> 150 %	> 150 %	Dated cut point[a]		Y	< 63 %	< 66 %	< 80 %
ID# 1										78
3						20.0				
4										
5	TC							47		
6										70
8	TC									
9							Y			71
10			212							
11							Y			
12									61	
13					16.0			59		
14										
15			301	151		17.0			39	
17		TC								
18								48		
22	TC									
24	TC									

[a]dated cut point for IgG high: ≥ 23 GPL (before 10/31/12); ≥ 15 (after 11/1/12)
dated cut point for IgM high: ≥ 10 MPL (before 4/30/12); ≥ 13 (after 5/1/12)

gene heterozygote, 2 had high Factor VIII, 1 had high Factor XI, 2 were positive for the lupus anticoagulant, 3 had low protein S, 2 had low Free S, 3 had low antithrombin III, and 3 had high ACLA, Table 3.

Cancer was associated with PE in 78 patients, 22 % of the cohort (45 women [23 % of women], 33 men [21 % of men], Table 1, Fig. 1). None of the cancer patients took either TT or ET, Table 1. Of the 33 men and 45 women with PE and concurrent cancer (Fig. 1), hospital based coagulation measures (Factor V Leiden, homocysteine, lupus anticoagulant, anticardiolipin antibody IgG and IgM, proteins C, S, and antithrombin III) were obtained in 17 (9 men, 8 women, Tables 4 and 5). Thrombophilia was rare in the 17 cancer patients with PE, with exception of homocysteine, which was high in 40 % of cancer patients, marginally more common than in the 24 hormone users (13 %, p = .063), Tables 4 and 5.

Of the 237 patients hospitalized with PE, free of cancer and free of TT or ET supplementation, 116 had thrombophilia measures, Tables 4 and 5. These 116 cases did

Table 4 Coagulation disorders in 24 cases (6 men [on testosterone] and 18 women [on estrogen]) who had testosterone/hormone therapy before PE, compared to 116 cases with PE but no hormone, no cancer (62 men, 54 women), and compared to 17 cancer cases (9 men, 8 women)

	Factor V	PTG	MTHFR	PAIG	Homocysteine[a]	Lupus anticoagulant	ACLA IgG	ACLA IgM
Abnormal range	TC,TT	TC,TT	TT	4G4G	umol/l	Positive	Dated[b]	Dated[c]
Hormone Cases (n = 24,6 men on TT, 18 women on ET)	4/24 (17 %)	2/24 (8 %)	1/24 (4 %)	1/24 (4 %)	3/24 (13 %)	2/24 (8 %)	2/24 (8 %)	2/24 (8 %)
PE_no hormone, no Cancer (n = 116, 62 men, 54 women)	15/105 (14 %)	7/71 (10 %)			18/43 (42 %) **	17/68 (25 %)	1/61 (2 %)	5/58 (9 %)
Cancer (n = 17,9 men, 8 women)	0/15 (0 %)				6/15 (40 %)	1/17 (6 %)	0/15 (0 %)	1/17 (6 %)

**p < .025, comparing with Hormone cases by Fisher's test
[a]dated cut point for Homocysteine high: ≥ 15 (11/15/08-12/2/14); ≥10.4 (after 12/3/14)
[b]dated cut point for IgG high: ≥ 23 GPL (before 10/31/12); ≥ 15 (after 11/1/12)
[c]dated cut point for IgM high: ≥ 10 MPL (before 4/30/12); ≥ 13 (after 5/1/12)

Table 5 Coagulation disorders in 24 cases (6 men [on testosterone] and 18 women [on estrogen]) who had testosterone/hormone therapy before PE, compared to 116 cases with PE but no hormone, no cancer (62 men, 54 women), and compared to 17 cancer cases (9 men, 8 women)

	Factor VIII	Factor XI	Protein C	Protein S	Free S	Antithrombin III
Abnormal range	> 150 %	> 150 %	< 73 %	< 63 %	< 66 %	< 80
Hormone Cases (n = 24,6 men on TT,18 women on ET)	3/24 (13 %)	1/23 (4 %)	2/24 (8 %)	5/24 (21 %)	4/24 (17 %)	3/24 (13 %)
PE_no hormone, no Cancer (n = 116, 62 men, 54 women)			27/90 (30 %)*	8/77 (10 %)	11/74 (15 %)	8/80 (10 %)
Cancer (n = 17,9 men, 8 women)			1/16 (6 %)	1/16 (6 %)		1/14 (7 %)

* $p < .05$, comparing with Hormone cases by Fisher's test

not differ (p > 0.4) from the 24 hormone using cases, except for high homocysteine (42 % vs 13 %, $p < .025$) and low protein C (30 % vs 8 %, $p < .05$), Tables 4 and 5.

Discussion

Increased risk of VTE in women using combined oral contraceptives has been known for at least 52 years [26], and is well recognized for hormone replacement therapy [27]. By comparison, the association of VTE in men [1] and women [4, 6] using TT has only recently been described, as of 2011 and 2013–2015 respectively [1–6, 8]. Previously, in 596 men hospitalized for DVT-PE, we reported that 7 (1.2 %) had taken TT before and at time of their admission [3], and all 5 men who had evaluation of thrombophilia-hypofibrinolysis were found to have previously undiagnosed procoagulants. Separately, we studied 147 men hospitalized for DVT-PE, finding 2 (1.4 %) with antecedent TT use, both of whom had previously undiagnosed thrombophilia [5].

In the current study, of 154 men hospitalized for PE, 8 (5 %) used TT, and of 193 women, 24 (12 %) used ET. congruent with previous studies [26, 27]. Congruent with our previous reports [3, 5], all of the men with PE after TT in the current study were found to have familial-acquired thrombophilia, as were 16/18 women (89 %) with PE after ET. Thrombophilia in the 24 cases using TT and ET was comparable to that in 116 cases not using TT or ET. As in the current study, when TT or ET are given to patients with previously undiagnosed thrombophilia, thrombosis commonly occurs [8].

In the current study, thrombophilia was rare in patients whose PE was associated with cancer, in agreement with the report by Fiaz et al. [28] who reported that thrombophilia was more common among VTE patients without cancer than in those with cancer.

Health [9, 10] and cost [29–31] ramifications of a PE, either unprovoked or after TT or ET are significant. After PE, there is a high cost of hospitalization, rehospitalization, and post-PE care [29]. As summarized by Reitsma [32], "...the one-year mortality is 20 % after a first VTE. Of the surviving patients, 15–25 % will experience a recurrent episode of VTE in the three years after the first event. Primary and secondary prevention is key to reducing death and disability from VTE."

Selective coagulation screening based on prior VTE history, if applied to our 347 patients hospitalized for PE, had low sensitivity, and would have identified only 25 % of men with PE on TT, and only 4 % of women with PE on estrogen-progestin oral contraceptives-HRT. However, cost-effectiveness studies [33, 34] suggest that selective coagulation screening based on prior VTE history is more cost-effective than universal screening.

Limitations of our study include its retrospective observational nature, and a limited sample size of patients who took TT or ET and had coagulation screening. Our study is further limited by not having coagulation data on patients admitted with PE who died before coagulation measures were obtained.

Conclusions

Of 154 men hospitalized for PE, 8 (5 %) used TT, and of 193 women, 24 (12 %) used ET. Our data suggests that PE is an important complication of TT in men and ET in women, in part reflecting an interaction between familial and acquired thrombophilia and exogenous hormone use.

Our findings may have important clinical ramifications, because VTE risk is an important determinant of the benefit risk ratio of both TT and ET. In women, PE accounts for about one third of the incidence of potentially fatal VTE events associated with HRT [35], and HRT increases the risk of VTE by 2- to 3-fold [36].

Reitsma [32] has concluded that "...for primary prevention of VTE, genetic testing is not likely to play a role in the future." However, as the cost of screening for familial and acquired thrombophilias falls over time, with the development of multilocus genetic risk scores to improve classification, we believe that coagulation studies before starting TT, ET, and oral contraceptive therapy should be done as an approach to primary prevention of VTE, including at least PCR studies of the Factor V Leiden and Prothrombin gene mutations, Factors VIII and XI, homocysteine, and the lupus anticoagulant.

Abbreviations
PE: Pulmonary embolism; TT: Testosterone therapy; ET: Estrogen therapy; VTE: Venous thromboembolism; DVT: Deep venous thrombosis; BCP: Birth control pills; HRT: Hormone replacement therapy; ACLA: Anticardiolipin antibodies.

Competing interests
The authors declare that they have no competing interests.

Authors' contributions
MP acquired data, drafted and revised manuscript and helped with coordination. CG designed the study, drafted and revised the manuscript as well as interpreted the data. PS acquired data and revised the manuscript. AK acquired data and revised the manuscript. MG acquired data and revised the manuscript. MR acquired data and revised the manuscript. NM acquired data and revised the manuscript. VJ acquired data and revised the manuscript. KL acquired data and revised the manuscript. PW analyzed and interpreted the data, provided statistical analysis and revised the manuscript. All authors read and approved the final manuscript.

Authors' information
MP is a PGY-2 MD at the Jewish hospital of Cincinnati, Ohio involved in many projects. CG is an MD and the medical director of the Cholesterol, Metabolism, and Thrombosis center of Jewish hospital. PS is a MD and current researcher at the Cholesterol, Metabolism, and Thrombosis center. AK is a current second year college student working with Dr Glueck. MG is a current second year college student working with Dr Glueck. MR is a PGY-2 MD at the Jewish hospital of Cincinnati, Ohio. NM is a PGY-2 MD at the Jewish hospital of Cincinnati, Ohio. VJ is a MD and current researcher at the Cholesterol, Metabolism, and Thrombosis center. KL is a PGY-2 MD at the Jewish hospital of Cincinnati, Ohio. PW is a PhD and statistician at the Cholesterol, Metabolism, and Thrombosis center.

Acknowledgements
No other individuals to acknowledge.

References
1. Glueck CJ, Goldenberg N, Budhani S, Lotner D, Abuchaibe C, Gowda M, et al. Thrombotic events after starting exogenous testosterone in men with previously undiagnosed familial thrombophilia. Transl Res. 2011;158:225–34.
2. Glueck CJ, Wang P. Testosterone therapy, thrombosis, thrombophilia, cardiovascular events. Metabolism. 2014;63:989–94.
3. Glueck CJ, Richardson-Royer C, Schultz R, Burger T, Bowe D, Padda J, et al. Testosterone therapy, thrombophilia-hypofibrinolysis, and hospitalization for deep venous thrombosis-pulmonary embolus: an exploratory, hypothesis-generating study. Clin Appl Thromb Hemost. 2014;20:244–9.
4. Freedman J, Glueck CJ, Prince M, Riaz R, Wang P. Testosterone, thrombophilia, thrombosis. Transl Res. 2015;165:537–48.
5. Glueck CJ, Friedman J, Hafeez A, Hassan A, Wang P. Testosterone therapy, thrombophilia, and hospitalization for deep venous thrombosis-pulmonary embolus, an exploratory, hypothesis-generating study. Med Hypotheses. 2015;84:341–3.
6. Glueck CJ, Bowe D, Valdez A, Wang P. Thrombosis in three postmenopausal women receiving testosterone therapy for low libido. Womens Health (Lond Engl). 2013;9:405–10.
7. Glueck CJ, Richardson-Royer C, Schultz R, Burger T, Labitue F, Riaz MK, et al. Testosterone, thrombophilia, and thrombosis. Clin Appl Thromb Hemost. 2014;20:22–30.
8. Glueck CJ, Prince M, Patel N, Patel J, Shah P, Mehta N, et al. Thrombophilia in 67 Patients With Thrombotic Events After Starting Testosterone Therapy. Clin Appl Thromb Hemost. 2015.
9. Kearon C. Natural history of venous thromboembolism. Circulation. 2003; 107:I22–30.
10. White RH. The epidemiology of venous thromboembolism. Circulation. 2003;107:I4–8.
11. Bertoletti L, Quenet S, Laporte S, Sahuquillo JC, Conget F, Pedrajas JM, et al. Pulmonary embolism and 3-month outcomes in 4036 patients with venous thromboembolism and chronic obstructive pulmonary disease: data from the RIETE registry. Respir Res. 2013;14:75.
12. Lidegaard O, Lokkegaard E, Svendsen AL, Agger C. Hormonal contraception and risk of venous thromboembolism: national follow-up study. BMJ. 2009;339:b2890.
13. Lidegaard O, Nielsen LH, Skovlund CW, Skjeldestad FE, Lokkegaard E. Risk of venous thromboembolism from use of oral contraceptives containing different progestogens and oestrogen doses: Danish cohort study, 2001–9. BMJ. 2011;343:d6423.
14. Davey DA. Update: estrogen and estrogen plus progestin therapy in the care of women at and after the menopause. Womens Health (Lond Engl). 2012;8:169–89.
15. Merriman L, Greaves M. Testing for thrombophilia: an evidence-based approach. Postgrad Med J. 2006;82:699–704.
16. Xin-Guang C, Yong-Qiang Z, Shu-Jie W, Lian-Kai F, Hua-Cong C. Prevalence of the Factor V E666D Mutation and Its Correlation With Activated Protein C Resistance in the Chinese Population. Clin Appl Thromb Hemost. 2015;21:480–3.
17. Zavala-Hernandez C, Hernandez-Zamora E, Martinez-Murillo C, Majluf-Cruz A, Vela-Ojeda J, Garcia-Chavez J, et al. Risk Factors for Thrombosis Development in Mexican Patients. Ann Vasc Surg. 2015;29:1625–32.
18. Siegerink B, Maino A, Algra A, Rosendaal FR. Hypercoagulability and the risk of myocardial infarction and ischemic stroke in young women. J Thromb Haemost. 2015;13:1568–75.
19. Phillippe HM, Hornsby LB, Treadway S, Armstrong EM, Bellone JM. Inherited Thrombophilia. J Pharm Pract. 2014;27:227–33.
20. Glueck CJ, Bell H, Vadlamani L, Gupta A, Fontaine RN, Wang P, et al. Heritable thrombophilia and hypofibrinolysis. Possible causes of retinal vein occlusion. Arch Ophthalmol. 1999;117:43–9.
21. Glueck CJ, Freiberg RA, Fontaine RN, Tracy T, Wang P. Hypofibrinolysis, thrombophilia, osteonecrosis. Clin Orthop Relat Res. 2001;19–33.
22. Glueck CJ, Wang P, Bell H, Rangaraj V, Goldenberg N. Associations of thrombophilia, hypofibrinolysis, and retinal vein occlusion. Clin Appl Thromb Hemost. 2005;11:375–89.
23. Glueck CJ, Wang P. Ocular vascular thrombotic events: a diagnostic window to familial thrombophilia (compound factor V Leiden and prothrombin gene heterozygosity) and thrombosis. Clin Appl Thromb Hemost. 2009;15:12–8.
24. Schenk JF, Stephan B, Zewinger S, Speer T, Pindur G. Comparison of the plasminogen activator inhibitor-1 4G/5G gene polymorphism in females with venous thromboembolism during pregnancy or spontaneous abortion. Clin Hemorheol Microcirc. 2008;39:329–32.
25. Jeon YJ, Kim YR, Lee BE, Choi YS, Kim JH, Shin JE, et al. Genetic association of five plasminogen activator inhibitor-1 (PAI-1) polymorphisms and idiopathic recurrent pregnancy loss in Korean women. Thromb Haemost. 2013;110:742–50.
26. Tyler ET. Oral contraception and venous thrombosis. JAMA. 1963;185:131–2.
27. Perez Gutthann S, Garcia Rodriguez LA, Castellsague J, Duque Oliart A. Hormone replacement therapy and risk of venous thromboembolism: population based case–control study. BMJ. 1997;314:796–800.
28. Faiz AS, Khan I, Beckman MG, Bockenstedt P, Heit JA, Kulkarni R, et al. Characteristics and Risk Factors of Cancer Associated Venous Thromboembolism. Thromb Res. 2015;136:535–41.
29. Fernandez MM, Hogue S, Preblick R, Kwong WJ. Review of the cost of venous thromboembolism. Clinicoecon Outcomes Res. 2015;7:451–62.
30. LaMori JC, Shoheiber O, Mody SH, Bookhart BK. Inpatient resource use and cost burden of deep vein thrombosis and pulmonary embolism in the United States. Clin Ther. 2015;37:62–70.
31. Raskob GE, Angchaisuksiri P, Blanco AN, Buller H, Gallus A, Hunt BJ, et al. Thrombosis: a major contributor to global disease burden. Arterioscler Thromb Vasc Biol. 2014;34:2363–71.
32. Reitsma PH. Genetics in thrombophilia. An update. Hamostaseologie. 2015; 35:47–51.
33. Wu O, Robertson L, Twaddle S, Lowe G, Clark P, Walker I, et al. Screening for thrombophilia in high-risk situations: a meta-analysis and cost-effectiveness analysis. Br J Haematol. 2005;131:80–90.
34. Wu O, Robertson L, Twaddle S, Lowe GD, Clark P, Greaves M, et al. Screening for thrombophilia in high-risk situations: systematic review and

cost-effectiveness analysis. The Thrombosis: Risk and Economic Assessment of Thrombophilia Screening (TREATS) study. Health Technol Assess. 2006;10: 1–110.

35. Beral V, Banks E, Reeves G. Evidence from randomised trials on the long-term effects of hormone replacement therapy. Lancet. 2002;360:942–4.
36. Canonico M, Plu-Bureau G, Lowe GD, Scarabin PY. Hormone replacement therapy and risk of venous thromboembolism in postmenopausal women: systematic review and meta-analysis. BMJ. 2008;336:1227–31.

Effect of malaria infection on hematological profiles of people living with human immunodeficiency virus in Gambella, southwest Ethiopia

Tsion Sahle[1†], Tilahun Yemane[2] and Lealem Gedefaw[2*†]

Abstract

Background: Malaria and human immunodeficiency virus are the two most devastating global health problems causing more than two million deaths each year. Hematological abnormalities such as anemia, thrombocytopenia and leucopenia are the common complications in malaria and HIV co-infected individuals. The aim of this study was to determine the effect of malaria infection on hematological profiles of people living with HIV attending Gambella Hospital ART clinic, Southwestern Ethiopia.

Objective: To determine the effect of malaria infection on hematological profiles of people living with HIV attending Gambella Hospital ART clinic, Southwestern Ethiopia.

Methods: A facility based comparative cross-sectional study was conducted from May 25 to November 11, 2014 in Gambella Hospital. A total of 172 adult people living with HIV (86 malaria infected and 86 malaria non-infected) participants were included in the study. Demographic, anthropometric and clinical data were collected. Venous blood samples and stool specimen were collected for laboratory analysis. Microscopic examination of peripheral blood films was done for detection of malaria parasites. Descriptive statistics, student T- test, bivariable and multivariable analyses were performed using SPSS V-20. Statistical significance was set at $p < 0.05$.

Results: A total of 172 adult people living with HIV were included in the study. The prevalence of anemia, thrombocytopenia and leucopenia in malaria and HIV co-infected participants were 60.5%, 59.3%, and 43.0%, respectively. Resident (AOR: 4.67; 95% CI: 1.44, 15.14), malaria infection (AOR: 2.42; 95% CI: 1.16, 5.04) and CD_4^+ count were predictors for anemia. A predictor for thrombocytopenia was malaria infection (AOR: 9.79; 95% CI: 4.33, 22.17). Malaria parasitic density (AOR: 0.13; 95% CI: 0.03, 0.57) and CD_4^+ count (AOR: 4.77; 95% CI: 1.23, 18.45) were predictors of leucopenia.

Conclusions: Findings suggest that the prevalence of anemia and thrombocytopenia were significantly higher in the malaria and HIV coinfected participants than the HIV mono-infected participants. Mean values of hematological profiles were significantly different in the two groups. Future prospective studies with larger sample size from other settings are needed to substantiate the findings.

Keywords: Malaria, Anemia, HIV, Gambella

* Correspondence: lealem.gedefaw@ju.edu.et
[†]Equal contributors
[2]Department of Medical Laboratory Science and Pathology, Jimma University, Jimma, Ethiopia
Full list of author information is available at the end of the article

Background

Hematological abnormalities are the common complications in malaria infection and they play a major role in malaria pathophysiology. These changes involve the major cell lines, such as red blood cells, leucocytes and thrombocytes and the abnormalities such as anemia, thrombocytopenia and leukocytosis or leucopenia [1–5]. Hematological abnormalities such as anemia [6], neutropenia [7], and thrombocytopenia [8] are commonly reported abnormalities associated with HIV infection. HIV has effects on the systemic inflammatory response, causing activation and/or apoptosis in a variety of immune cells as well as elevated levels of proinflammatory cytokines and chemokines in plasma and lymph nodes. This immune activation is also a potential means by which HIV affects the disease course and outcome in other infections, such as malaria [9].

Malaria and HIV are the two most devastating global health problems of our time, causing more than two million deaths each year [10, 11] and greatest medical challenges facing Africa today [12]. Both malaria and HIV are diseases of poverty and can exert further poverty by affecting young adults in the work force, and this contributes to less productivity in the development of local economy [9].

Both malaria and HIV can cause hematological abnormalities independently. Those hematological abnormalities: anemia, thrombocytopenia and leucopenia have been documented as strong, independent predictors of morbidity and mortality in malaria co -infected HIV positive individuals than mono infected HIV positive individuals.

Beside this HIV infection is associated with a twofold higher risk of severe malaria in adults, and a six to eightfold increase in the risk of death [13].

Immunological complications are common in HIV infection, besides these hematological abnormalities have been documented as strong independent predictors of morbidity and mortality in HIV-infected individuals [14]. Although from hematological abnormalities cytopenia is the most frequent one but it is rare in the early stages of HIV infection [15]. Although malaria and HIV are known to be the most common public health problems in Ethiopia [16], yet limited study has been done, which evaluates the extent of hematological changes in malaria and HIV co-infected individuals particularly in this study area. Therefore, this study was intended to determine the effect of malaria infection on hematological profiles of people living with HIV attending Gambella Hospital ART clinic, Southwestern Ethiopia.

Methods

Study area and study period

A facility based comparative cross sectional study was conducted in the Gambella Hospital from May 25 to November 11, 2014. Gambella Hospital is located in Gambella Town which is located 777 Km Southwest of Addis Ababa, Ethiopia. Gambella Hospital is the only hospital in the region and offers services for nearly 200,000 people.

All HIV positive adults attending in the Gambella Hospital ART Clinic for routine follow up and/or treatment during the study period and willing to participate were included consecutively. HIV positive adults on any anti-malarial treatment during the study period were excluded from the study.

The sample size was calculated by using a statistical formula for comparison of two populations mean obtained from previously conducted study in Gondar University Hospital, Ethiopia [17]. Accordingly, a total of 172 (86 malaria positive and 86 malaria negative) HIV positive participants were included in the study.

Data collection and processing

The participant socio-demographic and anthropometric data were collected using structured questionnaire and clinical data of each participant were collected from the existing ART logbook by the clinician who work in ART clinic.

Four ml of venous blood sample was collected using an EDTA containing vacutainer tube from each participant for laboratory investigation. For the detection of malaria both thick and thin blood films were prepared, stained with 10% Giemsa solution and examined with a light microscope. The malaria parasitic density was calculated by counting the number of parasites in thick blood film against 200 or 500 WBCs. The number of parasites per μl of blood was calculated [18].

The remaining blood sample was used for hematological analysis (CBC) and for the $CD_4{}^+$ lymphocyte count. Hematological parameters: red blood cell count (RBC), hemoglobin (Hgb), hematocrit (HCT), mean cell volume (MCV), mean cell hemoglobin (MCH), mean cell hemoglobin concentration (MCHC), total white blood cell count (WBC), differential neutrophil (NEUT), MID (Eos, Bas and Mon), differential lymphocyte count (LYM) and platelet count (PLT), were determined using the automated blood cell analyzer CELL DYNE 1800® (Abbott Laboratories Diagnostics Division, USA). $CD_4{}^+$ lymphocyte count was assayed using the BD FACS® COUNT (Becton Dickenson California, USA). Anemia, thrombocytopenia and leucopenia were defined as; Hgb <12 g/dl for female and Hgb <13 g/dl for male [19], platelet count $< 150 \times 10^9$/l and WBC count $< 4.0 \times 10^9$/l, respectively [20]. Stool specimen was collected and examined directly using both wet mount smear preparations and formol-ether concentration technique. To get reliable data training was given for data collectors. To assure the quality of the laboratory data standard operating procedure for each test was followed. Reagents were checked for their expiry date and prepared according to the manufacturer's instruction. Quality control procedures were performed daily according to the laboratory's protocol. Control samples were used for hematology analyzer and for the FACS count machine. Malaria slides were checked by two experienced laboratory technologist.

Data analysis and interpretation

The data were checked for completeness before analysis. The descriptive statistics was used to see the distribution of the socio-demographic, anthropometric and clinical characteristics of the participants. For the continuous variables mean, standard deviation and 95% confidence interval were determined in each group. Student's t - test was used to compare the mean value of hematological parameters between malaria infected and non-infected participants. Multivariable logistic regression was used to test the degree of association between dependent and independent variables. The variables with p-value ≤ 0.25 in bivariable analysis were nominated for multivariable analysis. All variables with p-value < 0.05 were considered as statistically significant. Data were analyzed using SPSS Version 20 (IBM Corporation, Chicago, USA) software for windows.

Results

General characteristics of the study participants

In a total of 172 participants with the mean age of 31.95 (±7.6) years, the majority were females (60.5%) with normal BMI (68.6%) and on HAART medication (82.6%). Among malaria and HIV infected participants 81 (94.2%), 3 (3.5%) and 2 (2.3%) of study participants were infected with *P. falciparum, P. vivax* and mixed infection, respectively. The malaria parasitic density ranges from 110 to 179,705 with a median of 4134 parasites/μl.

Of the total study participants, 16 (9.3%) had opportunistic infections. From these; four participants had tuberculosis, three participants had pneumocystis pneumonia and the other three participants had herpes zoster virus while the remaining six study participants had oesophageal candidiasis, tinea capitis, cryptococcal meningitis each account for two participants. The overall prevalence of intestinal parasites was 7.6%. *Giardia lamblia* ten (76.9%) was the most frequent parasite, followed by *Entamoeba histolytica/dispar* one (7.7%), *Hook worms* one (7.7%) and *Ascaris lumbricoides* one (7.7%).

Hematological profiles of HIV and malaria co-infected participants

From a total of 172 participants, 89 (51.7%) had anemia, 61 (35.5%) had thrombocytopenia, and 68 (39.5%) had leucopenia. Among malaria and HIV co-infected study participants 52 (60.5%), 51 (59.3%), and 37 (43.0%) had anemia, thrombocytopenia and leucopenia, respectively. From malaria non-infected study participants 37 (43.0%), 10 (11.6%) and 31 (36.0%) had anemia, thrombocytopenia leucopenia, respectively. A statistically significant difference was observed in the prevalence of anemia ($P = 0.022$) and thrombocytopenia ($P < 0.001$) between the two groups (Fig. 1).

There was a significant mean difference with respect to Hgb, HCT, lymphocyte, neutrophil, and platelet values. However, no significant difference observed in values of RBC, MCV, MCH, MCHC, WBC, MID and CD_4^+ count (Table 1).

Factors associated with abnormal hematological profiles in PLWHA

Malaria infected study participants were two times more likely to be anemic than malaria non-infected study participants (AOR: 2.42; 95% CI: 1.16, 5.04) (Table 2). Study participants who were malaria infected had ten times more likely to be thrombocytopenic than malaria none infected study participants (AOR: 9.79, 95% CI: 4.33, 22.17) (Table 3). Malaria parasitic density ≥10,000 parasites/μl (AOR: 0.13; (95% CI: 0.03, 0.57) and CD_4^+ count ≤ 200 cells/μl (AOR: 4.77; 95% CI: 1.23, 18.45) were predictors of leucopenia (Table 4).

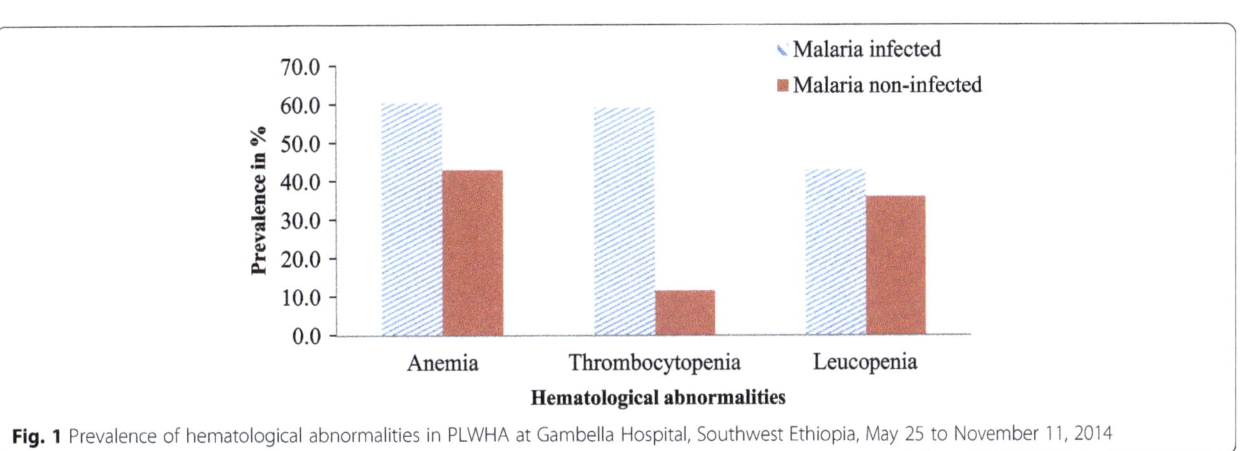

Fig. 1 Prevalence of hematological abnormalities in PLWHA at Gambella Hospital, Southwest Ethiopia, May 25 to November 11, 2014

Table 1 Comparison of hematological profiles between malaria infected and malaria non- infected participants

Hematological Profiles	Malaria infected Mean ± SD	Malaria non- infected Mean ± SD	t- value	*P*-value
RBC ($\times 10^{12}$/L)	3.88 ± 0.69	4.08 ± 0.66	−1.914	0.057
Hgb (g/dL)	11.77 ± 1.80	12.69 ± 2.03	−3.120	0.002
HCT (%)	34.60 ± 5.44	37.23 ± 5.59	−3.116	0.002
MCV (FL)	88.99 ± 10.86	91.10 ± 12.33	−1.190	0.236
MCH (pg)	30.53 ± 3.38	31.36 ± 4.12	−1.443	0.151
MCHC (g/dL)	34.08 ± 1.38	33.74 ± 3.08	0.921	0.359
WBC ($\times 10^{9}$/L)	4.66 ± 2.19	5.09 ± 3.57	−0.944	0.346
LYM (%)	35.76 ± 14.24	48.17 ± 12.95	−5.974	<0.0001
MID (%)	14.42 ± 7.81	13.89 ± 22.80	0.204	0.838
NEUT (%)	49.11 ± 17.41	40.34 ± 12.03	3.842	<0.0001
PLT ($\times 10^{9}$/L)	148.72 ± 77.91	236.88 ± 75.02	−7.559	<0.0001
CD_4^+ (cell/μl)	434.36 ± 292.41	460.63 ± 230.24	−0.655	0.513

*SD- Standard deviation, RBC-Red blood cell, HCT-Hematocrit, Hgb-Hemoglobin, MCV-Mean cell volume, MCH-Mean cell hemoglobin, MCHC-Mean cell hemoglobin concentration, WBC-White blood cell, LYM-Lymphocyte, MID - Average of basophils, eosinophil and monocyte, NEUT-Neutrophil, PLT- Platelets and CD_4^+-cluster of differentiation

Discussion

The current study has attempted to provide information on the effect of malaria on the hematological profiles of PLWHA. The major observations are: the prevalence of anemia, thrombocytopenia and leucopenia were higher in malaria infected participant than malaria non-infected participants. The mean hematological profiles were lower in participants with malaria infection than without malaria infection. Residence, malaria infection and CD_4^+ count were identified as predictors for anemia. Malaria infection was significantly associated with thrombocytopenia, whereas malaria parasitic density and CD_4^+ count were significantly associated with leucopenia.

In this study the prevalence of anemia was higher (60.5%) in malaria and HIV co-infected participants than those HIV mono-infected participants (43.0%). This finding was in agreement with other studies [17, 21–23]. However, the prevalence of anemia in malaria and HIV co-infected participants was lower as compared to studies conducted in Ghana (2012), Nigeria (2006) and Gondar (2013) which reported 97.1%, 66.7% and 71.3%, respectively [17, 21, 22]. The difference might be due to variation in methods according to sample size they use a small sample size and clinical condition like HAART status and immune status of the participants. Anemia due to malaria infection can occur through different mechanisms; include RBC lysis, organ sequestration, phagocytosis of uninfected and infected RBCs, and dyserythropoiesis [3].

The second prevalent hematological abnormality in malaria and HIV co-infected study participants was thrombocytopenia (59.3%) and in HIV mono-infected study participants (11.6%). This shows there is a significant association between malaria infection and thrombocytopenia, which is supported by a study done in Nigeria (60%) (2006) [21]. The possible causes of thrombocytopenia in malaria infection was increased sequestration and highly elevated levels of platelet bound immunoglobulin that leads to increased peripheral destruction [4].

Among malaria and HIV co-infected participants, 43.0% had leucopenia and among HIV mono-infected participants 36.0% had leucopenia. There was no statistically significant difference between the two groups. In contrary, the study done in Nigeria (2006) reported that the occurrence of leucopenia were more than two times higher in malaria and HIV co-infected participants than HIV mono-infected participants [21]. This difference might be due to variation in the method used for investigation of hematological profiles, In Nigeria the white cell counting was done manually where as in the current study cell count was done using Cell Dyne 1800 hematology analyzer. The cut off values they used for the leucopenia was $\leq 3 \times 10^9$/l but in our case leukopenia was defined as WBC count $< 4.0 \times 10^9$/l. Sometimes, reduction in the leukocyte counts is attributed to hypersplenism or sequestration in the spleen rather than actual depletion [5].

Our result showed that the prevalence of *Plasmodium falciparum* (94.2%) was higher than the prevalence of *Plasmodium vivax* (3.5%) in malaria and HIV co-infected participants. It is consistent with the studies conducted in Gondar (2013) and Nigeria (2006) [17, 21] but contradicts to the study done in India (2012) [24]. This difference might be due to geographical and climatic variations of the study area. *Plasmodium falciparum* is highly prevalent in Sub-Saharan country than Asia and Latin America [25].

The mean value of Hgb, HCT, platelet and lymphocyte count were lower in malaria and HIV co-infected

Table 2 Predictors of anemia

Variables	Anemia		COR (95% CI)	*P*- value	AOR (95% CI)	*P*-value
	Yes *n* (%)	No *n* (%)				
Age						
18–29	35 (58.3)	25 (41.7)	1		1	
30–39	39 (47.0)	44 (53.0)	0.63 (0.32–1.24)	0.181	0.58 (0.27–1.23)	0.157
40–49	11 (47.8)	12 (52.2)	0.65 (0.25–1.72)	0.390	0.73 (0.25–2.12)	0.563
≥ 50	4 (66.7)	2 (33.3)	1.43 (0.24–8.41)	0.693	1.79 (0.23–13.68)	0.571
Sex						
F	55 (52.9)	49 (47.1)	1.12 (0.61–2.07)	0.711		
M	34 (50.0)	34 (50.0)	1			
Resident						
Urban	75 (49.0)	78 (51.0)	1		1	
Rural	14 (73.7)	5 (26.3)	2.91 (1.00–8.48)	0.050	4.67 (1.44–15.14)	0.010
BMI						
< 18.5	23 (52.3)	21 (47.7)	0.73 (0.18–2.95)	0.659		
18.5–24.99	60 (50.8)	58 (69.2)	0.69 (0.18–2.57)	0.580		
> 25	6 (60.0)	4 (40.0)	1			
HAART status						
Yes	70 (49.3)	72 (50.7)	1		1	
No	19 (63.3)	11 (36.7)	1.77 (0.79–4.00)	0.165	1.87 (0.71–4.91)	0.203
Opportunistic infection						
Yes	7 (43.8)	9 (56.2)	0.70 (0.25–1.98)	0.503		
No	82 (52.6)	74 (47.4)	1			
Intestinal parasite						
Yes	8 (61.5)	5 (38.5)	1.54 (0.48–4.91)	0.465		
No	81 (50.9)	78 (49.1)	1			
Malaria infection						
Yes	52 (60.5)	34 (39.5)	2.02 (1.10–3.72)	0.023	2.42 (1.16–5.04)	0.018
No	37 (43.0)	49 (57.0)	1		1	
Parasitic density of malaria						
1–999	12 (57.1)	9 (42.9)	1			
1000–9999	26 (60.5)	17 (39.5)	0.76 (0.22–2.59)	0.664		
≥ 10,000	14 (63.6)	8 (36.4)	0.87 (0.30–2.53)	0.804		
$CD_4{}^+$ count (cells/μl)						
≤ 200	18 (69.2)	8 (30.8)	1.62 (0.61–4.30)	0.328	1.34 (0.45–3.94)	0.596
200–499	35 (41.7)	49 (58.3)	0.52 (0.26–1.00)	0.051	0.37 (0.17–0.77)	0.009
≥ 500	36 (58.1)	26 (41.9)	1		1	

*COR-Crude odd ratio, AOR-Adjusted odd ratio, CI-Confidence interval, 1-indicator and Statistical significant at $p < 0.05$

participants than malaria non-infected participants. This finding is consistent with the previous studies done in Nigeria (2006 and 2013) [21, 26]. However, this result contradicts to the study from Cameroon in 2012 [27]. This difference might be due to a small number of study participants involved in Cameroon study. In contrary, in our study there was no significant difference in the mean value of RBC, MCV, MCH and MCHC in malaria infected and non-infected PLWHA. This finding is supported by a study done in Cameroon (2012) [27]. This might be due to normocytic normochromic (NCNC) nature of anemia in both malaria and HIV infections.

Multivariable logistic regression analysis of this study showed that: those study participants live in rural area were more likely to be anemic than participants live in urban areas. It might be due to the type of food the rural

Table 3 Predictors of thrombocytopenia

Variables	Thrombocytopenia		COR (95% CI)	*P*-value	AOR (95% CI)	*P*-Value
	Yes *n* (%)	No *n* (%)				
Age						
18–29	19 (31.7)	41 (68.3)	1			
30–39	32 (38.6)	51 (61.4)	1.35 (0.67–2.72)	0.397		
40–49	8 (34.5)	15 (65.5)	1.15 (0.42–3.17)	0.786		
≥ 50	2 (33.3)	4 (66.7)	1.08 (0.18–6.41)	0.933		
Sex						
F	37 (35.6)	67 (64.4)	1.05 (0.56–1.99)	0.868		
M	24 (35.3)	44 (64.7)	1			
HAART status						
Yes	45 (31.7)	97 (68.3)	1		1	
No	16 (53.3)	14 (46.7)	0.41 (0.18–0.90)	0.027	1.46 (0.59–3.59)	0.407
Opportunistic infection						
Yes	5 (31.2)	11 (68.8)	0.81 (0.27–2.45)	0.712		
No	56 (35.9)	100 (64.1)	1			
Malaria infection						
Yes	51 (59.3)	35 (40.7)	11.07 (5.04–24.33)	<0.001	9.79 (4.33–22.17)	<0.001
No	10 (11.6)	76 (88.4)	1		1	
Malaria parasitic density						
1–999	12 (57.1)	9 (42.9)	1			
1000–9999	26 (60.5)	17 (39.5)	1.15 (0.39–3.30)	0.799		
≥ 10000	13 (59.1)	9 (40.9)	1.08 (0.32–3.64)	0.897		
CD_4^+ count (cells/μl)						
≤ 200	16 (61.5)	10 (38.5)	3.36 (1.29–8.71)	0.013	2.69 (0.90–8.05)	0.076
200–499	25 (29.8)	59 (70.2)	0.89 (0.44–1.80)	0.747	0.79 (0.33–1.80)	0.589
≥ 500	20 (32.3)	42 (67.7)	1		1	

*COR-Crude odd ratio, AOR-Adjusted odd ratio, CI-Confidence interval, 1-indicator and statistically significant at $p < 0.05$

community consume, lack of frequent follow up and other factors which could cause anemia. Malaria infected PLWHA were two times more likely to be anemic than malaria non-infected PLWHA. This result is consistent with the study done in Nigeria (2012) [23]. Likewise, malaria infected study participants were ten times more likely to be thrombocytopenic than malaria non-infected PLWHA.

Participants who had CD_4^+ count ≤ 200 cells/μl were nearly five times more likely to have leucopenia than those who had CD_4^+ count ≥ 500 cells/μl PLWHA. This finding is consistent with other studies done in India (2012), Brazil (2011) and Uganda (2014) [28–30]. Another predictor of leucopenia in this study was malaria parasitic density. Those study participants who had a higher malaria parasitic density were 13% less likely to be leucopenic than those having the lowest parasitic density. However, in contrast to this a study from Cameroon (2012) reported that parasite density is not significantly associated with any hematological parameters [27].

Malaria and HIV are highly prevalent infection in the developing countries, especially in sub-Saharan Africa. They cause hematological abnormalities which decrease the immune response and increase adult mortality. Therefore, assessment of hematological abnormalities in malaria HIV co-infection individuals has remarkable benefit to prevent HIV malaria co-morbidity [31].

In general, this study was a comparative cross sectional study which tried to identify independent factors of hematological profiles in HIV and malaria co infected individuals. The limitations of the study are: first this study is limited by its cross sectional design, not longitudinal, preventing assessment of cause and effect relationship. Second, we did not consider the malaria seasonality and species identification using PCR.

Table 4 Predictors of leucopenia

Variables	Leucopenia		COR (95% CI)	*P*-value	AOR (95% CI)	*P*-Value
	Yes *n* (%)	No *n* (%)				
Sex						
F	41 (39.4)	63 (60.6)	0.98 (0.53–1.84)	0.970		
M	27 (39.7)	41 (60.3)	1			
Age						
18–29	23 (38.3)	37 (61.7)	1			
30–39	35 (42.2)	48 (57.8)	1.17 (0.59–2.31)	0.645		
40–49	7 (30.4)	16 (69.6)	0.70 (0.25–1.97)	0.504		
≥ 50	3 (50.0)	3 (50.0)	1.61 (0.23–8.65)	0.580		
HAART status						
Yes	56 (39.4)	86 (60.6)	1			
No	12 (40.0)	18 (60.0)	1.02 (0.46–2.28)	0.954		
Opportunistic infection						
Yes	5 (31.2)	11 (68.8)	0.67 (0.22–2.02)	0.479		
No	63 (40.4)	93 (59.6)	1			
Malaria infection						
Yes	37 (43.0)	49 (57.0)	1.34 (0.73–2.47)	0.350		
No	31 (36.0)	55 (64.0)	1			
Malaria parasitic density (parasite/μl)						
1–999	13 (61.9)	8 (38.1)	1		1	
1000–9999	20 (46.5)	23 (53.3)	0.53 (0.18–1.55)	0.250	0.55 (0.18–1.69)	0.303
≥ 10000	4 (18.2)	18 (81.8)	0.14 (0.34–0.55)	0.005	0.13 (0.03–0.57)	0.007
CD_4^+ count (cells/μl)						
≤ 200	16 (61.5)	10 (38.5)	7.12 (2.58–19.61)	<0.001	4.77 (1.23–18.45)	0.023
200–499	25 (29.8)	59 (70.2)	3.11 (1.47–6.57)	0.003	2.85 (0.94–8.62)	0.064
≥ 500	20 (32.3)	42 (67.7)	1		1	

*COR-Crude odd ratio, AOR-Adjusted odd ratio, CI-Confidence interval, 1- indicator and statistically significant at $p < 0.05$

Conclusions

Findings suggest that the prevalence of anemia and thrombocytopenia were significantly higher in the malaria and HIV coinfected patients than the HIV mono-infected patients. Mean values of hematological profiles were significantly different in the two groups. Future prospective studies with larger sample size from other settings are needed to substantiate the findings.

Acknowledgement
We would like to thank our data collectors for their invaluable effort. Our deep gratitude also goes to our study subjects who were volunteered and took their time to give us all the relevant information for the study.

Funding
The study was funded by Jimma University. The funder has no role in the design of the study and collection, analysis, and interpretation of data and in writing the manuscript.

Authors' contribution
TS, TY and LG conceived the study, participated in the design and data analysis. TS, LG and TY involved in data acquisition, laboratory work and drafted the manuscript. LG critically reviewed the manuscript. All authors read and approved the manuscript.

Competing interests
We declare that we have no competing interests.

Author details
[1]Department of Clinical Laboratory, Gambella Hospital, Gambella, Ethiopia. [2]Department of Medical Laboratory Science and Pathology, Jimma University, Jimma, Ethiopia.

References

1. Maina NR, Walsh D, Gaddy C, Hongo G, Waitumbi J, Otieno L, Jones D, Ogutu BR. Impact of Plasmodium falciparum infection on hematological parameters in children living in Western Kenya. Malar J. 2010;9(3):1–11.
2. Crawley J. Reducing the burden of anemia in infants and young children in malaria-endemic countries of Africa: from evidence to action. Am J Trop Med Hyg. 2004;71 Suppl 2:25–34.
3. Lamikanra AA, Brown D, Potocnik A, Casals-pascual C, Langhorne J, Roberts DJ. Malarial anemia : of mice and men. Blood. 2007;110(1):18–28.
4. Iqbal W. Hematological manifestations in malaria. Haematol Updat. 2010; 2010:35–7.

5. Mckenzie FE, Prudhomme WA, Magill AJ, Forney JR, Permpanich B, Lucas C, GasserJr RA, Wondsrichanalai C. White blood cell counts and malaria. J Infect Dis. 2005;192(2):323–30.
6. Sullivan PS, Hanson DL, Chu SY, Jones JL, Ward JW, Sullivan BPS. Epidemiology of anemia in human immunodeficiency virus (HIV)-infected persons: results from the multistate adult and adolescent spectrum of HIV disease surveillance project. Blood. 1998;91(1):301–8.
7. Kuritzkes DR. Neutropenia, neutrophil dysfunction, and bacterial infection in patients with human immunodeficiency virus disease : the role of granulocyte colony-stimulating factor. Clin Infect Dis. 2000;30(2):256–60.
8. Sullivan PS, Hanson DL, Chu SY, Jones JL, Ciesielski CA. Surveillance for Thrombocytopenia in Persons Infected With HIV: Results From the Multistate Adult and Adolescent Spectrum of Disease Project. J Acquir Immune Defic Syndr. 1996;14(4):374–9.
9. Hochman S, Kim K. The impact of HIV and malaria co-infection: what is known and suggested venues for further study. Interdiscip Perspect Infect Dis. 2009;2009:1–8.
10. World vision and Roll Back malaria. The link between malaria and HIV and AIDS. http://www.wvi.org/sites/default/files/HIV_and_Malaria_flyer_English.pdf. Accessed 30 May 2015.
11. World Health Organization (WHO). Malaria in HIV/AIDS patients. http://www.who.int/malaria/areas/high_risk_groups/hiv_aids_patients/en/. Accessed 30 May 2015.
12. World Health Organization (WHO). Malaria and HIV interactions and their implications for public health policy. Geneva: WHO; 2004.
13. Grimwade K, French N, Mbatha DD, Zungu DD, Dedicoat M, Gilks CF. HIV infection as a cofactor for severe falciparum malaria in adults living in a region of unstable malaria transmission in South Africa. AIDS. 2004;18(3):547–54.
14. Kirchhoff F, Silvestri G. Is Nef the elusive cause of HIV-associated hematopoietic dysfunction ? J Clin Invest. 2008;118(5):1622–5.
15. Coyle TE. Hematological complications of human immuno deficiency virus infection and the acquired immuno deficiency syndrome. Med Clin North Am. 1997;81(2):449–70.
16. Kassa D, Petros B, Messele T, Admassu A, Adugna F, Wolday D. Parasito-hematological features of acute Plasmodium falciparum and P.vivax malaria patients with and without HIV co-infection at Wonji Sugar Estate, Ethiopia. Ethiop J Health Dev. 2005;19(2):132–9.
17. Wondimeneh Y, Ferede G, Atnafu A, Muluye D. HIV-Malaria Co-infection and their immunohematological profiles. Eur J Exp Biol. 2013;3(1):497–502.
18. Ethiopian health and nutrition research institute (EHNRI). Manual for the Laboratory Diagnosis of Malaria. first edit. Addis Ababa: Ethiopia federal ministery of health (EFMOH); 2012. p. 40.
19. World Health Organization (WHO). Worldwide prevalence of anemia 1993-2005. Geneva: WHO; 2008.
20. Hoffbrand AV, Catovsky D, Tuddenham EG, Green AR, editors. Postgraduate hematology. Sixth edit. Blackwell Publishing Ltd. 2011. p. 956.
21. Erhabor O, Babatunde S, Uko KE. Some hematological parameters in Plasmodial parasitized HIV-infected Nigerians. Niger J Med. 2006;15(1):52–5.
22. Tagoe DN, Boachie J. Assessment of the impact of malaria on CD_4^+ T Cells and haemoglobin levels of HIV-malaria co-infected patients. J Infect Dev Ctries. 2012;6(9):660–3.
23. Akinbo FO, Omoregie R. Plasmodium falciparum infection in HIV-infected patients on highly active antiretroviral therapy (HAART) in Benin City. Nigeria J Res Heal Sci. 2012;12(1):15–8.
24. Bharti AR, Saravanan S, Madhavan V, Smith DM, Sharma J, Balakrishnan P, Letendre SL, Kumarasamy N. Correlates of HIV and malaria co-infection in Southern India. Malar J. 2012;11(306):2–5.
25. Quintero JP, Siqueira AM, Tobón A, Blair S, Moreno A, Arévalo-herrera M, Guimaraes Lacerda MV, Valencia SH. Malaria-related anemia : a Latin American perspective. Mem Inst Oswaldo Cruz. 2011;106(1):91–104.
26. Etusim PE, Ihemanma CA, Nduka FO, P.E. M, Ukpai O. Comparative study on the hematological characteristics of malaria infected and malaria non-infected persons referred to Art/HIV laboratory, Abia State University Teaching Hospital, Aba, Abia State. J Sci Multidiscip Res. 2013;5(1):100–12.
27. Tchinda GG, Atashili J, Achidi EA, Kamga HL, Njunda AL, Ndumbe PM. Impact of malaria on hematological parameters in people living with HIV/AIDS attending the Laquintinie Hospital in Douala, Cameroon. PLoS One. 2012;7(7):e40553.
28. Parinitha SS, Kulkarni MH. Hematological changes in HIV infection with correlation to CD_4 cell count. Australas Med J. 2012;5(3):157–62.
29. De Santis GC, Brunetta DM, Vilar FC, Brandao RA, De Albernaz Munizb RZ, de Lima GMN. Amorelli chacel ME, Covas DT, Machado AA. Hematological abnormalities in HIV-infected patients. Int J Infect Dis. 2011;15(12):808–11.
30. Kyeyune R, Saathoff E, Ezeamama AE, Löscher T, Fawzi W, Guwatudde D. Prevalence and correlates of cytopenias in HIV-infected adults initiating highly active antiretroviral therapy in Uganda. BMC Infect Dis. 2014;14(496):1–10.
31. Berg A, Patel S, Aukrust P, David C, Gonca M, Berg ES, Dalen I, Langeland N. Increased severity and mortality in adults co-infected with malaria and HIV in Maputo, Mozambique : A prospective cross-sectional study. PLoS One. 2014;9(2):e88257.

Randomized double-blind safety comparison of intravenous iron dextran versus iron sucrose in an adult non-hemodialysis outpatient population

Martha L. Louzada[1,2], Cyrus C. Hsia[1,2,6*], Fatimah Al-Ani[2], Fiona Ralley[2,3], Anargyros Xenocostas[1,2], Janet Martin[2,4], Sarah E. Connelly[2,4], Ian H. Chin-Yee[1,2], Leonard Minuk[1,2] and Alejandro Lazo-Langner[1,2,5]

Abstract

Background: Intravenous iron therapy is a treatment option for iron deficient patients who are intolerant to oral iron or where oral iron is ineffective, but with possible adverse effects. Currently, prospective studies comparing different intravenous iron formulations are needed to determine safety and efficacy of these agents.

Methods: We conducted a prospective, double-blind, randomized controlled trial (RCT) to assess the feasibility of a trial comparing the safety of high molecular weight intravenous iron dextran, Infufer®, with intravenous iron sucrose, Venofer®, in non-hemodialysis adult outpatients. Primary outcome was the occurrence of immediate severe drug reactions.

Results: We enrolled 143 patients in a one-year period. Overall, 45/143 (31.5 %) patients (20 iron dextran, 25 iron sucrose) developed 48 infusion reactions (14 immediate, 28 delayed, and 3 both). The risk of an immediate reaction was similar in both groups, 9/73 (12.3 %) iron dextran versus 8/70 (11.4 %) iron sucrose, RR = 0.93 (95 % CI; 0.38 to 2.27). The risk of a delayed reaction was significantly higher in the iron sucrose group 22/70 (31.4 %) versus the iron dextran group 9/73 (12.3 %), RR = 2.55 (95 % CI; 1.26 to 5.15; $p = 0.0078$).

Conclusion: In this limited feasibility study, no major differences in immediate reactions were seen, but a significantly higher number of delayed reactions were seen in the iron sucrose group. Further, under our assumptions and design a full RCT to evaluate the safety of different intravenous iron preparations is not feasible. Future studies should consider modifying the clinical outcomes, utilize multiple centers, and consider other emerging parenteral iron formulations. (ClinicalTrials.gov NCT005936197 January 3, 2008).

Keywords: Intravenous iron, Iron dextran, Iron sucrose, Safety, Feasibility, Randomized controlled trial

* Correspondence: cyrus.hsia@lhsc.on.ca
Martha L. Louzada and Cyrus C. Hsia shared first authorship.
[1]Department of Medicine, Division of Hematology, London, ON, Canada
[2]University of Western Ontario, London, ON, Canada
Full list of author information is available at the end of the article

Background

Iron deficiency is the most common cause of anemia worldwide affecting up to 50 % of children under 5 years of age and up to 20 % of women under the age of 50 [1–3]. Use of oral iron supplementation is the standard first line treatment; however, it is associated with several side effects that may lead to lack of compliance. Adverse drug reactions (ADRs) to oral iron can be as high as 70 % with associated non-adherence rates of 70 % [4]. Intravenous iron may be an alternative for patients intolerant or unresponsive to oral iron formulations and is most widely used in patients with chronic kidney disease on hemodialysis [5–8]. It is also frequently used preoperatively with or without erythropoietin to augment hemoglobin levels prior to surgery, in patients with iron deficiency anemia secondary to gastrointestinal bleeding or pre-dialysis patients with chronic kidney disease where oral iron supplementation is insufficient [5, 9].

In the non-hemodialysis setting there is evidence to support the effectiveness of intravenous iron but relatively little evidence comparing the safety of different intravenous iron formulations. A few observational studies and randomized trials comparing the adverse reactions of iron dextran to iron sucrose have suggested the development of more frequent and serious ADRs in patients using iron dextran [9–15]. A previous retrospective study conducted at our centre showed higher incidence rates of adverse events and severe reactions in patients receiving iron dextran compared to iron sucrose [16]. However, these findings are difficult to interpret because different doses of intravenous iron have been used in studies and different formulations exist for the same agent (e.g., high versus low molecular weight iron dextran).

Due to extensive intravenous iron utilization in hospitals, the need of prospective randomized trials to inform clinical decisions in selection of appropriate intravenous iron formulations is increasing. In this study, we sought to evaluate the feasibility of a randomized trial to compare the safety of a high molecular weight iron dextran with iron sucrose in non-hemodialysis adult outpatients.

Methods

Participants

The study was conducted at the London Health Sciences Centre, a University-affiliated academic center in London, Ontario Canada. We included adult (18 years of age or older (outpatients with iron deficiency anemia eligible to receive intravenous iron as a part of their clinical management. Iron deficiency anemia was defined as hemoglobin less than 130 g/L and a ferritin of less than 50 μg/L. This hemoglobin level was chosen because our perioperative blood conservation program identifies potential surgical patients with hemoglobin values between 100 and 130 g/L for possible intravenous iron to reduce the exposure to allogeneic blood products. Patients were excluded if they were on hemodialysis, had previous exposure to any form of intravenous iron or were unable to provide written informed consent.

Study design and sample size

The primary objective of this study was to assess the feasibility and to inform details for the design of a future randomized controlled trial to be conducted at our centre comparing the safety of equal doses of intravenous iron dextran or iron sucrose in non-hemodialysis adult patients. Based on the results of our previous retrospective study of adverse reactions to intravenous iron [16], we calculated that we would need to enrol 213 patients per group to demonstrate a 5 % difference between groups for the main outcome at the 95 % level of significance with a power of 80 %. In order for such a trial to be considered feasible we would need to enrol approximately 100 patients per year. Based on our clinical volumes we anticipated that we could identify 120 potential patients per year. If 90 % agreed to participate, then we would be able to complete accrual for the full trial within 4 years.

The study was designed as a double-blinded randomized controlled trial comparing equal doses of intravenous iron dextran with intravenous iron sucrose. Randomization sequences were computer-generated via a third party (IBM, San Jose, California, USA) and stratified by site (2 sites), in blocks of 8. Randomization tables were only accessible by our central pharmacy requiring this information for concealment of iron products. Participants could choose to stop the study any point during the study or be unblinded at the discretion of the treating physician if it was felt that continuing would harm the patient. Subsequently, crossover to the other agent could be done at the discretion of the treating physician. The study complied with the Declaration of Helsinki, Health Canada and the international conference on harmonization – good clinical practice (ICH-GCP) guidelines. The study protocol was approved by the Research Ethics Board of the University of Western Ontario (HSREB 13767). Written informed consent was obtained from all participants. This study was registered at ClinicalTrials.gov with number NCT00593619 January 8, 2008.

Interventions

Patients were randomized to receive either intravenous iron dextran with an estimated molecular weight of 200 kDa (Infufer®, Sandoz Canada Inc., Montreal, Canada) or iron sucrose (Venofer®, Luitpold Pharmaceuticals Inc., Shirley, New York, USA) at a dose of 300 mg given in 250 mL of normal saline and administered over 2 h with the first 25 mg over 10 min as a test dose. Each study drug was concealed and had a unique study label. No premedications were permitted. Before and after iron infusion, samples were obtained for complete blood count and serum ferritin.

Study outcomes

The primary feasibility outcome of the study was enrollment of at least 100 patients per year. The primary clinical outcome of the study was the occurrence of immediate severe adverse reactions (ADRs). Secondary outcomes were the occurrence of: immediate and delayed serious ADRs; immediate anaphylactic/anaphylactoid ADRs, immediate combined mild and moderate ADRs, delayed ADRs, all-cause mortality; mean time physicians spent managing ADRs; mean time nurses spent managing ADRs; and absolute difference in hemoglobin, platelet and ferritin. We also planned to collect costing data for a cost effectiveness analysis. ADRs were recorded including the onset (in minutes from initial administration), duration and description of symptoms/signs, intervention(s) applied, and any additional nursing time required to manage the reaction. ADRs were considered immediate if they occurred during the infusion time or delayed if occurred within the first 24 h post-infusion (Fig. 1). All patients were contacted at home via telephone after 24 h by a member of the research team for assessment of delayed reactions. The severity of ADRs was classified according to the National Cancer Institute (NCI) Common Terminology Criteria for Adverse Events v3·0 guidelines: (Table 2). Three blinded assessors (2 Hematologists and 1 Cardiologist), blinded to patient allocation, reviewed the ADRs and independently adjudicated the type and severity of ADRs. Discrepancies were resolved by consensus with a fourth investigator.

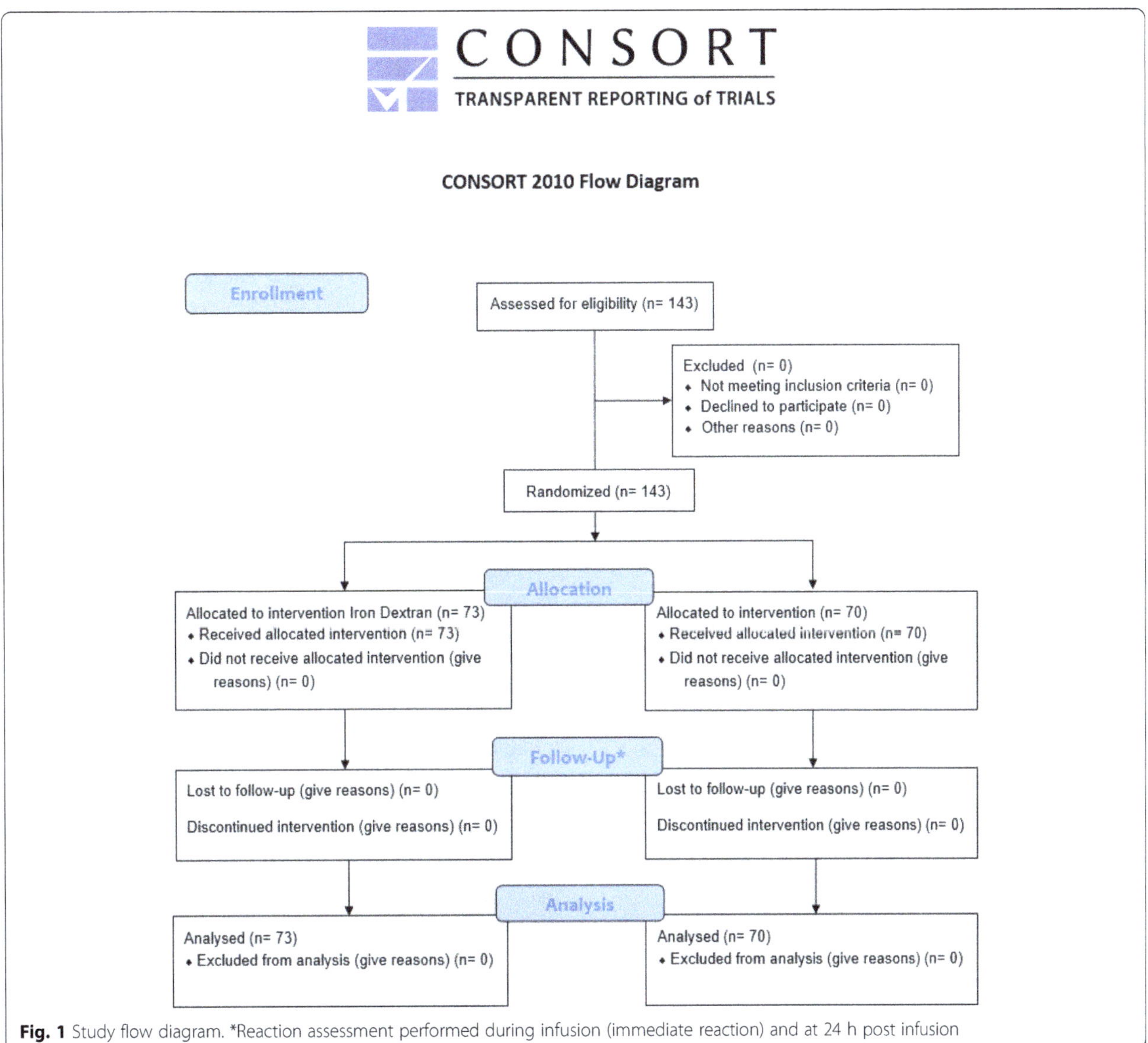

Fig. 1 Study flow diagram. *Reaction assessment performed during infusion (immediate reaction) and at 24 h post infusion

Statistical analysis

All statistical analyses were performed on an intention-to-treat basis. Baseline characteristics of participants, primary and secondary outcomes were analyzed by means of descriptive statistics. For comparison between groups we used Fisher's exact test for categorical variables and unpaired t-test for continuous variables. We calculated relative risk (RR) and 95 % confidence intervals (95 % CI) for primary and secondary outcomes, using the iron sucrose group as reference. *P*-values <0.05 were considered statistically significant.

Results

Between January 2008 and January 2009 we enrolled 143 patients. The study was terminated early after an interim analysis found four severe ADRs occurred. All potentially eligible patients were approached and agreed to participate in the study (Fig. 1). No participants withdrew consent or were lost to follow-up. Patient characteristics are shown in Table 1. Of the participants, 46/143 (32.2 %) were males, the median age was 68 years (standard deviation 17.6) and the most frequent indication for intravenous iron therapy was pre-operative iron supplementation in 117/143 (81.8 %).

Table 1 Baseline characteristics of included patients

Characteristics	Iron dextran N = 73	Iron sucrose N = 70	P
Female sex (%)	45 (61.6)	52 (74.3)	0.112
Age, years (sd)	70 (17.6)	66 (17.4)	0.872
IV iron indication [n(%)]			
Pre-operative			
Cardiovascular surgery	18 (25)	14 (20)	
Gastrointestinal surgery	10 (14)	8 (11)	
Orthopedic surgery	32 (44)	36 (51)	
Other surgeries	1 (1)	1 (1)	
Bleeding			
Menorrhagia	2 (3)	2 (3)	
Acute GI bleed	4 (5)	5 (5)	
Chronic GI Bleed	3 (5)	1 (3)	
Other			
Malignancy	2 (3)	2 (3)	
Indication not available	1 (2)	1 (3)	
Other characteristics [n(%)]			
Chronic kidney disease	7 (10)	2 (3)	0.167
Previous treatment [n(%)] (available data)	68	57	
PO iron	53 (73)	50 (71)	
IM iron	3 (4)	0 (0)	
Erythropoietin (EPO)	2 (3)	1 (2)	
Both iron & EPO	33 (45)	30 (43)	
None	10 (14)	6 (4)	

Abbreviations: *GI* gastrointestinal, *IM* intramuscular Iron, *PO* oral, *sd* standard deviation

Overall, 45/143 (31.5 %) patients developed 48 infusion reactions (14 immediate, 28 delayed, and 3 with both). The risk of an immediate reaction was similar in both groups: 9/73 (12.3 %) iron dextran and 8/70 (11.4 %) iron sucrose (RR = 0.93, 95 % CI; 0.38 to 2.27, $p = 0.873$). However, the risk of a delayed reaction was significantly higher in the iron sucrose group [22/70 (31.4 %)] versus 9/73 (12.3 %) in the iron dextran group (RR = 2.55, 95 % CI; 1.26 to 5.15; $p = 0.0078$).A detailed list of immediate and delayed reactions are provided in Table 2. The reactions were classified into four major categories (musculoskeletal, cardiovascular, allergic, and gastrointestinal) in Fig. 2 and highlight that there were more musculoskeletal and gastrointestinal delayed adverse reactions with iron sucrose.

After infusion start, the mean time for the occurrence of immediate reactions was 32 min (range 2 to 120). All of the immediate and delayed reactions were transient and self-limited with deaths reported. There were nine immediate reactions (6 iron dextran and 3 iron sucrose) that occurred within the first 10 min that can be considered reactions within the "test dose" period of time. Eighteen patients required medical intervention with no significant difference between the dextran or sucrose arms. While most of the ADRs were mild in severity (Grade 1 or 2), a total of four patients (2.7 %) were considered to have severe grade 3 or 4 ADRs and were sent to the emergency department for appropriate management, two in each study arm, and were unblinded at the request of the treating physicians. A Data Safety Monitoring committee stopped the trial due to these events. Only one patient was crossed over to the other product (from iron sucrose to iron dextran) at the discretion of the treating physician without any further complications.

Hematologic parameters including hemoglobin, platelet count and ferritin were evaluated before and after the first intravenous iron infusion. There were no significant differences between groups (data not shown). Finally, although we planned to estimate resource utilization and costs, unfortunately this data was not accurately recorded and therefore it is not reported.

Discussion

We conducted a study to evaluate the feasibility of a randomized controlled trial comparing the safety of two parenteral iron formulations in previously untreated non-dialysis iron deficient patients. The study was stopped prematurely due to the occurrence of 4 severe ADRs requiring physician assessment and intervention. Although we were able to exceed our recruitment target with a total of 143 patients enrolled in a one-year period, with the

Table 2 Adverse drug reactions and severity classified according to the National Cancer Institute Common Toxicity Criteria

	Sex	Iron formulation	Reaction (Grade of severity)
Immediate reactions			
1.	F	Sucrose	Back pain (2), tachycardia (1), nausea (1)
2.	F	Sucrose	[a]Allergic Reaction (3)
3.	F	Dextran	Chest pain (2)
4.	F	Dextran	Pruritus (1)
5.	F	Sucrose	Taste alteration (1)
6.	M	Sucrose	Headache (2), Tachycardia (1)
7.	F	Dextran	Dyspnea (1), Flushed (1), Abdominal distension/bloating (3)
8.	F	Dextran	[a]Urticaria (3)
9.	F	Sucrose	Abdominal distension/bloating (1)
10.	M	Dextran	Dyspnea (2)
11.	F	Sucrose	Urticaria (2)
12.	F	Sucrose	Flushing (2)
13.	F	Sucrose	[a]Hypotension (3), back pain (2)
14.	F	Dextran	Hypotension (2), Urticaria (2), Chills (1)
15.	F	Dextran	Nausea (1)
16.	F	Dextran	[a]Allergic Reaction (3)
17.	F	Dextran	Neuropathy - sensory (2)
Delayed reactions			
1.	M	Sucrose	Arthralgia (1), Myalgia (1)
2.	F	Dextran	Nausea (1), Headache (1), Chills (1), Abdominal distension (1)
3.	F	Sucrose	Fatigue (1)
4.	F	Dextran	Headache (1), Fatigue (1)
5.	F	Dextran	Presyncope (2)
6.	F	Sucrose	Arthralgia (1), Myalgia (1), Chills (1)
7.	F	Sucrose	Diarrhea (1), Abdominal distension (1), Headache (2)
8.	F	Dextran	Headache (1)
9.	F	Sucrose	Headache (2), flushes (1)
10.	F	Dextran	Pruritus (1)
11.	F	Sucrose	Urticaria (2), Fever (2), Presyncope (2)
12.	M	Dextran	Back pain (2)
13.	F	Sucrose	Fatigue (1), Arthralgia (1)
14.	M	Sucrose	Headache (1), Abdominal distension (1)
15.	F	Sucrose	Abdominal distension (1), Fever (1)
16.	F	Sucrose	Fever (1), Headache (2)
17.	F	Sucrose	Diarrhea (1)
18.	F	Sucrose	Headache (1), Back pain (1)
19.	F	Sucrose	Pruritus (1)
20.	F	Dextran	Urticaria (2)
21.	F	Sucrose	Urticaria (1)
22.	F	Sucrose	Edema limbs (1)
23.	F	Sucrose	Headache (1)
24.	F	Sucrose	Abdominal distension (1), Diarrhea (1)

Table 2 Adverse drug reactions and severity classified according to the National Cancer Institute Common Toxicity Criteria *(Continued)*

25.	F	Sucrose	Abdominal distension (1)
26.	F	Dextran	Arthralgia (1), Myalgia (1), Back pain (1)
27.	F	Sucrose	Chills (1), Generalized muscle weakness (1), Nausea (1)
28.	M	Sucrose	Nausea (1), Headache (1), Abdominal pain (1)
29.	F	Dextran	Nausea (1), Headache (1), Presyncope (2)
30.	F	Sucrose	Nausea (1)
31.	F	Sucrose	Arthralgia (1), Myalgia (1), Chills (1)

[a]Patients who required further intervention including transfer to emergency department
Severity of events according to the National Cancer Institute Common Toxicity Criteria
0 = No adverse event or within normal limits
1 = Mild adverse event
2 = Moderate adverse event
3 = Severe and undesirable adverse event
4 = Life-threatening or disabling adverse event
5 = Death related to adverse event

observed rate of severe immediate reactions, a randomized trial designed to detect a 2 % difference in immediate ADRs would not be feasible as a single centre study. The design of the study with a one point in time evaluation and a short follow up that did not require extra hospital visits or blood tests were attractive features that maximized patients' participation.

With respect to the clinical outcomes of the study, we found no significant difference in the incidence of total or immediate ADRs between iron dextran group and iron sucrose group. However, the risk of a delayed reaction was significantly higher in the iron sucrose group. The incidence of the overall number of reactions is much higher than previously reported. Our data is congruent with previously published available literature with respect to the incidence of severe adverse reactions of high molecular weight iron dextran and iron sucrose. Overall, studies have reported extremely low rates of serious adverse reactions with different preparations of intravenous iron. In particular, anaphylactoid reactions and death are extremely rare. Studies performed before 2000, using high molecular weight dextran suggest an incidence of severe ADRs of about 1 % [11, 13, 17]. A small study compared the safety of low molecular weight iron dextran with iron sucrose in patients with chronic kidney disease and showed that the incidence of side effects associated with iron-dextran was not different than that of iron-sucrose [18].

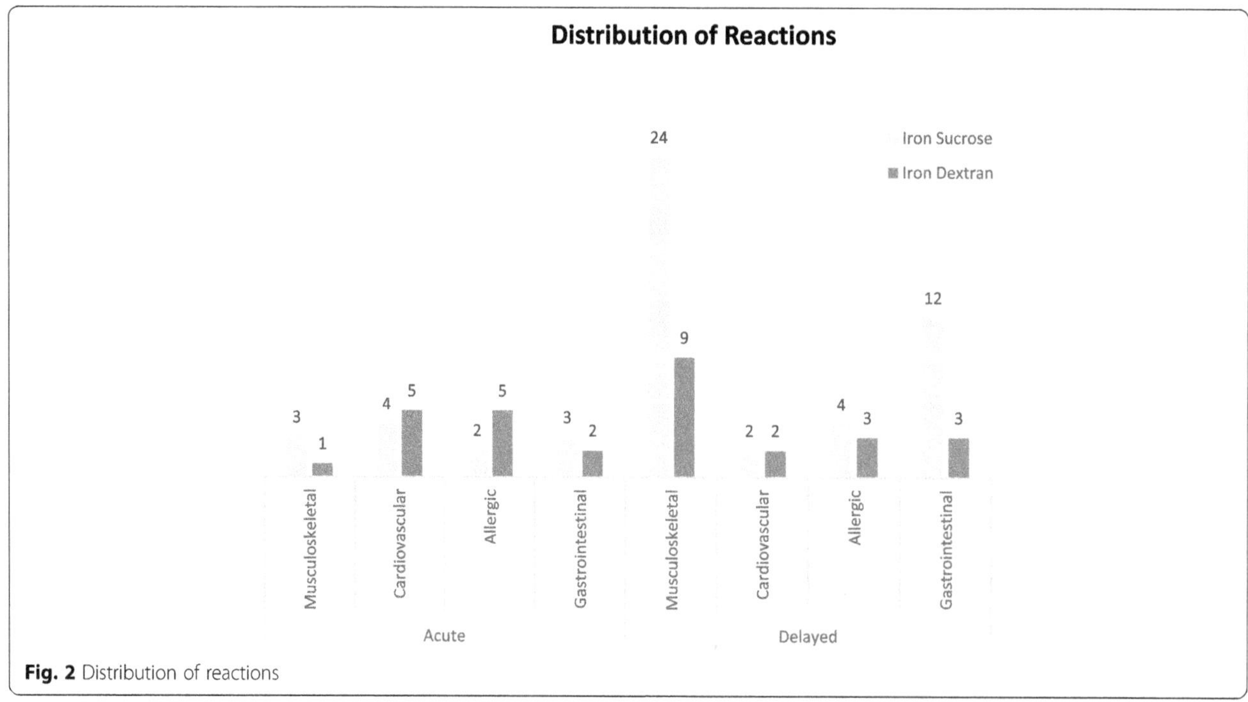

Fig. 2 Distribution of reactions

A recent single institution retrospective study of 619 unique patients showed that no serious ADRs were associated with intravenous iron use in patients receiving low molecular weight iron dextran, iron sucrose, ferric gluconate and high molecular weight dextran. Regarding the incidence of ADRs, low molecular weight dextran and ferric gluconate were similar and both caused less ADRs than iron sucrose. High molecular weight dextran, although used in a small number of patients (only nine patients in that study), was associated with a high rate of ADRs (44.4 %) [19] and other studies suggest that high molecular weight iron dextran formulation has a higher incidence of adverse outcomes compared to iron sucrose [6, 7, 10, 20, 21].

Whereas in our earlier retrospective study, we found that the risk of severe ADRs was 7-fold higher with Infufer® compared to Venofer® [16], in our current study, we were not able to show a difference. We found similar incidence rates of acute reactions and severe ADRs, but a surprising significant increase in delayed ADRs in the sucrose group ($p = 0.078$). Of particular note, when reactions were categorized there appeared to be more musculoskeletal and gastrointestinal delayed reactions with iron sucrose. However, we cannot completely rule out that the lower incidence of delayed ADRs in the iron sucrose group in our previous study may have been due to reporting bias. Further, the majority of our patients, 81 to 83 %, received intravenous iron in the pre-operative setting limiting the generalizability of this data to patients with iron deficiency in general routine practice.

In this study, we did not aim to collect markers of oxidative stress or other markers to determine the mechanisms of these reactions. In addition to our study's early termination another limitation of our study is that we were not able to evaluate the risk of adverse reactions with subsequent intravenous iron infusions. Nevertheless, studies suggest that up to 70 % of ADRs occur during or right after the first intravenous iron infusion [11–13]. Further, we used iron sucrose at a dilution of 1.2 mg/mL (a lower end of dilution for this product) and dilution of nanoparticle colloidal suspensions such as intravenous iron formulations leads to reduced stability due to ionic shielding. However, both products were administered using the same dilution at our commonly used iron sucrose concentration of 1.2 mg/mL (that was also used in our previous study).

Conclusion

We conducted a randomized controlled trial (RCT) to evaluate the feasibility for accrual and to inform the design of a future trial comparing the safety of intravenous iron dextran versus iron sucrose in non-hemodialysis adult patients at a single center. Whereas accrual was possible under our assumptions in the first year, it was stopped early. With the limited data, we found no significant difference in the incidence of immediate ADRs and a rate of delayed reactions that was significantly higher in the sucrose group. Given these findings we conclude that under our assumptions and design that a full RCT is not feasible to be conducted at a single center. Future studies should consider modifying the clinical outcomes, utilize multiple centers, and consider other emerging parenteral iron formulations.

Abbreviations

ADR: adverse drug reaction; ICH-GCP: international conference on harmonization – good clinical practice; NCI: National Cancer Institute; RCT: randomized controlled trial; RR: relative risk.

Competing interests

The authors declare that they have no competing interests.

Authors' contributions

CCH designed the research, performed research, analyzed data, wrote and revised the paper. MLL and FAA analyzed data and wrote the paper. IHC-Y and FR designed the research, analyzed data, and revised the paper. J.M. and S.C. designed the research and revised the paper. LM helped perform research. AL-L and AX analyzed data and revised the paper. All authors read and approved the final manuscript.

Acknowledgements

We are indebted to Pam Psutka, Pharmacist, for her role in initiating and implementing the project. We thank Donna Berta and Valerie Binns, nurses on the Blood Conservation Program and OnTRAC for their assistance in getting perioperative patients on intravenous iron and recruiting patients for the study. We also acknowledge the tireless work and excellent patient care provided by our IV therapy clinic nurses, Katrina Ormond and staff.

Author details

[1]Department of Medicine, Division of Hematology, London, ON, Canada. [2]University of Western Ontario, London, ON, Canada. [3]Department of Anesthesia and Perioperative Medicine, London, ON, Canada. [4]Department of Pharmacy, London Health Sciences Centre, London, ON, Canada. [5]Department of Epidemiology & Biostatistics, London, ON, Canada. [6]London Health Sciences Centre, Department of Medicine, Division of Hematology. Rm E6-219A, Victoria Hospital, 800 Commissioners Road E., London, ON N6A 5W9, Canada.

References

1. 2014 Annual Results Report: Nutrition. New York: UNICEF; 2015. p. 23. http://www.unicef.org/publicpartnerships/files/2014_Annual_Results_Report_Nutrition.pdf. Accessed 10 March 2016.
2. Christofides A, Schauer C, Zlotkin SH. Iron deficiency anemia among children: addressing a global public health problem within a Canadian context. Paediatr Child Health. 2005;10(10):597–601.
3. McClung JP, Marchitelli LJ, Friedl KE, Young AJ. Prevalence of iron deficiency and iron deficiency anemia among three populations of female military personnel in the US Army. J Am Coll Nutr. 2006;25(1):64–9.
4. Kruske S, Ruben A, Brewster D. An iron treatment trial in an aboriginal community: improving non-adherence. J Paediatr Child Health. 1999;35:153.
5. Auerbach M, Rodgers GM. Intravenous iron. N Engl J Med. 2007;357(1):93–4.
6. Faich G, Strobos J. Sodium ferric gluconate complex in sucrose: safer intravenous iron therapy than iron dextrans. Am J Kidney Dis. 1999;33(3):464–70.
7. Auerbach M, Ballard H. Clinical use of intravenous iron: administration, efficacy, and safety. Hematol Am Soc Hematol Educ Program. 2010;2010:338–47.
8. Barton J, Barton E, Bertoli L, Gothard C, Sherrer J. Intravenous iron dextran therapy in patients with iron deficiency and normal renal function who failed to respond to or did not tolerate oral iron supplementation. Am J Med. 2000;109(1):27–32.

9. Laman CA, Silverstein SB, Rodgers GM. Parenteral iron therapy: a single institution's experience over a 5-year period. J Natl Compr Canc Netw. 2005;3(6):791–5.
10. Burns DL, Pomposelli JJ. Toxicity of parenteral iron dextran therapy. Kidney Int Suppl. 1999;69:S119–24.
11. Fishbane S, Ungureanu VD, Maesaka JK, Kaupke CJ, Lim V, Wish J. The safety of intravenous iron dextran in hemodialysis patients. Am J Kidney Dis. 1996;28(4):529–34.
12. Fishbane S. Safety in iron management. Am J Kidney Dis. 2003;41(5 Suppl):18–26.
13. Hamstra RD, Block MH, Schocket AL. Intravenous iron dextran in clinical medicine. JAMA. 1980;243(17):1726–31.
14. Prakash S, Walele A, Dimkovic N, Bargman J, Vas S, Oreopoulos D. Experience with a large dose (500 mg) of intravenous iron dextran and iron saccharate in peritoneal dialysis patients. Perit Dial Int. 2001;21(3):290–5.
15. Fishbane S, Lynn R. The efficacy of iron dextran for the treatment of iron deficiency in hemodialysis patients. Clin Nephrol. 1995;44(4):238–40.
16. Hsia CC, Ormond K, Chin-Yee IH, Xenocostas A. A retrospective review of adverse reactions to intravenous iron in non-hemodialysis patients. J Public Health Pharm. 2008;1(1):57–69.
17. Fishbane S. Safety issues with iron sucrose. Am J Kidney Dis. 2003;41(4):899.
18. Sav T, Tokgoz B, Sipahioglu MH, Deveci M, Sari I, Oymak O, et al. Is there a difference between the allergic potencies of the iron sucrose and low molecular weight iron dextran? Ren Fail. 2007;29(4):423–6.
19. Okam M, Mandell E, Hevelone N, Wentz R, Ross A, Abel G. Comparative rates of adverse events with different formulations of intravenous iron. Am J Hematol. 2012;87(11):E123–124.
20. Critchley J, Dunbar Y. Adverse events associated with intravenous iron infusion (low-molecular weight iron dextran and iron sucrose): a systematic review. Transfus Altern Transfus Med. 2007;9:8–36.
21. Moniem K, Bhandari S. Tolerability and efficacy of parenteral iron therapy in hemodialysis patients, a comparison of preparations. Transfus Altern Transfus Med. 2007;9:37–42.

17

Alterations in hematologic indices during long-duration spaceflight

Hawley Kunz[1], Heather Quiriarte[2], Richard J. Simpson[3], Robert Ploutz-Snyder[4], Kathleen McMonigal[5], Clarence Sams[5] and Brian Crucian[5*]

Abstract

Background: Although a state of anemia is perceived to be associated with spaceflight, to date a peripheral blood hematologic assessment of red blood cell (RBC) indices has not been performed during long-duration space missions.

Methods: This investigation collected whole blood samples from astronauts participating in up to 6-months orbital spaceflight, and returned those samples (ambient storage) to Earth for analysis. As samples were always collected near undock of a returning vehicle, the delay from collection to analysis never exceeded 48 h. As a subset of a larger immunologic investigation, a complete blood count was performed. A parallel stability study of the effect of a 48 h delay on these parameters assisted interpretation of the in-flight data.

Results: We report that the RBC and hemoglobin were significantly elevated during flight, both parameters deemed stable through the delay of sample return. Although the stability data showed hematocrit to be mildly elevated at +48 h, there was an in-flight increase in hematocrit that was ~3-fold higher in magnitude than the anticipated increase due to the delay in processing.

Conclusions: While susceptible to the possible influence of dehydration or plasma volume alterations, these results suggest astronauts do not develop persistent anemia during spaceflight.

Keywords: Spaceflight, Red blood cells, Anemia, Platelets

Background

A number of physiologic changes are known to occur during prolonged spaceflight. The combined effects of microgravity, radiation, physical and psychological stressors, altered nutrition, disrupted circadian rhythms, and other factors have impacts on many of the body's systems, including vision, the musculoskeletal system, and the immune system [1]. Another marked alteration in physiology is the redistribution of fluids upon entering microgravity, which in turn may influence various hematologic parameters.

Without constant gravitational force, an almost immediate shift of fluids toward the head occurs, resulting in a "puffy" face and a reduced leg volume. An "acute plethora" of blood surrounds the central organs as peripheral blood is no longer held in the extremities by gravity [2–4]. While there is relevant existing information regarding red blood cells and spaceflight, it is primarily associated with short-duration Space Shuttle missions. Hematocrit, red blood cell (RBC) count, hemoglobin and plasma volume have been measured during short-duration spaceflight. RBC count and hemoglobin were found to be elevated throughout a 14-day mission, while plasma volume was found to be decreased 17% within the first 24 h immediately after launch, and remained depressed when measured at flight day 8 [2, 4]. In the same subjects, RBC mass was measured, but only immediately after landing, at which time a reduction in RBC mass was found [2–4]. The authors ascribed the likely cause of the reduction in RBC mass to be the "acute plethora" of RBCs resulting from fluid shifts during flight. These reductions in RBC mass following spaceflight have been observed throughout the history of spaceflight [3, 5]. During 10 to 14-day space missions, average losses of 10% to 15% of RBC mass immediately on landing are consistently reported, corresponding to a loss of approximately 1% RBC mass per day

* Correspondence: brian.crucian-1@nasa.gov
[5]NASA Johnson Space Center, 2101 E NASA Parkway, Houston, TX 77058, USA
Full list of author information is available at the end of the article

[3, 5]. These summary alterations result in an approximate 10% decrease in total blood volume [1] following short duration flight. Similar reductions have been observed in post-flight samples obtained after long-duration spaceflight [3, 5–7]. A reduction in RBC mass during spaceflight, termed "spaceflight anemia," is therefore a generally accepted phenomenon and appears to be a normal adaptation to microgravity [3, 5].

A majority of the studies examining alterations in RBC mass have been limited to post-flight evaluations. The few in-flight evaluations have been limited to short-duration flights, throughout which physiologic adaptations to microgravity are likely to still be occurring. Findings during short-duration flight may therefore not accurately reflect the in-flight condition during long-duration flight. As hematology indices generally do not tolerate freezing and ambient blood samples are rarely returned from space, there is a dearth of in-flight hematologic indices during long-duration spaceflight. The evidence that does exist for long-duration spaceflight appears to indicate that the reductions in RBC mass may actually be less severe for longer missions [7]. Further, very little information regarding the effects of spaceflight on platelets is available [3]. Therefore, additional data describing the in-flight hematologic condition as the body adapts to long-duration spaceflight are needed.

Here we report RBC and platelet indices on blood collected before, *during*, and after long-duration spaceflight as a subset of a two parent investigations of the effects of long-duration spaceflight on the immune system [8]. In-flight samples were collected in conjunction with crew returns and returned to the laboratory within 48 h, enabling an examination of ambient blood samples collected on board the International Space Station (ISS). A standard complete blood count (CBC) was performed on all samples. Alterations in the bulk leukocyte subsets during spaceflight, including in- and post-flight elevations of white blood cell and granulocyte concentrations, were previously reported alongside additional white blood cell functional data [8]. Here, in-flight hematologic indices were examined in an effort to better understand in-flight alterations in RBC and platelet parameters during long-duration spaceflight. To accurately interpret the data and to determine the impact of the processing delay resulting from the time required to transport ambient blood from the International Space Station (ISS) to the laboratory, a stability study examining the effects of room-temperature blood storage on these indices was also performed.

Methods

Subjects

Thirty-one astronaut crewmembers (25 males, 6 females, mean age 52 years, range 38–61) participated in one of two parent investigations, the National Aeronautics and Space Administration (NASA) 'Integrated Immune' and the University of Houston 'Salivary Markers' studies onboard the ISS. Of the 31 crewmembers, 24 flew on the Russian Soyuz capsule and completed missions of approximately 6 months. The remaining 7 crewmembers rotated to the ISS via the United States Space Shuttle. Of those 7, 5 completed missions lasting greater than 100 days, and 2 had mission durations of less than 60 days.

To determine the effects of room temperature storage on hematologic indices, 20 healthy, adult, non-astronaut subjects (12 males, 8 females, mean age 45 ± 13 years, range 26–65) were recruited for a stability study by the NASA Johnson Space Center (JSC) Test Subject Facility. For all astronaut and stability study subjects, approval was obtained from the JSC Institutional Review Board and written informed consent was obtained from all subjects.

Blood sampling

For both the flight study and the stability study, peripheral blood was collected into a 10.0 mL ethylenediaminetetraacetic acid (EDTA) spray-coated blood collection tube (BD, Franklin Lakes, NJ, USA). Pre-flight samples were collected at approximately 180 days (L-180) and 45 days (L-45) prior to launch. In-flight, samples were collected within the first 2 weeks of flight (early), between months 2 and 4 of the mission (mid), and approximately 6 months into the mission, immediately prior to return (late). For those astronauts completing shorter duration missions, only 2 samples were collected and corresponded to the "early" and "mid" time points. Post-flight, samples were collected within 3–8 h post-landing (R + 0) and 30 days post-flight (R + 30). Stability subject samples consisted of a single 10.0 mL EDTA spray-coated blood collection tube (BD), sampled as indicated following.

Processing

All CBCs were performed using calibrated, automated hematology analyzers (JSC processing: Coulter LH750, Miami, FL, USA; Kennedy Space Center (KSC) processing: Coulter Gen-S, Miami, FL, USA; Star City, Russia processing: ABX Pentra, Horiba Medical, Irvine, CA, USA; University of Houston Processing: Mindray BC3200, Mindray, Shenzhen, China). Upon arrival to the laboratory, a 1.0 mL aliquot was removed for CBC analysis. All pre- and post-flight astronaut blood samples were immediately processed at JSC; however, the analysis of samples collected in-flight was delayed up to 48 h as a result of the time required to transport the ambient blood from the ISS to the laboratory. Briefly, blood samples were collected from each participating crewmember onboard the ISS (Fig. 1) approximately 10 h prior to hatch closure of the returning vehicle (either Shuttle or Soyuz). Collected blood samples were stored in customized blood pouches and transferred to the returning vehicle for return to Earth. Processing of in-flight samples was performed at JSC or the University of Houston, KSC, or at Star city, Russia, depending on the mission landing site.

To examine the effects of the processing delay on the in-flight samples, sterile syringes were used to obtain 1.0 mL aliquots from the 10.0 mL EDTA-coated blood collection tubes collected from healthy donors. The first CBC was run immediately following blood collection from each stability study subject. Subsequently, blood was stored in the dark at room temperature, and 1.0 mL aliquots were removed and analyzed at 24, 48, and 72 h post-collection. All stability samples were processed and analyzed at JSC.

Statistical analysis

This was a longitudinal, repeated-measures study examining the effects of spaceflight on multiple hematologic parameters. Each astronaut served as his/her own control and all in-flight and post-flight time points were compared to the astronaut's baseline sample. The L-180 time point was considered baseline, as pre-mission stressors may have influenced the L-45 time point. The distribution of each parameter was tested for normality using the Shapiro-Wilk Normality Test. Non-normal data were transformed logarithmically and outliers were removed for analysis. For all RBC indices, mixed-effects linear models were used to compare each subsequent time point to the L-180 baseline. A random intercept was used to account for the repeated-measures design of the study. Statistical analysis was performed using STATA statistical software (v14, StataCorp LP, College Station, TX, USA). Significance was set at $p < 0.05$.

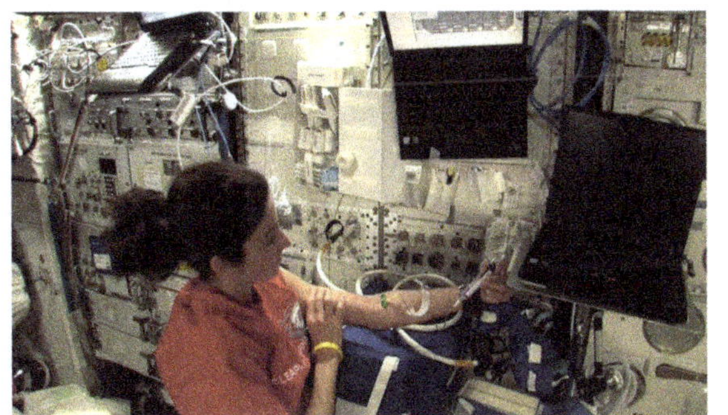

Fig. 1 Blood collection onboard the ISS. Astronaut Nicole Stott performs phlebotomy on the ISS. Samples were collected ~10 h prior to return vehicle undocking (Space Shuttle or Soyuz). Blood samples were returned to the laboratory for analysis within 48 h of collection

To determine the stability of the hematologic indices, two one-sided tests of equivalency for dependent samples were performed on the data from the 20 healthy stability study subjects, comparing each of the aged samples to the corresponding Day 0 baseline sample. The within-person coefficient of variation for each hematologic parameter reported by Lacher et al. [9] was used to define the equivalence bounds for the two one-sided tests. Significant results ($p < 0.05$) in the two one-sided tests indicate that the aged samples and the baseline sample are practically equivalent. Results from the stability study were used to inform results from the astronaut study and assist with interpretation, but no direct comparisons were made between the astronauts and the stability study subjects. The stability study statistical calculations were performed using Microsoft Excel and the spreadsheet developed by Lakens [10].

Results

Of the RBC and platelet indices included in a CBC, the hematology analyzers measure RBC count, mean corpuscular volume (MCV), hemoglobin, and platelet concentration. All other parameters are calculated from these measurements. Only the RBC count, hemoglobin, mean corpuscular hemoglobin (MCH), and platelet concentration remained stable for 48 h at room temperature (Fig. 2a-c, f). Parameters were considered stable if, when compared to the baseline sample, they were significantly within the pre-defined equivalent bounds ($p < 0.05$) at the 24 and 48 h time points. At both 24 and 48 h after collection, when compared to the baseline sample, the platelet concentration fell within the pre-defined equivalent bounds ($p < 0.05$); however, at 72 h after collection, the platelet concentration was no longer significantly practically equivalent to the baseline sample ($t(19) = -1.554$, $p = 0.068$). Both hematocrit and MCV steadily increased over the 72 h of storage at room temperature (Fig. 2d and e). Compared to baseline, MCV was not within the equivalent bounds at 24 h ($t(19) = 6.337$, $p = 1.000$). While elevated at 24 h, hematocrit was significantly within the equivalent bounds ($t(19) = -1.885$, $p = 0.037$); however, hematocrit was not significantly within the equivalent bounds by 48 h ($t(19) = 0.75$, $p = 0.\ 076$). Given the relationship between hematocrit, MCV, and RBC count (hematocrit = [MCV × RBC count]/10) alterations in MCV will necessarily affect the hematocrit values. The elevations in hematocrit over the 72 h therefore reflect the elevations in MCV. Additional parameters that were measured but not included in any subsequent analysis due to instability following delayed processing include red cell distribution width, mean corpuscular hemoglobin concentration, and mean platelet volume (data not shown).

All astronaut samples drawn on the ISS were returned to the lab within 48 h, and the majority of samples were returned by ~37 h post-collection.

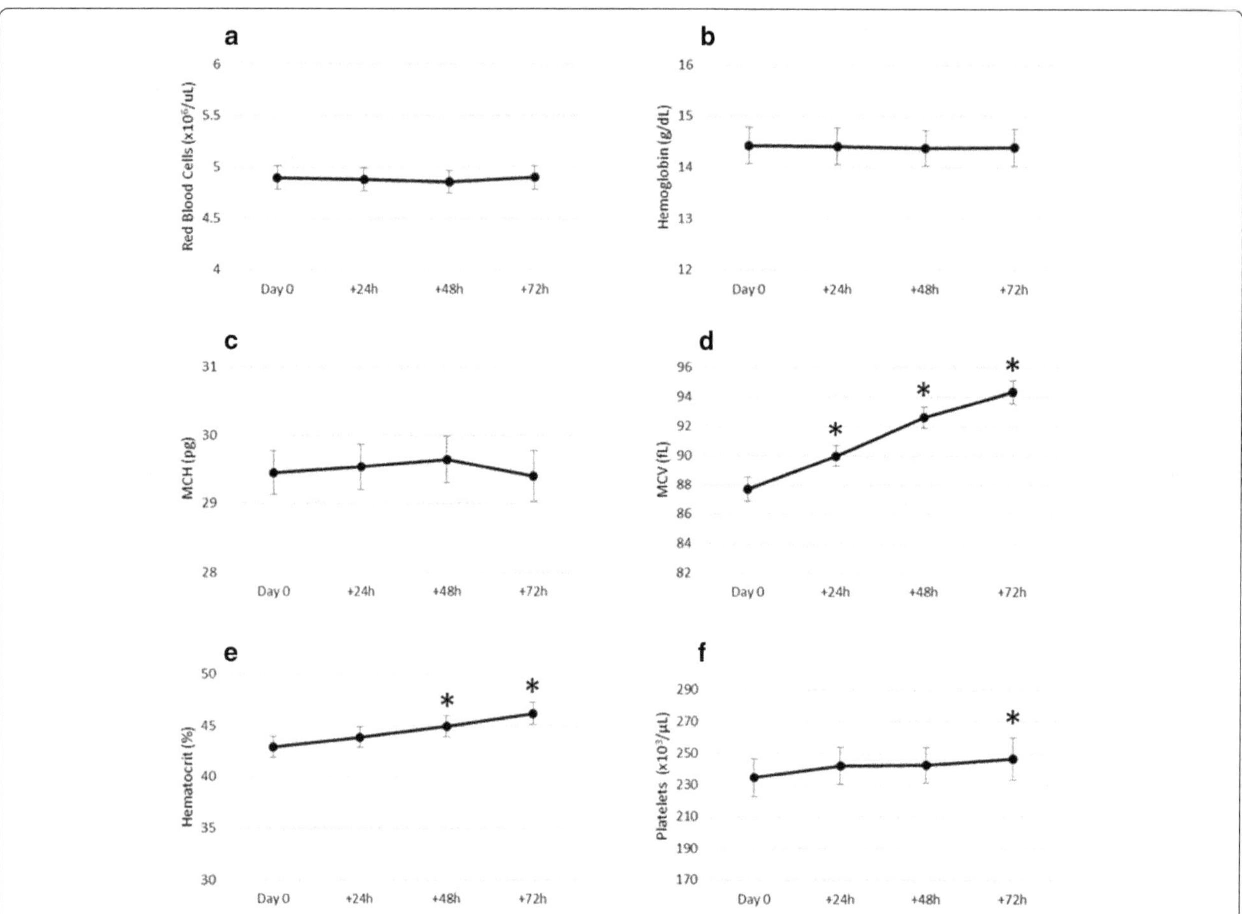

Fig. 2 Hematologic indices evaluated immediately following blood collection, and 24, 48, and 72 h after collection. All aged samples were compared to the baseline sample analyzed immediately post-collection using two one-sided tests for dependent samples. Data are presented as mean ± standard error. Samples that were not statistically considered equivalent to the baseline sample ($p > 0.05$) are indicated with *. **a** Red blood cell concentration ($\times10^6$ cells/μL); **b** hemoglobin concentration (g/dL); **c** mean corpuscular hemoglobin (MCH; pg); **d** mean corpuscular volume (MCV; fL); **e** hematocrit (%); and **f** platelet concentration ($\times10^3$ cells/μL). All parameters were measured using calibrated automated hematology analyzers

Therefore, only parameters that remained stable at 48 h were included in the analysis of the effects of long-duration spaceflight on hematologic indices, with the exception of hematocrit and MCV, discussed below. The effects of long-duration spaceflight on the analyzed hematologic indices are presented in Fig. 3a-f. All parameters remained consistent prior to flight, with no significant differences between the L-180 and L-60 time points. RBC concentration was significantly elevated at all three in-flight time points compared to the L-180 baseline time point (Fig. 3a; L-180: mean 4.4 ± 0.4, range 3.5–5.1; Early: mean 4.8 ± 0.5, range 3.9–5.7; Mid: 4.7 ± 0.4, range 3.9–5.4; late: 4.7 ± 0.4, range 4.1–5.6). Hemoglobin was elevated early in flight compared to L-180, but returned to pre-flight values as the mission progressed (Fig. 3b; L-180: mean 14.1 ± 1.4, range 11.0–17.8; Early: mean 15.0 ± 1.9, range 10.7–17.5). Throughout the mission, MCH decreased, and was significantly lower than the L-180 baseline by the late-flight time point (Fig. 3c; L-180: mean 31.7 ± 1.6, range 28.8–36.4; Late: 31.3 ± 1.9, range 26.3–34.0). While hemoglobin fell below L-180 baseline values on landing day (Fig. 3b; L-180: mean 14.1 ± 1.4, range 11.0–17.8; R + 0: mean 13.5 ± 1.4, range 10.1–15.9), RBC count and MCH returned to pre-flight values upon re-entry, and by R + 30, all indices were at pre-flight levels.

Significant increases in MCV observed in flight (3.9%, 4.6%, and 4.2% increases in mean values compared to the L-180 baseline at early, mid, and late, respectively; Fig. 3d), reflect the changes observed following the 48 h processing delay (5.6% increase in mean values from baseline to +48 h; Fig. 2d). Therefore, we do not identify any MCV variations attributable to spaceflight. As noted previously, elevations in MCV will also manifest as elevations in hematocrit. Although hematocrit values increased when subjected to processing delays and were significantly elevated at 48 h after collection (Fig. 2e), the alterations in hematocrit during spaceflight were striking (Fig. 3e). The significant ($p < 0.05$) elevations in hematocrit observed in flight were of greater magnitude

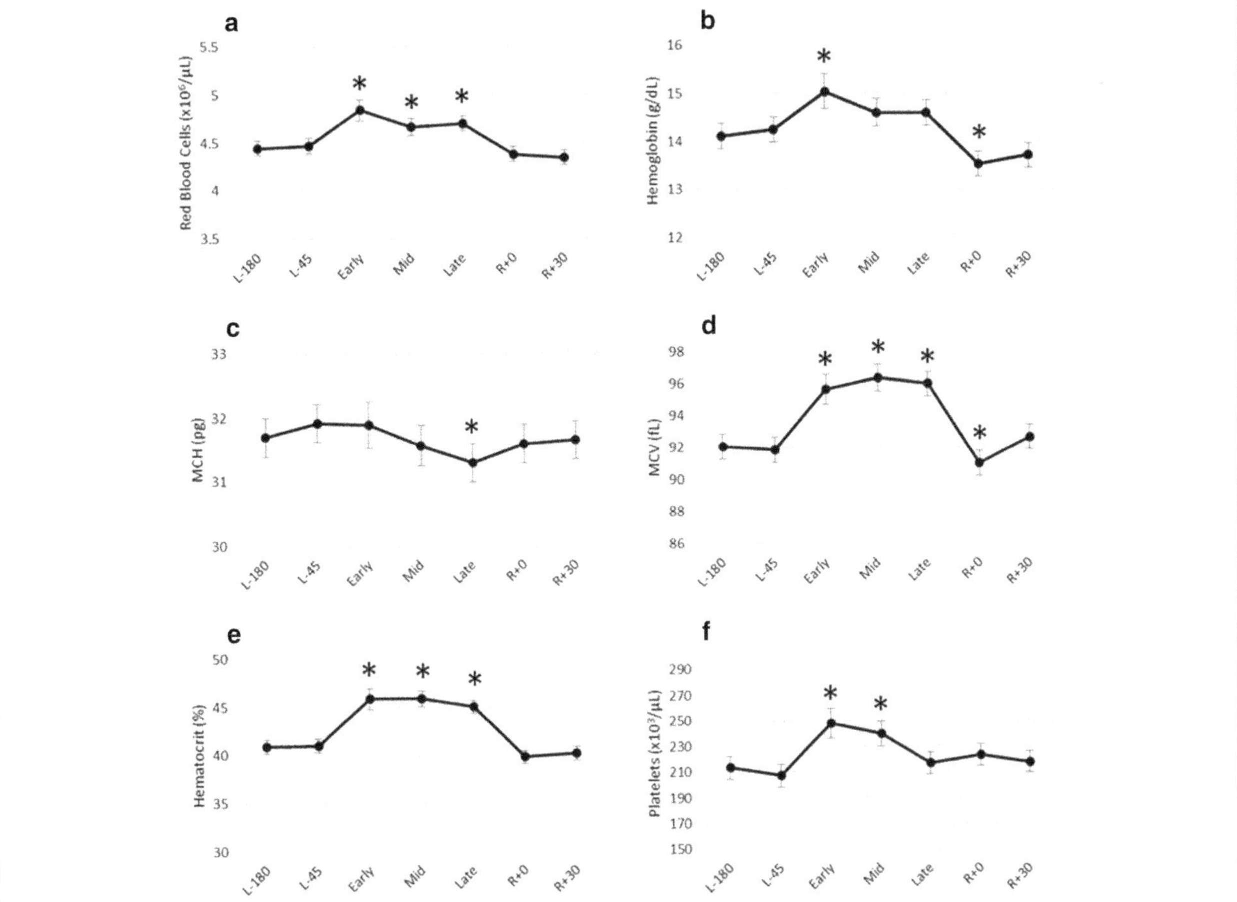

Fig. 3 Hematologic indices evaluated before, during, and after spaceflight. All samples were compared to the L-180 baseline time point using a linear mixed model with random intercept. Data are presented as mean ± standard error. Significant differences from the L-180 baseline ($p < 0.05$) are indicated with *. **a** Red blood cell concentration ($\times 10^6$ cells/µL); **b** hemoglobin concentration (g/dL); **c** mean corpuscular hemoglobin (MCH; pg); **d** mean corpuscular volume (MCV; fL); **e** hematocrit (%); and **f** platelet concentration ($\times 10^3$ cells/µL). All parameters were measured using calibrated automated hematology analyzers

than those observed simply from the elevations in MCV as a result of the processing delay. A 4.7% increase in the mean hematocrit was observed after the 48 h processing delay (Day 0), while the percentage increases in mean hematocrit at the early, mid, and late time points compared to the L-180 time point were 12.2%, 12.2%, and 10.0%, respectively (L-180 mean 40.9 ± 3.9, range 33.1–48.0; Early: mean 45.9 ± 4.7, range 38.2–52.1; Mid: 45.9 ± 5.5, range 38.9–58.3; Late: 45.0 ± 2.5, range 38.9–49.9). These in-flight elevations are therefore most likely due to a combination of a true in-flight increase in RBC count and an artifactual increase in MCV resulting from the processing delay.

Platelet concentration was elevated early in flight. While tracking toward recovery, platelet concentration remained significantly elevated at the mid-flight time point, but was not significantly higher than pre-flight by the late time point (Fig. 3f). The concentration remained stable upon landing and during recovery.

Discussion

While spaceflight anemia has been consistently reported post-flight and during short-duration flight [3, 5], little is known about the in-flight condition during long-duration missions. In this study, we observed statistically significant elevations in the concentrations of RBCs, platelets, and hemoglobin, and we interpret an apparent increase in hematocrit at multiple time points during long-duration spaceflight.

The alterations associated with spaceflight observed in this study are in accordance with previous findings of elevated RBC indices in-flight. RBC concentration, hemoglobin, and hematocrit have been shown to be elevated during the first few days of flight [2, 4, 11]; however, here we show that RBC concentration remains elevated even after the initial period of adaptation to microgravity. Although previous findings suggest that RBC mass is decreased in association with spaceflight [2–4, 7], alterations in cell mass and concentration need not track together. While the observed elevations in RBC concentration and hematocrit may simply be due to greater losses in plasma volume than in RBC mass, it is possible that RBC mass is partially restored as the body adjusts to the absence of gravity as flight duration extends, and the losses in RBC mass are less severe during long-duration spaceflight. In a review of literature on RBC mass and spaceflight, Tavassoli et al. [3] noted that in the first 3 weeks of flight, length of flight and losses in RBC mass were positively correlated, with greater losses in RBC mass occurring in longer flights; however, in the studies performed on the longer-duration Skylab 2, 3 and 4 missions (28, 59, and 84 days, respectively), the longer missions were actually associated with smaller decreases in RBC mass [3, 7]. Therefore it has been previously postulated that during prolonged exposure to microgravity a new RBC mass homeostasis is reached, and the early reductions in RBC mass are abrogated [5, 12].

The observed reduction in MCH late in-flight may be reflected in the relationship between RBC concentration and hemoglobin, as RBC concentration remained elevated throughout the flight while hemoglobin was significantly elevated only early in the flight. A reduced requirement for oxygen-carrying capabilities and easier delivery of oxygen to tissues while in microgravity may drive some of these changes [5, 6].

Previous post-flight findings are varied, as both elevations [7, 13] and depressions [7, 11] in RBC count, hemoglobin, and hematocrit have been reported. Here we found significant post-flight decreases in hematocrit and MCV, while all other parameters rapidly returned to baseline upon re-entry. Interestingly, immediately after the 28-day Skylab 2 mission RBC count, hemoglobin concentration and hematocrit fell below pre-flight values, and while RBC count had recovered by day 7 post-flight, hematocrit and hemoglobin concentration were still below pre-flight levels at 18 days post-flight [7]. In contrast, on the Skylab 3 and 4 missions (59 and 84 days, respectively) RBC count, hemoglobin concentration, and hematocrit were elevated immediately upon landing, but subsequently began to decline and were significantly lower than pre-flight values 3 days after landing, returning to normal in the 3 week testing period following the flights [7]. With the dependence of these indices on plasma volume, the timing of the sample and the conditions of the return may have a large impact. Both dehydration and plasma volume shifts upon re-entry into gravity can significantly affect these parameters. Plasma volume has been shown to be rapidly restored upon re-entry [14, 15], which may account for the rapid return to baseline values of RBC count observed in this study, given the in-flight elevations in these parameters; however, without an accurate measure of plasma volume, it is difficult to make any conclusive statements. Additional sampling between the R + 0 and the R + 30 samples may be beneficial in determining the erythrokinetics post-flight. Depressions in RBC count, hemoglobin concentration, and hematocrit in the weeks after spaceflight were reported after the Skylab missions and by others [2, 7, 11, 14] and were interpreted as potential depressions in red blood cell mass during spaceflight that were slower to recover upon return to Earth than the depressions in plasma volume. Monitoring the RBC indices in the days following flight in the current study would have provided interesting information, given the observed in-flight elevations, and not depressions, in various hematologic indices.

Little data exist regarding in-flight platelet concentrations [3]; however, the reports that do exist suggest that microgravity and simulated microgravity actually induce a state of thrombocytopenia [16, 17]. In contrast, the elevations in platelet concentration observed in this investigation at the early and mid-flight time points may be due to reductions in plasma volume without any true increase in platelet numbers. The gradual return toward baseline of platelet concentration over the course of the 6-month mission may be indicative of a homeostatic mechanism that serves to counteract elevations in platelet concentration resulting from reduced plasma volume. Interestingly, BE Crucian, SR Zwart, S Mehta, P Uchakin, HD Quiriarte, D Pierson, CF Sams and SM Smith [18] recently reported that plasma thrombopoietin, which stimulates platelet production and is generally elevated when platelet levels are low, was elevated throughout 6-months of orbital spaceflight; however, vascular endothelial growth factor (VEGF) and C-X-C motif chemokine 5 (CXCL5), both of which are platelet-derived and positively correlated with platelet concentration [19, 20], were also elevated throughout the 6-month missions [18]. The elevations in plasma VEGF and CXCL5 [16], in conjunction with the finding that platelet concentration was also elevated, appears to indicate that long-duration spaceflight does not induce thrombocytopenia; however, the discrepant finding that thrombopoietin was also elevated [16] warrants further investigation.

Although the performance of a CBC on samples collected during spaceflight generated novel information, these findings must be interpreted with caution. The cellular concentrations are dependent on plasma volume, and therefore the observed elevations may be influenced by reductions in plasma volume without any real increase in cellular mass. Indeed, plasma volume has been shown to decrease by approximately 17% within the first 24 h of spaceflight [2]; however, like changes in RBC mass, the alterations in plasma volume have been primarily observed during short-duration flight or post-flight, and little evidence exists describing changes in plasma volume during long-duration spaceflight. The reductions in plasma volume observed between flight days 8 and 12 by Alfrey et al. [2], while still significant, were smaller than the reductions observed on the first flight day, indicating there may be a continued trend toward plasma volume recovery as time on board the ISS progresses. In a comparison of short and long-duration flights, the average loss in plasma volume for 5 long-duration astronauts was marginally lower than the average loss in 29 short-duration astronauts, though this was not statistically significant [21]. To fully interpret the alterations presented in the current study, plasma volume must also be assessed during long-duration space flight.

The measurement of erythropoietin (EPO) in-flight would also aid in the interpretation of the reported findings; unfortunately EPO was not determined as part of the parent immune investigations. EPO controls RBC mass by regulating the rate of division of RBC progenitors in the bone marrow, and it has also been postulated to play a role in the neocytolysis process by which newly released RBCs are selectively destroyed upon entering into microgravity [12, 15, 22]. EPO has been shown to be reduced early in-flight but elevated following short-duration flight [4], indicating that homeostatic mechanisms attempt to reduce RBC mass upon entering microgravity and restore it upon landing. However, to our knowledge, EPO has not been measured during long-duration flight. The measurement of EPO in future studies of prolonged spaceflight may help to explain the present findings of elevated RBC count throughout long-duration flight.

The delay in processing for the in-flight blood samples is also a limitation of the study. RBC, hemoglobin and platelet concentration have all been shown to be stable for up to 72 h when blood samples collected with EDTA are stored at 4 °C [23]; however, blood samples for our investigations were returned at ambient temperature. Despite the recommendations that samples be refrigerated, results of the stability tests indicate that RBC count, hemoglobin concentration, MCH values, and platelets remain stable for at least 48 h, even at room temperature. The elevations in hematocrit and MCV reported here are in accordance with other study findings. MCV begins to increase within 6–12 h of blood collection, which, in turn, causes an elevation in hematocrit without any alterations in RBC concentration or plasma volume, even in refrigerated samples [23]. While the elevations in hematocrit and MCV hinder our analysis of the in-flight data, the stability of RBC count, hemoglobin, MCH, and platelet concentration over 48 h indicates that the observed alterations in these parameters are likely caused by factors associated with space-flight, and are not the result of delayed sample processing.

Conclusions

Spaceflight anemia is a widely reported phenomenon; however, the vast majority of evidence demonstrating reductions in RBC mass has been collected post-flight. To our knowledge, this is one of the first studies to examine hematologic parameters on blood samples collected during long-duration spaceflight. The data suggest that spaceflight anemia may be less of a concern during long-duration spaceflight. However, as previously noted, the fluctuations in these concentration-dependent variables are influenced by changes in plasma volume. Despite this limitation, the sustained elevation of RBC and platelet concentrations throughout a 6-month mission on board the ISS reported here seems to warrant further investigation, and accurate in-flight assessments of plasma volume during long-duration spaceflight would aid in the interpretation of the findings of this study.

Abbreviations

CBC: Complete blood count; CXCL5: C-X-C motif chemokine 5; EDTA: Ethylenediaminetetraacetic acid; EPO: Erythropoietin; ISS: International Space Station; JSC: Johnson Space Center; KSC: Kennedy Space Center; MCH: Mean corpuscular hemoglobin; MCV: Mean corpuscular volume; NASA: National Aeronautics and Space Administration; RBC: Red blood cell; VEGF: Vascular endothelial growth factor

Acknowledgements

The authors thank the ISS crewmembers for participating in this study. The authors also acknowledge the support provided by the JSC Clinical Laboratory, the JSC Mission Integration Team, and the KSC Baseline Data Collection Facility during this study. The authors are particularly grateful for operational support provided by Mimi Shao at KSC and Matt Roper at JSC. The authors also acknowledge discussions with Ms. Jennifer Crucian MT(ASCP), Hematology Department, Methodist St. John Hospital, Houston, Texas, which supported preparation of this manuscript.

Funding

This work was supported by a grant from the NASA Human Research Program's Human Health and Countermeasures Element to CS/BEC (SMO-015) and NASA grant NNJ10ZSA003N awarded to RJS.

Authors' contributions

HK performed data analysis and contributed to the writing of the manuscript. HQ contributed to the data collection. RJS oversaw data collection for ISS astronauts and provided edits to the manuscript. RPS provided assistance with the data analysis and interpretation. KM assisted with data collection, clinical interpretation of the findings and in manuscript development. CS supervised all study procedures, execution of the flight investigations, and manuscript preparation. BEC contributed to data collection for the ISS astronauts, data analysis, and wrote portions of the manuscript. All authors read and approved the final manuscript.

Competing interests

The authors declare that they have no competing interests.

Author details

[1]KBRwyle, 2400 NASA Parkway, Houston, TX 77058, USA. [2]Louisiana State University, Baton Rouge, Louisiana 70803, USA. [3]University of Houston, 4800 Calhoun Rd, Houston, TX 77004, USA. [4]University of Michigan School of Nursing, 400 North Ingalls Building, Ann Arbor, MI 48109, USA. [5]NASA Johnson Space Center, 2101 E NASA Parkway, Houston, TX 77058, USA.

References

1. Williams D, Kuipers A, Mukai C, Thirsk R. Acclimation during space flight: effects on human physiology. Can Med Assoc J. 2009;180(13):1317–23.
2. Alfrey CP, Udden MM, Leach-Huntoon C, Driscoll T, Pickett MH. Control of red blood cell mass in spaceflight. J Appl Physiol. 1996;81(1):98–104.
3. Tavassoli M. Anemia of spaceflight. Blood. 1982;60(5):1059–67.
4. Udden MM, Driscoll TB, Pickett MH, Leach-Huntoon CS, Alfrey CP. Decreased production of red blood cells in human subjects exposed to microgravity. J Lab Clin Med. 1995;125(4):442–9.
5. Smith SM. Red blood cell and iron metabolism during space flight. Nutrition. 2002;18(10):864–6.
6. De Santo NG, Cirillo M, Kirsch KA, Correale G, Drummer C, Frassl W, Perna AF, Di Stazio E, Bellini L, Gunga HC. Anemia and erythropoietin in space flights. Semin Nephrol. 2005;25(6):379–87.
7. Kimzey SL. Hematology and immunology studies. In: Johnston RS, Dietlein LF, editors. Biomedical results from Skylab. Washington, D.C.: NASA; 1977. p. 249–82.
8. Crucian BE, Stowe RP, Mehta SK, Quiriarte H, Pierson DL, Sams CF. Alterations in adaptive immunity persist during long-duration spaceflight. Npj. Microgravity. 2015;2015:1.
9. Lacher DA, Barletta J, Hughes JP. Biological variation of hematology tests based on the 1999–2002 National Health and nutrition examination survey, In: National Health Statistics Reports: Centers for Disease Control and Prevention, vol. 2012. p. 54.
10. Lakens D. Equivalence tests: a practical primer for t tests, correlations, and meta-analyses. Soc Psychol Personal Sci. 2017; doi:10.1177/1948550617697177.
11. Leach CS, Johnson PC. Influence of spaceflight on erythrokinetics in man. Science. 1984;225(4658):216–8.
12. Risso A, Ciana A, Achilli C, Antonutto G, Minetti G. Neocytolysis: none, one or many? A reappraisal and future perspectives Front Physiol. 2014;5:54.
13. Leach CS. Biochemical and hematologic changes after short-term space flight. Microgravity Q. 1992;2(2):69–75.
14. Alfrey CP. The influence of space flight on erythrokinetics in man, Space life sciences missions 1 and 2. Experiment E261 final report. Washington, D.C.: NASA; 1995.
15. Alfrey CP, Udden MM, Huntoon CL, Driscoll T. Destruction of newly released red blood cells in space flight. Med Sci Sports Exerc. 1996;28(10 Suppl):S42–4.
16. Davis TA, Wiesmann W, Kidwell W, Cannon T, Kerns L, Serke C, Delaplaine T, Pranger A, Lee KP. Effect of spaceflight on human stem cell hematopoiesis: suppression of erythropoiesis and myelopoiesis. J Leukoc Biol. 1996;60(1):69–76.
17. Kalandarova MP. Changes in hematologic indicators in personnel testing during 370-day anti-orthostatic hypokinesia. Kosm Biol Aviak Med. 1991; 25(3):15–8.
18. Crucian BE, Zwart SR, Mehta S, Uchakin P, Quiriarte HD, Pierson D, Sams CF, Smith SM. Plasma cytokine concentrations indicate that in vivo hormonal regulation of immunity is altered during long-duration spaceflight. J Interf Cytokine Res. 2014;34(10):778–86.
19. Feng X, Scheinberg P, Samsel L, Rios O, Chen J, McCoy JP Jr, Ghanima W, Bussel JB, Young NS. Decreased plasma cytokines are associated with low platelet counts in aplastic anemia and immune thrombocytopenic purpura. J Thromb Haemost. 2012;10(8):1616–23.
20. Gunsilius E, Petzer AL, Gastl G. Space flight and growth factors. Lancet. 1999; 353(9163):1529.
21. Meck JV, Reyes CJ, Perez SA, Goldberger AL, Ziegler MG. Marked exacerbation of orthostatic intolerance after long- vs. short-duration spaceflight in veteran astronauts. Psychosom Med. 2001;63(6):865–73.
22. Alfrey CP, Rice L, Udden MM, Driscoll TB. Neocytolysis: physiological down-regulator of red-cell mass. Lancet. 1997;349(9062):1389–90.
23. Zini G. International Council for Standardization in H. Stability of complete blood count parameters with storage: toward defined specifications for different diagnostic applications. Int J Lab Hematol. 2014;36(2):111–3.

The impact of helicobacter pylori eradication on platelet counts of adult patients with idiopathic thrombocytopenic purpura

Sara Aljarad[1], Ahmad Alhamid[3], Ahmad Sankari Tarabishi[3], Ameen Suliman[1] and Ziad Aljarad[2*]

Abstract

Background: Idiopathic (immune) thrombocytopenic purpura (ITP) is an acquired disorder characterized by autoantibodies against platelet membrane antigens. Several studies found an association between Helicobacter Pylori infection and the incidence of ITP. So far, It is still unclear whether *H. pylori* eradication will increase platelet counts in adult ITP patients. We conduct this study to investigate platelet recovery in ITP patients after *H. pylori* eradication.

Methods: This is a prospective study. The diagnostic criterion for Idiopathic thrombocytopenic purpura is: isolated thrombocytopenia, with no evidence of any underlying causes like drugs, TTP, SLE, hepatitis, HIV,CLL and… etc. We examined blood smears of all patients. We have diagnosed Helicobacter pylori infection by histological examination of several biopsies obtained from stomach and duodenum by esophagogastroduodenoscopy (EGD). If EGD was not applicable due to patient's poor situation or platelet count, H.pylori infection was diagnosed by the positivity of serum antibodies or respiratory urease test. We treated infected patients with triple therapy (omeprazole 40 mg once daily, amoxicillin 1000 mg twice daily and clarithromycin 500 mg twice daily) for 14 days. Uninfected patients did not receive any treatment. We did platelet quantification at the beginning of the study, at the end of the first month, at the end of the third month and at the end of the sixth month.

Results: This study involved 50 patients with chronic ITP, 29 males (58%) and 21 females (42%). Participants ages range between18 and 51 years (mean age = 28.60 years). We diagnosed *H. pylori* in 36 patients (72%), who were treated with triple therapy. At the end of the sixth month, 10 of them (27.77%) showed complete response, and 18 of them (50%) showed partial response. The 14 uninfected patients, who did not receive any treatment, did not show neither complete nor partial response. Patient sex and age were not associated with achieving response, while baseline platelet count and H.pylori infection did.

Conclusion: Helicobacter pylori eradication significantly increases platelet counts in adult ITP patients.

Keywords: Idiopathic thrombocytopenic purpura, Helicobacter pylori, Platelet disorders

* Correspondence: dr.ziad-aljarad@hotmail.com
[2]Department of Gastroenterology, Aleppo University Hospital, Aleppo, Syria
Full list of author information is available at the end of the article

Background

Idiopathic (immune) thrombocytopenic purpura (ITP) is an acquired disorder characterized by autoantibodies against platelet membrane antigens [1].

There are considerable differences in the clinical manifestations among ITP patients. The onset may be acute and sudden or may be insidious, and may result in significant mortality and morbidity. Patients may be asymptomatic, and symptoms in symptomatic patients range from easy bruising to severe bleeding [1].

Incidence rate of ITP is about 50–100 new cases per million per year, half of them are children. At least 70% of cases diagnosed in childhood will recover completely within six months, even without treatment [2, 3]. A third of the remaining chronic cases will completely recover during follow-up [4, 5], another third will end up with only mild thrombocytopenia (platelet count above 50×10^9/L) [6].

Thrombocytopenia Purpura is usually chronic in adults [7], and the probability of complete remission is 20–40. Male to female ratio in the adult group clearly differs in most age groups (children approximately have equal incidence in both sexes. The average age at diagnosis in adults is 56–60 years [8].

Helicobacter pylori (*H. pylori*) is a gram-negative microaerophilic bacterium that colonizes in the stomach. *H. pylori* is implicated in the development of active chronic gastritis, gastric ulcers, and duodenal ulcers.

H. pylori is a cofactor in the development of both gastric adenocarcinoma and mucosa-associated lymphoid tissue lymphoma. Recently, It has been discovered that *H. pylori* is implicated in various autoimmune disorders, including pernicious anemia and idiopathic thrombocytopenic purpura (ITP) [9], linked to the development of peptic ulcers in stomach and gastric carcinoma. Approximately 50% of the world's population are infected with *H. pylori*, making it the most prevalent bacterial infections in the world. Its prevalence is greater in low-income countries than in developed ones [10]. The exact route of infection is still unknown, but fecal-oral and oral-oral routes seem to be the most likely [10].

No enough evidence is available to determine the impact of H.pylori eradication on platelet count in ITP patients. We also have not found in the medical literature a study in our region about the prevalence of *H. pylori* infection among ITP patients, and the effect of *H. pylori* eradication on ITP patients in our country, as related studies differ in their results from country to another. The objective of this research is to:

1. Determine the prevalence of *H. pylori* infection in ITP patients.

2. Evaluate the response of ITP patients to *H. pylori* eradication.

Methods

This prospective study was conducted at the University of Damascus, Division of Hematology at Al-Mouwasat University Hospital and Al Assad University Hospital-Department of Internal Medicine, between October 2016 and October 2017. The study included all adult patients of both sexes, who were diagnosed with ITP according to the American Society of Hematology as follows:

- General platelet count is less than 100×10^9/L.
- Exclusion of the secondary causes of thrombocytopenia (e.g. drugs, hepatitis C virus, Human Immunodeficiency virus, pseudothrombocytpenia, malignancies). We examined blood smears of all patients.

Exclusion criteria

- Patients younger than 14 years old.
- Patients with life-threatening bleeding or an active hemorrhage requiring immunosuppression or other therapeutic options to increase platelet count.
- Patients with secondary causes of thrombocytopenia, including any drugs that are suspected of developing thrombocytopenia.
- Taking antibiotics, proton pump inhibitors or H2 blockers a month before screening for *H. pylori*, because these lead to false negatives.
- Any previous *H. pylori* eradication program.

If platelet count and patient status allowed, We diagnosed H.pylori infection was by histological examination of different biopsies obtained from different areas of stomach and duodenum (including the gastric antrum) via esophagogastroduodenoscopy (EGD). IF EGD is not applicable, We diagnosed *H. pylori* infection by the positivity of serum antibodies or urease breath test. We first did serological testing. If the serology was positive, we considered the patient infected. If serology was negative, we did urease breath test. Infected patients were then given triple therapy for H.pylori (omeprazole 40 mg once daily, amoxicillin 1000 mg twice daily, clarithromycin 500 mg twice daily) for 14 days. They were not given any additional ITP treatment to raise platelet count. Patients who were not infected with H.Pylori did not receive any treatment that aimed to increase platelet count during the follow-up period. This method helps to ensure that differences in outcomes are more likely to result from H.pylori eradication rather than other confounding treatments.

Patients had chronic ITP, which means that patients have taken several treatment lines like corticosteroids, splenectomy, IVIG and danazol before detecting HP but without. In addition, no life-threatening bleeding happened during the follow-up period. So, we did not give

Table 1 Prevalence of infection with H. Pylori and diagnostic methods used

H.pylori infection:	Number of cases (%):	Diagnostic method used:
H. pylori positive (Hp^+) Patients	36 (72%)	• Positivity of serum antibodies or urease breath test in 20 patients (55.56%). • Histological examination of gastric and duodenal biopsies obtained by EGD in 16 patients (44.44%).
H. Pylori negative (Hp^-) Patients	14 (28%)	• The Respiratory Urease test and serum antibodies in 4 patients (28.5%). • Histological examination of gastrointestinal lesions from the gastrointestinal tract in 10 patients (71.5%).

any therapeutic agent that may causes rising platelet count to avoid confounding differences in results between Hp positive and Hp negative patients.

Patients were followed up for 6 months. We did baseline platelet quantification, at the end of the first month, at the end of the third month and at the end of the sixth month.

No loss to follow-up or data missing happened.

Response criteria

As several similar studied did, We adopted the following definitions of response:

Complete response: Platelet count of more than $150 \times 10^9/L$ (within the normal range).

Partial response: Elevation of Platelet count from $50 \times 10^9/L$ to $50 \times 10^9/L$, or twice the baseline platelet count.

Statistical study

We performed statistical analyses with SPSS (Version 22.0; SPSS Inc.: Chicago, IL, USA). We used P- value to evaluate statistical significance of differences between groups. The level of significance is $P < 0.05$. Categorical variables were described using frequencies and percentages. Numerical variables were described using (mean or median standard deviation). In order to examine the significance of difference between groups, we conducted Chi-square test and Fisher exact test for categorical variables, and Student T test and the Mann-Whitney U test for numerical variables.

Results

The final sample of the study included 50 patients, 29 of them were males (58%), and 21 were females (42%). Participants ages were between 18 and 51 years (mean age = 28.60 years), with a standard deviation of 8.75 years.

The prevalence of H.pylori infection was as following:

Thirty six patients (72%) were diagnosed with *H. pylori* infection.

H. pylori infection was diagnosed by the positivity of both respiratory urease test or serum antibodies in 20 patients (55.56%), and by histological examination of gastric and duodenal biopsies in 16 patients (44.44%), as shown in (Table 1) and (Fig. 1).

Platelet counts at the beginning of the study

At the beginning of the study, platelet counts in Hp^+ Patients ranged from $22 \times 10^9/L$ to $88 \times 10^9/L$, and the mean value was $46.25 \times 10^9/L$ (SD = 17.724). Platelet counts in Hp^- Patients ranged from $12 \times 10^9/L$ to $42 \times 10^9/L$ and the mean value was $25.21 \times 10^9/L$ (SD = 8.469). Independent sample T test shows that the mean platelet count of Hp $^-$ patients is significantly less than the mean platelet count of the Hp^+ Patients (P (0.001). Table 2).

Platelet counts at the end of the first month

In Hp^+ patients, platelet counts ranged from $17 \times 10^9/L$ to $215 \times 10^9/L$, and the mean value was $67.94 \times 10^9/L$ (SD = 39.51). Platelet count increased in 23 patients (63.88%) compared to baseline counts, and decreased in 13 patients (36.12%). Only two patients (5.55%) achieved complete response (platelet count $150 \times 10^9/L$), and 10 patients (27.77%) achieved partial response (platelet count elevation from to $50 \times 10^9/L$, or twice the baseline platelet count). Overall response achieved in 12 patients (33.33%).

In Hp^- patients, platelet counts ranged from $21 \times 10^9/L$ to $36 \times 10^9/L$, and the mean value was $28.28 \times 10^9/L$ (SD = 4.71). Independent sample T test shows that the mean platelet count at the end of the first month of the study in Hp $^-$ patients is significantly less than the mean platelet count of the Hp^+ Patients (P (0.001) Table 2). Platelet count slightly increased in 6 patients (42.85%), but they did not achieve neither complete nor partial response.

Platelet counts at the end of the third month

In Hp^+ patients, platelet counts ranged from $22 \times 10^9/L$ to $357 \times 10^9/L$, and the mean value was $112.13 \times 10^9/L$ (SD = 84.06). Platelet count increased in 27 patients

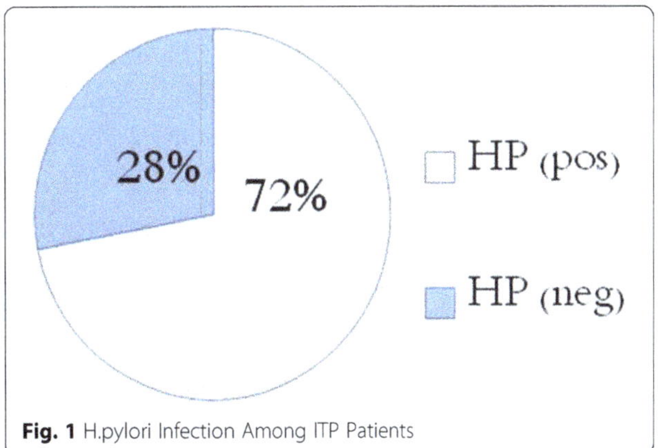

Fig. 1 H.pylori Infection Among ITP Patients

Table 2 Platelet Count during the study

Groups		Range of platelet counts (10^9/L)	The mean value	Standard deviation	*P* value
Platelet Count at the beginning of the study	HP (+)	22–88	46.25	17.724	0.001
	HP (−)	12–42	25.21	8.469	
Platelet counts at the end of the first month	HP (+)	17–215	67.94	39.51	0.001
	HP (−)	21–36	28.28	4.71	
Platelet counts at the end of the third month	HP (+)	22–357	112.13	84.06	0.001
	HP (−)	15–42	28.42	6.489	
Platelet counts at the end of the sixth month:	HP (+)	15–212	98.66	59.54	0.001
	HP (−)	15–41	26.42	7.50	
difference in platelet counts between the end of the sixth month and baseline platelet count (platelet count at the end of the sixth month – baseline platelet count)	HP (+)	(− 37)-(187)	52.42	37.66	0.001
	HP (−)	(−27) −(19)	1.21	4.63	

(75%) compared to baseline counts, and decreased in 9 patients (25%). 8 patients (22.22%) achieved complete response, and 16 patients (44.44%) achieved partial response. Overall response achieved in 26 patients (72.22%).

In Hp^- patients, platelet counts ranged from 15 x 10^9/L to 42 x 10^9/L, and the mean value was 28.42 x 10^9/L (SD = 6.489). Independent sample T test shows that the mean platelet count at the end of the third month of the study in Hp^- patients is significantly less than the mean platelet count of the Hp^+ Patients (P (0.001 Table 2)). Platelet count increased in 8 patients (57.15%), but they did not achieve neither complete nor partial response.

Platelet counts at the end of the sixth month

In Hp^+ patients, platelet counts ranged from 25 x 10^9/L to 212 x 10^9/L, and the mean value was 98.66 x 10^9/L (SD = 59.54). Platelet count increased in 34 patients (94.44%) compared to baseline counts, and decreased in two patients (5.56%). 10 patients (27.77%) achieved complete response, and 18 patients (50%) achieved partial response. Overall response achieved in 28 patients (77.77%).

In Hp^- patients, platelet counts ranged from 15 x 10^9/L to 41 x 10^9/L, and the mean value was 28.42 x 10^9/L. Independent sample T test shows that the mean platelet count at the end of the sixth month of the study in Hp^- patients is significantly less than the mean platelet count of the Hp^+ Patients (P (0.001) Table 2). Platelet count increased in 5 patients (25.71%) compared to baseline, but they did not achieve neither complete nor partial response.

We notice a slight decrease in the mean platelet count of Hp^+ group at the end of the sixth month compared to that of the third month, so do the difference in means between Hp^+ and Hp^- groups. But the mean platelet count of Hp^+ group at the end of the sixth month is still greater than that at the beginning of the study and at the end of the first month, so do the difference in means between Hp^+ and Hp^- groups .

Mean platelet count in Hp^+ group at the end of the sixth month is still greater than the mean platelet count of Hp^- group at all stages. Furthermore, number of responding patients increased at the end of the sixth month.

Figure 2 shows the changes in mean platelet count in Hp^+ and Hp^- groups.

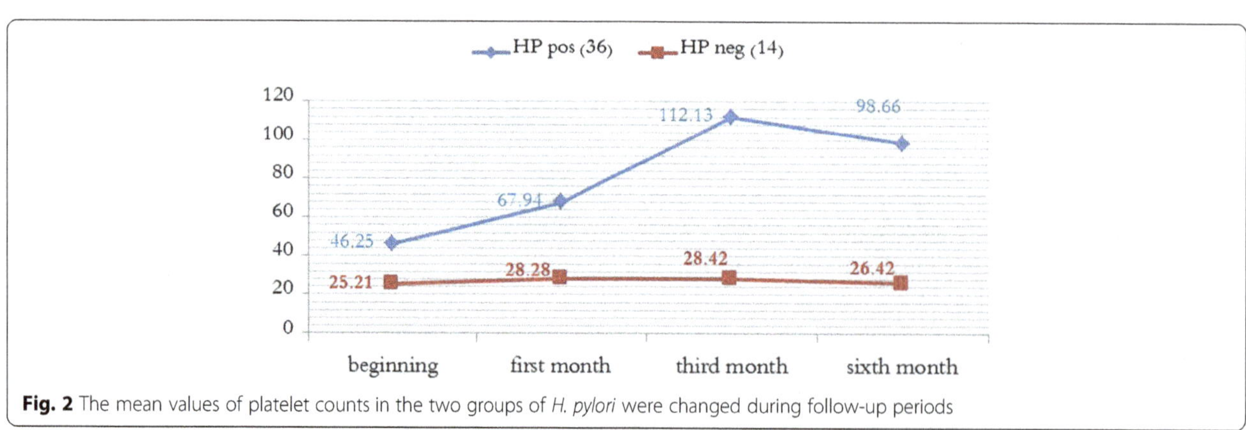

Fig. 2 The mean values of platelet counts in the two groups of *H. pylori* were changed during follow-up periods

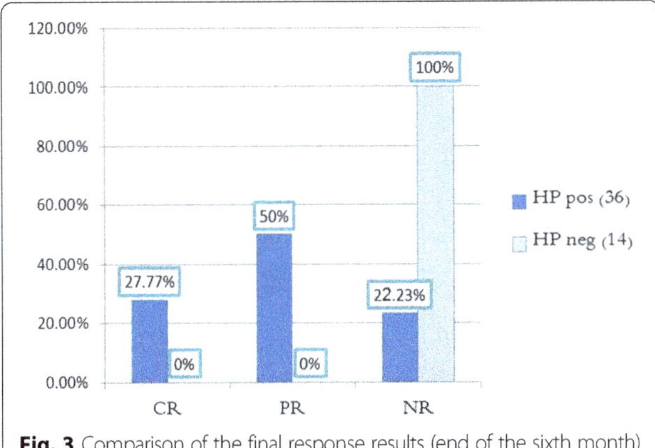

Fig. 3 Comparison of the final response results (end of the sixth month) between the two groups of *H. pylori*

We conclude from Fig. 2 that: Although the mean baseline platelet count is greater in Hp^+ group, the difference between Hp^+ and Hp^- groups is getting greater in the subsequent follow-up visits, as indicated by the gradually increased space between the curves. All that confirms the significant difference of platelet counts between the two groups (Table 2).

In conclusion, 10 Hp^+ patients (27.77%) achieved complete remission, and 18 Hp^+ patients (50%) achieved partial response. All responding patients are Hp^+ (who received triple therapy for H.pylori). 8 Hp^+ patients (22.23%) achieved no response. All the 14 (100%) Hp– patients (who received no treatment) did not achieve neither complete nor partial response (Fig. 3), even though some patients showed a slight increase in platelet count (Table 3). In other words, it is possible to say that treatment of *H. pylori* has effectively increased platelet count, and this improvement was not spontaneous.

Comparison between complete response, partial response and no response groups

After obtaining the final results of patients at the end of the sixth month, they were divided into three groups according to the response:

- Complete response group, including 10 patients.
- Partial response group, including 18 patients.
- No-response group, including 22 patients.

We will compare the three groups in terms of age distribution, sex distribution, baseline mean platelet count, H.pylori infection status.

First: Comparison of the mean age

The mean age of complete response group, partial response group, and no response group is 24.40, 28.95 years and 30.50 years, respectively as shown in (Fig. 4). One way ANOVA shows no statistically significant difference between these values. This means that age is not an effective factor in response Table 4.

Second: Comparison of the primary platelet count

The mean value of baseline platelet count in complete response group, partial response group and no response group is 40.50 × 10^9/L, 52. × 10^9/L and 30.41 × 10^9/L, respectively as shown in (Fig. 5). One way ANOVA test indicates a statistical significance of these differences as shown in (p) Table 4.

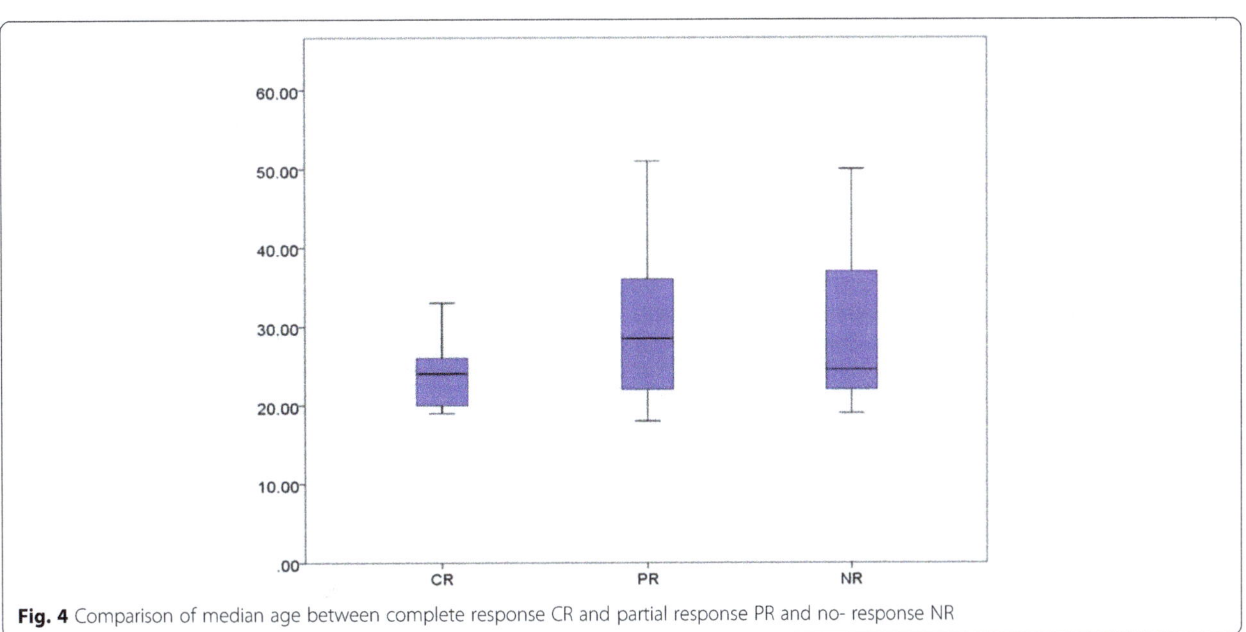

Fig. 4 Comparison of median age between complete response CR and partial response PR and no- response NR

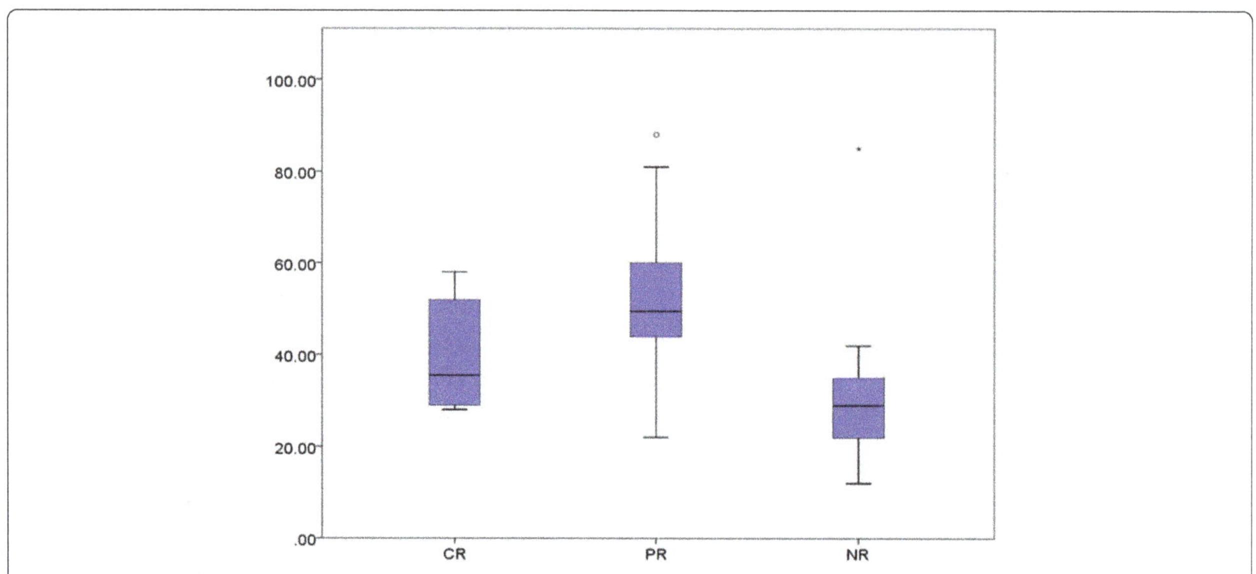

Fig. 5 Comparison of the median value of platelet count at the start of the study between complete response cases CR and partial response PR and non-response NR

Third: Comparison of sex distribution

The complete response group included 6 males (60%) and 4 females (40%). The partial response group included 9 males (50%) and 9 females (50%). No response group included 14 males (63.6%) and 8 females (36.4%) as shown in (Fig. 6). Fisher Exact test indicates that there is no statistically significant difference between these ratios. Therefore, patient's sex was not an effective factor to achieve response. As shown in Table 4.

Fourth: Comparison of *H. pylori* infection status

All cases of complete and partial response were Hp^+. Out of the 22 cases of the no response group, 8 patients (36.4%) were Hp^+, and 14 patients (63.6%) were Hp^- as shown in (Fig. 7). Chi-square test indicates a statistically significant difference between these groups in H.pylori infection status. In other words, the response cases were more common among the HP (+) patients. That means *H. pylori* eradication increased platelet count, because no other treatment was given. As shown in Table 5.

Discussion

We gave Triple therapy to Hp^+ patients with no additional treatment, and Hp^- were monitored without any treatment. Mean baseline platelet count was significantly higher in Hp^+ group. Mean platelet count of Hp^+ patients was also significantly higher than that of Hp^- at the end of the first, third and sixth month. Mean platelet count markedly improved in Hp^+ group, and the difference in mean platelet count was gradually getting greater in subsequent follow-up visits at the end of the first month and third month.

We notice a slight decrease in the mean platelet count of Hp^+ group at the end of the sixth month compared to that of the third month, so do the difference in means between Hp^+ and Hp^- groups. But the mean platelet count of Hp^+ group at the end of the sixth month is still greater than that at the beginning of the study and at the end of the first month, so do the difference in means between Hp^+ and Hp^- groups. Mean platelet count in Hp^+ group at the end of the sixth month is still greater than the mean platelet count of Hp^- group at all stages.

Table 3 Comparison of the end result of the response (end of the sixth month) between the two groups of H. Pylori

	HP (+) (36)	HP (−) (14)	*P* value
Complete response	10 (27.77%)	0 (0%)	
Partial response	18 (50%)	0 (0%)	0.001
No response	8 (22.23%)	14 (100%)	0.001

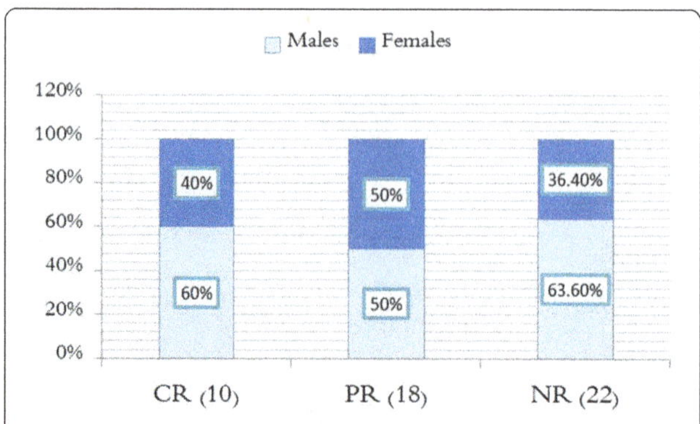

Fig. 6 Comparison of sex distribution between complete response CR and partial response PR and non-response NR

Table 4 Comparison of the platelet count, and the patient's sex, and the median age, by type of response

		Platelet count	Males	Females	Median age
Complete response	HP(+) (36)	40.50	6 (60%)	4 (40%)	24.40
	HP(−) (14)				
Partial response	HP(+) (36)	52.44	9 (50%)	9 (50%)	28.95
	HP(−) (14)				
No response	HP(+) (36)	30.41	14 (63.6%)	8 (36.4%)	30.50
	HP(−) (14)				

The difference between mean baseline platelet count and mean platelet count at the end of the sixth month was significantly higher in Hp^+ group.

Patients who achieved complete or partial response were all Hp^+, while Hp^- patients did not achieve neither complete nor partial response. The previous findings indicate that the improvement noticed in Hp^+ group is often due to H.pylri eradication, not a spontaneous improvement.

Age and sex are not related to achieving response, while baseline platelet count and H.pylori infection status do.

Scientific explanation of this improvement

The pathogenic role of *H. pylori* infection in the development of ITP is still unclear, several mechanisms are suggested: *H. pylori* may modify the balance of Fc-receptors on the surface of monocytes. This modification leads to activation of these receptors, which makes monocytes attack platelets. Bacterial antigens and glycoprotein platelet surface antigens express some similarity. When antibodies are produced against these bacterial antigens, they interact with the glycoprotein Platelet surface antigens, thus lead to decrease platelet count. Some strains of *H. pylori* induce platelet activation mediated by *H. pylori*-bound vWF interacting with GPIb, and supported by IgG. [11–15].

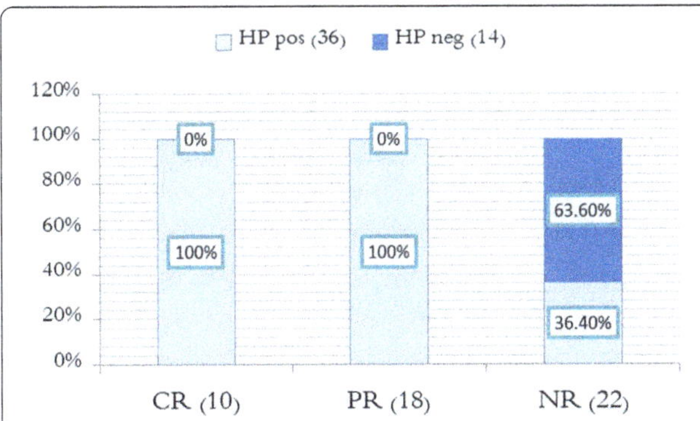

Fig. 7 Comparison of the percentages of the *H. pylori* infection with complete response CR and partial response PR and non-response NR

Table 5 Comparison the percentages of the H. Pylori infection by type of response

Group	HP (+) (36)	HP (−) (14)	*P* value
Complete response(10)	10 (100%)	0 (0%)	Less than 0.001
Partial response (18)	18 (100%)	0 (0%)	
No-response (22)	8 (36.4%)	14 (63.6)	

Study limitations include the small sample size due to the rarity of ITP. Another limitation is the absence of a control group consisted of healthy asymptomatic participants to compare the prevalence of H.pylori infection between ITP patients and the healthy population.

Conclusion

- *H. pylori* eradication in ITP patients Leads to significant Improvement of peripheral blood platelet count in most patients.

Recommendations

- To investigate for *H. pylori* infection in ITP patients, even in the absence of gastrointestinal symptoms.
- To consider the triple anti-H.pylori therapy as a first therapeutic option for Hp^+ ITP patients, with periodic monthly monitoring of platelet count during the first 6 months to confirm the response.
- To conduct a large-scale well-controlled case-control studies to confirm the relationship between H.pylori infection and the development of ITP.
- To conduct randomized controlled trials to confirm the benefit of H.pylori eradication in Hp^+ ITP patients.
- To conduct a systematic review and meta-analysis of the available literature.

Abbreviations

H. pylori: Helicobacter pylori; HCV: hepatitis C virus; HIV: human immunodeficiency virus; HP: Helicobacter pylori; ITP: Idiopathic Thrombocytopenic Purpura; IVIG: Intravenous immunoglobulin; SLE: Systemic lupus erythematous; SPSS: a statistical package for the social sciences; TTP: thrombotic thrombocytopenic purpura

Author's contribution

Conception and design: ZA, AST, AA.Analysis and interpretation of the data: ZA, SA, AS.Drafting of the article: ZA, SA, AST, AA.Critical revision of the article for important intellectual content: SA, AS. All authors read and approved the final version of the manuscript.

Competing interests

The authors declare that they have no competing interest.

Author details

[1]Department of Hematology, Al Mouwasat University Hospital, Damascus, Syria. [2]Department of Gastroenterology, Aleppo University Hospital, Aleppo, Syria. [3]Medical student, Faculty of Medicine, University of Aleppo, Aleppo, Syria.

References

1. Terrell DR, Beebe LA, Neas BR, et al. Prevalence of primary immune thrombocytopenia in Oklahoma. Am J Hematol. 2012 Sep;87(9):848–52.
2. Rodeghiero F, Stasi R, Gernsheimer T, et al. Standardization of terminology, definitions and outcome criteria in immune thrombocytopenic purpura of adults and children. Report from an international working group. Blood. 2009 Mar 12;113(11):2386–93.
3. Kuhne T, Imbach P, Bolton Maggs PH, et al. Newly diagnosed ITP in the children an observational study. Lancet. 2001;358(9299):2122–5.
4. Toltl LJ, Arnold DM. Pathophysiology and management of chronic immune thrombocytopenia: focusing on what matters. Br J Haematol. 2011 Jan; 152(1):52–60.
5. Franchini M, Veneri D. Helicobacter pylori –associated immune thrombocytopenia. Am J Hematology. 2012 Jul;38(5):463–8.
6. Neunert C, Lim W, Crowther M, et al. The American Society of Hematology 2011 evidence-based practice guideline for immune thrombocytopenia. Blood. 2011 Apr 21;117(16):4190–207.
7. Cines DB. Blanchette . "immune thrombocytopenic purpura". N Engl J Med. 2002;346(13):995–1008.
8. Cines DB, Bussel JB (2005). how I treat idiopathic thrombocytopenic purpura (ITP). Blood 2012;120(5):960–969.
9. Tan HJ, Goh KL. Extragastrointestinal manifestations of helicobacter pylori infection: facts or myth? A critical review. J Dig Dis. 2012 Jul;13(7):342–9.
10. Weiss AA. Helicobacter pylori treatment and eradication. In: Sands MD BE, editor. "MOUNT SINAI EXPERT GUIDES gastroenterology" textbook. 1st ed; 2015. p. 180–93.
11. Campuzano-Maya G. Proof of an association between helicobacter pylori and idiopathic thrombocytopenic purpura in Latin America. Helicobacter. 2007 Jun;12(3):265–73.
12. Gerhard M, Rad R, Prinz C, Naumann M. Pathogenesis of helicobacter pylori infection. Helicobacter. 2002;7(Suppl 1):17–23.
13. Cines DB. ITP: time to "bug off"? Blood. 2007;110(12):3818–9.
14. Byrne MF, Kerrigan SW, Corcoran PA, et al. Helicobacter pylori binds von Willebrand factor and interacts with GPIb to induce platelet aggregation. Gastroenterology. 2003 Jun;124(7):1846–54.
15. Stasi R, Rossi Z, Stipa E, Amadori S, Newland AC, Provan D. Helicobacter pylori eradication in the management of patients with idiopathic thrombocytopenic purpura. Am J Med. 2005 April;118(4):414–9.

Pregnant mothers are more anemic than lactating mothers, a comparative cross-sectional study, Bahir Dar, Ethiopia

Berhanu Elfu Feleke[1*] and Teferi Elfu Feleke[2]

Abstract

Background: Information on the hemoglobin status of pregnant and lactating mothers was scarce. The objectives of this study were to determine the burden and determinants of anemia in the pregnant and lactating mother.

Methods: A comparative cross-sectional study was conducted. Descriptive statistics were used to identify the prevalence of anemia. Binary logistic regression and multiple linear regressions were used to identify the predictors of anemia.

Results: The prevalence of anemia in lactating and pregnant women was 43.00% (95% CI {confidence interval}, 41% - 45%) and 84% of anemia was microcytic and hypocromic anemia. Anemia in lactating and pregnant women was positively associated with malaria infection [AOR{adjusted odds ratio} 3.61 (95% CI: 2.63–4.95)], abortion [AOR 6.63 (95% CI: 3.23–13.6)], hookworm infection [AOR 3.37 (95% CI: 2.33–4.88)], tea consumption [AOR 3.63 (95% CI: 2.56–5.14)], pregnancy [AOR 2.24 (95% CI: 1.57–3.12)], and Mid-upper arm circumference [*B* 0.36 (95% *CI:* 0.33, −0.4)]. Anemia in pregnant and lactating mother was negatively associated with urban residence [AOR 0.68, (95% CI: 0.5–0.94)], iron supplementation during pregnancy [AOR 0.03 (95% CI, 0.02–0.04)], parity [*B* -0.18 (95% CI: -0.23, −0.14)], age [B -0.03 (95% *CI:* -0.04, −0.03)].

Conclusion: The burden of anemia was higher in pregnant women than lactating women.

Keywords: Anemia, Determinants, Lactation, Pregnancy, Prevalence

Background

Anemia is a condition in which the hemoglobin concentration of a woman is less than 11 g/dl (gram per deciliter). World health organization report indicated that 20–50% of the world population was affected by iron deficiency anemia [1, 2]. Anemia was one of the great public health burdens for pregnant women affecting 56 million pregnant women globally [3, 4]. In the developed countries, 18% of pregnant women were anemic but in developing countries, 35–75% of pregnant women were anemic [5, 6].

Anemia during pregnancy has many adverse outcomes for the mother and her child. Globally, anemia resulted in the death of 115,000 mothers and 591,000 perinatal mortality annually [7–12]. Anemia during pregnancy predisposes mother to prolonged labor, abnormal delivery, increases the risk of hemorrhage [13–15]. Also, anemia increases the risk of infection to pregnant women due to its effect on the immune system [11, 16–20]. Newborns receive a number of complications as a result of maternal anemia. Among others, maternal anemia increases the risk of perinatal mortality and morbidity, preterm deliveries, low birth weight baby, intrauterine growth retardation (IUGR) [21–31].

The burden of anemia varies from country to country; in Germany, 51% of pregnant women were anemic, in Trinidad and Tobago 15%, in Nepal 72.6% and 58% in India [32–35]. In Africa, more than 60% of pregnant women were anemic: in Ghana 44% of pregnant women, in Benin 24.3% of pregnant women, in Kenya 69.1% of pregnant women and in eastern Sudan 80.3% of pregnant women were anemic [36–42]. Ethiopia is among country highly affected by anemia: the prevalence of anemia among pregnant women ranges from 15%-63%, in lactating mothers the prevalence of anemia was 22.3% [4, 43–49].

Finding from different scholars globally revealed that anemia in pregnancy was associated with gestational age, iron supplementation during pregnancy, wealth quintile,

* Correspondence: elfufeleke@gmail.com
[1]Department of Epidemiology and Biostatistics, University of Bahir Dar, Bahir Dar, Ethiopia
Full list of author information is available at the end of the article

Table 1 Socio-demographic characteristics of study participants ($n = 1651$)

SN	Population profile		Frequency	Percentage
1.	Age	16–25	1279	77.5
		26–35	316	19.1
		36–45	56	3.4
2.	Residence	Urban	865	52.4
		Rural	786	47.6
3.	Religion	Orthodox	1596	96.7
		Muslim	45	2.7
		Protestant	10	0.6
4.	Ethnicity	Amhara	1488	90.1
		Agaw	110	6.7
		Oromo	13	0.8
		Tigray	23	14
		Others	17	1
5.	Educational status	Illiterate	40	2.4
		Elementary	408	24.7
		Secondary	318	19.3
		Certificate	399	24.2
		Diploma	242	14.7
		First degree	227	13.7
		Second degree	17	1
6.	Occupation	Housewife	814	49.3
		Government employee	306	16.5
		Merchants	161	9.8
		Farmers	156	9.4
		NGO employee	157	9.5
		Others	57	3.5

gravidity, mid-upper arm circumference (MUAC), age, residence, history of malaria infection, hookworm infection, parity, history of abortion, chronic inflammatory disorders, use of insecticide-treated bed net, tea consumption and use of animal product [33, 34, 39, 41, 42, 48–55].

Even if anemia resulted in these entire adverse outcomes for pregnant mother and their children, information on hemoglobin status of pregnant and lactating mothers are scarce. Due to lack of information decision makers are not capitalizing on the problem of anemia in pregnancy and lactating mother. This study is designed to attempt to fill these gaps. The objectives of this study were to compare the prevalence of anemia among pregnant and lactating women. Furthermore, the study attempted to identify the determining factors of anemia in pregnant and lactating mother and these aims were achieved successfully.

Methods

Health facility-based comparative cross-sectional study was conducted. The study was conducted in the city of Bahir dar, the capital of the Amhara regional state, located at the geographical coordinates of 11° 38′ north latitude and 37° 15′ east longitude, which is located approximately 560 km (km) northwest of Addis Ababa. The target populations were all pregnant and lactating mother in the city of Bahir dar and the study population were those presenting themselves for medical help. Pregnant or lactating mother unable to communicate were excluded from the study. The sample size was calculated using Epi-info software version 7 using the assumption of 95% confidence interval, pregnant to lactating mother ratio of 2:1, the proportion of anemia among lactating mother 22.3% [46], a power of 90%, an odds ratio of 1.5 and a non-response rate of 10%. Finally, the estimated sample size was 567 pregnant women and 1133 lactating women. Study participants were selected from health facilities of Bahir dar city. Stratified sampling technique was used to select study participants from each health facility. The data were collected from November 2014–May 2015. The data collection procedures contained two parts, exit interview and collecting blood and stool samples. For the interview part, first, the questionnaire was prepared in English then translated to Amharic (local language) then back to English to keep its consistency. The interview was conducted by 10 nurses professional and supervised by 3 health officers. The blood and stool samples were collected by 5 first degree holder laboratory technologists and supervised by two second degree holder laboratory technologists. From each woman, one gram stool sample was collected in 10 ml (ML) SAF (sodium acetate- acetic acid-formalin solution). Concentration technique was used. The stool sample was well mixed and filtered using a funnel with gauze then centrifuged for one minute at 2000 RPM (revolution per minute) and the supernatant was discarded. 7 ML normal saline was added, mixed with a wooden stick, 3 ML ether was added and mixed well then centrifuged for 5 min at 2000 RPM. Finally, the supernatant was discarded and the whole sediment was examined for parasites [56]. 1 ML blood sample was collected from each woman following standard operational procedures to measure their hemoglobin level and red blood cell indices using Mindray hematology analyzer. To maintain the quality of the data; pretest was conducted in 50 parents, training was given to data collectors and supervisors and the whole data collection process was closely supervised by the investigator and supervisors. The collected data were checked for completeness. The data were entered into the computer using Epi-info software and analyzed using statistical package for social sciences (SPSS) software. Descriptive statistics were used to estimate the prevalence of anemia among pregnant and lactating women. Binary logistic regression and multiple linear

Table 2 Binary logistic regression output of determinants of anemia during pregnancy ($n = 550$)

Variables		*Anemia*		*COR[95% CI]*	*AOR[95% CI]*	*p-value*
		Yes	*No*			
Residence	Urban	32	261	0.08 [0.05–0.13]	0.14 [0.08–0.25]	<0.01
	Rural	155	102			
History of malaria	Yes	83	63	3.8 [2.51–5.76]	2.84[1.65–4.92]	<0.01
	No	104	300			
History of abortion	Yes	27	9	6.64 [2.9–15.59]	4.44 [1.58–12.05]	0.01
	No	160	354			
Hookworm infection	Present	78	20	12.27 [6.97–21.78]	5.97 [3.03–11.76]	<0.01
	Absent	109	343			
Iron supplementation during pregnancy	Supplied	141	343	0.18 [0.1–0.32]	0.12 [0.06–0.25]	<0.01
	Not supplied	46	20			
Tea consumption	Yes	110	68	6.2 [4.11–9.37]	2.88 [1.54–5.38]	<0.01
	No	77	295			
Occupation	Government employ	22	96	0.37 [0.22–0.63]	0.35 [0.18–0.69]	<0.01
	Others	165	267			

COR crude odds ratio, *AOR* adjusted odds ratio

regressions were used to identify the determinants of anemia.

Ethical clearance was granted from Amhara National Regional State Health Bureau ethical committee. Legal permission was obtained from each health center. Written informed consent was obtained from each study participant. The confidentiality of the data was kept at all steps. Women with intestinal parasites or low hemoglobin concentration (<11 g/dl) were referred to the nearby health center for further management.

Results

A total of 1651 women was included giving a response rate of 97.12%. The mean age of the respondents was 22.65 years (SD [standard deviation] 5.12 years). Orthodox Christian constituted 96.7% (1596) of study participants, 90.1% of study participants were Amhara by ethnicity, 52.7% of women were from urban areas, and 49.3% of study participants were house wife by their occupation (Table 1).

Table 3 linear regression output for determinants of hemoglobin concentration in pregnancy (dependent variable = hemoglobin concentration in g/dl)

Variables	*B coefficient [95% CI]*	*t*	*p-value*
MUAC	0.37 [0.32, 0.41]	15.55	<0.01
Gravidity	−0.35[−0.42,-0.29]	−10.91	<0.01
Age of pregnant mother	0.03 [0.02,0.03]	6.69	<0.01
Gestational age	−0.02[−0.03,-0.01]	−3.73	<0.01

B beta coefficient

Anemia in pregnant women

A total of 550 pregnant women was included giving a response rate of 97%. The mean age of pregnant women was 26.88 years (SD = 5.82 years). After adjusting for women's residence, history of abortion, history of malaria, occupation, hookworm infection, tea consumption and iron supplementation during pregnancy: the risk of anemia increases in rural women, history of abortion or malaria, hookworm infection, and tea consumptions. The risk of anemia was lower in women with government employer, in women that were supplied by iron during pregnancy (Table 2).

On linear regression anemia in pregnancy was associated with age, gravidity, mid-upper arm circumferences (MUAC) and gestational age (Table 3).

The degree of anemia defers with the gestational age of pregnant mothers, per one week increase in the age of gestation her hemoglobin concentration will decrease by 0.02 g/dl. That means the higher the gestational age the risk of becoming anemic will also become high.

Anemia in lactating women

A total of 1101 lactating women were included with a response rate of 97.18%. The mean age of the lactating women was 20.54 years (SD 3.12 years). On binary logistic regression after adjusting for residence, history of malaria, history of abortion, hookworm infection, iron supplementation, tea consumption: anemia in lactating women was associated with a residence, history of malaria, history of abortion, iron supplementation and tea consumption (Table 4).

Table 4 Logistic regression output of determinants of anemia in lactating women ($n = 1101$)

Variables		Anemia		COR[95% CI]	AOR[95% CI]	p-value
		Yes	No			
Residence	Urban	228	344	0.53 [0.41–0.67]	4.03 [2.3–7.03]	<0.01
	Rural	295	234			
History of malaria	Yes	274	122	4.11 [3.13–5.40]	4.73 [3.02–7.41]	<0.01
	No	249	456			
History of abortion	Yes	50	9	4.62 [2.16–10.18]	7.44 [2.3–24.09]	<0.01
	No	569	473			
Iron supplementation during pregnancy	Supplied	45	494	0.02 [0.01–0.02]	0.007 [0.004–0.013]	<0.01
	Not supplied	478	84			
Tea consumption	Yes	184	108	2.37 [1.78–3.15]	2.32 [1.48–3.64]	<0.01
	No	338	470			

On linear regression hemoglobin concentration in pregnancy was associated with MUAC, parity, age, and frequency of breastfeeding per 24 h (Table 5).

Anemia in pregnant and lactating women

The prevalence of anemia in lactating and pregnant women was 43% (95% CI, 41%-45%), 84% of anemia was microcytic hypocromic, 4.54% of anemia was macrocytic hypercromic, and 5.82% of anemia was normocytic normocromic (Table 6).

After adjusting for residence, pregnancy, history of malaria, history of abortion, hookworm infection, iron supplementation during pregnancy, tea consumption, occupation and educational status; anemia in pregnant or lactating mother were associated with a residence, pregnancy, history of malaria, history of abortion, hookworm infection, iron supplementation during pregnancy and tea consumption (Table 7).

On linear regression determinants of anemia in pregnant or lactating women were associated with mid-upper arm circumferences, age, and parity of pregnant or lactating women (Table 8).

Discussion

The prevalence of anemia in lactating and pregnant women was 43% (95% CI, 41%-45%) and 84% of anemia was iron deficiency anemia followed by normocytic normocromic anemia This finding is lower when compared to findings from eastern Ethiopia [48] Germany [32], Nepal [33], India [35], eastern Sudan [40], Kenya [41]; agrees with findings from Ghana [39]and higher than finding from northern Ethiopia [49] southern Ethiopia [45] Trinidad and Tobago [34], Benin [42]. These might be due to the reason that different distribution of determinants of anemia across different social, cultural or geographical areas.

The risk of anemia in rural Lactating or pregnant women was 32% higher as compared to urban lactating or pregnant women [AOR 0.68, (95% CI: 0.5–0.94)]. This finding agrees with finding from northern Ethiopia [49]. This is due to the reason that women in the rural areas are in low socio-economic status so that they have no access to use iron rich foods [48].

Malaria infected women had 3.61 folds higher risk of anemia as compared to women with no history of malaria infection [AOR 3.61(95% CI: 2.63–4.95)]. This finding agrees with finding from north Ethiopia [49], Nepal [33], Ghana [52]. This is due to the fact that Plasmodium species ingests the red blood cells of the host and finally decreases the number of red blood cells.

Abortion increases the risk of anemia by 6.63 folds higher [AOR 6.63 (95% CI: 3.23–13.6)]. This finding agrees with finding from Trinidad and Tobago [34]. This is due to the reason that abortion increases the risk of hemorrhage.

Table 5 Linear regression output for determinants of hemoglobin concentration in lactating mothers (dependent variable = hemoglobin concentration in g/dl) ($n = 1101$)

Variables	B coefficient [95% CI]	t	P-value
MUAC	0.25 [0.21, 0.29]	11.08	<0.01
Parity	−0.14 [−0.21, −0.06]	−3.64	<0.01
Age of lactating mother	−0.03[−0.05, −0.01]	−3.43	<0.01
Frequency of breast feeding	−0.28 [−0.33, −0.24]	−12.96	<0.01

Table 6 The red blood cell indices of anemic women ($n = 705$)

Mean corpuscular volume (MCV)	Mean corpuscular hemoglobin concentration (MCHC)			Total
	Normocromic	Hypocromic	Hypercromic	
Normocytic	41	2	3	46
Microcytic	13	592	12	617
Macrocytic	6	4	32	42
Total	60	598	47	705

Table 7 Logistic regression output of determinants of anemia in pregnant and lactating women (n = 1651)

Variables		*Anemia*		*COR[95%CI]*	*AOR[95%CI]*	*P-value*
		Yes	*No*			
Residence	Urban	260	605	0.32 [0.26–0.40]	0.68 [0.5–0.94]	0.02
	Rural	450	336			
History of malaria	Yes	357	185	4.13 [3.3–5.17]	3.61 [2.63–4.95]	<0.01
	No	353	756			
History of abortion	Yes	77	18	6.24 [3.61–10.91]	6.63 [3.23–13.6]	<0.01
	No	633	923			
Hookworm infection	Present	228	119	3.27 [2.53–4.22]	3.37 (2.33–4.88)	<0.01
	Absent	482	822			
Iron supplementation during pregnancy	Supplied	186	837	0.04 [0.03–0.06]	0.03 [0.02–0.04]	<0.01
	Not supplied	524	104			
Tea consumption	Yes	295	176	3.09 [2.46–3.88]	3.63 [2.56–5.14]	<0.01
	No	415	765			
Pregnant/lactating	Pregnant women	187	363	0.57 [0.46–0.71]	2.24 [1.57–3.12]	<0.01
	Lactating women	523	578			

Hookworm infection increases the risk of anemia by 3.37 folds higher [AOR 3.37 (95% CI: 2.33–4.88)]. This finding agrees with findings from northern Ethiopia [49], Nepal [33]. This is due to the fact that hookworm causing parasites significantly depletes the red blood cell of the host.

Iron supplementation during pregnancy decreases the risk of anemia by 97% [AOR 0.03 (95% CI: 0.02–0.04)]. The main reason for not receiving iron during pregnancy was unavailability of the drug. This finding agrees with finding from eastern Ethiopia [48]. This is due to the reason that iron act as a predominant role in the production of red blood cells.

Tea consumption increases the risk of anemia 3.63 folds higher [AOR 3.63 (95% CI: 2.56–5.14)]. This finding agrees with finding from Ethiopia [55]. This is because the fact that tea contains chemicals that inhibit the absorption of iron [57].

Pregnant mother had 2.24 folds higher risk of anemia than lactating mother [AOR 2.24 (95% CI: 1.57–3.12)]. This is due to the reason that after the delivery the mother has access to foods, especially animal products so that they can get more foods than when she was pregnant. In addition, mother can be treated for hookworm after delivery; during pregnancy, hookworm was not treated because the drug has a teratogenic effect.

Table 8 Linear regression output for determinants of hemoglobin in lactating or pregnant mothers (dependent variable = hemoglobin level in g/dl) (n = 1651)

Variables	*B coefficient [95% CI]*	*t*	*p-value*
MUAC	0.36 [0.33, −0.4]	21.66	<0.01
Parity	−0.18 [−0.23, −0.14]	−7.69	<0.01
Age of lactating/pregnant mother	−0.03[−0.04, −0.03]	−7.59	<0.01

MUAC had a positive relationship with hemoglobin concentration. Mid-upper arm circumference (MUAC) increase the hemoglobin concentration of women will also increase [***B*** 0.36 (95% *CI:* 0.33, −0.4)]. This finding agrees with finding from eastern Ethiopia [48] signaling that MUAC can be used to evaluate the nutritional level of pregnant or lactating women.

As the parity of women increases their hemoglobin concentration decreases [***B*** -0.18 (95% CI: -0.23, −0.14)].

This finding agrees with finding from the republic of Seychelles [53], Trinidad and Tobago [34], Benin [42]. This is due to the reason that as the number of pregnancy increases the risk of ante-partum hemorrhage and postpartum hemorrhage for the women became high.

The age of the women and her hemoglobin concentration had negative relationships. As the age increases the risk of becoming anemic would be high [B -0.03 (95% *CI:*-0.04, −0.03)]. This finding agrees with finding from Benin [42], northern Ethiopia [49]. This is due to the reason that as the age of the mother increases her parity wills also increases.

The main limitation of this study might be recall bias, but the interview was conducted using a structured questionnaire and the interviewers were trained health professionals they can probe and make the respondents remember the issues.

Conclusion

Both pregnant and lactating mothers were affected by anemia and the burden of anemia is higher in the pregnant mother than the lactating mother and iron deficiency anemia is the most common type of anemia. Anemia in pregnancy and lactation was determined by a history of malaria, history of abortion, hookworm infection, tea consumption, MUAC, residence, iron supplementation during pregnancy, parity, and age.

Recommendation

Iron supplementation should be given both to pregnant and lactating mothers. Iron supplementation should be included as part of malaria treatment in women with malaria. Women are advised to avoid tea during their pregnancy and lactation period. Scholars should consider MUAC as an alternative tool to detect nutritional defects in pregnancy.

Abbreviation

AOR: Adjusted Odds Ratio; B: Beta Coefficients; CI: Confidence Interval; COR: Crude Odds Ratio; G/DL: Gram per Deciliter; IUGR: Intra Uterine Growth Retardation; KM: Kilometer; MCHC: Mean Corpuscular Hemoglobin Concentration; MCV: Mean Corpuscular Volume; ML: Milliliter; MUAC: Mid Upper Arm Circumference; RPM: Revolution per Minute; SAF: Sodium Acetate- Acetic Acid-Formalin Solution; SD: Standard Deviation; SPSS: Statistical Package for Social Science

Acknowledgements

Our heartfelt appreciation goes to federal democratic republic of Ethiopia ministry of health for their financial support. We would like to acknowledge the Amhara national regional state health bureau for their unreserved support during this work. We would like to acknowledge staffs in the health center of Bahir dar for their cooperation during the data collection period. At last but not least we would like to acknowledge all institutions and organization that had input for this work.

Funding

This research work was financially supported by federal democratic republic of Ethiopia ministry of health. The funder has no role in design of the study and collection, analysis, and interpretation of data and in writing the manuscript.

Authors' contributions

BEF conceived the experiment; BEF and TEF performed the experiment, plan the data collection process, analyzed and interpreted the data. BEF and TEF wrote the manuscript and approved the final draft for publication.

Competing interests

The authors declares that they have no competing interests.

Author details

[1]Department of Epidemiology and Biostatistics, University of Bahir Dar, Bahir Dar, Ethiopia. [2]Departement of pediatrics, saint paulose hospital, Addis Ababa, Ethiopia.

References

1. Gopalan C. Strategies for combating under nutrition: lessons learned for the future. In: Nutrition in developmental transition in Southeast Asia. New Delhi: World Health Organization; 1992. p. 109–11.
2. Patterson A, Brown W, Roberts D. Dietary and supplement treatment of iron deficiency results in improvements in general health and fatigue in Australian women of childbearing age. J Am Coll Nutr. 2001;20(4):337–42.
3. Balarajan Y, Ramakrishnan U, Ozaltin E, Shankar A, Subramanian V. Anaemia in low-income and middle-income countries. Lancet. 2011;378(9809):2123–35.
4. WHO: World wide prevalence of anaemia 1993–2005, vol. 1. Atlanta CDC; 2008.
5. WHO: The prevalence of anaemia in women: a tabulation of available information. In. Geneva: World Health Organization; 1992.
6. WHO: World Health Organization, Centers for Disease Control and Prevention. Worldwide Prevalence of Anemia:. In: WHO Global Database of Anemia. 2008.
7. Salhan S, Tripathi V, Singh R, Gaikwad H. Evaluation of hematological parameters in partial exchange and packed cell transfusion in treatment of severe anemia in pregnancy. Anemia. 2012;2012:1–7.
8. DeBenoist B, McLean E, Egli I, Cogswell M: Worldwide prevalence of anaemia 1993-2005. In: *WHO Global database on anaemia*. World health Organization; 2008.
9. Weiss G, Goodnough L. Anemia of chronic disease. N Engl J Med. 2005;352: 1011–23.
10. Bernard B, Mohammad H, David P. An analysis of anemia and pregnancy-related maternal mortality. J Nutr. 2001;131:604S–15S.
11. Megan OB, Roland K, Gernard M, Elmar S, David H, Wafaie F, Anemia I. An independent predictor of mortality and immunologic progression of disease among women with HIV in Tanzania. J Acquir Immune Defic Syndr. 2005;40(2):219–26.
12. Allen L. Anemia and iron deficiency: effects on pregnancy outcome. Am J Clin Nutr. 2000;71(5 Suppl):1280S–12804S.
13. Malhotra M, Sharma J, Batra S, Sharma S, Murthy N, Arora R. Maternal and perinatal outcome in varying grades of anemia. Int J Gynaecol Obstet. 2002; 79(2):93–100.
14. Meuris S, Piko B, Eerens B, Vanbellinghen P, Dramaix A, Hennart P. Gestational malaria: assessment of its consequences on fetal growth. Am J Tropical Medicane and Hygiene. 1993;48:603–9.
15. Kumar A. National nutritional anaemia control programme in India. Indian J Public Health. 1999;43:3–5.
16. Stephen O. Iron and its relation to immunity and infectious disease. J Nutr. 2001;131:616S–35S.
17. Allen L. Anemia and iron deficiency: effects on pregnancy outcome. Am J Clin Nutr. 2000;71(5 Suppl):S1280–4.
18. Ramussen K. Is there a causal relationship between iron deficiency or iron deficiency anaemia and weight at birth, length of gestation and perinatal mortality? J Nutr. 2001;131(2 Suppl):S590–603.
19. Letsky E. Maternal anaemia in pregnancy, iron and pregnancy – a haematologist's viewpoint. Fetal Matern Med Rev. 2001;12:159–75.
20. Elise L. Maternal hemoglobin concentration and pregnancy outcome: a study of the effects of elevation in el alto. **Bolivia** *MJM*. 2010;13(1):47–55.
21. WHO. Nutritional anaemias. In: *World Health Organ Tech Rep Ser*. vol. 405. Geneva: World Health Organization; 1968.
22. CDC: Recommendations to prevent and control iron deficiency in the United States. In: *MMWR Morb Mortal Wkly Rep*. vol. 47: Centers for Disease Control and Prevention; 1998: 1–29.
23. Steer P. Maternal hemoglobin concentration and birth weight. Am J Clin Nutr. 2000;71(suppl):1285S–7S.
24. Goldenberg R, Tamura T, DuBard M, Johnston K, Copper R, Neggers Y. Plasma ferritin and pregnancy outcome. Am J Obstet Gynecol. 1996;175:1356–9.
25. Luke B. Nutritional influences on fetal growth. Clin Obstet Gynecol. 1994; 37(3):538–49.
26. Ashok K, Arun KR, Sriparna B, Debabrata D, Jamuna SS. Cord blood and breast milk iron status in maternal anemia. Pediatrics. 2008;121(3):673–80.
27. Ismail M, Ordi J, Menendez C, Ventura P, Aponte J, Kahigwa E, Hirt R, Cardesa A, Alonso A. Placental pathology in malaria: a histological, immunohistochemical, and quantitative study. Hum Pathol. 2000;31:85–93.
28. Verhoeff F, Brabin B, Van-Buuren S, Chimsuku L, Kazembe P, Wit J, Broadhead R. An analysis of intra-uterine growth retardation in rural Malawi. Eur J Clin Nutr. 2001;55:682–9.
29. Yarlini B, Subramanian S, Fawzi W. Maternal iron and folic acid supplementation is associated with lower risk of low birth weight in India. J Nutr. 2013;143:1309–15.

30. Adam I, Babiker S, Mohmmed A, Salih M, Prins M, Zaki Z. Low body mass index, anaemia and poor perinatal outcome in a rural hospital in eastern Sudan. J Trop Pediatr. 2008;54:202–4.
31. Brabin B, Piper C. Anaemia and malaria attributable low birth weight in two populations in Papua New Guinea. Ann Hum Biol. 1997;24:547–55.
32. Bergmann R, Gravens-Muller L, Hertwig K, Hinkel J, Andres B, Bergmann K. Iron deficiency is prevalent in a sample of pregnant women at delivery in Germany. Eur J Obstet Gynecol Reprod Biol. 2002;102(2):155–60.
33. Michele D, Rebecca S, Jaya S, Elizabeth P, Steven L, Subarna K, Sharada S, Joanne K, Marco A, Keith W. Hookworms, malaria and vitamin a deficiency contribute to anemia and iron deficiency among pregnant women in the plains of Nepal. J Nutr. 2000;130:2527–36.
34. Uche-Nwachi E, Odekunle A, Jacinto S, Burnett M, Clapperton M, David Y, Durga S, Greene K, Jarvis J, Nixon C, et al. Anaemia in pregnancy: associations with parity, abortions and child spacing in primary healthcare clinic attendees in Trinidad and Tobago. Afr Health Sci. 2010;10(1):66–70.
35. Balarajan Y, Fawzi W, Subramanian S. Changing patterns of social inequalities in anaemia among women in India: cross sectional study using nationally representative data. BMJ Open. 2013;3:e002233.
36. Vanden-Broek N, White S, Neilson J. The relationship between asymptomatic human immunodeficiency virus infection and the prevalence and severity of anemia in pregnant Malawian women. Am J Trop Med Hyg. 1998;59:1004–7.
37. Massawe S, Urassa E, Lindmark G. Anaemia in pregnancy: a major health problem with implications for maternal health care. Afr J Health Sci. 1996;3:126–32.
38. Massawe S, Urassa E, Lindmark G. Effectiveness of primary level antenatal care in decreasing anemia at term in Tanzania. Acta Obstet Gynecol Scand. 1999;78:573–9.
39. Frank M, Birgit R, Matthias G, Stefknie B, Holger T, Elisabeth K, William T, Ulrich B. Anaemia in pregnant Ghanaian women: importance of malaria, iron deficiency, and haemoglobinopathies. Transactions Ofthe Royal Society Of Tropical Medicine And Hygiene. 2000;94:477–83.
40. Ishraga A, Gamal A, Ahmed M, Magdi S, Naji A, Mustafa E, Ishag A. Anaemia, folate and v itamin B12 deficiency among pregnant women in an area of unstable malaria transmission in eastern Sudan. Trans R Soc Trop Med Hyg. 2009;103:493–6.
41. Peter O, Anna V-E, Mary H, Monica P, John A, Kephas O, Piet K, Laurence S. Malaria and anaemia among pregnant women at first antenatal clinic visit in Kisumu, western Kenya. Trop Med Int Health. 2007;12(12):1515–23.
42. Od S"I, Ghislain K, Manfred A, Florence B-L, Achille M, Michel C. Maternal Anemia at First Antenatal Visit: Prevalence and Risk Factors in a Malaria-Endemic Area in Benin. AmJTropMedHyg. 2012;87(3):418–24.
43. Jemal H, Rebecca P. Iron deficiency anemia is not a rare problem among women of reproductive ages in Ethiopia: a community based cross sectional study. BMC Blood Disorders. 2009;9(7):1–8.
44. Gies S, Brabin B, Yassin M, Cuevas L. Comparison of screening methods for anaemia in pregnant women in Awassa, Ethiopia. Trop Med Int Health. 2003; 8(4):301–9.
45. Gibson R, Abebe Y, Stabler S, Allen RH, Westcott JE, Barbara JS, Nancy FK, MH K. Zinc, gravida, infection, and iron, but not vitamin B-12 or folate status, predict hemoglobin during pregnancy in southern Ethiopia. J Nutr. 2008;138:581–6.
46. Haidar J, Nelson M, Abiud M, Ayana G. Malnutrition and iron deficiency Anaemia in urban slum communities form Addis Ababa, Ethiopia. East Afri Med J. 2003;80(4):191–4.
47. Umeta M, Haidar J, Demissie T, Akalu G, Ayana G. Iron deficiency Anaemia among women of reproductive age in nine administrative regions of Ethiopia. EthiopJHealth Dev. 2008;22(3):252–8.
48. Alene KA, Dohe AM. Prevalence of anemia and associated factors among pregnant women in an urban area of eastern Ethiopia. Anemia. 2014;2014:1–8.
49. Alem M, Enawgaw B, Gelaw A, Kena T, Seid M, Olkeba Y. Prevalence of anemia and associated risk factors among pregnant women attending antenatal care in Azezo health center Gondar town, Northwest Ethiopia. J Interdiscipl Histopathol. 2013;1(3):137–44.
50. Mbonye AK, Bygbjerg I, Magnussen P. Intermittent preventive treatment of malaria in pregnancy: a community-based delivery system and its effect on parasitemia, anemia and low birth weight in Uganda. Int J Infect Dis. 12(1):22–9.
51. Nynke B, Elizabeth L. Etiology of anemia in pregnancy in south Malawi. Am J Clin Nutr. 2000;72(suppl):247S–56S.
52. Lena H, Christa V-O, George B-A, Ville H, Patrick A, Teunis E, Ulrich B, Frank M. Decline of placental malaria in southern Ghana after the implementation of intermittent preventive treatment in pregnancy. Malar J. 2007;6(144)
53. Emeir D, Maxine B, Julie W, Chin-Kuo C, Paula R, Gary M, Philip D, Thomas C, Conrad S, Strain J. Iron status in pregnant women in the Republic of Seychelles. Public Health Nutr. 2009;13(3):331–7.
54. MacLeod C: Intestinal nematode infections. In: Parasitic Infections in Pregnancy and the Newborn New York: MacLeod, C. L., ed; 1988.
55. Haidar J. Prevalence of Anaemia, deficiencies of iron and folic acid and their determinants in Ethiopian women. J Health Popul Nutr. 2010;28(4):359–68.
56. Institute S: Methods in Parasitology. In: Sodium acetate-acetic acid-formalin solution method for stool specimen. Basel: Swiss TPH: Swiss Tropical Institute; 2005: 1–18.
57. Iron Deficiency Anemia: Nutritional Considerations [http://www.nutritionmd.org/consumers/hematology/iron_anemia_nutrition.html].

Rapid access clinic for unexplained lymphadenopathy and suspected malignancy: prospective analysis of 1000 patients

Andrea Kühnl[1], David Cunningham[1], Margaret Hutka[1], Clare Peckitt[2], Hamoun Rozati[1], Federica Morano[1], Irene Chong[1], Angela Gillbanks[1], Andrew Wotherspoon[3], Michelle Harris[1], Tracey Murray[1] and Ian Chau[1*]

Abstract

Background: In patients presenting with peripheral lymphadenopathy, it is critical to effectively identify those with underlying cancer who require urgent specialist care.

Methods: We analyzed a large dataset of 1000 consecutive patients with unexplained lymphadenopathy referred between 2001 and 2009 to the Royal Marsden Hospital (RMH) rapid access lymph node diagnostic clinic (LNDC).

Results: Cancer was diagnosed in 14% of patients. Factors predictive for malignant disease were male sex, age, supraclavicular and multiple site involvement. Cancer-associated symptoms were present for a median of 8 weeks. The median time from referral to start of cancer therapy was 53 days. Fine needle aspiration (FNA) was performed in 83% of patients with malignancies. Sensitivity and specificity of FNA were limited (50 and 87%, respectively for any malignancy; 30 and 79%, respectively for lymphoma). The vast majority of cancer patients received diagnostic biopsies on the basis of suspicious clinical and ultrasound findings; the FNA result contributed to establishing the diagnosis in only 4 cases.

Conclusions: In conclusion, we demonstrate that Oncologist-led rapid access clinics are successful concepts to assess patients with unexplained lymphadenopathy. Our data suggest that a routine use of FNA should be reconsidered in this setting.

Keywords: Lymphadenopathy, Rapid access clinic, Cancer diagnosis

Background

Peripheral lymphadenopathy has a wide range of infectious, neoplastic and inflammatory differential diagnoses. When assessing patients with unexplained lymphadenopathy, the main challenge is to identify patients with malignancy or other critical conditions requiring urgent specialist care. In addition, the diagnostic work-up should minimize unnecessary procedures and avoid prolonged hospitalization in the interest of cost-effectiveness and patients' satisfaction.

To optimize management of patients with lymphadenopathy and suspicion of cancer, rapid access lump clinics have been implemented throughout the UK, allowing quick referral routes and close collaboration between hemato-oncologists, radiologists, ENT specialist and surgeons [1]. Similarly, quick diagnosis units have been successfully introduced in other European countries [2] and were recently proposed as suitable diagnostic services for the US healthcare system [3]. However, the optimal set-up of these clinics remains a matter of debate given the difficult task of dealing with a magnitude of distinct conditions in an effective way. Data on performance and outcome of rapid access clinics are therefore essential to further improve this service and to define the most adequate diagnostic pathways for patients with unexplained lymphadenopathy.

* Correspondence: ian.chau@rmh.nhs.uk
[1]Department of Medicine, Royal Marsden NHS Foundation Trust, Downs Road, Sutton, Surrey SM2 5PT, UK
Full list of author information is available at the end of the article

Lymphomas are among the most common malignant diagnoses in patients with unclear lymphadenopathy, with the incidence anticipated to rise in the next decades. Lymphomas comprise a heterogeneous group of hematologic malignancies, the most common ones being diffuse large B cell lymphoma (DLBCL), follicular lymphoma (FL) and Hodgkin lymphoma (HL). Lymphoma patients often present with unspecific symptoms commonly seen in non-severe illnesses, which can cause significant delays to specialist referral [4]. Excision biopsy remains the gold standard for diagnosing lymphoma and the full histological work-up requires complex immunohistochemical analyses by an experienced histopathologist. Timely diagnosis and start of treatment is considered particularly important for DLBCL and HL patients who can be cured by multi-agent chemotherapies.

We have successfully established a rapid access multidisciplinary lymph node diagnostic clinic (LNDC) for unexplained lymphadenopathy at the Royal Marsden Hospital (RMH), a tertiary referral comprehensive cancer centre [5]. Here, we report on the outcome of 1000 consecutive patients referred from 2001 and 2009 to the LNDC with focus on patients diagnosed with lymphoma.

Methods

We analyzed 1000 consecutive patients referred between September 2001 and September 2009 to the RMH LNDC with available data. The analysis was performed as part of a designated service evaluation for this time period, but results are representative of the current standard in this clinic. The LNDC at RMH was established in 1996 as a rapid access clinic for patients with unexplained lymphadenopathy referred by their General Practitioners [5]. The clinic is held twice a week. The core clinical team comprises a consultant medical oncologist and a lymphoma clinical nurse specialist.

Depending on clinical presentation, diagnostic procedures were arranged as described before [5], including blood tests, microbiology assessments, ultrasound (US), computed tomography (CT) and fine needle aspiration (FNA). There were designated slots for US assessment and results were immediately available. FNA cytology results were available within 1 week and graded C0-C5 as described before [5]. Patients were referred for diagnostic biopsies if suspicion of malignancy was high.

Patients diagnosed with malignancies or benign tumors that required surgical intervention were referred internally to the respective RMH units. Patients with non-malignant conditions for specific treatment were referred to other hospitals as appropriate. Patients with benign reactive lymphadenopathy or self-limiting diseases were discharged from RMH, either immediately or after follow-up clinic visits.

Clinical data, diagnostic results and details on patient management were retrospectively collected on the RMH Electronic Patient Record system. An experienced histopathologist reviewed all lymph node biopsies where a final diagnosis of lymphoma was made. The date of diagnosis for malignant disease was defined as the date of final histological diagnosis. Lymph node areas involved were compared between patient groups using the chi-square test. Multivariate analysis for prediction of malignancy was performed using a stepwise logistic regression model including the following variables: age, gender, ethnicity (white vs. non-white) and site of lymphadenopathy (cervical, axillary, inguinal, extranodal, multiple sites). Data analysis was performed using stata version 13.1.

Results

Characteristics and diagnoses of study patients

We analyzed 1000 patients referred between 2001 and 2009 to the RMH LNDC. Patients had a median age of 41 years (range 16–94), were mainly Caucasians (83%) and predominantly female (63%). Malignant disease was diagnosed in 138 (14%) patients (81 with lymphoma (median age 55 years) and 55 with solid tumors (median age 58 years); Table 1). Ninety-one patients had benign neoplasms (median age 50 years) and 89 patients were diagnosed with specific infectious or inflammatory diseases (median age 37 years). The majority of cases (62%) either had reactive/unspecific lymphadenopathy ($n = 510$; median age 37 years), normal tissue/anatomical variants (e.g. prominent muscle; $n = 46$; median age 47 years) or no palpable lesion ($n = 61$; median age 46 years; Table 1). The category reactive/

Table 1 Diagnostic categories

Category	no.
Malignant tumor	138
Lymphoma	81
Other hematological malignancy	2
Solid tumor	55
Benign tumor	91
Non-neoplastic, non-infectious lesion	111
Cyst	47
Vascular malformation	3
Hematoma	4
Normal tissue/variant	46
Goiter	4
Hernia	3
Other	4
Infectious/inflammatory disease	89
Reactive/unspecific lymphadenopathy	510
Nothing palpable	61

Diagnostic categories of the total study cohort ($n = 1000$)

unspecific lymphadenopathy included cases with normal lymph nodes. Of 510 patients with reactive/unspecific lymphadenopathy, 247 (48%) had lymph nodes less than 1 cm in size and 52 (10%) had symptom duration of less than 6 weeks.

Table 2 shows specific tumor subtypes and infectious/inflammatory diseases diagnosed. Forty-four percent of lymphomas were potentially curable subtypes (HL, DLBCL, Burkitt lymphoma). The most common lymphoma subtype was FL ($n = 31$). Among solid tumors, squamous cell carcinomas (SCC) of the head and neck ($n = 20$) and metastatic melanoma ($n = 8$) were most frequently diagnosed.

Clinical presentation of cancer patients

All patients diagnosed with malignant disease presented with nodes/lumps of more than 1.5 cm in size. Cancer-associated symptoms were present for a median of 8 weeks (range 0–832). Of 35 patients with HL or DLBCL, 15 (43%) had elevated LDH levels and 5 (14%) had B-symptoms as indicators for highly proliferative disease. Median duration of symptoms in these patients was 7 weeks (range 1–104).

Patients with malignant disease presented significantly more often with supraclavicular nodes and lymphadenopathy involving multiple sites compared to non-malignant cases (Table 3). Frequency of extranodal involvement was significantly lower in malignant vs. non-malignant conditions ($P = 0.009$). Axillary involvement was more frequently seen in solid tumors as compared to lymphomas (16% vs. 5%; $P = 0.03$). Lymphomas presented significantly more often with multiple site involvement (22% vs. 5%; $P = 0.008$) in comparison to solid tumors.

In multivariate analyses, supraclavicular and multiple site involvement were significantly predictive of malignancy, whereas extranodal involvement was an independent predictor of non-malignant disease (Table 4). In addition, higher age and male sex were predictive of malignant disease.

Cancer treatment and waiting times

Time to final diagnosis and treatment was assessed in 122 cancer patients with available data. The median time from first clinic visit to full histological diagnosis was 22 days (range 1–924), 28 days for lymphomas (range 7–356) and 19 days for solid tumors (range 1–924). The main reason for diagnostic delays in lymphoma cases was presence of mild/intermittent symptoms, leading to prolonged monitoring of patients before a diagnostic biopsy was arranged.

Seventy-five (56%) patients with malignant disease received systemic treatment, 19 (14%) received initial radiotherapy and 20 (15%) primary surgery. Four patients with metastatic solid tumors received best supportive care only. In 16 patients diagnosed with indolent lymphoma a watch

Table 2 Specific diagnoses

Lymphoma subtypes (no.), $n = 81$	
Hodgkin lymphoma (incl. 1 PTLD)	19
Diffuse large B cell lymphoma	16
Mantle cell lymphoma	4
Burkitt lymphoma	1
Follicular lymphoma	31
Small lymphocytic lymphoma	7
Marginal zone lymphoma	1
Lymphoplasmacytic lymphoma	2
Solid tumors (no.), $n = 55$	
Breast	6
Head and neck (SCC)	20
Thyroid	1
Salivary gland	4
Upper GI adenocarcinoma (1 oesophageal, 1 gastric)	2
Cervix/ovarian	2
Skin (8 Melanoma, 1 SCC, 1 Merkel cell)	10
Prostate	1
Lung (non-small cell)	1
Renal	1
Olfactory neuroblastoma	1
Unknown Primary	6
Benign tumors (no.), $n = 91$	
Angioma/angiofibroma	2
Lipoma	44
Fibroadenoma	6
Pilomatrixoma	2
Pleomorphic salivary gland adenoma	15
Warthin's tumor	18
Granular cell tumor	1
Follicular adenoma (thyroid)	1
Schwannoma	1
Not specified	1
Infectious/inflammatory diseases (no.), $n = 89$	
Chronic sialadenitis/tonsillitis	12
Dermatopathic lymphadenopathy	12
Local inflammation/abscess	8
Sarcoidosis/granuloma	13
Kikuchi's disease	2
Specific acute infections	42
Toxoplasmosis	14
Tuberculosis	13
Epstein-Barr virus	6
Human immunodeficiency virus	5
Syphilis	1

Table 2 Specific diagnoses *(Continued)*

Lymphoma subtypes (no.), $n = 81$	
Mumps	1
Bartonella infection	2

PTLD indicates post -transplant lymphoproliferative disorder; SCC indicates squamous cell carcinoma
Specific diagnoses assigned to patients on the study ($n = 1000$)

and wait policy was adopted. The median time from referral to start of therapy was 53 days (range 21–930; 56 days for lymphomas and 50 days for solid tumors), including watch and wait and best supportive care as therapies. After exclusion of cases delayed due to patients' decision, the median times to therapy were 50 days (lymphomas) and 48 days (solid tumors).

Rapid and streamline pathways for diagnosis and therapy might be of particular importance for potentially curable lymphomas, such as HL and DLBCL. Median time from referral to start of therapy in HL was 48 days (range 26–202) and 45 days for DLBCL (range 22–116). Median time from referral to start of therapy has improved since implementing specific cancer waiting time targets in the UK in 2005, with a median time of 38 days between 2005 and 2009 compared to 51 days between 2001 and 2004 (Additional file 1: Figure S1).

Diagnostic procedures

96% of patients with malignancy and all lymphoma patients had a core or excision biopsy as diagnostic procedure. Six solid tumor cases were diagnosed with FNA only (5 did not have a biopsy, 1 had a non-diagnostic biopsy). FNA was performed in 423 of 1000 cases, in 114/138 (83%) of malignancies and in 63/81 (78%) of lymphomas.

FNA results were inadequate (C0/C1) in 94/423 (22%) of patients, which was similar with US guidance [68/316 (22%)] and without [26/107 (24%)]. FNA raised suspicion of cancer (C3–5 cytology) in 57/114 (50%) of all malignancies and in 19/81 (24%) of lymphomas. Benign cytology (C2) was seen in 44/114 (39%) malignancies, the majority of which were lymphomas ($n = 39$). Sensitivity of US and FNA was 93 and 50% to detect any malignancy, and 88 and 30% to detect lymphoma, respectively. Specificity was 96% (US) and 87% (FNA) for detection of all malignancies, and 91% (US) and 79% (FNA) for detection of lymphoma.

Given the limited sensitivity and specificity of FNA as diagnostic tool, we analyzed which diagnostic finding actually prompted the LNDC team to arrange a biopsy in malignant cases ($n = 133$; Table 5). Most patients ($n = 129$) were referred to biopsy on the basis of high clinical suspicion with or without additional abnormal findings in US performed on the day of clinic visit. Only in 2 cases with cancer of unknown primary and 1 Burkitt lymphoma patient, the FNA C5 result led to referral for biopsy. In 1 patient with lymphoplasmacytic lymphoma, the FNA result (C3) was the only finding that raised suspicion of malignancy and prompted a diagnostic biopsy. In 10 patients with solid tumors (5 head and neck, 3 breast, 1 salivary gland, 1 unknown primary), the FNA C4/5 result was important to decide on doing a core rather than excision biopsy. In 11 patients with minor symptoms (10 lymphoma cases and 1 salivary gland carcinoma), the diagnostic biopsy was delayed due to FNA C2 results, with a median time from first visit to diagnosis of 79 days (range 47–212). Thus, FNA was of limited value for establishing the diagnosis in the majority of malignant diseases in our series.

Most non-malignant cases [539/862 (63%)] did not have either biopsy or FNA. Among 310 non-malignant cases undergoing FNA, 81 (26%) were inadequate, 190 (61%) showed benign cytology and 13 (4%) raised suspicion of malignancy. In 26 cases the FNA result was diagnostic for the non-malignant condition (11 pleomorphic salivary gland adenomas, 6 Warthin's tumors, 3 branchial cysts, 2 tuberculosis cases, 1 abscess, 1 toxoplasmosis, 1 hematoma, 1 pilomatrixoma). Biopsies were not performed in 742/862 (86%) of non-malignant cases, mainly guided by clinical examination and US (Additional file 1: Figure S2). In 152/742 (20%) cases with non-malignant disease, the FNA result helped to establish the diagnosis and to avoid a more invasive biopsy.

Discussion

Implementation of rapid access diagnostic clinics for patients with unexplained lymphadenopathy facilitates early diagnosis of cancer. Here, we provide a detailed report on

Table 3 Anatomical areas involved

Areas involved	Malignant ($n = 138$) no. (%)	Non-malignant ($n = 862$) no. (%)	*P*
Cervical	71 (51)	518 (60)	0.055
Supraclavicular	11 (8)	26 (3)	0.004
Axillary	13 (9)	119 (14)	0.158
Inguinal	19 (14)	77 (9)	0.073
Multiple sites	21 (15)	47 (5)	< 0.001
Extranodal	3 (2)	75 (9)	0.008

Sites of nodal- and extranodal involvement in malignant and non-malignant cases

Table 4 Multivariable analysis for prediction of malignant disease ($n = 1000$)

Variables	OR	95% CI	P
Age (years)	1.04	1.03–1.06	< 0.001
Male sex	2.84	1.92–4.21	< 0.001
Supraclavicular	2.41	1.10–5.31	0.03
Multiple sites	4.02	2.20–7.34	< 0.001
Extranodal	0.17	0.05–0.58	0.004

OR indicates odds ratio, *CI* indicates confidence interval

1000 consecutive patients seen in the multidisciplinary LNDC at RMH between 2001 and 2009.

The pick-up rate for malignant diseases in our study was 14% which is in line with previous findings at our [5] and other institutions [6] and similar to results from neck lump clinics [7–10]. However, a recent Spanish study investigating 372 patients with unexplained lymphadenopathy referred from primary health care centers to an internist-led quick diagnosis unit reported a cancer rate of 32% [2]. The study excluded patients without palpable lesion at the time of clinic visit, which was found in 6% of our cases. In addition, they had a lower incidence of reactive nodes (42%) and only 4 cases with benign tumors. In contrast, reactive and benign findings accounted for 71% of referrals in our series. Given the set-up of our clinic in a tertiary care cancer center involving assessment by a consultant medical oncologist and a lymphoma clinical nurse specialist, a better selection of patients who require urgent assessment would be preferable.

Most cancer referral guidelines suggest referral of patients with unclear lymphadenopathy or lumps greater than 1-2 cm in size [1, 11]. Our findings support adherence to a minimum size limit. Half of reactive nodes but no case of malignancy presented with sub-centimeter lymphadenopathy in our cohort. The use of calipers for exact nodal measurements might help to increase the quality of referrals. In addition, extranodal lumps (not in the breast or head and neck) that are unchanged in size for many years should not be subject to an urgent referral pathway.

Table 5 Indication for biopsy in malignant cases ($n = 133$)

Indication for biopsy in malignant cases	Reason for US/FNA not impacting on decision-making
Clinical suspicion ($n = 68$)	No US performed ($n = 63$)
	US inconclusive/not suspicious ($n = 5$)
	No FNA performed ($n = 19$)
	FNA results inconclusive/not suspicious/ not awaited ($n = 49$)
Clinical and US suspicion ($n = 61$)	No FNA performed ($n = 5$)
	FNA results inconclusive/not suspicious/ not awaited ($n = 56$)
Clinical suspicion and FNA C5 ($n = 2$)	No US performed ($n = 2$)
FNA C3 result ($n = 1$)[a]	No US performed ($n = 1$)
Clinical and US suspicion, FNA C5 ($n = 1$)	Not applicable

[a]No clinical suspicion of malignancy
Diagnostic findings that led to performing a confirmatory biopsy in patients with malignant disease ($n = 133$)

Our study shows that by far the most important diagnostic tool is examination/evaluation by an experienced clinician, taking into account several factors to estimate the probability of malignancy, such as size, texture and site of the lump, symptoms, risk factors, and examination of loco-regional and disease-related sites. The majority of non-malignant cases did not undergo any invasive investigation and could therefore efficiently be assessed outside a specialist center. Thus, some form of local Hemato-oncology involvement or remote Specialist triaging, alongside improved communication and guidance between primary care and specialist centers might further assist appropriate patient selection. This would allow for a more effective use of resources and would spare low-risk patients the psychological burden of being assessed for cancer.

We and others have identified clinical factors in patients with unexplained lymphadenopathy that predict for malignancy [5, 6] Here, we validate our previous findings identifying male sex, age, as well as supraclavicular and multiple site involvement as independently predictive for malignant disease. Presence of these features in patients with unexplained lymphadenopathy should alert clinicians to the possibility of underlying cancer.

Referrals of patients with lymphomas and solid tumors occurred in a timely manner with median symptom duration of only 8 weeks at the time of presentation in our clinic. Particularly lymphoma-related symptoms are often not indicative of malignant disease or serious illness, which usually leads to a longer time to seeking medical help compared to other cancers [4]. Howell et al. [12] reported a median time of 10 weeks from onset of lymphoma-related symptoms to seeking medical help and Summerfield et al. [13] observed a mean time of 16 weeks. The shorter intervals in our series might indicate an increasing public awareness about the need to investigate an unexplained change in health. Referred patients were seen promptly in our clinic (mean waiting time of 7 days). A median time from referral to start of treatment of 53 days in patients diagnosed with cancer still warrants improvement. Similar to previous findings [12], main delays occurred after the first clinic appointment, and were predominantly "diagnostic delays" for lymphoma patients (mainly indolent lymphomas) and "therapy delays" in solid tumors (mainly palliative treatment).

Indolent lymphomas typically present with diffuse, mild symptoms and have a high false-negative rate in FNA assessment. Accordingly, the main reason for delay in the diagnosis of indolent lymphomas was an initially observational approach, in some cases supported by benign FNA results. To diagnose indolent lymphomas quicker, cases without high clinical suspicion of malignancy would generally have to undergo early biopsies. This would significantly increase the rate of invasive procedures for non-cancer patients.

FNA assessment on the day of clinic visit in patients with suspicion of malignancy is part of our LNDC set-up. This is in line with national recommendations for rapid access head and neck lump clinics. However, lymphomas are usually the most common malignancies diagnosed in clinics for general lymphadenopathy or head and neck lumps and FNA is not regarded an appropriate tool for lymphoma diagnosis. Limitations of FNA in lymphoma are well documented [14–16]. Our findings further support these data with the sensitivity of FNA being only 30%. Accuracy of FNA is better for solid tumors, but significantly depends on the exact site of disease as shown for head and neck lumps [16]. A rapid access LNDC deals with a variety of cancer types and routine use of FNA for every patient might not be optimal in this regard.

FNA as primary diagnostic tool should have a minimal rate of inadequate and false-negative samples and should decrease the need for diagnostic biopsies. This however highly depends on the clinic setting: local FNA performance, clinical expertise, availability/quality of US assessment and frequency of cancer types. The utility of FNA is certainly higher in cytologist-led one-stop clinics were samples can be immediately assessed and retaken if necessary. In addition, accuracy of FNA for lymphoma, particularly high-grade NHL, can be improved by flow cytometry [17, 18], but this is an expensive technique only available at specialist centers. Of note, even if FNA is indicative/diagnostic for lymphoma, this will not substitute for a surgical biopsy to allow the full range of tests needed for exact diagnosis. Also in solid tumors, the majority of patients still require a biopsy after FNA to establish the diagnosis and to provide sufficient material for molecular and immunohistochemical testings. In view of the increasing use of targeted therapies, the need for adequate tissue to assess predictive biomarkers will further grow. In our series, only 5 patients with solid tumors were diagnosed with FNA only. In a further few cancer cases, FNA results were important to decide on performing a biopsy. In the majority of malignant cases, indication for biopsy was guided by clinical suspicion and US features. In addition, many patients required repeat aspirations (data not shown), which involves additional costs and follow-up visits. Repeat false-negative results (including inadequate samples) are not only misleading for clinicians, but also impose significant stress on patients.

US is highly sensitive to distinguish malignant from non-malignant lumps and can provide important information about the type of malignancy. US is cheap, safe and widely available. Our data indicate that if an integrated US service and a highly experienced clinical team is available, pre-selection of patients for FNA should be more stringent. For example, FNA should be performed if there is high suspicion of SCC of the head and neck. Or, if there is low suspicion of malignancy and a benign FNA result is regarded sufficient to rule out malignancy. On the other hand, FNA should be avoided if lymphoma is suspected (e.g. age, B-symptoms, typical US features).

Conclusions

In conclusion, this is the largest dataset of a rapid access clinic for patients with unclear lymphadenopathy. Our results provide valuable insights into the successful performance of our LNDC and build a basis for further improvement of this diagnostic service model.

Abbreviations

CT: Computed tomography; DLBCL: Diffuse large B-cell lymphoma; FL: Follicular lymphoma; FNA: Fine needle aspiration; HL: Hodgkin lymphoma; LDH: Lactate dehydrogenase; LNDC: Lymph node diagnostic clinic; RMH: Royal Marsden Hospital; SCC: Squamous cell carcinoma; US: Ultrasound

Acknowledgements

All authors would like to acknowledge National Health Service funding to the National Institute for Health Research Biomedical Research Centre at the Royal Marsden NHS Foundation Trust and The Institute of Cancer Research.

Authors' contributions

AK: retrospective data collection, analysis and interpretation of data, writing of the manuscript; DC: clinical lead of LNDC, editing and review of the manuscript; CP: statistical analyses; MH, HR, FM, ICho: retrospective data collection and interpretation; AG: data management; AW: lead histopathologist of LNDC; MH, TM: prospective data collection and data management; ICha.: conception of the study, analysis and interpretation of data, editing and review of the manuscript. All authors have read and approved the final manuscript.

Competing interests

D.C. has received research funding from Amgen, Astra Zeneca, Bayer, Celgene, Medimmune, Merrimack, Merck Serono and Sanofi. The authors declare that they have no competing interests.

Author details

[1]Department of Medicine, Royal Marsden NHS Foundation Trust, Downs Road, Sutton, Surrey SM2 5PT, UK. [2]Department of Computing, Royal Marsden NHS Foundation Trust, London, Surrey, UK. [3]Department of Histopathology, Royal Marsden NHS Foundation Trust, London, Surrey, UK.

References

1. (NICE) NI for CE. Improving outcomes in Haematological cancers. London: Natl Inst Clin Excell; 2003.
2. Bosch X, Coloma E, Donate C, et al. Evaluation of unexplained peripheral lymphadenopathy and suspected malignancy using a distinct quick diagnostic delivery model: prospective study of 372 patients. Med. 2014; 93(16):e95.
3. Gupta S, Sukhal S, Agarwal R, Das K. Quick diagnosis units-an effective alternative to hospitalization for diagnostic workup: a systematic review. J Hosp Med. 2014;9(1):54–9. https://doi.org/10.1002/jhm.2129.
4. Howell DA, Smith AG, Roman E. Help-seeking behaviour in patients with lymphoma. Eur J Cancer Care. 2008;17(4):394–403.
5. Chau I, Kelleher MT, Cunningham D, et al. Rapid access multidisciplinary lymph node diagnostic clinic: analysis of 550 patients. Br J Cancer. 2003; 88(3):354–61.
6. Vassilakopoulos TP, Pangalis GA. Application of a prediction rule to select which patients presenting with lymphadenopathy should undergo a lymph node biopsy. Med. 2000;79(5):338–47.
7. Al Hamarneh O, Liew L, Shortridge RJ. Diagnostic yield of a one-stop neck lump clinic. Eur Arch Otorhinolaryngol. 2013;270(5):1711–4.
8. Williams MV, Drinkwater KJ, Jones A, O'Sullivan B, Tait D. Waiting times for systemic cancer therapy in the United Kingdom in 2006. Br J Cancer. 2008; 99(5):695–703.
9. Williams C, Byrne R, Holden D, Sherman I, Srinivasan VR. Two-week referrals for suspected head and neck cancer: two cycles of audit, 10 years apart, in a district general hospital. J Laryngol Otol. 2014;128(8):720–4.
10. Vowles RH, Ghiacy S, Jefferis AF. A clinic for the rapid processing of patients with neck masses. J Laryngol Otol. 1998;112(11):1061–4.
11. (NICE) NI for CE. Referral guidelines for suspected cancer. London: Natl Inst Clin Excell; 2005.
12. Howell DA, Smith AG, Roman E. Lymphoma: variations in time to diagnosis and treatment. Eur J Cancer Care. 2006;15(3):272–8.
13. Summerfield GP, Carey PJ, Galloway MJ, Tinegate HN. An audit of delays in diagnosis and treatment of lymphoma in district hospitals in the northern region of the United Kingdom. Clin Lab Haematol. 2000;22(3):157–60.
14. Nikonova A, Guirguis HR, Buckstein R, Cheung MC. Predictors of delay in diagnosis and treatment in diffuse large B-cell lymphoma and impact on survival. Br J Haematol. 2015;168(4):492–500.
15. Hehn ST, Grogan TM, Miller TP. Utility of fine-needle aspiration as a diagnostic technique in lymphoma. J Clin Oncol. 2004;22(15):3046–52.
16. Howlett DC, Harper B, Quante M, et al. Diagnostic adequacy and accuracy of fine needle aspiration cytology in neck lump assessment: results from a regional cancer network over a one year period. J Laryngol Otol. 2007; 121(6):571–9.
17. Zeppa P, Vigliar E, Cozzolino I, et al. Fine needle aspiration cytology and flow cytometry immunophenotyping of non-Hodgkin lymphoma: can we do better? Cytopathology. 2010;21(5):300–10.
18. Bangerter M, Brudler O, Heinrich B, Griesshamnuer M. Fine needle aspiration cytology and flow cytometry in the diagnosis and subclassification of non-Hodgkin's lymphoma based on the World Health Organization classification. Acta Cytol. 2007;51(3):390–8.

Seroprevalence and trends of transfusion transmitted infections at Harar blood bank in Harari regional state, Eastern Ethiopia: eight years retrospective study

Zelalem Teklemariam, Habtamu Mitiku and Fitsum Weldegebreal*

Abstract

Background: The use of unscreened blood exposes the patient to many transfusion transmitted infections including Hepatitis B Virus (HBV), Hepatitis C virus (HCV), Human Immunodeficiency Virus (HIV), and syphilis, among others. Thus, blood transfusion demands for meticulous pre-transfusion testing and screening. Trends of transfusion transmitted infections are important to take appropriate measures on blood bank services. Therefore the aim of this study was to assess seroprevalence and trends of transfusion transmitted infections at Harar blood bank in Harari regional state, Eastern Ethiopia from 2008 to 2015.

Methods: A retrospective cross-sectional study was employed to review blood donors' history and laboratory tests records from November 16–December 31, 2017. All records of blood donors having vividly documented history and laboratory tests were reviewed by data collectors. All data were entered into EPI data version 3.1. It was exported and analyzed with Statistical Package for the Social Sciences version 16 soft ware.

Result: A total of 11, 382 blood donors' history and laboratory tests records were reviewed. Majority of them were males (82.6%), 57.6 % were in the age group of 17 to 25 years and 99.9% donors donated blood for the first time. The overall seroprevalence of transfusion transmitted infections (HBV, HIV, HCV and syphilis combined) was found to be 6.6%. The prevalence of HBV, HIV, HCV and syphilis were found to be 4.4%, 0.6%, 0.8% and 1.1%, respectively. The trend in prevalence of syphilis and HCV was statistical significant by year ($p < 0.05$). Those donors in the age group of 26–35 years (AOR: 2.1; 95% CI: 1.2,3.6), 36–45 years (AOR: 4.1; 95% CI: 2.4,7.1) and greater than 46 years (AOR:4.6; 95% CI: 2.3,9.1) were more likely to be infected with syphilis compared to the age group of 17–25 years. Male were more likely to be infected with HBV (AOR: 1.9; 95% CI: 1.4, 2.5) than females.

Conclusions: The magnitude of transfusion transmitted infections was lower than the previous studies conducted in Ethiopia. However, the decline in trends of transfusion transmitted infections has not been significant for some pathogens. Therefore, strict adherence with the criteria of preliminary blood donor selection should be implemented to reduce the amount of blood being withdrawn from transfusion after collection and screening.

Keywords: Transfusion transmitted infections, Hepatitis B virus, Hepatitis C virus, Human immunodeficiency virus, Syphilis, Blood bank, Harar, Eastern Ethiopia

* Correspondence: fwmlab2000@gmail.com
College of Health and Medical Sciences, Department of Medical Laboratory Sciences, Haramaya University, P.O. Box 235, Harar, Ethiopia

Background

Blood transfusion services (BTS) are transfusion of blood components. This saves millions of patients from death and morbidity each year worldwide [1]. There were reports that a quarter of a million mothers deaths globally due to obstetric bleeding. Furthermore, anemia causes 15% of child death in Africa [2]. Ethiopia is a country with high number of maternal mortality [3], motor accident and population non-immune to malaria. All the above cases required safe blood transfusion [2]. Blood transfusion corrects different conditions of patients like anemia, deficiency of plasma clotting factor, thrombocytopenia, hypoalbuminia and other [4].

It is known that blood can be vehicle for number of blood pathogens. Transfusion of unscreened blood to the patient has risk of acquiring Transfusion Transmitted Infections (TTIs) like Hepatitis B Virus (HBV), Hepatitis C Virus (HCV), Human Immunodeficiency Virus (HIV), syphilis, malaria and other. Despite uncertainty in the exact rates of transmission, blood transfusion is still considered to be a contributing mode of viral transmission in parts of Africa. Proportion of new HIV infections might ranges from 5 to 10% [5]. Similarly, 12.5% of patients at risk of post transfusion hepatitis [6]. HBV is the highly known potential infectious virus which is associated with complications like cirrhosis, portal hypertension and hepatocellular carcinoma [7].

Several Studies had been conducted to assess the prevalence and trends of TTIs among blood donors in different parts of the world. They found out an increase or decrease of trends TTIs [8–13]. Thus, blood transfusion units of each health institutions should have major role to screen, monitor and control TTIs. This practice also give some clues about the magnitude of TTIs in healthy populations' [1, 8].

Selection of blood donors with low TTIs risk was followed by effective laboratory screening in major work of blood transfusion units [14, 15]. These activities have been extremely effective but transmission of diseases still occurs. Because of the inability of the laboratory test to detect those persons with an infection in the window period, lack of budget for all standard laboratory for TTIs testing and trained manpower, presence of immunologically variant viruses, presence non-seroconverting silent carriers, laboratory testing errors and poor quality control of laboratory tests [9, 16–18].

There were few studies on the seroprevalence and trends of TTIs among blood donors in Ethiopia, which found with variable findings [11, 19–23]. A study conducted among Ethiopian blood donors in 1995 showed that the seroprevalence of HIV-1, syphilis and HBV was 16.7%, 12.8% and 14.4%, respectively [23]. In another retrospective study conducted in Gondar from January 2003 and December 2007 showed a seroprevalence of HIV, HBV, HCV and syphilis of 3.8%, 4.7%, 0.7%, and 1.3% respectively. And significantly declining trends of seroprevalence of HIV, HCV and syphilis was observed [19]. There was no published report about the prevalence and trends of TTIs among blood donors in Harari region. Hepatitis B Virus (HBV), Hepatitis C Virus (HCV), Human Immunodeficiency Virus (HIV) and syphilis are the four major Transfusion Transmitted Infections (TTIs) which have been routinely screened from all blood donated at Harar Blood Bank. Therefore we sought to assess the trends in donor seroprevalence of HBV, HCV, HIV and syphilis over an 8 year period (2008–2015).

Methods

Study area and period

The study was conducted from November 16- December 31, 2017 in Harar blood bank, Harari Regional State. Harar town is the capital city of Harari People Regional state, which is one of the most historical towns, located in the eastern part of Ethiopia. It is found at 525 km east of Addis Ababa, the capital city of Ethiopia. The blood bank was established in 1976/77 by Ethiopian Red Cross society. It has been collecting blood from donors by undergoing campaign in different institutes, routinely screens the collected blood for the presence of four major TTIs (HIV, HCV, HBV and syphilis) and provides screened blood to recipients in need at hospitals in the regional state. In addition, they prepare different blood components including platelet, and plasma as well as providing voluntary counseling for all blood donors after testing their blood sample.

Study design

A retrospective cross-sectional study was employed to review blood donors' history and laboratory tests records.

Sample size and sampling techniques

The sample size for prevalence and trends of transfusion transmitted infections was determined by using single population proportion formula considering the seroprevalence of HIV, HBV, HCV and syphilis found as 3.8%, 4.7%, 0.7%, and 1.3%, respectively from blood donors at Gondar University Teaching Hospital, Northwest Ethiopia [19]. Sample sizes for estimating seroprevalence of HIV, HBV, HCV and syphilis in the above-mentioned study were 351, 430, 67 and 123, respectively. Even if the largest sample size from the previous study (i.e. 430) would have been taken as the final sample size for this study. But, for greater point estimate and power of the analysis, all ($n = 11{,}382$) blood donors' history and laboratory tests records were reviewed at Harar Blood bank from 2008 to 2015.

Method of data collection

Blood donors were either volunteers, or replacement remunerated or mobile (donates blood during campaign). In the blood bank, all blood donors are required pass through a panel of questions on previous illnesses and medical conditions and physical examination for blood donation eligibility according to the national blood donation criteria. The eligibility criteria were age between 17 and 65 years, body weight > 45 kg, no history of high-risk sexual behavior and practice, blood transfusion, jaundice, hepatitis, surgery, and hypertension, and current fever. The medical and socio-demographic histories of the donors were recorded on each individual blood donor history record and venous blood was collected from each donor by laboratory technologists following standard procedures.

All blood donors' history and laboratory tests records documented at Harar Blood bank from 2008 to 2015 were reviewed by trained nurses working in the blood bank. Information such as age, sex, marital status, occupation status, residence, blood donor types (replacement (family, remunerated), volunteer and mobile (donates blood during campaign)), frequency of donation and laboratory examination results were reviewed.

Laboratory examination

All blood donors samples were tested for HBsAg, anti-HCV and HIV using Wantai AiD™ HBsAg Enzyme Linked Immuno Sorbant Assay (ELISA),Wantai AiD™ anti-HCV ELISA and WANTAI HIV 1 + 2 Ag/Ab ELISA test kit respectively developed by Beijing Wantai Biological Pharmacy Enterprise Co., Ltd. China Laboratory diagnosis. And for syphilis: using DIALAB ELISA developed by Nora Kampitsch, MSc, India. The anti-syphilis Ab ELISA test is a one-step enzyme immunoassay for the qualitative detection of antibodies to *Treponema Pallidum* in human serum or plasma. All the positive blood samples tested were repeated in duplicate before labeling them as seropositive by the same tests. Confirmatory test about active infection was not performed.

Operational definition

Voluntary donors: donor gives blood of his or her own free will and receives no payment, either in the form of cash or in kind.

Replacement donors: donors of blood who replace blood used by their relatives or friends from blood bank stocks.

Mobile donors: a donors who gave blood only once during blood donation campaign made at people gathering in school, in community or other institution for their own activities.

Transfusion Transmitted Infections (TTI): infectious agents including HBV, HIV, HCV and Syphilis.

Data quality control

Those blood donors' history and laboratory tests records with complete study variables were included in this study. Training was given to two nurses before actual data collection in order to assure the quality of data. Each data collected by data collectors was checked for completeness at end of each day by principal investigator. Preset of data collection tool was made at Dire Dawa blood bank.

Data analysis

Data were coded, entered into EPi data version 3.5.1 and exported to Statistical Package for the Social Sciences (SPSS) version 16 for analysis. To define the prevalence of TTIs, the number of TTI-positive donations during each year was divided by the total number of blood donations that year with 95% confidence interval (CI). The prevalence across different years and socio –demographic variables was compared using the Chi-square test. Regression analysis was done to assess the association between each TTIs with some socio–demographic variables. The Cochran–Armitage trend test (Z) was used to determine any significant trends in the rates of infected donations over time. Statistical significance was set at $p < 0.05$.

Result

In this study, a total 11,382 blood donors' history and laboratory tests records were reviewed. The mean age of the blood donors were 27 years with standard deviation of ±8.8 and range of 18–65 years. Majority of them were male (82.6%) in sex and in the age group of 17–25 years (57.6). Most of the blood was collected from mobile donors (56.0%), and those who donated blood for first time (99.9%). Majority of the blood donors had blood group O (45.1%) and Rhesus factor (RH) positive (93.4%) (Table 1).

Seroprevalence of transfusion transmitted infections

The overall seroprevalence of TTIs (total seroprevalence of HBV, HIV, HCV and Syphilis) was 6.6% (95% CI: 6.2–7.2%). The seroprevalence HBV, HIV, HCV and syphilis were 4.4%, 0.6%, 0.8% and 1.1%, respectively. A total of 0.2% (24/11382) blood donor had coinfections. From whom, HBV-syphilis (45.8%) (11/24) and HBV-HIV (20.8%) (5/24) coinfections were the dominant ones (Table 2).

Trend of HIV, HBV, HCV and syphilis

The prevalence of HBV, HIV, HCV and syphilis was the highest in the year 2008 (6.3%), 2008 (1.2%), 2012 (3.1%) and 2015(2.6%), respectively. The prevalence of HBV and HIV was not statistical significant different by year. However, the prevalence of HCV declined in most years, but it started to increase by the year 2009 and 2012. While, the prevalence of syphilis declined in most years except the highest record in 2015. The difference in prevalence of syphilis and HCV was statistical significant

Table 1 Characteristics of blood donor who donated blood from 2008 to 2015 in Harari regional state blood bank in Eastern Ethiopia

Variables	No (%)
Sex	
Male	9403 (82.6)
Female	1979 (17.4)
Age	
17–25	6555 (57.6)
26–35	2934 (25.8)
36–45	1402 (12.3)
≥ 46	490(4.3)
Occupation	
Farmer	1081 (9.5)
Military	1956(17.2)
Government employed	1896 (16.7)
Daily laborer	163(1.4)
Driver	222(2.0)
Factory worker	154 (1.4)
House wife	110(1.0)
Student	4079(35.8)
Private employed	1259(11.1)
Unemployed	132(1.2)
Other	330(2.9)
Donor type	
Mobile	6376 (56.0)
Replacement	4089(35.9)
Voluntary	917 (8.1)
Number of donation	
First time	11,369 (99.9)
Repeated	13 (0.1)
Blood group	
A	3151 (27.7)
B	2434 (21.4)
AB	661 (5.8)
O	5136 (45.1)
RH type	
Positive	10,634 (93.4)
Negative	748 (6.6)
Donor address Region	
Harari	6217(54.6)
Oromiya	3214(28.2)
Dire Dawa	919(8.1)
Somali	887(7.8)
Other(Addis Ababa, Afar, Amahar, Benishangaul, Southern Nations, Nationalities, and Peoples', Tigray)	144(1.3)

Table 2 Prevalence of co-infections of HIV, HBV, HCV and syphilis among blood donors from 2008 to 2015 in Harari regional state blood bank in Eastern Ethiopia

Coinfections	No (%)
HBV/ HIV	5 (0.04)
HBV/HCV	4 (0.04)
HBV/Syphilis	11 (0.1)
HCV/syphilis	2 (0.02)
HIV/syphilis	2 (0.02)
Total ($n = 11,382$)	24 (0.2)

by year ($p < 0.05$). But, the overall difference in the prevalence in TTIs ((total seroprevalence HBV, HIV, HCV and Syphilis), was not statically significant by year ($p > 0.05$) (Table 3).

Seroprevalence and associated factors of transfusion transmitted infections

Blood donors who were in the age group of 26–35 years, 36–45 years and greater than 46 years were two times (AOR:2.1; 95% CI: 1.2,3.6), 4 times (AOR: 4.1; 95% CI: 2.4,7.1) and more than four times (AOR: 4.6; 95 CI: 2.3,9.1) more likely to be infected with syphilis than those who were in the age group of 17–25 years. Regarding occupational status, students (AOR: 0.2; 95% CI: 0.04, 0.8) and private employees (AOR: 0.2; 95% CI: 0.03, 0.9) were 80% less likely to be infected with syphilis than non-employees. Replacement blood donors were 70% less likely to be infected with syphilis than voluntary donors (AOR: 0.3; 95% CI: 1.6, 6.7) (Table 4).

Looking at the association of predictor variables with viral hepatitis (HBV and HCV), males were two times more likely (AOR: 1.9; 95% CI: 1.4, 2.5) to be infected with HBV than females. Besides, government employees (AOR: 0.4; 95 CI: 0.2, 0.7) and students (AOR: 0.4; 95% CI: 0.2, 0.8) were 60% less likely to be infected than non-employees. While, those blood donors in the age group of ≥ 46 years (1.8%) were more than two times more likely to be infected with HCV than in the age group of 17–25 years (0.6%) (AOR: 2.7; 95 CI: 1.2, 6.2) (Table 5).

Discussion

The overall seroprevalence of transfusion transmitted infection was 6.6% in this study. This result did not include TTIs during the window period, which is serological negative. This still pose a threat to blood safety in environments. Thus, there might be higher rate of transfusion-transmissible infection in the community. However, the current study finding was higher than report from Eritrea (3.8%) [24] but lower than studies conducted in Jigjiga, eastern Ethiopia (11.5%) [25], Gondar, Ethiopia (9.5%) [19] and Sudan (13.1%) [26]. The difference might be due to difference in study area, study

Table 3 Trends of seropositivity of HBV, HIV, HCV and Syphilis among blood donors from 2008 to 2015 in Harari regional state blood bank in Eastern Ethiopia

Year	Total screened	HBV positive No(%)	HIV positive No(%)	HCV positive No (%)	Syphilis positive No(%)
2008	253	16(6.3)	3 (1.2)	2 (0.8)	4 (1.6)
2009	239	10(4.2)	1(0.4)	3 (1.3)	–
2010	581	28(4.8)	5 (0.9)	4(0.7)	7(1.2)
2011	984	52(5.3)	8 (0.8)	5(0.5)	3 (0.3)
2012	1146	41(3.6)	3 (0.3)	35(3.1)	1(0.1)
2013	1549	76 (4.9)	8(0.5)	6(0.4)	1 (0.1)
2014	2523	110 (4.4)	10 (0.4)	23(0.9)	–
2015	4107	167 (4.1)	25 (0.6)	14(0.3)	107 (2.6)
Total	11,382	500(4.4)	63 (0.6)	92 (0.8)	123 (1.1)
P value of linear regression trend		0.101	0.361	0.001	0.000

period (as there might change in the awareness of donors), socio demography of the study participants, strength of preliminary screening of donors and method of laboratory diagnosis used for screening of blood.

Majority of TTIs occurred in this study in the first time donors. This is similar to other study [19]. This can be due to replacement or mobile donors who are less likely to express about previous exposure and pass the primary screening and donate blood. In other words, there is low number of voluntary donors who seem to have low risk. There are a number of studies which indicate the prevalence rates of transfusion-transmissible infections that are found to be higher among replacement donors than voluntary donors [8, 9, 24]. These imply

Table 4 Characteristics of blood donors associated with HIV and Syphilis sero positivity from 2008 to 2015 in Harari regional state blood bank in Eastern Ethiopia

Characteristics	HIV positive No (%)	Crude odd ratio 95% CI	Adjusted odds ratio 95% CI	Syphilis positive No (%)	Crude odd ratio 95% CI	Adjusted odds ratio 95% CI
Sex						
Male	51/9403(0.5)	1		108/9403(1.1)	1	1
Female	12/1979(0.6)	0.9(0.5,1.7)	0.6(0.3,1.1)	15/1979(0.8)	1.5(0.9,2.6)	0.9(0.5,1.5)
Age						
17–25	21/6555(0.3)	0.5(0.1,1.4)	2.2(0.7,7.3)	34/6555(0.5)	1	1
26–35	28/2934(1.0)	1.3(0.4,3.7)	0.8(0.3,2.3)	36/2934(1.2)	2.4(1.5,3.8)	2.1(1.2,3.6)**
36–45	10/1402 (0.7)	0.9(0.3,2.9)	1.1(0.4,3.6)	38/1402(2.7)	5.3(3.4,8.5)	4.1(2.4,7.1)**
≥ 46	4/490 (0.8)	1	1	15/490(3.1)	6.1(3.3,11.2)	4.6(2.3,9.1)**
Occupation						
Farmer	10/1081(0.9)	1.1(0.1,8.6)	0.9(0.1,7.4)	22/1081(2.0)	1.4(0.3,5.8)	1.4(0.3,6.2)
Military	12/1956(0.6)	0.9(0.1,6.9)	1.1(0.1,8.9)	40/1956(2.0)	1.4(0.3,5.7)	0.6(0.1,2.5)
Government employed	11/1896(0.6)	0.6(0.8,4.8)	1.6(0.2,12.9)	31/1896(1.6)	1.1(0.3,4.6)	0.5(0.1,2.1)
Driver	1/222(0.5)	0.5(0.03,8.5)	1.9(0.1,31.4)	1/222(0.5)	0.3(0.03,3.3)	0.3(0.02,2.8)
Student	12/4079(0.3)	0.6(0.7,4.5)	1.8(0.2,14.5)	14/4079(0.3)	0.2(0.05,1.0)	0.2(0.04,0.8)**
Private employed	12/1259(1.0)	1.1(0.1,8.3)	0.9(0.1,7.4)	5/1259(0.4)	0.7(0.2,3.3)	0.2(0.03,0.9)**
Others*	4/757(0.5)	0.5(0.1,4.7)	1.9(0.2,17.9)	8/757(1.1)	3.9(0.7,20.1)	0.4(0.08,2.0)
Unemployed	1/132(0.8)	1		2/132(1.5)	1	1
Donor type						
Mobile	29/6376(0.5)	0.7(0.3,1.7)		82/6376(1.3)	0.9(0.5,1.6)	1.3(0.7,2.5)
Replacement	28/4089(0.7)	1.1(0.4,2.5)		28/4089(0.7)	0.5(0.3,0.9)	0.3(1.6,6.7)**
Voluntary	6/917(0.7)	1		13/917(1.4)	1	1

*Others: merchant, teacher, NGO, daily laborer, factory and housewife
**To indicate stastical significant

Table 5 Characteristics of blood donors associated with Hepatitis B and C virus seropositivity from 2008 to 2015 in Harari regional state blood bank in Eastern Ethiopia

Characteristics	Hepatitis B positive No (%)	Crude odd ratio 95% CI	Adjusted odds ratio 95% CI	Hepatitis C positive No (%)	Crude odd ratio 95% CI	Adjusted odds ratio 95% CI
Sex						
Male	448/9403 (4.8)	1.9(1.4,2.5)	1.7(1.3,2.3)**	80/9403(0.9)	1.4(0.8,2.5)	1.1(0.6,2.2)
Female	52/1979 (2.6)	1	1	12/1979(0.6)	1	1
Age						
17–25	267/6555 (4.1)	0.9(0.6,1.3)		40/6555(0.6)	1	1
26–35	144/2934(4.9)	1.1(0.7,1.6)		28/2934(1.0)	1.6(1.0,2.6)	1.5(0.8,2.7)
36–45	66/1402(4.7)	1.0(0.6,1.6)		15/1402(1.1)	1.8(1.0,3.2)	1.6(0.8,3.2)
≥ 46	23/490(4.7)	1		9/490(1.8)	3.1(1.5,6.3)	2.7(1.2,6.2)**
Occupation						
Farmer	57/1081(5.3)	0.6(0.3,1.2)	0.6(0.3,1.1)	15/1081(1.4)	1.8(0.8,3.9)	1.5(0.7,3.5)
Military	104/1956(5.3)	0.6(0.3,1.2)	0.6(0.3,1.1)	17/1956 (0.9)	1.1(0.5,2.4)	1.3(0.5,3.0)
Government employed	64/1896(3.4)	0.4(0.2,0.8)	0.4(0.2,0.7)**	12/1896(0.6)	0.8(0.3,1.8)	0.8(0.3,1.9)
Driver	11/222(5.0)	0.6(0.2,1.4)	0.5(0.2,1.3)	3/222(1.4)	1.7(0.5,6.3)	1.7(0.5,6.4)
Student	144/4079(3.5)	0.4(0.2,0.8)	0.4(0.2, 0.8)**	24/4079(0.6)	0.7(0.4,1.6)	1.1(0.5,2.7)
Private employed	59/1259(4.7)	0.5(0.3,1.1)	0.5(0.3,1.0)	10/1259(0.8)	1	
Others*	50/757(6.6)	0.8(0.4,1.5)	0.8(0.4,1.6)	11/889(1.2)	1.6(0.7,3.7)	1.5(0.7,3.7)
Unemployed	11/132(8.3)	1	1		1	1
Donor type						
Mobile	251/6376(3.9)	0.9(0.6,1.2)		44/6376(0.7)	1.1(0.5,2.5)	1.3(0.5,3.1)
Replacement	207/4089(5.1)	1.1(0.8,1.6)		42/4089(1.0)	1.6(0.7,3.7)	1.4(0.6,3.4)
Voluntary	42/917(4.6)	1		6/917(0.7)	1	1

*others: merchant, teacher, NGO, daily laborer, factory, housewife and unemployed
**To indicate statistical significant

there is need on increasing the number of voluntary donor through creating awareness among the population. This might gradually abolish the replacement or mobile donations; thereby ensuring the safety of blood transfusion. However, in this study area, there is low number of voluntary donors. Thus, blood bank made campaigns in community, school, universities and other institution in order to increase number of blood donors in (personal communication from blood bank). This donor might have some risk of TTIS. There is need for rigorous screening. Otherwise this might increase the number unsafe blood to be disposed which can increases costs laboratory examination and disposal.

The highest TTI in this study was HBV (4.4%). This is slightly lower than in Gondar, Ethiopia (4.7%) [19]. This was lower than report of a study conducted in Jigjiga (10.9%) [26] and in Bahir Dar Hospital (6%) [21] in Ethiopia and other African countries like Tanzania (8.8%) [11] and Congo, Kinshasa (5.4%) [13]. This result is higher than a report from Eritrea (2.58%) [24] and Dessie and Mekelle, Ethiopia (3%) [21]. The difference might due to difference risky behaviors at different, geographical location, capacity of the primary screening test, method laboratory diagnostic and other. In this study, all laboratory tests to screen TTIs are based on ELISA principles which have potentially high sensitivity and specificity. Males were more likely to be infected with HBV. This is similar to study conducted in Gondar [19] and in Jigjiga [26], Ethiopia. This difference prevalence might be due to sex differences in behavioral risk factors such as having multiple sex partners and alcohol drinking. However, government employed and students were less likely to be infected with HBV than unemployed. This was different compared to study conducted in Gondar [19] which found farmers were more likely to be infected with HBV. The difference might be due to difference in awareness of individuals about HBV or difference in exposure practices.

Hepatitis B Virus infection was the most common reason for donor disqualification from donating blood in this study. This is similar to studies conducted elsewhere [8, 9, 11, 12, 27]. The current prevalence of HBV was categorized the study area as high intermediate endemic transmission area [28]. Hepatitis B Virus infection is known as the most serious blood borne pathogen which can cause chronic infection resulting in cirrhosis of the liver, liver cancer, liver failure and death. Persons with chronic infection can also remain a carrier for HBV transmission [29]. Thus, there is need for further assessment of potential risk factors in the community and strengthening the preventive measures like vaccine in order to prevent further transmission.

The second most TTIs in this study were syphilis (1.1%). This was higher than a report from Eritrea (0.49%) [24] and Jigjiga, Ethiopia (0.1%) [26]. This was slightly lower than study conducted in Gondar, Ethiopia (1.7%) [19], Tanzania (4.7%) [11] and Congo, Kinshasa (3.7%) [13]. In this study the prevalence syphilis is more likely to be increased with age. This is similar to report from Tanzania [24]. But it is not consistent with the study conducted in Gondar [19] and Jigjiga [26], Ethiopia. A similar higher prevalence HCV was detected in those study participants in the age group ≥ 46 in this study. Thus there is need to assess potential risk factors of syphilis and HCV among this higher age groups. Those, students were less likely to be infected with syphilis in this study. This is similar to report from Gondar [19]. The main reasons might be due student might acquire information about sexual transmitted infection through their school and might follow different prevention methods of sexually transmitted infection.

Hepatitis B virus and Syphilis area the most common coinfection in this study. However, HIV –syphilis and HIV-HBV were the most common co infection detected in Gondar study [19]. The difference might be due decrease in the prevalence of HIV through different effort. The above overlap in co infection might indicate, they are following similar transmission.

The seroprevalence of HIV was detected at 0.6% in this study which was lower than 2.8% reported in the general population in the Harari Region [29]. This was higher than a report from blood donors in Jigjiga (0.1%) [26] and Eretria (0.18%) [24]. But, it was lower than a report from Gondar, Ethiopia by Diro et al. (4.5%) [20] and Tessema et al. (3.8%) [19] and other studies conducted in Tanzania (3.8%) [11], Congo, Kinshasa (4.7%) [13]. The basic difference might be due to; difference in prevention measures taken and their effectiveness in different geographical location; risk of transmission; awareness peoples about HIV transmission and preventions.

In general, the prevalence of HCV and syphilis decline significantly. The prevalence of HBV and HIV decline, but the decline was not statistical significant in this study. However, significantly declining trends of HIV, HCV and syphilis seropositivity were observed in the Gondar study [19]. The overall decline in TTs in this study was not significant. Thus, there is need for more intervention on screening and other measures on the blood donors and the community for further the reduction all TTIs transmission in community.

This study has some limitations. It is a retrospective blood donation card review which might not include some variables. All test result did not give positive serological result during the window period. But, detailed preliminary risk factors assessment was made by trained health professionals in the blood bank unit before donation based on blood donors screening guideline. The method laboratory analysis doesn't include molecular analysis which is more confirmatory test. However, this study tried to give better information on magnitude, trends and some associated factors of TTIs since it used large sample size and long year of blood donors' history and laboratory tests records retrieved.

Conclusion

The magnitude TTIs was lower than the previous studies conducted in Ethiopia. However, the study area has high intermediate endemic transmission. Majority of TTIS occurred among first time blood donors. Those students, private employed and government employed were less likely to be infected with syphilis and hepatitis B virus. Male were more likely to infected with HBV. There was significantly decline in the prevalence of HCV and Syphilis infection, but not for HIV and HBV. The prevalence of syphilis and HCV also increases with age. Therefore, strict adherence with the criteria of preliminary blood donor selection should be implemented to reduce the amount of blood being withdrawn from transfusion after collection and screening. It is also important to increase the number of repeated voluntary donors through promotion of blood bank activity. In addition, further study should be conducted to identify the gaps in the failure of preliminary screening in removing the donor before blood donation and feasible way increasing voluntary donors. There is also an assessment and taking measures on the potential risk factors of major TTI in the community.

Abbreviations

BTS: Blood Transfusion Services; HBV: Hepatitis B Viruses; HCV: Hepatitis C Viruses; HIV: Human Immunodeficiency Virus; TTIs: Transfusion Transmitted Infections; WHO: World Health Organization

Acknowledgements

First, we thank to Haramaya University Research affairs for launching this grant for staffs of the university. It is also our great pleasure to thank Harar blood bank staff for giving us information in order to finalize this research project.

Funding

This study was funded by Haramaya University Research affairs staffs' grant.

Authors' contributions

ZT, HM and FM designed the study, participated in data collection, analysis, interpretation, and write-up, drafted the manuscript and critically revised the manuscript. All authors read and approved the final manuscript.

Competing interests
The authors declare that they have no competing interests.

References

1. Khan ZT, Asim S, Tariz Z, Ehsan IA, Malik RA, Ashfaq B, et al. Prevalence of transfusion transmitted infections in healthy blood donors in Rawalpindi District, Pakistan–a five year study. Int J Pathol. 2007;5:21–5.
2. WHO African Region (2006). Ethiopia 2006 /Regional training workshop on blood donor recruitment: pre and post donation counseling.
3. Centeral Statistics Agency. ICF MacroCalverton. Addis Ababa: Ethiopia demographic and health survey 2011; 2011.
4. Talib VH, Khuana SK .Hematology for students 1996, 1 Ed 415–416.
5. Morar MM, Pitman JP, McFarland W, Bloch EM. The contribution of unsafe blood transfusion to human immunodeficiency virus incidence in sub-Saharan Africa: reexamination of the 5% to 10% convention. Transfusion. 2016;6(12):3121–32.
6. Fasola FA, Otegbayo IA. Post-transfusion hepatitis in sickle cell anaemia; retrospective-prospective analysis. Nig J Clin Pract. 2002;5:16–9.
7. UNAIDS. Joint United Nations program on HIV /AIDS. In: Prospect of Hepatitis B Virus infection; 2002. p. 15–6.
8. Pallavi P, Ganesh CK, Jayashree K, Manjunath GV. Seroprevalence and trends in transfusion transmitted infections among blood donors in a university hospital blood Bank:a 5 year study. Indian J Hematol Blood Transfus. 2011; 27(1):1–6. https://doi.org/10.1007/s12288-010-0047-x.
9. Fernandes H, D'souza PF, D'souz PM. Prevalence of transfusion transmitted infections in voluntary and replacement donors. Indian J Hematol Blood Transfus. 2010;26(3):89–91. https://doi.org/10.1007/s12288-010-0044-0.
10. Sube KLL, Seriano OF, Gore RP, Jaja S, Loro RL, Lino EO, Seriano OA, Wani SN, Alex LJ, Jack KR, Abraham IW. Prevalence of HIV among blood donors at juba teaching hospital blood Bank, South Sudan. South Sudan Med J. 2014;7(4):76–80.
11. Matee MI, Magesa PM, Lyamuya EF. Seroprevalence of human immunodeficiency virus, hepatitis B and C viruses and syphilis infections among blood donors at the Muhimbili National Hospital in Dar Es Salaam, Tanzania. BMC Public Health. 2006;6:21. https://doi.org/10.1186/1471-2458-6-21.
12. Patel S, Popat C, Mazumdar V, Shah M, Shringarpure Mehta KG, Gandhi A. Seroprevalence of HIV, HBV, HCV and syphilis in blood donors at a tertiary hospital (blood bank) in Vadodara. Int J Med Sci Public Health. 2013;2(3):747–50.
13. Batina A, Kabemba S, Malengela R. Infectious markers among blood donors in Democratic Republic of Congo (DRC). Rev Med Brux. 2007;28(3):145–9.
14. Dodd RY. Current risk for transfusion transmitted infections. Curr Opin Hematol. 2007;14:671–6.
15. Maresch C, Schluter PJ, Wilson AD, Sleigh A. Residual infectious disease risk in screened blood transfusion from a high-prevalence population: Santa Catarina, Brazil. Transfusion. 2008;48:273–81.
16. World Health Organization. Universal access to safe blood transfusion. Geneva: World Health Organization; 2008.
17. Jayaraman S, Chalabi Z, Perel P, Guerriero C, Roberts I. The risk of transfusion-transmitted infections in sub-Saharan Africa. Transfusion. 2010;50:433–42.
18. Gebreselassie L. Occurrence of HIV, HBV and HCV in blood donors of Addis Ababa. Ethiopia Ethiopian Med J. 1986;24:63–5.
19. Tessema B., Yismaw G., Kassu A, Amsalu A, Mulu A, Emmrich F, Sack U. Seroprevalence of HIV, HBV, HCV and syphilis infections among blood donors at Gondar University teaching hospital, Northwest Ethiopia: declining trends over a period of five years. BMC Infect Dis 2010, 10:111 http://www.biomedcentral.com/1471-2334/10/111.
20. Diro E, Alemu S, G/Yohannes A. Blood safety & prevalence of transfussion transmissible viral infections among donors at the red cross blood bank in Gondar University hospital. Ethiop Med J 2008;46(1):7–13.
21. Baye G, Yohannis M. The prevalence of HBV, HCV and malaria parasite among blood donors in Amhara and Tigray regional states. EthiopJ Health Dev. 2007;22(1):3–7.
22. Tsega E. Epidemiology, Prevention and treatment of viral hepatitis with emphasis on new developments. Review article Ethiopian Med J. 2000;38:131–41.
23. Rahlenbeck SI, Yohannes G, Molla K, Reifen R, Assefa A. Infection with HIV, syphilis and hepatitis B in Ethiopia: a survey in blood donors. Int J STD AIDS. 1997;8:261–4.
24. Fessehaye N, Naik D, Fessehaye T. Transfusion transmitted infections – a retrospective analysis from the National Blood Transfusion Service in Eritrea. Pan African Med J. 2011;9:40.
25. Mohammed Y, Bekele A. Seroprevalence of transfusion transmitted infection among blood donors at Jijiga blood bank, eastern Ethiopia: retrospective 4 years study. BMC Res Notes. 2016;9:129.
26. Abdallah TM, Ali AAA. Sero-prevalence of transfusion-transmissible infectious diseases among blood donors in Kassala. eastern Sudan J Med Sci. 2012; 3(4):260–2.
27. Sehgal S, Shaiji PS, Kaur Brar R. Seroprevalence and trends of transfusion transmissible infections in blood donors in Andaman and Nicobar Islands-an institutional retrospective study. J Clin Diagn Res. 2017;11(4):EC21–4.
28. World Health Organization. Guidelines for the prevention, care and treatment of persons with chronic hepatitis B infection. Geneva; 2015.
29. Center for Disease Control (CDC). A comprehensive immunization strategy to eliminate transmission of hepatitis B virus infection in the United States. Morb Mortal Wkly Rep. 2006;55(RR16):1–25.

22

Systematic review of azacitidine regimens in myelodysplastic syndrome and acute myeloid leukemia

Roman M. Shapiro[1] and Alejandro Lazo-Langner[2,3,4*]

Abstract

Background: 5-Azacitidine administered as a 7-day dosing regimen (7–0-0) is approved in high risk IPSS myelodysplastic syndrome (MDS) patients. Alternative regimens such as a 5-day (5–0-0) or 7-day with a weekend break (5–2-2) are commonly used. No randomized controlled trial has been done directly comparing all three dosing regimens. The objective of this study was to compare the efficacies of the 5–0-0, 5–2-2, and 7–0-0 regimens in MDS and AML.

Methods: A systematic review was conducted using MEDLINE, EMBASE and CENTRAL. Eligible studies were randomized controlled trials (RCTs), observational prospective and retrospective studies. The primary clinical outcomes were Objective Response Rate (ORR) defined as the sum of complete response (CR), partial response (PR), and hematological improvement (HI) as defined by the IWG 2006 criteria. A meta-analysis of simple proportions was conducted using a random effects model with weights defined according to Laird and Mosteller. Comparisons between groups were not attempted due to the heterogeneity of study designs.

Results: The only RCT directly comparing alternative azacitidine regimens showed no difference in ORR between the 5–0-0 and 5–2-2 regimens. All other RCTs compared a dosing regimen to conventional care. The pooled proportion of ORR was 44.8% with 95% CI (42.8%, 45.5%) for 7–0-0, 41.2% with 95% CI (39.2%, 41.9%) for 5–0-0, and 45.8% with 95% CI (42.6%, 46.4%) for 5–2-2.

Conclusions: Indirect comparison of alternative azacitidine dosing regimens in MDS and AML shows a benefit for the 7-day regimen in attaining ORR. Additional RCTs are required to definitively address this comparison.

Keywords: Azacitidine, Dosing, Myelodysplastic, Leukemia

Background

Azacitidine has become the standard of care for patients with high risk myelodysplastic syndrome (MDS) when a hematopoietic stem cell transplant is not an option. In the CALGB 9221 randomized clinical trial, azacitidine administered at 75 mg/m^2 for 7 continuous days resulted in an objective response rate of 16% compared to no response in the control group [1, 2]. This response rate included improvement in peripheral cytopenias resulting in transfusion independence as well as a reduction in the bone marrow blast percentage [2]. The subsequent international phase III open label randomized controlled trial (RCT) AZA-001 comparing azacitidine to conventional care that included low dose cytarabine, best supportive care or intensive chemotherapy showed a statistically significant survival benefit as well as a doubling in the time to progression to AML with azacitidine. The results of the AZA-001 clinical trial led to the FDA extending a survival benefit to the use of the drug in intermediate-2/high risk MDS by international prognostic scoring criteria (IPSS), CMML with 10–30% blasts, and AML with 20–30% blasts [3].

The standard approved dose cycle of azacitidine has been 75 mg/m^2 for 7 continuous days (7–0-0), according to the AZA-001 and CALGB clinical trials [2, 3].

* Correspondence: alejandro.lazolangner@lhsc.on.ca
[2]Department of Medicine, Division of Hematology, Western University, London, ON, Canada
[3]Department of Epidemiology & Biostatistics, Western University, London, ON, Canada
Full list of author information is available at the end of the article

However, due to difficulties with administration of weekend doses, many centres either administer the same dose on a 5-day schedule (5–0-0), or a 5-day schedule followed by a weekend break followed by an additional 2 days (5–2-2) [4]. There has been no formal randomized clinical trial comparing the efficacy and tolerability of the alternative azacitidine doses, and the assumption has been that they are equivalent [5]. However, there are several important pharmacologic points that may challenge this assumption.

The active form of azacitidine binds both RNA and DNA, exerting its cytotoxic effect via interference with RNA transcription and DNA methyltransferase I activity in actively proliferating cells [1, 6]. In studies of azacitidine pharmacokinetics, the drug was undetectable in daily pretreatment blood samples, suggesting a rapid elimination and no accumulation [1]. Therefore, as the drug is only active in proliferating cells and does not accumulate, shorter durations of therapy within each cycle are less likely to have the drug encounter all malignant clones in their S-phase [1, 5]. This would conceptually argue for the increased efficacy of longer duration of treatment per cycle [5]. However, this argument does not discount interrupted courses of therapy such as 5–2-2. Since the benefit of azacitidine has most definitively been demonstrated in RCT using the 7–0-0 schedule, it becomes important to collect efficacy data on the alternative dosing schedules in order to ensure they are at least as equally effective as 7–0-0 [7]. The objective of the current systematic review is to evaluate the efficacy and tolerability of the 5–0-0, 5–2-2, and 7–0-0 azacitidine dosing regimens in MDS patients.

Methods

The primary outcome was objective response rate (ORR) calculated as the combination of complete response (CR), partial response (PR), and hematological improvement (HI) as per the IWG 2006 criteria [8]. Due to the heterogeneity of the reporting of outcome data, the ORR was determined to be the outcome that could be extracted from the greatest number of articles and abstracts describing azacitidine treatment. Due to the inability to separate the treatment outcomes of AML patients that were included in retrieved studies of azacitidine therapy in MDS, these patients were included in the analysis of ORR.

Search strategy

A systematic literature search was conducted in November 2014 and updated in October 2015 using the OVID interface and included MEDLINE, EMBASE, and Cochrane Central Register of Controlled Trials (Central) databases. The full methodology is described below with no additional review protocol or registration. No language restrictions were applied.

A sensitive search strategy was based on combination of subject headings and text-words using alternative spellings and word endings, such as but not limited to the search terms 'AZA', 'azacitidine', 'azacytidine', 'vidaza', 'ladakamycin', 'myelodysplastic syndrome', 'myelodysplasia', and 'MDS'. Modifications to the search strategy were made for each database using appropriate thesaurus terms and fields. The Medline search strategy is indicated in Additional file 1. Articles were evaluated for inclusion based on the title and abstract. If an abstract was not available, an attempt was made to retrieve the full article for evaluation. Any articles retrieved with the search that included AML and CMML patients were included in the subsequent analysis if they met inclusion criteria.

Assessment of study quality and data extraction

Articles meeting inclusion criteria were retrieved for full data extraction. The inclusion criteria were as follows: randomized clinical trials, observational prospective, and observational retrospective studies evaluating the clinical response of patients with myelodysplastic syndrome to azacitidine. Studies were excluded if they were phase I clinical trials, review articles, case series, or abstracts that were subsequently published in full form. Studies assessing AML and CMML patients retrieved with the search strategy were included in the analysis. Relevant data from included articles was extracted using a data collection form, and encompassed the disease characteristics of patients included in selected studies, vidaza dosing regimens used, and outcome variables. The primary outcome was objective response rate (ORR) calculated as the combination of complete response (CR), partial response (PR), and hematological improvement (HI) as per the International Working Group (IWG) criteria. In those publications where the ORR was directly reported as is defined by the IWG criteria, this ORR was recorded. In those publications which did not directly report the ORR but did report CR, PR, and/or HI as defined by the IWG, the ORR was calculated as the sum of available data. If the ORR could not be calculated from an abstract and/or article, then this publication was not included in the data analysis. Articles that reported objective response based on the IWG 2000 criteria were included in the analysis, with the justification based on the overall similarity in objective response using the two criteria as is shown in Additional file 2: Table S3. Articles that included only AML patients had objective response defined as CR + CRi + PR + HI, where HI referred to patients who did not attain the response criteria for CR/CRi or PR. Articles that reported on MDS and AML patients where the objective response could not be separated based on disease type were included in the analysis. If the outcome results reported in a publication could not be attributed to a particular dosing regimen of azacitidine, an attempt was made to contact the corresponding author in order to obtain this data. The quality of RCT, including any possible degree of bias in the study, was assessed according to the criteria proposed by Jadad et al. [9] Non-randomized observational studies were assessed with respect to attrition bias and reporting bias using the Cochrane Bias Assessment Tool [10].

Statistical analysis

A meta-analysis of effect sizes of the articles meeting inclusion criteria was planned but could not be performed as there were insufficient RCT directly comparing the efficacy of various azacitidine dosing regimens. A pooled proportion analysis using a random effects model was conducted as previously described [11, 12]. The primary outcomes of interest were objective response rate and complete response as per IWG [8]. A z-test was used to assess for differences between effects, with a *p*-value <0.05 considered statistically significant. A sensitivity analysis was done evaluating the pooled proportion of ORR in subgroups of patients retrieved with the search strategy.

Results

Results of the search strategy from the systematic review

The search strategy from all databases identified 1690 articles and abstracts after duplicates were removed, from which 47 articles and 90 abstracts met inclusion criteria for full study evaluation (Fig. 1). Of the 47 articles, there were 6 that did not report outcomes corresponding to individual azacitidine dosing regimens thereby excluding these articles from the final analysis. One article was excluded because the dosing regimen did not correspond to any of 5–0-0, 5–2-2, or 7–0-0, and another two articles were excluded because ORR could not be calculated. The remaining 38 articles along with the 90 abstracts were included in the pooled proportions analysis. As there were no randomized controlled trials directly comparing alternative dosing schedules of azacitidine, a meta-analysis of effects could not be performed. For most domains, studies had an unclear or a high risk of bias (Fig. 2). References to studies not cited in the article text but included in the data analysis are shown in Additional file 3.

Characteristics of included studies

Of the 128 articles and abstracts meeting inclusion criteria, there were a total of 3 articles detailing randomized controlled trials (RCT) with one of the three articles summarizing data from three previous CALGB clinical trials (Table 1) [13]. Two of the RCTs evaluated the 7–0-0 regimen and one of the RCTs evaluated the 5–0-0 and 5–2-2 regimens, with all RCTs comparing azacitidine to conventional care that includes one or more of best supportive care, therapy with Ara-C, or intensive chemotherapy. The remainder of the articles were observational studies with either prospective (11/38) or retrospective (24/38) design.

A summary of the patient characteristics of included studies is shown in Additional file 2: Table S1. There were a total of 7520 patients, with 5545 patients receiving the 7–0-0 regimen, 1207 receiving the 5–0-0 regimen, and 768 receiving the 5–2-2 regimen. The median age of all patients was 70. The median age of all patients

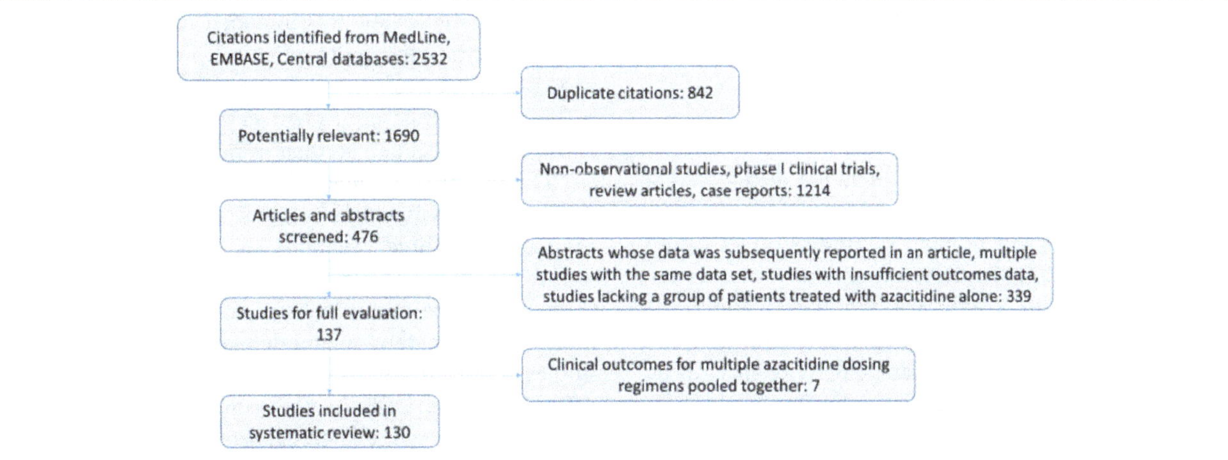

Fig. 1 Flow diagram for the systematic review. The screening strategy resulted in the inclusion of only abstracts and articles for which objective response rate (ORR) as defined by the IWG 2006 criteria was either reported or could be calculated from the reported data for each particular dosing strategy. Seven studies that met all screening criteria were excluded from the final analysis because they reported ORR that was a pooled outcome for several different dosing regimens, and the raw outcome data for each particular dosing regimen could not be attained from the authors

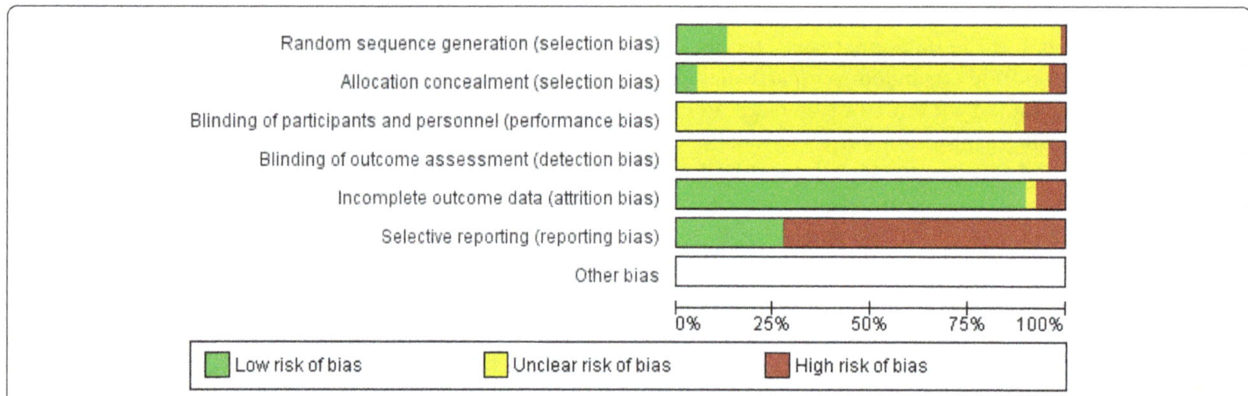

Fig. 2 Risk of bias graph showing review authors' judgements about each risk of bias item presented as percentages across all included studies. Every publication included in the systematic review was assessed for its risk of bias based on the reporting of data. Randomized clinical trials had the lowest risk of bias. The large amount of unclear risk of selection, performance, and detection bias reflects the relatively large number of non-randomized observational studies in the systematic review. The relatively high risk of reporting bias is a reflection of data acquired from conference abstracts that were judged to have a higher risk of selective reporting than full literature articles

reported in articles with the 5–0-0, 5–2-2, and 7–0-0 regimens was 66, 72, and 69, respectively. The mean number of cycles received by patients treated with the 5–0-0, 5–2-2, and 7–0-0 regimens was 6, 6.7, and 5.5, respectively. An r by c chi square test was done showing that it was statistically more likely for patients receiving the 7–0-0 treatment regimen to have IPSS high risk than it was for the other treatment groups $\chi^2(2, N = 2050) = 13.33$, $p = 0.0013$. Similarly, it was statistically more likely for patients receiving the 7–0-0 treatment regimen to have a diagnosis of AML $\chi^2(2, N = 2760) = 121.4$, $p < 0.000001$. For articles that reported ECOG values, those articles reporting on patients treated with the 5–0-0, 5–2-2, and 7–0-0 regimens had 80%, 75%, and 80% of their patients in an ECOG <= 1 group, respectively. An r by c chi square test was done showing that there was no statistically significant association between the proportion of patients with ECOG score ≤ 1 and treatment regimen $\chi^2(2, N = 1825) = 0.681$, $p = 0.7114$.

Direct comparison of dosing regimens

The outcomes from the articles included in the systematic review are summarized in Additional file 2: Table S2. There was a small number of studies directly comparing the different azacitidine regimens. There were two studies directly comparing the 5–0-0 and 5–2-2 dosing regimens. One was a randomized controlled trial showing no statistically significant difference in ORR between the 5–0-0 and 5–2-2 dosing regimens [14]. The other was an observational retrospective study that also showed no difference in ORR between the two regimens [15]. There were also two studies directly comparing the 5–0-0 and 7–0-0 regimens, both of which are observational retrospective studies that showed no statistically significant difference in ORR between the two regimens [15, 16]. Due to methodological heterogeneity, we did not conduct a direct comparison between groups.

Results of the pooled proportions analysis

The pooled proportion of ORR was 44.8% (95% CI 42.8% to 45.5%) for the 7–0-0 dosing regimen, 41.2% (95% CI 39.2% to 41.9%) for the 5–0-0 regimen, and 45.8% (95% CI 42.6% to 46.4%) for the 5–2-2 regimen. A sensitivity analysis was done evaluating the pooled proportion of ORR in subgroups of patients such as those strictly reported to have a diagnosis of MDS, to have higher risk disease based on the IPSS, and based on the type of study that was performed (observational prospective, observational retrospective, RCT). Results of the sensitivity analysis are shown in Table 2.

Discussion

This systematic review was intended to test the hypothesis of whether the more practically convenient 5–0-0 and 5–2-2 azacitidine dosing regimens used to treat MDS have at least equivalent efficacy to the approved 7–0-0 dosing regimen studied in randomized clinical trials. The number of studies directly comparing the alternative dosing regimens was small, and no study directly compared all three regimens to each other. In those studies where a comparison of alternative regimens was made, they were found to be equivalent in terms of the ORR. Unfortunately, methodological heterogeneity of studies prevented a meta-analysis of effects.

The choice of ORR as the primary outcome variable was made due to the heterogeneity of the reporting of outcome data in articles describing azacitidine therapy. The ORR was determined to be able to pool data from the greatest amount of published literature on the subject of azacitidine dosing. Due to the heterogeneity of the reporting of survival data and to the substantial

Table 1 Characteristics of full studies reported in literature articles included in the systematic review

Study ID	Design	N	Inclusion criteria	Schedule	Cycles	Comparator	Concomitant therapy
Fenaux et al. [3]	RCT^	179	adults > = 18 with FAB diagnosis high risk MDS	7-0-0	9	CCR*: BSC, Ara-C, intensive chemo	none
Silverman et al. [13]	RCT	309	those used for the 3 clinical trials	7-0-0	3	BSC	none
Lyons et al. [14]	RCT	151	age > =18 with FAB‡ diagnosis RA/RARS/RAEB/ RAEB-T/CMML and life expectancy >7 months	5-0-0, 5-2-2, 5-2-5	6	none	none
Xicoy et al. [15]	OR^^	107	MDS patients older than 75 treated with AZA	5-0-0, 5-2-2, 7-0-0	8	none	none
Garcia-Delgadoa et al. [16]	OR	200	age > =18 with either WHO-defined MDS or confirmed diagnosis of de novo/secondary AML with 20-30% blasts according to WHO who received at least 1 cycle of AZA	5-0-0, 7-0-0, 5-2-2	6, 8, 8	none	none
Sadashiv et al. [24]	OP^*	15	newly diagnosed AML who were deemed poor candidates for induction therapy and had an ECOG ≤2	5-0-0	5	none	none
Minoia et al. [25]	OR	18	therapy related MDS and AML not eligible for intensive chemotherapy	7-0-0	6	none	none
Drummond et al. [26]	OP	30	CMML-2 or CMML-1 patient with symptomatic marrow failure or proliferative disease	5-2-2	7	none	none
Fianchi et al. [27]	OR	31	consecutive patients receiving 5-aza	7-0-0	4	none	none
Ballya et al. [28]	OR	62	patients with diagnosis of MDS, CMML, or AML treated with AZA	7-0-0	8	none	none
Breccia et al. [29]	OP	38	WHO-diagnosed MDS patients treated with AZA† outside clinical trial	5-2-2	5	none	none
Breccia et al. [30]	OP	60	unselected WHO†‖-diagnosed MDS/CMML	5-2-2	6	none	none
Douvali et al. [31]	OR	42	intermediate-2/high risk MDS patients with normal hepatic function, ECOG 0-2	7-0-0	5.5	none	G-CSF
Duong et al. [32]	OR	84	patients with diagnosis of MDS or AML previously treated with chemotherapy having received at least 1 dose of AZA	7-0-0	4.5	none	none
Ettou et al. [33]	OR	169	consecutive patients treated with AZA between 2005 and 2011	7-0-0	6	none	none
Fianchi et al. [34]	OR	50	patients with therapy-related myeloproliferative neoplasms	7-0-0	4	none	ESA†* (8%), AML IC†** (12%)
Fil et al. [35]	OP	32	age > =18 with IPSS†† low/int-1 MDS and one or more of: (i) symptomatic anemia requiring RBC transfusion-supportive therapy, previously unresponsive to EPO or not expected to respond to EPO, (ii) thrombocytopenia requiring platelet transfusion, (iii) > 3 months ANC** less than 1.5	5-0-0	8	none	none
Gryna et al. [36]	OR	48	MDS patients, previous cytokine therapy allowed, ECOG <2 included	7-0-0	6	none	none
Itzykson et al. [37]	OR	86	MDS and AML patients treated with AZA	7-0-0	6	none	none
Itzykson et al. [38]	OR	282	IPSS Int-2/hi MDS patients as well as AML patients with blasts <30%	7-0-0, 5-0-0	6	none	none
O'Reilly et al. [23]	OR	47	elderly AML patients	5-0-0	5	none	none
Lee et al. [39]	OR	75	MDS patients treated with AZA	7-0-0	5	Decitabine	none
Lee et al. [40]	OR	203	patients needed to have an International Prognostic Scoring System (IPSS) lower risk score (IPSS low or intermediate-1) with significant cytopenia, or a higher risk score (IPSS intermediate-2 or high)	7-0-0	5	Decitabine	none
Al-Ali et al. [41]	OP	40	patients >18, life expectancy >2 months, with WHO-defined AML	5-0-0	3	none	none
Martin et al. [42]	OP	22	age > =18 with diagnosis of MDS based on FAB criteria, ECOG status <=2, adequate renal and hepatic function, no chemotherapy withing 4 weeks of enrollment	5-0-0	4.5	none	none

Table 1 Characteristics of full studies reported in literature articles included in the systematic review *(Continued)*

Study ID	Design	N	Inclusion criteria	Schedule	Cycles	Comparator	Concomitant therapy
Moon et al. [43]	OR	129	MDS patients treated with Azacitidine	7-0-0	3	none	G-CSF, EPO
Muller-Thomas et al. [44]	OR	32	MDS and sAML patients treated with Azacitidine	7-0-0	4	none	RA†***, VA in 2 patients
Muller-Thomas et al. [45]	OP	100	MDS patients treated with Azacitidine	7-0-0	4	none	none
O'Reilly et al. [46]	OR	32	consecutive treatment-naïve patients treated with AZA between 2006 and 2012	5-0-0	9	none	none
Ozbalak et al. [47]	OR	25	MDS, AML, and CMML patients not eligible for chemotherapy treated with azacitidine	7-0-0	8	none	none
Papoutselis et al. [48]	OR	87	late-stage MDS, ECOG 0–2	7-0-0	6	BSC	G-CSF
Pierdomenico et al. [49]	OR	50	consecutive patients treated with AZA between 2005 and 2011	5-0-0	7.5	none	none
Tobiasson et al. [50]	OP	30	age greater than 18 with IPSS low/int-1 or mixed MDS/myeloproliferative disorder, CMML less than 10% marrow blasts or RARS	5-0-0	6	none	none
Diamantopoulos et al. [51]	OR	44	higher risk MDS or AML with 20–30% bone marrow blasts	7-0-0	5	none	none
Passweg et al. [24]	OP	45	elderly or frail patients with AML not eligible for intensive chemotherapy	5-0-0	4	none	none
van der Helm et al. [25]	OR	55	newly diagnosed AML receiving upfront treatment with 5-aza	7-0-0	6	none	none
van der Helm et al. [26]	OR	26	newly diagnosed AML	7-0-0	6	none	none

Note. Studies reported in abstracts were not included in this table. Refer also to Additional file 3
^RCT: randomized controlled trial, ^^OR: objective restrospective, ^*OP: objective prospective *CCR: conventional care regimen, BSC: best supportive care, **ANC: absolute neutrophil count, ***BM: bone marrow, †AZA: azacitidine, ‡FAB: French-American-British classification, ††IPSS: International Prognostic Scoring System, †‖WHO: World Health Organization, †* Erythropoiesis stimulating agents, †** Intensive chemotherapy, †*** Retinoic acid, ††* Valproic acid

number of articles and abstracts that did not report overall survival, this outcome could not be used in the pooled proportions analysis. Other outcome variables commonly reported in studies of azacitidine, including CR, PR, HI, and transfusion dependence were independently evaluated as potential primary outcome variables for the pooled proportions analysis, and none encompassed as many studies as the ORR. Only the reporting of CR was similar to that of the ORR, with far more heterogeneity of reporting noted for the other outcome variables. Similarly to ORR, the attainment of stable disease has been found to have a correlation with overall survival in MDS, and was considered for inclusion in the pooled proportion analysis [17]. However, stable disease as an outcome was reported in a total of 42% of articles and abstracts. The exclusion of all articles and abstracts not reporting on stable disease would result in a greater degree of bias affecting the interpretation of the outcomes.

The definition of ORR did undergo an update in 2006, resulting in differences in the way this value was calculated from patient data compared to preceding years [8, 18]. Although this is a limitation of choosing the ORR as an outcome variable, the majority (75%) of the ORR used in the pooled proportions analysis was determined using the IWG 2006 criteria. Furthermore, due to the significant similarities between the IWG 2000 and IWG 2006 definitions of ORR, the relatively small number of articles and abstracts included in this review that reported the ORR using the IWG 2000 definition is unlikely to significantly affect the pooled proportions analysis. Additional file 2: Table S3 compares the IWG 2000 and IWG 2006 criteria for ORR.

The inclusion of CMML and AML patients in this systematic review was required because it was not possible to separate the outcomes of these patients from the MDS patients in most studies. Excluding any study that reported on CMML or AML in addition to MDS would have resulted in a substantial reduction in the total number of studies and patients as is shown in the sensitivity analysis (Table 2). For studies that reported on AML patients included in the review, response outcomes were reported allowing for the determination of ORR [19, 20–22]. Two studies of AML patients retrieved with the search strategy that did not report on HI were excluded from the pooled proportion and sensitivity analyses because ORR could not be calculated.

A pooled proportions analysis of the different dosing regimens across both randomized and observational studies was performed. Understanding the inherent limitation of this analysis [11, 12], it was found that the 7–0-0, 5–2-2, and 5–0-0 regimens had pooled ORR of 44.8%,

Table 2 Sensitivity analysis of objective response rate of azacitidine in MDS

	Objective Response Rate Random Effects Model	
	Pooled rate (%)	CI
All patients (N^* = 7520)		
7-0-0 (N = 5545)	44.8	(42.8, 45.5)
5-0-0 (N = 1207)	41.2	(39.2, 41.9)
5-2-2 (N = 768)	45.8	(42.6, 46.4)
MDS patients only (N = 2966)		
7-0-0 (N = 2187)	45.9	(44.1, 46.7)
5-0-0 (N = 536)	39.9	(36.8, 40.5)
5-2-2 (N = 243)	50.6	(48.7, 51.3)
IPSS int-2/hi patients (N = 1180)		
7-0-0 (N = 926)	46.8	(44.9, 47.3)
5-0-0 (N = 112)	54.6	(53.8, 55.0)
5-2-2 (N = 142)	60.7	(59.0, 61.5)
Randomized Controlled Trials (N = 883)		
7-0-0 (N = 440)	43.5	(43.0, 43.7)
5-0-0 (N = 320)	38.0	(35.4, 38.2)
5-2-2 (N = 123)	48.2	(48.0, 48.6)
Prospective Observational Studies (N = 1131)		
7-0-0 (N = 401)	45.9	(44.2, 46.9)
5-0-0 (N = 481)	39.3	(35.8, 40.1)
5-2-2 (N = 249)	40.0	(34.0, 40.5)
Retrospective Observational Studies (N = 4930)		
7-0-0 (N = 3910)	46.8	(44.4, 47.5)
5-0-0 (N = 624)	46.2	(44.9, 47.0)
5-2-2 (N = 396)	49.8	(47.5, 50.6)

*N refers to the number of patients included in a study

45.8%, and 41.2%, respectively. Interestingly, the confidence intervals of the 7–0-0 and 5–0-0 regimens do not overlap in a random effects model of pooled proportions, suggesting the possibility that the 7–0-0 may have somewhat greater efficacy in terms of the ORR than the 5–0-0 regimen. This as an indirect comparison of pooled ORR, but lends support to the idea that total time of exposure to azacitidine does play a role in clinical efficacy [6]. The same outcome is noted for the indirect comparison of the ORR of the 5–2-2 regimen and 5–0-0 regimen, also suggesting the possibility that a longer exposure to azacitidine has clinical benefit. Indirect comparison of the 7–0-0 and 5–2-2 regimens yielded overlapping confidence intervals, suggestive of the equal efficacy of these regimens in terms of ORR. What seems to be consistent is that a total course of 7 days (with or without a weekend break) of treatment with azacitidine has a statistically significant higher pooled ORR than a 5-day course.

It is important to note that the pooled set of patients receiving the 7–0-0 treatment regimen had a greater proportion of patients with IPSS high risk score and a diagnosis of AML than the other two treatment regimens. This likely reflected the fact that the 7–0-0 regimen was studied in clinical trials and is the regimen receiving clinical approval. How this impacted the pooled ORR for this group of patients across all studies is not clear because the IPSS is a prognostic score predictive of survival in MDS, not objective response rate [23]. To determine whether the higher proportion of AML patients treated with the 7–0-0 regimen affected the outcome of the pooled proportion analysis, a sensitivity analysis was performed assessing the response of patients with a diagnosis of MDS only (studies assessing any patients with a diagnosis of AML or CMML were excluded). It yielded the same outcome in that the pooled ORR with the 7–0-0 and 5–2-2 regimens were higher than the pooled ORR with the 5–0-0 regimen. The slightly higher ORR of the 7–0-0 in relation to the 5–0-0 regimen in an indirect pooled proportional analysis was consistent in similar sensitivity analyses focusing on patients assessed in randomized clinical trials, and on patients assessed in prospective observational studies (Table 2). The clinical significance of this finding is uncertain, however, without a direct comparison of the different dosing regimens in a clinical trial.

An important limitation of the current systematic review is that due to a paucity of randomized controlled trials in directly comparing the alternative azacitidine dosing regimens, most of the articles and abstracts included in this systematic review refer to observational prospective and retrospective studies. With a lack of randomization, blinding, and allocation concealment in these studies, there is a substantial risk of selection, performance, and detection bias as summarized in Fig. 2 [10]. However, with the consistency of the finding that the pooled ORR for a total of 7 days of azacitidine exposure is higher that the pooled ORR for 5 days of exposure, a randomized clinical trial is required for direct comparison and a definitive answer. If a trial is not performed, a standardization of outcome data reporting in the literature would facilitate the update of the sort of analysis done in this study with the inclusion of stable disease and survival as outcomes.

Conclusions

In summary, this systematic review of alternative azacitidine dosing regimens in MDS and AML patients has highlighted an important deficiency in the literature regarding outcome reporting. Based on a small number of studies directly comparing alternative dosing regimens, there is no difference in efficacy of the 7–0-0, 5–2-2, and 5–0-0 dosing regimens in attaining ORR. However, an indirect comparison of the dosing regimens in the form of a pooled proportions analysis encompassing all studies on the subject yielded a slightly higher ORR for a total of 7 days of exposure to azacitidine as compared to 5 days. A prospective randomized clinical trial directly comparing the three dosing regimens is required to definitively address this comparison. Furthermore, a standardization of the reporting of outcomes of azacitidine treatment would facilitate future indirect comparisons of dosing regimens if a randomized trial is not preformed.

Acknowledgements
Authors are kindly indebted to Alla Iansavitchene, BSc, MLIS, Library Services, London Health Science Centre, Western University, Ontario, Canada, for her help with the development and conduct of the literature search.
We thank Dr. Antonio Medina Almeida for providing the raw data from his retrospective study. We thank Dr. Maria Teresa Voso for providing us with her manuscript on azacitidine dosing.

Funding
Not applicable

Authors' contributions
The systematic review was conceived and planned by ALL and RS. The literature search was performed by ALL and RS. Articles were reviewed and data was extracted by RS. Data analysis and interpretation was done by ALL and RS. The manuscript was written by ALL and RS. Both authors read and approved the final manuscript

Competing interests
Dr. Alejandro Lazo-Langner is the Hemostasis, Thrombosis and Vascular Biology Section Editor for BMC Hematology.

Author details
[1]Department of Medicine, Western University, London, ON, Canada. [2]Department of Medicine, Division of Hematology, Western University, London, ON, Canada. [3]Department of Epidemiology & Biostatistics, Western University, London, ON, Canada. [4]Hematology Division, London Health Sciences Centre, 800 Commissioners Rd E, Rm E6-216A, London, ON N6A 5W9, Canada.

References

1. AMS M, Florek M. 5-Azacytidine. In: Small molecules in oncology. 2nd ed. New York: Springer Heidelberg; 2014. p. 299–324.
2. Silverman LR, Demakos EP, Peterson BL, Kornblith AB, Holland JC, Odchimar-Reissig R, Stone RM, Nelson D, Powell BL, DeCastro CM, Ellerton J, Larson RA, Schiffer CA, Holland JF. Randomized controlled trial of Azacitidine in patients with the Myelodysplastic syndrome: a study of the cancer and leukemia group B. J Clin Oncol. 2002;20:2429–40.
3. Fenaux P, Mufti GJ, Hellstrom-Lindberg E, Santini V, Finelli C, Giagounidis A, Schoch R, Gattermann N, Sanz G, List A, Gore SD, Seymour JF, Bennett JM, Byrd J, Backstrom J, Zimmerman L, McKenzie D, Beach CL, Silverman LR, for the International Vidaza High-Risk MDS Survival Study Group. Efficacy of azacitidine compared with that of conventional careregimens in the treatment of higher-risk myelodysplasticsyndromes: a randomised, open-label, phase III study. Lancet Oncol. 2009;10:223–32.
4. Frame D. Alternative dosing schedules for methylation inhibitors in MDS treatment. Managed Care. 2009;18(11):S15–20.
5. Saunthararajah Y. Key clinical observations after 5-azacytidine and decitabine treatment of myelodysplastic syndromes suggest practical solutions for better outcomes. Hematology. 2013; https://doi.org/10.1182/asheducation-2013.1.511.
6. Keating GM. Azacitidine. Drugs. 2012;72(8):1111–36.
7. Santini V, Prebet T, Fenaux P, Gattermann N, Nilsson L, Pfeilstocker M, Vyas P, List AF. Minimizing risk of hypomethylating agent failure in patients with higher-risk MDS and practical management recommendations. Leuk Res. 2014;38:1381–91.
8. Cheson BD, Greenberg PL, Bennett JM, Lowenberg B, Wijermans PW, Nimer SD, Pinto A, Beran M, de Witte TM, Stone RM, Mittelman M, Sanz GF, Gore SD, Schiffer CA, Kantarjian H. Clinical application and proposal for modification of the international working group (IWG) response criteria in myelodysplasia. Blood. 2006;108(2):419–25.
9. Jadad AR, Moore RA, Carroll D, et al. Assessing the quality of reports of randomized clinical trials: is blinding necessary? Control Clin Trials. 1996;17:1–12.
10. JPT H, Altman DG, Sterne JAC. Chapter 8: assessing risk of bias in included studies. In: JPT H, Green S, editors. Cochrane handbook for systematic reviews of interventions. Version 5.1.0 [updated march 2011]. The Cochrane collaboration; 2011. http://handbook-5-1.cochrane.org/. Accessed 1 June 2016.
11. Stukel TA, Demidenko E, Dykes J, Karagas MR. Two-stage methods for the analysis of pooled data. Statist Med. 2001;20:2115–30.
12. Lazo-Langner A, Rodger MA, Barrowman NJ, Ramsay T, Wells PS, Coyle DA. Comparing multiple competing interventions in the absence of randomized trials using clinical risk-benefit analysis. BMC Med Res Methodol. 2012;12:3.
13. Silverman LR, McKenzie DR, Peterson BL, Holland JF, Backstrom JT, Beach CL, Larson RA. Further analysis of trials with Azacitidine in patients with Myelodysplastic syndrome: studies 8421, 8921, and 9221 by the cancer and leukemia group B. J Clin Oncol. 2006;24(24):3895–903.
14. Lyons RM, Cosgriff TM, Modi SS, Gersh RH, Hainsworth JD, Cohn AL, McIntyre HJ, Fernando IJ, Backstrom JT, Beach CL. Hematologic response to three alternative DosingSchedules of Azacitidine in patients with Myelodysplastic syndromes. J Clin Oncol. 2009;27(11):1850–6.
15. Xicoy B, Jiménez MJ, García O, et al. Results of treatment with azacitidine in patients aged 75 years included in the Spanish registry of Myelodysplastic syndromes. Leuk Lymphoma. 2014;55(6):1300–3.
16. García-Delgadoa R, de Miguelb D, Bailénc A, et al. Effectiveness and safety of different azacitidine dosage regimens inpatients with myelodysplastic syndromes or acute myeloid leukemia. Leuk Res. 2014;38:744–50.
17. Gore SD, Fenaux P, Santini V, et al. A multivariate analysis of the relationship between response and survival among patients with higher-risk myelodysplastic syndromes treated within azacitidine or conventional care regimens in the randomized AZA-001 trial. Haematologica. 2013;98:1062–72.
18. Cheson BD, Bennett JM, Kantarjian H, et al. Report of an international working group to standardize response criteria for myelodysplastic syndromes. Blood. 2000;96:3671–4.

19. O'Reilly MA, McHale C, Almazmi A, et al. A 5-day outpatient regimen of azacitidine is effective and well tolerated in patients with acute myeloid leukemia unsuitable for intensive chemotherapy. Leuk Lymphoma. 2014; 55(12):2950–1.
20. Passweg JR, Pabst T, Blum S, et al. Azacytidine for acute myeloid leukemia in elderly or frail patients: a phase II trial (SAKK 30/07). Leuk Lymphoma. 2014;55(1):87–91.
21. van der Helm LH, Veeger NJGM, M. Kooy VM, et al. Azacitidine results in comparable outcome in newly diagnosed AML patients with more or less than 30% bone marrow blasts. Leuk Res. 2013;37:877–82.
22. van der Helm LH, Scheepers ERM, Veeger NJGM, et al. Azacitidine might be beneficial in a subgroup of older AML patients compared to intensive chemotherapy: a single centre retrospective study of 227 consecutive patients. J Hematol Oncol. 2013;6:29–37.
23. Greenberg P, Cox C, LeBeau MM, et al. International scoring system for evaluating prognosis in myelodysplastic syndromes. Blood. 1997;89(6):2079–88.
24. Sadashiv SK, Hilton C, Khan C, et al. Efficacy and tolerability of treatment with azacitidine for 5 days in elderly patients with acute myeloid leukemia. Cancer Medicine. 2014;3(6):1570–8.
25. Minoia C, Sgherza N, Loseto G, et al. Azacitidine in the front-line treatment of therapy-related myeloid Neoplasms: a multicenter case series. Anticancer Res. 2015;35:461–6.
26. Drummond MW, Pocock C, Boissinot M, et al. A multi-centre phase 2 study of azacitidine in chronic myelomonocytic leukaemia. Leukemia. 2014;28:1570–2.
27. Fianchi L, Criscuolo M, Breccia M, et al. High rate of remissions in chronic myelomonocytic leukemia treated with 5-azacytidine: results of an Italian retrospective study. Leuk Lymphoma. 2013;54(3):658–61.
28. Ballya C, Adèsa L, Rennevilleb A, Seberta M, et al. Prognostic value of TP53 gene mutations in myelodysplasticsyndromes and acute myeloid leukemia treated with azacitidine. Leuk Res. 2014;38:751–5.
29. Breccia M, Loglisci G, Salaroli A, et al. 5-Azacitidine efficacy and safety in patients aged > 65 years with myelodysplastic syndromes outside clinical trials. Leuk Lymphoma. 2012;53(8):1558–60.
30. Breccia M, Loglisci G, Cannella L, et al. Application of French prognostic score to patients with InternationalPrognostic scoring system intermediate-2 or high risk myelodysplasticsyndromes treated with 5-azacitidine is able to predict overall survivaland rate of response. Leuk Lymphoma. 2012;53(5):985–6.
31. Douvali E, Papoutselis M, Vassilakopoulos TP, et al. Safety and efficacy of 5-azacytidine treatment in myelodysplastic syndrome patients with moderate and mild renal impairment. Leuk Res. 2013;37:889–93.
32. Duong VH, Lancet JE, Alrawi E, et al. Outcome of azacitidine treatment in patients with therapy-related myeloid neoplasms with assessment of prognostic risk stratification models. Leuk Res. 2013;37:510–5.
33. Ettou S, Audureau E, Humbrecht C, et al. Fas expression at diagnosis as a biomarker of azacitidine activityin high-risk MDS and secondary AML. Leukemia. 2012;26:2297–9.
34. Fianchi L, Criscuolo M, Lunghi M, et al. Outcome of therapy-related myeloid neoplasms treated with azacitidine. J Hematol Oncol. 2012;5:44.
35. Fili C, Malagola M, Follo MY, et al. Prospective phase II study on 5-days Azacitidine forTreatment of symptomatic and/or erythropoietin unresponsive patients with low/INT-1–risk Myelodysplastic syndromes. Clin Cancer Res. 2013;19(12):3297–308.
36. Gryna J, Zeigler ZR, Shadduck RK, et al. Treatment of myelodysplastic syndromes with 5-azacytidine. Leuk Res. 2002;26:893–7.
37. Itzykson R, Kosmider O, Cluzeau T, et al. Impact of TET2 mutations on response rate to azacitidine in myelodysplastic syndromesand low blast count acute myeloid leukemias. Leukemia. 2011;25:1147–52.
38. Itzykson R, Thépot S, Quesnel B, et al. Prognostic factors for response and overall survival in 282 patients with higher-risk myelodysplastic syndromes treated with azacitidine. Blood. 2011;117:403–11.
39. Lee JH, Choi Y, Kim SD, et al. Comparison of 7-day azacitidine and 5-day decitabine for treating myelodysplastic syndrome. Ann Hematol. 2013;92:889–97.
40. Lee YG, Kim I, Yoon SS, et al. Comparative analysis between azacitidine and decitabine forthe treatment of myelodysplastic syndromes. Br J Hematol. 2013;161:339–47.
41. Al-Ali HK, Jaekel N, Junghanss C, et al. Azacitidine in patients with acute myeloid leukemia medically unfit for or resistant to chemotherapy: a multicenter phase I/II study. Leuk Lymphoma. 2012;53(1):110–7.
42. Martin MG, Walgren RA, Procknow E, et al. A phase II study of 5-day intravenous azacitidine in patients with myelodysplastic syndromes. Am J Hematol. 2009;84:560–4.
43. Moon JH, Kim SN, Kang BW, et al. Predictive value of pretreatment risk group and baseline LDH levels in MDS patients receiving azacitidine treatment. Ann Hematol. 2010;89:681–9.
44. Müller-Thomas C, Schuster T, Peschel C, Götze KS. A limited number of 5-azacitidine cycles can be effective treatment in MDS. Ann Hematol. 2009;88: 213–9.
45. Müller-Thomas C, Rudelius M, Rondak IC, et al. Response to azacitidine is independent of p53 expression in higher-risk myelodysplastic syndromesand secondary acute myeloid leukemia. Haematologica. 2014;99:e179.
46. O'Reilly MA, McHale C, Almazmi A, et al. A 5-day: the favourable way? Ann Hematol. 2014;93:1619–20.
47. Ozbalak M, Cetiner M, Bekoz H, et al. Azacitidine has limited activity in 'real life' patientswith MDS and AML: a single centre experience. Hematol Oncol. 2012;30:76–81.
48. Papoutselis M, Douvali E, Papadopoulos V, et al. Has introduction of azacytidine in everyday clinical practice improved survival in late-stage Myelodysplastic syndrome? A single center experience. Leuk Res. 2014;38: 161–5.
49. Pierdomenico F, Esteves S, Almeida A. Efficacy and tolerability of 5-day azacytidine dose-intensified regimen in higher-risk MDS. Ann Hematol. 2013;92:1201–6.
50. Tobiasson M, Dybedahl I, Holm MS, et al. Limited clinical efficacy of azacitidine in transfusion-dependent, growth factor-resistant, low- and Int-1-risk MDS: results from the nordic NMDSG08A phase II trial. Blood Cancer J. 2014;4:1–7.
51. Diamantopoulos P, Zervakis K, Papadopoulou V, et al. 5-Azacytidine in the treatment of Intermediate-2 and high-risk Myelodysplastic syndromes and acute myeloid leukemia. A five-year experience with 44 consecutive patients. Anticancer Res. 2015;35:5141–8.

23

Diagnostic accuracy in field conditions of the sickle SCAN rapid test for sickle cell disease among children and adults in two West African settings: the DREPATEST study

Akueté Yvon Segbena[1^], Aldiouma Guindo[2], Romain Buono[3], Irénée Kueviakoe[1], Dapa A. Diallo[2], Gregory Guernec[3], Mouhoudine Yerima[4], Pierre Guindo[2], Emilie Lauressergues[5], Aude Mondeilh[5], Valentina Picot[6] and Valériane Leroy[3*]

Abstract

Background: Sickle cell disease (SCD) accounts for 5% of mortality in African children aged < 5 years. Improving the care management and quality of life of patients with SCD requires a reliable diagnosis in resource-limited settings. We assessed the diagnostic accuracy of the rapid Sickle SCAN® point-of-care (POC) test for SCD used in field conditions in two West-African countries.

Methods: We conducted a case-control study in Bamako (Mali) and Lomé (Togo). Known cases of sickle cell disease (HbSS, HbSC), trait (HbAS), HbC heterozygotes (HbAC) and homozygous (HbCC), aged ≥6 months were compared to Controls (HbAA), recruited by convenience. All subjects received both an index rapid POC test and a gold standard (high-performance liquid chromatography in Bamako; capillary electrophoresis in Lomé). Personnel conducting tests were blinded from subjects' SCD status. Sensitivity and specificity were calculated for each phenotype. Practicality was assessed by local healthcare professionals familiar with national diagnostic methods and their associated constraints.

Results: In Togo, 209 Cases (45 HbAS, 39 HbAC, 41 HbSS, 44 HbSC and 40 HbCC phenotypes) were compared to 86 Controls (HbAA). 100% sensitivity and specificity were observed for AA Controls and HbCC cases. Estimated sensitivity was 97.7% [95% confidence interval: 88.0–99.9], 97.6% [87.1–99.9%], 95.6% [84.8–99.5%], and 94.9% [82.7–99.4], for HbSC, HbSS, HbAS, and HbAC, respectively. Specificity exceeded 99.2% for all phenotypes. Among 160 cases and 80 controls in Mali, rapid testing was 100% sensitive and specific. Rapid testing was well accepted by local healthcare professionals.

Conclusion: Rapid POC testing is 100% accurate for homozygote healthy people and excellent (Togo) or perfect (Mali) for sickle cell trait and disease patients. In addition to its comparable diagnostic performance, this test is cheaper, easier to implement, and logistically more convenient than the current standard diagnostic methods in use. Its predictive value indicators and diagnostic accuracy in newborns should be further evaluated prior to implementation in large-scale screening programs in resource-limited settings where SCD is prevalent.

Keywords: Sickle cell disease, Diagnosis, Rapid diagnosis test, Sensitivity, Specificity, Performances, Africa

* Correspondence: Valeriane.Leroy@inserm.fr
^Deceased
[3]Inserm UMR 1027, Epidémiologie et analyses en santé publique : risques, maladies chroniques et handicaps, Université Paul Sabatier Toulouse 3, Faculté de Médecine Purpan, 37 Allées Jules Guesde, 31073 Toulouse Cedex 7, France
Full list of author information is available at the end of the article

Background

Sickle Cell Disease (SCD) is the most common inherited blood disorder worldwide, accounting for 5% of the mortality in African children < 5 years of age [1, 2]. In SCD, mutations occurring on the gene encoding for the hemoglobin (Hb) β chain are transmitted in a recessive way, with an impact on the structural, functional and rheological properties of the erythrocyte [3]. 75.5% of the SCD cases worldwide occur in Sub-Saharan Africa. The term "SCD" includes various Hemoglobin variants phenotypes responsible of the characteristic syndrome, but four are predominant in West Africa. The most common and severe form of SCD is the homozygous HbSS phenotype (sickle cell anaemia) inherited from both parents [2, 3]. Other forms of SCD include the compound heterozygotes HbSC disease and HbS/βthalassaemia [4]. HbC homozygotes and heterozygotes are usually well and these are not forms of sickle cell disease [5].

Under-five mortality is high in SCD patients and associated particularly with the HbSS phenotype in sub-Saharan Africa [6]. The cornerstone of care management is based on early diagnosis, ideally neonatal, of SCD to allow prompt parental education and counselling about disease complications, immunization and antibiotic prophylaxis [1, 7].

Thus, improving the care management and quality of life of patients with SCD requires establishing a reliable diagnosis feasible in resource-limited settings [1, 6, 7]. Currently, two tree gold standard approaches are validated for first-level neonatal screening and routine diagnosis: High Performance Liquid Chromatography (HPLC); Capillary Electrophoresis (CE) and Isoelectric focusing (IEF) [8–10]. Their sensitivity and specificity for detection of normal and common abnormal hemoglobin variants are close to perfect [10–12]. Moreover, a quantification of HbA2 and HbF is also possible, allowing the identification of β-thalassemia and hereditary persistence of fetal hemoglobin forms [10–12]. Whatever the technique used for first-level diagnosis, all international guidelines support the need to perform confirmatory tests using another method. However, these methods are neither rapid, nor easy to implement in resource-limited settings, since they require a consequent financial investment with constraints: time, regular restocking of reagent, availability of electricity, mobilization of dedicated and trained technicians, transport and storage of biological samples, and adherence to strict laboratory standards. They also suffer from high loss to follow-up risk, due to the long lag time between sample collection and the delivery of results that could excess 4 to 6 weeks.

Many devices, at different stages of development, among the novel Point-Of-Care (POC) tests for hemoglobin variants, have emerged as potential alternative tools for reliable and simple diagnosis of SCD in developing countries. Among these, we can cite: i) based on the difference of solubility of the HbA and HbS, the microfluidic paper-based analytical devices (μPADs) from Halcyon Biomedical [13]; ii) based on the difference of Red Blood Cells density from an aqueous multiphase system, the Daktari Sickle Cell developed by Daktari Diagnostics, iii) based on lateral flow immunoassay devices, the Hemotype SC from Silver Lake Research Corporation [14] and the Sickle SCAN® from BioMedomics. The latter, a sandwich format chromatographic immunoassay approach developed for the qualitative measurement of HbA, HbS and HbC in whole blood samples, has demonstrated excellent intrinsic performances to detect common Hb variants [13, 15].

As the Sickle SCAN test employs lateral flow immunoassay technology, it has a potential large-scale screening utility in resource-limited settings. The Sickle Scan® POC device has recently been assessed in field conditions in two studies in sub-Saharan Africa, with promising results [16, 17]. However, none of these studies provided information regarding the climate conditions. The aim of this study is to assess the diagnostic accuracy (sensitivity and specificity) of the Sickle SCAN® POC test and its acceptability to persons conducting the tests under field conditions (temperature and relative humidity) in children older than 6 months of age and adults, in Lomé (Togo) and Bamako (Mali), West Africa.

Methods

Study design

DREPATEST was a multicenter diagnosis accuracy study based on a case-control design (1 case for 2 controls), stratified on the two clinical sites (Bamako, Mali, and Lomé, Togo), and reported according to the Standard for Reporting Diagnosis Accuracy [18]. The study was conducted from May 23, 2016 to October 16, 2016.

Ethics approval and consent to participate

Approvals from ethical committees in both Togo (« Comité d'Ethique de la Recherche en Santé du Togo ») and Mali ("Comité d'Ethique Institutionnel du CRLD du Mali") were obtained in April and May 2016, respectively. Individual consent was obtained from each participant. The manuscript does not contain any individual person's identifiable data or information.

Population

In each site, we selected a convenience samples of patients with SCD (HbSS and HbSC), with sickle cell trait (HbAS) and/or patients homozygous and heterozygous for HbC (HbCC, HbAC), and compared these each to two healthy controls (HbAA) at the same site. Due to their high prevalence in Togo, patients homozygous for HbC (HbCC) can only be recruited in CHU Campus in Lomé.

Subjects were recruited either during their initial diagnosis visit or during a follow-up visit at the Centre de Recherche et de Lutte contre la Drépanocytose (CRLD) of Bamako (Mali), or at the Unité d'Hématologie Clinique, Centre Hospitalier Universitaire Campus of Lomé (Togo). Eligibility criteria included: age > 6 months; no blood transfusion received in the last 3 months; absence of severe vaso-occlusive pain episodes; an informed consent form signed either by the participant or his/her guardian (for children). All the subjects were tested using both the index POC test and the reference standard test in their respective country: HPLC in Bamako [19] and CE in Lomé [9]. In Mali, for all subjects previously diagnosed using the gold standard, a blood drop was collected and used to perform the POC test. Otherwise, in Togo or newly diagnosed Malian subjects, a venipuncture sample collected in EDTA and stored at 4 °C until analysis, providing the blood needed to conduct both the rapid test (immediately) and the standard test (within the 24 h). All the SickleSCAN® tests were performed during the consultation.

Sample size

PASS 14·0 software was used to calculate the sample size for each assumed parameter of sensitivity and specificity, with a two-sided test following a normal distribution. A total sample size of 240 (which includes at least 158 cases with an abnormal phenotype) achieves 76% power to detect a change in sensitivity from 0.99 to 0.96 using a two-sided binomial test and 19% power to detect a change in specificity from 0.85 to 0.8 using a two-sided binomial test [20]. This corresponds to a total of 280 Togolese subjects, including 200 cases (40 of each of the five Hb abnormal expected phenotypes: HbAS, HbAC, HbSS, HbSC, HbCC) and 80 controls (to be compared with each phenotype), and a sample size in Mali of 240 subjects, including 160 Cases (40 of each of the four Hb phenotypes: HbAS, HbAC, HbSS, HbSC) and 80 controls.

Procedures

The hemoglobin type was determined using either a high-performance liquid chromatography (D-10 instrument; Bio-Rad) in Mali, or a Capillaris Electrophoresis (MinicapR; Sebia) in Togo to perform the reference test. Sickle SCAN™ is a qualitative lateral flow immunoassay that indicates the presence of HbA, HbS, and HbC in whole blood samples using the sandwich format chromatographic immunoassay approach with colorimetric detector nanoparticles conjugated to antibodies. The rapid test was performed according to the BioMedomics protocol, with 5 μl of blood from the finger or from the venipuncture added to the prefilled buffer solution. After mixing by inverting the bottle tree times, three drops were discarded and five other drops were dropped to the testing cartridge. Five minutes later, the result was read. The rapid test manufacturer-recommended temperature ranges for storage is between 2 °C and 30 °C, while there was no manufacturer-recommended humidity ranges recommended.

All POC tests have been assessed under field conditions including the specific conditions of expedition by plane, and storage to according to the local customs, either in Togo or Mali. The POC tests were stored under local temperatures and humidity conditions. These environmental parameters were recorded alongside the reading of test results, 5 min after a blood sample was obtained and loaded. A photo was taken of each test result, thereby allowing for a subsequent review of findings. Information and clinical care were provided to subjects whose SCD or trait were first diagnosed with the reference method. All POC providers were trained to perform and interpret the Sickle SCAN® tests.

The conduct of this study can be likened to a reversed-flow design with a reference standard diagnostic before the POC test [21]. To prevent any interpretation bias, clinical data were not available to personnel conducting the POC.

Data collection

A two-sided Case Report Form (CRF) linked by an anonymized subject number, served for data collection. The first part, which could only be accessed by the clinical investigators, documented subjects' socio-demographic and clinical characteristics, including the Hb phenotype obtained by the reference method, if known. The second part contained the results of the POC test and the temperature and humidity parameters recorded in the setting. Data were stored in Microsoft© Access 2013, specific queries guaranteed the detection of potential missing, inconsistent or duplicate data.

The acceptability of the rapid test to health care workers was assessed using a self-administered qualitative and descriptive survey, collecting: the perception of the user manual's clarity; perception of the time to obtain the result, and the complexity level felt to interpret the result.

Statistical analysis plan

Each investigation site's data were analyzed distinctly using R 3·2·5. Socio-demographic, medical, and site characteristics were described and compared between Hb phenotypes (HbSS, HbSC, HbCC, HbAS, HbAC) and controls (HbAA). Results are expressed with numbers and percentages for categorical variables, or with medians and interquartile ranges for continuous variables. Comparative analysis was conducted between the sum of cases and controls, using Fisher's exact test or Chi-Square tests for percentages and t-tests or F-tests for means. A type 1 error risk α equal to 0·05 was chosen for the set. For each Hb phenotype, sensitivity and specificity were evaluated with a 95% confidence interval assuming a binomial distribution. We used a logistic regression model to predict the Hb phenotype obtained by the reference method, including the SickleSCAN® test outcome as the main explanatory variable. Other variables included: age (years); sex; intake of anti-malarial therapy; iron and vitamin B9 supplementation; ambient temperature (°C); and relative humidity (%). A multivariate analysis was conducted with the variables having a P-value $< 0{\cdot}20$ in the univariate models. Continuous covariates were categorized when linearity assumption could not be checked before being integrated into the logistic models. Fitting of the adjusted final model was made using a backward elimination approach. Adjusted Odds Ratio (aOR) with their 95% confidence intervals (95% CI) were calculated for each variable. Receiver Operating Characteristic (ROC) curves were constructed and Areas Under the Curve (AUC) and their 95% CI were examined to compare the ability of different models to predict each Hb phenotype.

Results

Lomé study: POC versus CE

From May 23rd to June 30th 2016, 313 subjects were eligible in Togo (Fig. 1). Nine subjects failed to meet the required criteria, and six persons declined to participate. In addition, two blood samples were of insufficient quality to be used with the reference test. Of the 296 samples tested using the reference method (CE), only one gave an inconclusive result. Overall, the study was conducted among the remaining 295 subjects (94%): 209 abnormal phenotypes (45 AS, 39 AC, 41 SS, 44 SC and 40 CC phenotypes), and 86 Controls (AA).

There were significantly more men (73.3%) among abnormal phenotypes than in controls (58.4%) but no other statistically significant differences were noted (Table 1). Three children were younger than 1 year at inclusion. The POC devices have been stored during 60 to 73 days at a median ambient temperature of 29.5 degrees (range: 28.4 °C – 35 °C) and a median humidity of 72% (range: 62–77%).

Sixty-seven (22.7%) POC tests were performed under ambient temperature above the manufacturer-recommended maximum, ranging from 30·5 °C to 35·0 °C. Ninety-four (31.8%) tests were conducted at a relative humidity greater than 75%, the upper quartile.

All HbCC subjects and controls (HbAA) were correctly classified using the POC test according to the reference method (Table 2). Figure 2 provides the photos of the POC tests with representative results for each phenotype.

However, over the 295 tests, six misclassifications (2%) were reported among the HbAS, HbAC, HbSS and HbSC cases (Table 2). Out of these six misclassifications, none was observed among the three infants aged less than 12 months and five of them could be related to extreme ambient conditions: one was observed above the manufacturer-recommended temperature (at 30.5 °C) but under normal humidity, four were observed within the manufacturer-recommended temperature ranges, but above 75% of humidity. Two among the observed misclassifications conducted above 75% of humidity were also directly linked to the reading operator misinterpretation. For the last case misclassified observed under "normal

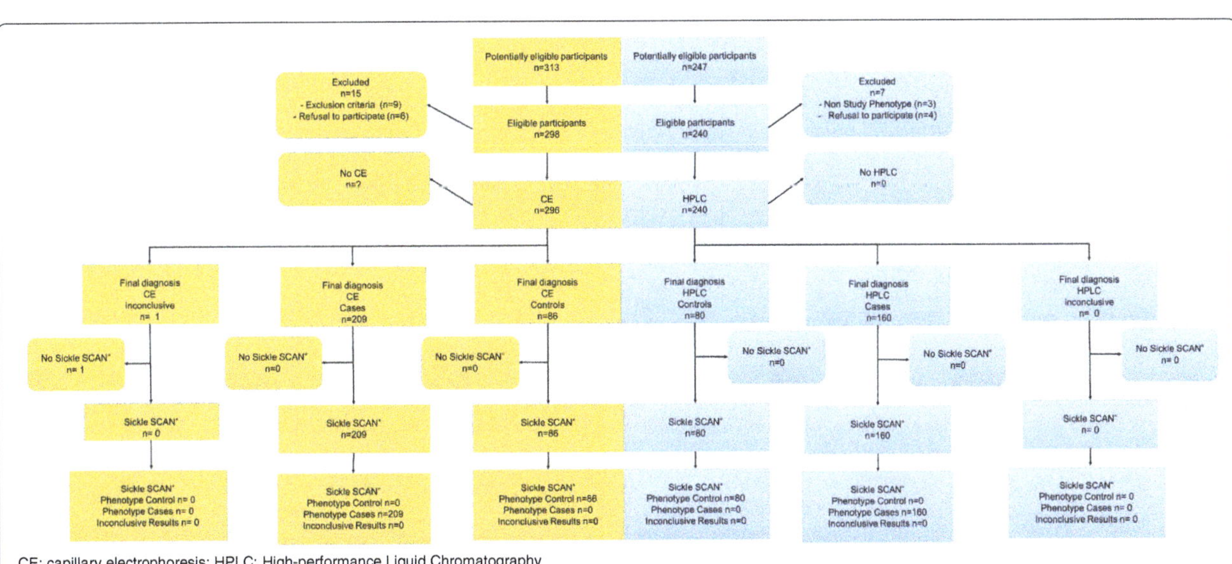

CE: capillary electrophoresis; HPLC: High-performance Liquid Chromatography

Fig. 1 Flow Chart of participants in Lomé (Togo), Mai-June 2016, ($n = 295$) (On the left side) and in Bamako (Mali), October 2016, ($n = 240$) (On the right side)

Table 1 Baseline characteristics between sickle cell anaemia and trait cases and controls in Lomé (Togo) and Bamako (Mali)

Haemoglobin Phenotype	Lomé (Togo), reference = Capillary electrophoresis ($n = 295$)							Bamako (Mali), Gold Standard = HPLC ($n = 240$)					
	Controls	Cases p[a]	AS	AC	SS	SC	CC	Controls	Cases p[a]	AS	AC	SS	SC
	$N = 86$ (%)	$N = 209$ (%)	$N = 45$ (%)	$N = 39$ (%)	$N = 41$ (%)	$N = 44$ (%)	$N = 40$ (%)	$N = 80$ (%)	$N = 240$ (%)	$N = 40$ (%)	$N = 40$ (%)	$N = 40$ (%)	$N = 40$ (%)
Age (year)		0·842							0·523				
Median	23·2	23·3	23·4	23·3	11·8	25·7	32·9	25·3	22·4	24·8	17·7	17.1	22·3
Q1-Q3	21·8–26·6	20·0–28·1	21·2–24·6	21·0–26·2	5·8–22·9	15·4–34·1	23·2–40·4	14·9–31·3	11·9–30·2	17·7–31·4	7·1–28·6	10·4–24·7	16·1–28·6
Sex		0·017						1					
Male	63 (73·3)	122 (58·4)	29 (64·4)	26 (66·7)	21 (51·2)	27 (61·4)	19 (47·5)	31 (38·8)	62 (38·8)	14 (35)	16 (40)	13 (32·5)	19 (47·5)
Site conditions													
Temperature (°C)		$< 10^{-3}$							–				
Minimum	28·8	28·4	29·5	28·4	28·8	28·4	28·4	25·6	25·6	–	–	–	–
Q1-Q3	29·5–29·7	28·8–29·7	29·5–30·5	29·5–30·5	28·8–29·5	28·8–28·8	28·4–28·9	25·6	25·6	–	–	–	–
Maximum	30·5	35·0	30·5	35·0	30·5	30·5	30·2	25·6	25·6	–	–	–	–
Relative Humidity (%)		0·36											
Minimum	65	62	65	65	62	62	62	32	32	–	–	–	–
Q1-Q3	70–77	70–76	65–77	65–77	70–75	75–76	72–75	32	32	–	–	–	–
Maximum	77	77	77	77	77	77	76	32	32	–	–	–	–

[a] Comparison between Controls (AA) and the total of Togolese Cases (AS, AC, SS, SC, CC) or Malian Cases (AS, AC, SS, SC)

Table 2 Aggregate confusion matrix between results achieved by two different reference methods and the Sickle SCAN® device, to determine the haemoglobin phenotype in Lomé (Togo), May–June 2016, ($n = 295$) (On the left side) and in Bamako (Mali), October 2016, ($n = 240$) (On the right side)

		Capillary Electrophoresis									High Performance Liquid Chromatography					
		AA	AS	AC	SS	SC	CC	Total			AA	AS	AC	SS	SC	Total
Sickle SCAN®	AA	86	0	0	0	0	0	86	Sickle SCAN®	AA	80	0	0	0	0	80
	AS	0	43	1	0	0	0	44		AS	0	40	0	0	0	40
	AC	0	1	37	0	1	0	39		AC	0	0	40	0	0	40
	SS	0	1	0	40	0	0	41		SS	0	0	0	40	0	40
	SC	0	0	0	1	43	0	44		SC	0	0	0	0	40	40
	CC	0	0	1	0	0	40	41								
	Total	86	45	39	41	44	40	295		Total	80	40	40	40	40	240

ambient conditions", photos suggest an unclear result, with the visual indicator corresponding to the HbA identification slightly marked when co-associated with other Hb variants (AS, AC).

Sensitivity and specificity estimates (and associated 95% CI) for each Hb phenotype are presented in Table 3. From perfect intrinsic performance for Controls, sensitivity increases between 97.6 and 100% for SCD patients. The lowest sensitivity is observed in HbAS and HbAC trait subjects with 94.9 and 95.6%, respectively. The specificity exceeded 99% in all cases.

In the final multivariate analysis, the only variable associated with the reference test outcome was the Hb phenotype determined by the Sickle SCAN® test. Indeed, association between this variable and the variable of interest was perfect for Controls and HbCC Cases and almost perfect for HbAS (aOR = 5353·5; 95%CI [475–60,336]), HbAC (aOR = 2349·5; 95% CI [321·2–17,188·9]), HbSS (aOR = 10,120; 95% CI [620·4–165,067·7]), and HbSC (aOR = 10,750; 95% CI [659·8–175,139·1]).

HbAA discriminating power model is perfect, with a maximum AUC value (Fig. 3). AUC values for the HbAS and HbAC models are 97.6% [95% CI: 94.5–100.0] and 97.1% [95% CI: 93.5–100.0], respectively.

Bamako: POC versus HPLC

The Mali flow chart is presented in Fig. 1. Among the 247 eligible patients, 98% met the inclusion criteria. There were no differences between cases and controls for the following variables: age, sex, hydroxycarbamide intake and iron supplementation. Vitamin B9 supplementation and antimalarial drug intake were overrepresented in Cases, particularly in HbSS and HbSC patients. Only, three children were younger than 1 year at inclusion. In Mali, all POC tests have been stored during 77 to 119 days and performed in an air-conditioned room at 25.6 °C and 32% of humidity.

For all 240 subjects, the Sickle SCAN® test yielded the same result as the HPLC gold standard, leading to sensitivity and specificity estimates of 100% (Table 2).

Acceptability to health care professionals

Twenty professionals (17 from Togo and three from Mali), all involved in SCD care, with high levels of clinical

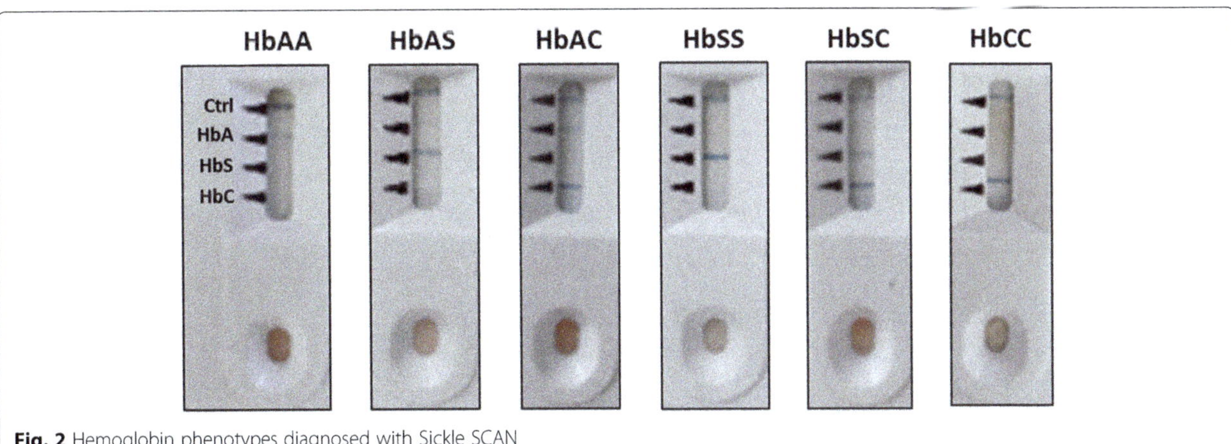

Fig. 2 Hemoglobin phenotypes diagnosed with Sickle SCAN

Table 3 Sensitivity and specificity for each haemoglobin phenotype identified using the reference standard method (Capillary Electrophoresis) in Lomé (Togo), May–June 2016. (*N* = 295)

Haemoglobin phenotype identified by Capillary Electrophoresis	N	Sensitivity (%)	95% CI[a]	Specificity (%)	95% CI[a]
AA	86	100	[93·8–100]	100	[97·4–100]
AS	45	95·6	[84·8–99·5]	99·6	[97·8–99·9]
AC	39	94·9	[82·7–99·4]	99·2	[97·2–99·9]
SS	41	97·6	[87·1–99·9]	99·6	[97·2–99·9]
SC	44	97·7	[88·0–99·9]	99·6	[97·8–99·9]
CC	40	100	[87·1–100]	100	[97·8–100]

[a] 95% Confidence Intervals (CI) have been computed using the binomial distribution

laboratory experience and expertise (two hematologists, one pharmacist, one biological engineer and fourteen biological technicians) completed the acceptability questionnaire: 90% perceived the user manual as either "reasonably clear" or "very clear." The time required to obtain the result was labelled "short" for 95%. All respondents found the interpretation of results to be either "simple" or "very simple." Each step required to perform the rapid test was described as "simple" or "very simple" to execute for at least 95% of the participants. Specific suggestions included: translating instructions into French; and improving the readability of the "HbA" line in the presence of HbAS or HbAC phenotypes to avoid confusion.

Discussion

This study is one of the first to evaluate the accuracy of the Sickle SCAN® test under clinical field conditions of a POC test in West Africa using two different gold standards, the HPLC and CE tests. Our study provides new insights into the African operational considerations of using this point-of-care (POC) device under real field conditions that could have been different from those recommended by the manufacturer. This study in different conditions is a necessity given to the difficulties in African settings. We have included operational results with POC device storage and temperature and hygrometry conditions recorded at the time of the testing, the POC performances, as well as a qualitative study to explore the acceptability of the device to a range of health care professionals supposed to use it. In Mali, using the HPLC reference test, sensitivity and specificity were both estimated to be 100%, regardless of the Hb phenotype. For a person expressing a particular Hb phenotype, the likelihood of being diagnosed with an identical Hb phenotype by the Sickle SCAN® test is 100%. This test was performed under favorable conditions of constant temperature and relative humidity, monitored by an air-conditioning system. In Togo, using

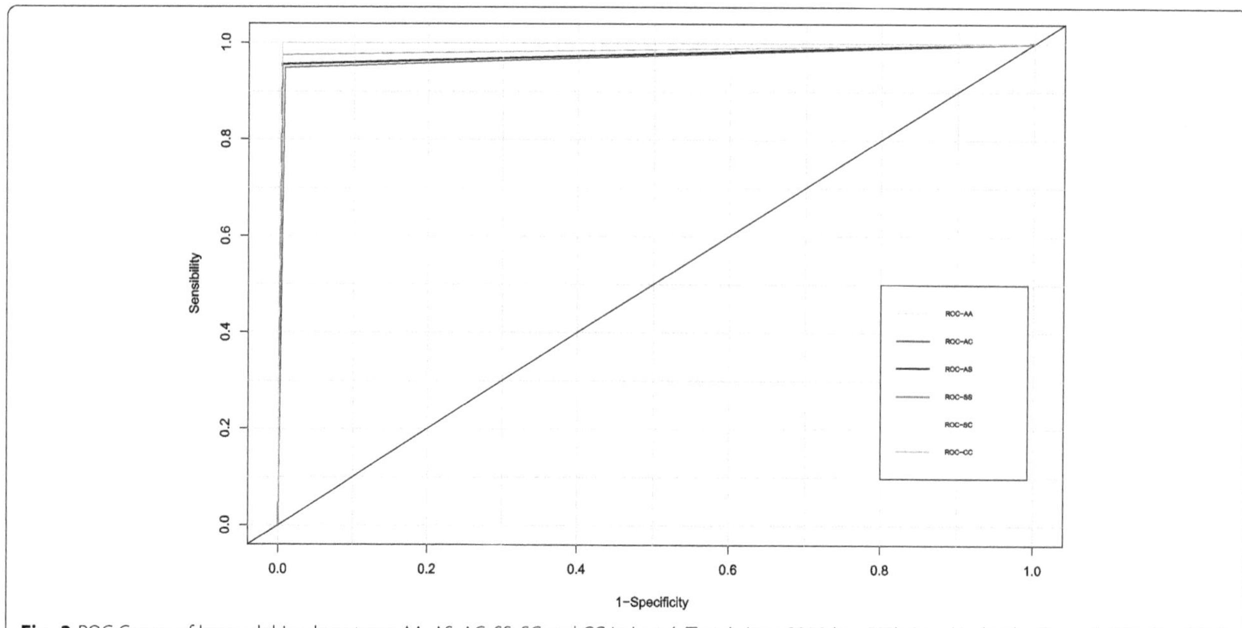

Fig. 3 ROC Curves of hemoglobin phenotypes AA, AS, AC, SS, SC and CC in Lomé (Togo), June 2016 (*n* = 295). Area Under the Curve (AUC): AS= 0·976 IC95% [0·945-1], AC= 0·9705 IC95% [0·935-1], AA= 1, SS = 0.9858 IC95% [0·9616-1], SC= 0·9866 IC95% [0·964-1], CC = 0·9866 IC95% [0·994-1]

the CE reference test, the POC test identifies and differentiates HbAA controls and HbCC perfectly. But, compared with the Malian samples, the estimated sensitivity declined for HbAS or HbAC phenotypes, reaching a minimum of 94.9% for HbAC patients. Specificity estimates for all cases were excellent, exceeding 99%. In Togo, among the six misclassifications on a total of 295 samples, five could have occurred under unfavorable ambient conditions (temperature/relative humidity), and one was related to an error of interpretation. Nevertheless, the Sickle SCAN® test allow to perfectly predict HbAA and HbCC phenotypes diagnosed by CE, and prediction is almost perfect for HbAS, HbAC, HbSS, and HbSC ($p < 10^{-5}$). For each model, the power discrimination was not improved after adjustment. Overall, the rate of misclassification is estimated to be 6/535 tests performed, i.e. 1.1%: this rate in a diagnosis strategy could be considered as acceptable, as it will be further confirmed. Thus, we conclude that this POC device is accurate and robust when used under field West-African conditions. But, it also emerges that the sensitivity and specificity of the Togo data with regard to the identification of carriers and patients are lower than the sensitivity and specificity demonstrated for the identification of healthy subjects. In addition, the use of this POC device was acceptable to health care professionals, who found it to be simple, easy to interpret, and yielding results in less than 5 min.

Validity of the study

All three diagnostic tests – the two comparator reference tests and the and POC index test – were performed and analyzed independently. The index POC test was not a component of the reference test. All tests were administered on a blinded basis; different providers conducted different tests. In addition, no clinical information was provided to persons conducting the Sickle SCAN® test. All subjects were initially diagnosed by a single national reference test, a strict monitoring process insuring control for verification bias. Our CRF contains dedicated space for ambiguous results, and after monitoring, no such results were reported during the study period. After test reading, each device was photographed to allow a control quality process. Finally, sensitivity and specificity estimates were precisely assessed for each phenotype. Thus, we conclude that our study findings are robust.

Based on the HPLC reference method, Kanter et al. found similar results in seventy-one US subjects aged 6 months to 72 years, diagnosed by HPLC for HbAA, HbAC, and SCD phenotypes [13] with 99% sensitivity and 99% specificity. We noted a 2% specificity differential for HbAC phenotype in their study [13], compared to our results in Mali.

Testing 139 blood samples issued from a pediatric and adult mixed population in USA, MacGann et al. found a sensitivity of 98.3% to 100% and specificity of 92.5–100% to detect the presence of HbA, HbS, and HbC compared to CE as a standard [15]: thus, a lower sensitivity and specificity rates in HbAA persons, with a discrepancy equal to − 1·7% and − 6·0%, respectively, and in HbCC patients. We found similar results in our study conducted in Togo. McGann et al. also described excellent inter-observer agreement [15]. Finally, two recent studies were conducted in field conditions in sub-Saharan countries. In a preliminary small sample-size study in Nigeria, it diagnosed SCD with 100% sensitivity and 98% specificity compared to HPLC as the standard in 57 adults and pediatric patients (including only one HbSS and one HbSC) [16]. In Tanzania, it diagnosed SCD with 98.1% sensitivity and 91.1% specificity compared to electrophoresis for un-experienced observers in 745 participants [17]. These results were very similar to ours.

Our study has three limitations. First, due to random variation, no case of S/β°thalassaemia was included in the cases of Bamako setting. But the principle of the test already suggests that such phenotypes cannot be recognized because their definition requires the determination of minor fractions of hemoglobin (HbF and HbA2), red cell indices, level of iron stores of body, and sometimes family and genetic studies [15]. Second, we did not assess test accuracy during the neonatal period, for logistical reasons but the accuracy assessment of the Sickle SCAN® test on fetal Hb forms remains of interest. Third, we were not able to estimate negative and positive predictive values for a given screening strategy; these performance measures will be further addressed in a separate study to be conducted in new-born. Finally, we were not able to provide more details on the cost of the current diagnosis methods used in Togo and Mali that are more complex to assess with both direct and indirect costs. In our study, the test price ranged from US$5 to US$6 (provided free of cost by manufacturer and excluding taxes in 2016), this relatively affordable test received positive feedback from health professionals regarding its ease of use and its speed and convenience. Elsewhere, the commercial costs alone can run to $5–10 per test in resource-limited setting and should more affordable with its regular use [22].

Conclusion

Thus, we conclude that the Sickle SCAN® test demonstrates excellent to perfect (HbAS, HbAC, HbSS, HbSC) or perfect (HbCC and HbAA) diagnostic accuracy, under both laboratory and field conditions. This rapid test demonstrates outstanding sensitivity and specificity when evaluated against existing gold standards. In addition, this test allows instrument- and electricity-free visual diagnostics, and requires minimal training to be performed. This rapid test is cheaper, easier to implement, and logistically more convenient than the current standard diagnostic methods in use in West Africa.

Further studies are now crucial to assess the predictive value indicators and the rate of true positive/negative among people receiving a Sickle SCAN® test result. More specially, there is a need to assess this POC device to detect SCD in the neonatal period, and fully measure the interaction with fetal hemoglobin, to inform the implementation of a neonatal screening strategy that could change the future of patients born with SCD.

While more research is needed to study the performances of the rapid test in the neonatal population, this study henceforth adds important new data to the growing evidence that this POC test could be used as first-line in a screening strategy to eliminate healthy subjects first before confirming remaining cases or indeterminate with a standard reference test. It has the potential to significantly impact the delay of diagnosis and improve the access to early care in patients living with SCD in resource-limited settings [13].

Abbreviations

aOR: Adjusted odds ratio; AUC: Area under the curve; CE: Capillary electrophoresis; CI: Confidence intervals; CRF: Case Report Form; Hb: Hemoglobin; HPLC: High Performance Liquid Chromatography; IEF: Isoelectric focusing; POC: Point-Of-Care; SCD: Sickle cell disease

Acknowledgements

We acknowledge all of the subjects and patients included in this study. We also thank the staff from all the participating centers, the investigators and coordinators contributing to the project. We warmly thank Béatrice Garrette, Jean-Paul Caubère (Pierre Fabre Foundation), Christophe Longuet (Mérieux Foundation) and Didier Ekouévi (Faculté des Sciences de la Santé, Lomé) for their support. Special thanks David Paltiel (Yale School of Public Health) for his efficient and courteous help in editing this paper. The funders had no role in study design, data collection and analysis, decision to publish, or preparation of the manuscript.

Funding

This study was funded by the Pierre Fabre and Mérieux Foundations. The funders had no role in study design, data collection and analysis, decision to publish, or preparation of the manuscript.

Authors' contributions

DD, AG, EL, VL, YAS and IK designed the study. VP trained the study staff and monitored the study. MY, AM, RB and PG conducted the study in the field. RB and GG conducted the analysis under VL supervision. VL and RB co-wrote the first draft of the manuscript. All authors have read and approved the final version.

Competing interests

The authors declare that they have no competing interests.

Author details

[1]CHU Campus, Lomé, Togo. [2]Centre de Recherche et Lutte contre la Drépanocytose, 03 BP: 186 BKO 03, Point G, Commune III, Bamako, Mali. [3]Inserm UMR 1027, Epidémiologie et analyses en santé publique : risques, maladies chroniques et handicaps, Université Paul Sabatier Toulouse 3, Faculté de Médecine Purpan, 37 Allées Jules Guesde, 31073 Toulouse Cedex 7, France. [4]Département de Santé Publique, Université de Lomé, Lome, Togo. [5]Pierre Fabre Foundation, Lavaur, France. [6]Mérieux Foundation, Lyon, France.

References

1. Ware RE, de Montalembert M, Tshilolo L, Abboud MR. Sickle cell disease. Lancet. 2017;17:30193–9
2. Piel FB, Patil AP, Howes RE, Nyangiri OA, Gething PW, Dewi M, Temperley WH, Williams TN, Weatherall DJ, Hay SI. Global epidemiology of sickle haemoglobin in neonates: a contemporary geostatistical model-based map and population estimates. Lancet. 2013;381(9861):142–51.
3. Rees DC, Williams TN, Gladwin MT. Sickle-cell disease. Lancet. 2010; 376(9757):2018–31.
4. Nagel RL, Fabry ME, Steinberg MH. The paradox of hemoglobin SC disease. Blood Rev. 2003;17(3):167–78.
5. Galacteros F. Sickle cell anemia. Physiopathology and diagnosis. Rev Prat. 1995;45(3):351–60.
6. Piel FB, Hay SI, Gupta S, Weatherall DJ, Williams TN. Global burden of sickle cell anaemia in children under five, 2010-2050: modelling based on demographics, excess mortality, and interventions. PLoS Med. 2013;10(7):e1001484.
7. Chaturvedi S, DeBaun MR. Evolution of sickle cell disease from a life-threatening disease of children to a chronic disease of adults: the last 40 years. Am J Hematol. 2016;91(1):5–14.
8. Housni HE, Vandesompele J, Vannuffel P, Gulbis B, Parma J, Cochaux P. Rapid and easy prenatal diagnosis of sickle cell anemia using double-dye LNA probe technology. Br J Haematol. 2007;136(3):509–10.
9. Mantikou E, Harteveld CL, Giordano PC. Newborn screening for hemoglobinopathies using capillary electrophoresis technology: testing the Capillarys Neonat fast Hb device. Clin Biochem. 2010;43(16–17):1345–50.
10. Bain BJ. Haemoglobinopathy diagnosis: algorithms, lessons and pitfalls. Blood reviews. 2011;25(5):205–13.
11. Ryan K, Bain BJ, Worthington D, James J, Plews D, Mason A, Roper D, Rees DC, de la Salle B, Streetly A, et al. Significant haemoglobinopathies: guidelines for screening and diagnosis. Br J Haematol. 2010;149(1):35–49.
12. Van Delft P, Lenters E, Bakker-Verweij M, de Korte M, Baylan U, Harteveld CL, Giordano PC. Evaluating five dedicated automatic devices for haemoglobinopathy diagnostics in multi-ethnic populations. Int J Lab Hematol. 2009;31(5):484–95.
13. Kanter J, Telen MJ, Hoppe C, Roberts CL, Kim JS, Yang X. Validation of a novel point of care testing device for sickle cell disease. BMC Med. 2015;13:225.
14. Quinn CT, Paniagua MC, DiNello RK, Panchal A, Geisberg M. A rapid, inexpensive and disposable point-of-care blood test for sickle cell disease using novel, highly specific monoclonal antibodies. Br J Haematol. 2016; 175(4):724–32.
15. McGann PT, Schaefer BA, Paniagua M, Howard TA, Ware RE. Characteristics of a rapid, point-of-care lateral flow immunoassay for the diagnosis of sickle cell disease. Am J Hematol. 2016;91(2):205–10.
16. Nwegbu MM, Isa HA, Nwankwo BB, Okeke CC, Edet-Offong UJ, Akinola NO, Adekile AD, Aneke JC, Okocha EC, Ulasi T, et al. Preliminary evaluation of a point-of-care testing device (SickleSCAN) in screening for sickle cell disease. Hemoglobin. 2017;41(2):77–82.
17. Smart LR, Ambrose EE, Raphael KC, Hokororo A, Kamugisha E, Tyburski EA, Lam WA, Ware RE, McGann PT. Simultaneous point-of-care detection of anemia and sickle cell disease in Tanzania: the RAPID study. Ann Hematol. 2018;97(2):239–46.
18. Vandenbroucke JP. Strega, Strobe, Stard, Squire, Moose, Prisma, Gnosis, Trend, Orion, Coreq, Quorom, Remark... and Consort: for whom does the guideline toll? J Clin Epidemiol. 2009;62(6):594–6.
19. Ou CN, Rognerud CL. Liquid chromatography in diagnosis of rare hemoglobin variant (Hb Chicago) and its combination with HB S: Hb Chicago/S trait and Hb Chicago/sickle cell disease. Clin Chem. 1996;42(5):774–6.
20. Machin D, Campbell MJ, Tan SB, Tan SH. Sample size tables for clinical studies. 3rd ed. Chichester: Wiley; 2008.
21. Rutjes AW, Reitsma JB, Vandenbroucke JP, Glas AS, Bossuyt PM. Case-control and two-gate designs in diagnostic accuracy studies. Clin Chem. 2005;51(8):1335–41.
22. Williams TN. An accurate and affordable test for the rapid diagnosis of sickle cell disease could revolutionize the outlook for affected children born in resource-limited settings. BMC Med. 2015;13:238.

Hematological profile of pregnant women at St. Paul's Hospital Millennium Medical College, Addis Ababa, Ethiopia

Angesom Gebreweld[1*], Delayehu Bekele[2] and Aster Tsegaye[3]

Abstract

Background: In pregnancy, hematological changes occur in order to meet the demands of the developing fetus and placenta, with major alterations in blood volume. Abnormal hematological profile affects pregnancy and its outcome. This study aimed to assess hematological profiles of pregnant women at a tertiary care teaching hospital.

Method: This cross sectional study was conducted among 284 consecutive pregnant women at St. Paul's Hospital Millennium Medical College. Socio-demographic characteristics were collected using pre-tested structured questionnaire. About 4 ml of venous blood was collected from each participant for hematological parameters analysis using Cell-Dyn1800 (Abbott Laboratories Diagnostics Division, USA) and peripheral blood film review.

Result: There were differences in mean hematological parameters between trimesters: specifically differences in mean values of WBC (1stand 3rd), Hb(1stand2nd and 1st& 3rd), HCT (1stand2nd), RDW (1stand2nd and 1stand3rd), neutrophil and lymphocyte (1stand 2nd and 1stand3^{rd,} for both) were statistically significant ($p < 0.05$). The prevalence rates of anemia and thrombocytopenia were 11.62 and 7.7%, respectively and were dominantly of mild type. On the bases of blood picture, we classified anemia's of pregnancy as microcytic hypochromic (51.5%), normocytic hypochromic (27.3%), normocytic normochromic (18.2%), and dimorphic (3%).

Conclusion: Significant changes in selected hematological parameters between trimesters, and an anemia and thrombocytopenia of mild type were documented in this study. The commonest morphologic features were mostly characteristic features of iron deficiency anemia. These warrant the need for monitoring hematological parameters of pregnant women at any stage of the pregnancy to avoid adverse outcomes.

Keywords: Pregnancy, Hematological profile, Anemia, Thrombocytopenia

Background

In pregnancy, hematological changes occur in order to meet the demands of the developing fetus and placenta, with major alterations in blood volume. The plasma volume increase by 40 to 45% on average, this increase is mediated by a direct action of progesterone and estrogen on the kidney causing the release of renin and thus an activation of the aldosterone renin-angio-tensin mechanism. This leads to renal sodium retention and an increase in total body water. This increase occurs faster in the late second trimester [1–3].

Red blood cell mass increases by 15–20% as a result of the increase in the production of erythropoietin. As the increase in red cell mass is relatively smaller than that of plasma volume, the net result of hemoglobin (Hb) concentration falls by 1–2 g/dl. This is termed the physiological anemia of pregnancy [3, 4].

In pregnancy, the peripheral blood count of white blood cell (WBC) is raised due to pregnancy induced physiological stress. Neutrophils contribute most to the overall higher WBC count. [5]. However, the platelet count decreases during pregnancy because of hemodilution, increased platelet activation and consumption, particularly in the third trimester [4, 5].

* Correspondence: afsaha@gmail.com
[1]Department of Medical Laboratory Science, College of Medicine and Health Science, Wollo University, Dessie, Ethiopia
Full list of author information is available at the end of the article

Although physiological in nature, abnormal hematological profile affects pregnancy and its outcome. One of the most important underlying cause of maternal mortality is due to underlying hematological complications. Anemia and thrombocytopenia are the most frequent hematologic complications during pregnancy [6, 7].

Anemia of pregnancy is said to occur when Hb concentration is less than 110 g/l [8], as per World Health Organization (WHO) recommendation. Global prevalence of anemia in pregnant women is 41.8%. Africa and Asia are the most heavily affected regions. Throughout Africa, about 56% of pregnant women are anemic. As documented in the WHO2008 report, this hematological disorder is a severe public health problem in Ethiopian pregnant women and the estimated prevalence was 62.7% [9, 10].

The functional consequences of anemia are serious and include an increased risk of maternal, fetal, and neonatal mortality. Poor pregnancy outcomes such as low birth weight and preterm birth; impaired cognitive development, reduced learning capacity, and diminished school performance in children; and decreased productivity in adults are among the consequences [11]. In neighboring Sudan, 20.3% of maternal deaths are associated with anemia [12].

Thrombocytopenia is one of the most common hematologic abnormalities encountered during pregnancy. About 8–10% of pregnant women are affected by thrombocytopenia (platelet count $< 150 \times 10^9$/L), particularly in the third trimester. Approximately 75% of these cases are due to a benign process of gestational thrombocytopenia which is mild and have no significance for mother or fetus. But, in some instances, thrombocytopenia can also be associated with a complex clinical disorder such as preeclampsia and hemolysis, elevated liver enzymes, low platelets (HELLP) syndrome (20%), or idiopathic thrombocytopenic purpura (ITP) (5%). There can also be profound and even life-threatening results for both mother and baby [13–15].

As several studies showed pregnancy may have effect on hematological parameter and essential to monitor these parameters at any stage of the pregnancy [16–18]. This study was, therefore, conducted to assess hematological profile of pregnant women at St. Paul's Hospital Millennium Medical College, Addis Ababa, Ethiopia. The study provided information about the magnitude of anemia, morphological type of anemia, thrombocytopenia and change of hematological values at different trimesters which is important to detect hematological complication early and to administer appropriate therapy.

Methods

Study design, area and setting

A cross sectional health facility based study was conducted at St. Paul's Hospital, Addis Ababa, Ethiopia from June to August 2014. St. Paul's Hospital Millennium Medical College (SPHMMC) is the second largest public hospital in Ethiopia, which is located in Gullele sub city in Addis Ababa and built by Emperor Haile Selassie in 1969. The hospital receives referrals from around the country and is under the guidance of the Ethiopian Federal Ministry of Health.

Population

A total of 284 consecutive pregnant women were enrolled from antenatal care clinic of obstetrics and gynecology Department of SPHMMC. Written informed consent was obtained from all. Pregnant women with bleeding problem, multiple pregnancies, Hepatitis B Virus infection, human immunodeficiency virus and less than 18 years of age were excluded from the study.

Data collection

A structured pre tested interviewer administered questionnaire (see Additional file 1) and medical records were used to collect socio-demographic and clinical data of the study participants. Venous blood specimen (4 ml) was taken from each pregnant woman by a senior laboratory professional for peripheral blood film and complete blood count. Cell-Dyn 1800 (Abbott Laboratories Diagnostics Division, USA) hematological analyzer was used to determine complete blood count. Peripheral blood smear were prepared and stained by Wright's stain to look at morphological characteristics of anemia. The peripheral smears were examined by a senior laboratory technologist and principal investigator independently. Standard operating procedures were strictly followed in each step to maintain quality of the laboratory results.

According to WHO, Anemia of pregnancy is said to occur when Hb concentration is less than 110 g/l. Anemic pregnant women were further categorized as women with mild anemia, moderate anemia and severe anemia which corresponds to Hb value 100–109 g/l, 70–99 g/l, and lower than 70 g/l respectively [8]. Thrombocytopenia is said to be present when the platelet count of the pregnant women is less than 150×10^9 / L. The platelet counts from 100 to 150×10^9/L is considered mild thrombocytopenia, levels ranging from 50 to 100×10^9/L are considered as moderate thrombocytopenia and levels less than 50×10^9/L are considered as severe thrombocytopenia [15].

Data analysis

The data was entered and analyzed using Statistical Package for the Social Science (SPSS) Version16 statistical software. Frequencies and means ± standard deviation (SD) were used to summarize descriptive statistics. One-way analysis of variance (ANOVA) was used in the analysis to compare the hematologic values among trimesters. P values < 0.05 were considered as statistically significant.

Ethical considerations

The study was approved by Departmental Research and Ethics Review Committee (DRERC) of the Department of Medical Laboratory Sciences, Addis Ababa University. After a letter of cooperation sent to St Paul's Hospital Millennium Medical College from the Department of Medical Laboratory Sciences the Institutional Review Board also approved the study. Then a letter informing the hospital administrators was written from the Institutional Review Board (IRB) and Permission obtained from St. Paul's Hospital Millennium Medical College to conduct the study. Individual consent was obtained before the questionnaires were administered and blood samples were collected. To ensure confidentiality, participants' data were linked to a code number. Any abnormal test results of participants were communicated to their attending physician.

Results

General characteristics of the study participants

A total of 284 pregnant women with a mean (SD) age of 27.3 ± 4.48 years (ranges from 18 to 40) were included in the study. About 170 (59.9%) were in their third trimester, 66 (23.2%) in second trimester, and 48 (16.9%) in first trimester. Majority of the study groups 118 (41.5%) were in the age range of 26–30 years and urban residents (261, 91.9%) (Table 1).

Table 1 Characteristics of Pregnant women ($N = 284$) at St. Paul's Hospital Millennium Medical College Addis Ababa, Ethiopia, June to August 2014

Variables		Frequency	Percentage (%)
Age group (years)	≤20	16	5.6
	21–25	93	32.7
	26–30	118	41.5
	31–35	43	15.1
	≥36	14	4.9
Occupation	Farmer	16	5.6
	Housewife	164	57.7
	Government	24	8.5
	Student	8	2.8
	Private	72	25.4
Educational status	Illiterate	42	14.8
	Elementary	115	40.5
	Secondary	54	19.0
	Preparatory	23	8.1
	University/college	50	17.6
Residence	Rural	23	8.1
	Urban	261	91.9
Trimester	1st trimester	48	16.9
	2nd trimester	66	23.2
	3rd trimester	170	59.9

Hematological profiles of the study participants

The overall mean (SD) of selected hematological parameters for the study participants were as follows: WBC count 7.93 ± 2.68 × 10^9/L, RBC count 4.58 ± 2.34 × 10^{12}/L, Hb130.1 ± 16.4 g/L, HCT 40.07 ± 4.15%, MCV 90.60 ± 6.59 fL, MCH 29.32 ± 2.72 pg, MCHC 32.33 ± 1.35%, and PLT 249.36 ± 80.08 × 10^9/L(Table 2).

When analyzed by trimester, the mean (SD) WBC values for the respective first, second and third trimester pregnant women were 7.02 ± 2.61, 7.83 ± 2.62, and 8.22 ± 2.68(× 10^9/L), respectively. The difference was statistically significant between those in1st and 3rd trimester ($P < 0.05$).The Mean Hb value of pregnant women in first trimester (136.5 ± 15.9 g/l) was significantly higher compared to those in second trimester (126.2 ± 17.2 g/l), and in third trimester (129.7 ± 15.8 g/l). Mean HCT value in the three pregnancy groups were 41.59 ± 4.47, 38.92 ± 4.47, and 40.08 ± 3.79 (%), with a statistically significant difference between those in 1st and 2nd trimesters ($P < 0.05$). Whereas the mean red cell indices (MCV, MCH and MCHC) and mean PLT values did not differ between the three trimester groups (Table 2).

Moreover, the mean RDW values of those in the 2nd and 3rd trimesters are higher than those in the 1st trimester. The neutrophil counts also follow the same increasing pattern while the lymphocyte counts in the 2nd and 3rd trimesters group are significantly lower than those in the 1st trimester ($P < 0.05$) (Table 2).

Hematological abnormalities

Using the WHO criterion of Hb < 110 g/dl as indicative of anemia, 33 (11.62%) pregnant mothers were anemic. Of them, 23 (69.70%) were mildly anemic (Table 3). Based on RBC morphologic classification of anemia, most of the anemic pregnant women had microcytic hypochromic 17 (51.5%) type of anemia (Fig. 1).

Thrombocytopenia (Platelet count < 150 × 10^9/L), was detected in 22 pregnant women giving a prevalence of 7.7%. Among them, most 20 (90.91%) were mildly thrombocytopenic (Table 4). The prevalence of thrombocytopenia was 4.2, 6.1 and 9.4% at first, second and third trimester groups, respectively (Table 5).

Discussion

The study reported herein aimed to determine the hematological profile of pregnant women visiting St. Paul's Hospital Millennium Medical College in Addis Ababa from June to August 2014.

The progressive increment of WBC from those in their first (7.02 ± 2.61) to those in their third (8.22 ± 2.68) trimester and the dominance of neutrophil in our study

Table 2 Hematological Profiles of pregnant women based on trimesters (Mean ± SD) in St. Paul's Hospital Millennium Medical College Addis Ababa, Ethiopia, June to August 2014

Parameters	Trimester				*P*-Value		
	Overall	1st trimester PW	2nd trimester PW	3rd trimester PW	1st&2nd	1st&3rd	2nd&3rd
WBC x 10^9/L	7.93 ± 2.68	7.02 ± 2.61	7.83 ± 2.62	8.22 ± 2.68	.246	.018	.580
RBC x 10^{12}/L	4.58 ± 2.34	4.61 ± 0.51	4.86 ± 4.78	4.46 ± 0.47	.836	.927	.475
Hb (g/l)	130.1 ± 16.4	136.5 ± 15.9	126.2 ± 17.2	129.7 ± 15.8	.002	.031	.275
HCT (%)	40.07 ± 4.15	41.59 ± 4.47	38.92 ± 4.47	40.08 ± 3.79	.002	.061	.126
MCV (fl)	90.60 ± 6.59	90.26 ± 5.68	91.24 ± 7.29	90.45 ± 6.56	.712	.982	.689
MCH (pg)	29.32 ± 2.72	29.58 ± 2.41	29.53 ± 3.16	29.16 ± 2.62	.995	.615	.618
MCHC %	32.33 ± 1.35	32.72 ± 1.42	32.30 ± 1.51	32.23 ± 1.24	.229	.070	.934
RDW (%)	13.99 ± 1.71	13.25 ± 1.22	14.51 ± 2.09	14.01 ± 1.59	.000	.017	.099
PLT x 10^9/L	249.36 ± 80.08	267.62 ± 100.89	254.02 ± 68.06	242.39 ± 77.29	.641	.131	.575
MPV (fl)	9.62 ± 1.37	9.48 ± 1.32	9.60 ± 1.61	9.66 ± 1.28	.888	.708	.957
Lymphocyte (%)	24.31 ± 8.64	28.42 ± 10.68	24.22 ± 8.16	23.18 ± 7.84	.025	.001	.674
MID WBC (%)	7.57 ± 2.34	8.07 ± 2.5	7.11 ± 2.12	7.61 ± 2.35	.986	.863	.707
Neutrophil (%)	67.72 ± 9.17	63.52 ± 11.27	67.91 ± 8.33	68.82 ± 8.52	.028	.001	.766

PW pregnant women, $P < 0.05$ is statically significant
MID WBC: which include Monocyte, eosinophile, basophile, and other midsized immature WBCs

is consistent with findings of Akinbami et al. (from 7.37 ± 2.38 to 8.31 ± 2.15) [19], Das et al. (from 6.14 ± 1.76 to 8.09 ± 4.12) [16], Osonuga et al. (from 6.22 ± 1.79 to 8.11 ± 4.13) [17] and Ifeanyi et al. (from4.8+/− 2.6 to 7.81 +/− 1.7) [18]. Physiologic stress induced by pregnancy [5] has been implicated as a possible mechanism for pregnancy associated leukocytosis. Besides, fetal immunity development pathways which include selective immune tolerance and modulation have also been suggested as possible explanations [20].

The finding of a significantly higher number of neutrophils in the second and third trimester pregnant women compared to the first trimester pregnant women in our study concurs with this scientific explanation. Neutrophils are the major type of WBC counts and their number can double during pregnancy compared to its postpartum values [5, 6].

In the present study, hemoglobin concentration and hematocrit values were highest in the first trimester, reach their lowest point in the second trimester and begin to raise again in the third trimester groups. This is consistent with a study conducted by James et al. (Hb127.3 ± 11.4114.1 ± 11.6, & 116.7 ± 11.8 g/l and HCT 37.05 ± 2.96, 33.12 ± 3.00 and 34.03 ± 2.97% for 1st, 2nd and 3rd trimesters respectively) [21] and Akinbami et al. (32.07 ± 6.80, 29.76 ± 5.21, and 33.04 ± 3.88%) [19] for hematocrit. While it contradicts with a study conducted by Ifeanyi et al. [18] and Osonuga et al. [17] in Nigeria which respectively showed low Hb and HCT in the first trimester, highest in the second trimester and drop in the 3rd trimester.

The decrease in hemoglobin concentration and packed cell volume from those in first trimester to those in second trimester may be due to hemodilution, hormonal changes, and increased iron demand [6, 16, 19]. Hormonal changes results production of rennin from kidneys to increase plasma volume during pregnancy. The increase

Table 3 Distribution of anemia by severity among the anemic pregnant women ($n = 33$), St. Paul's Hospital Millennium Medical College Addis Ababa, Ethiopia, 2014

Severity of anemia	Number	Percentage (%)
Mild anemia	23	69.7
Moderate anemia	10	30.3
Severe anemia	0	0
Total	33	100

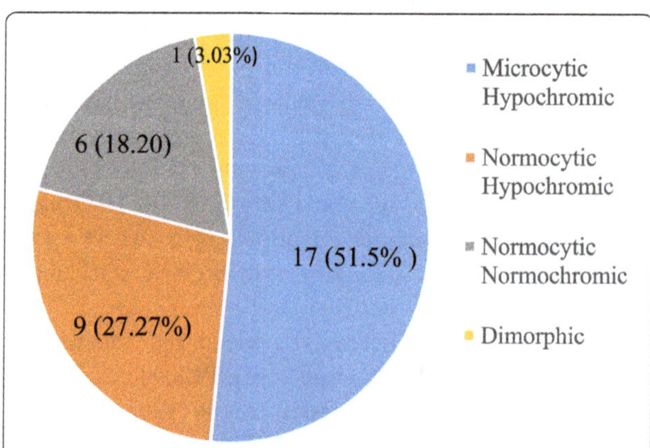

Fig. 1 Distribution of Morphologic Type of Anemia among the anemic pregnant women ($n = 33$), St. Paul's Hospital Millennium Medical College Addis Ababa, Ethiopia, 2014

Table 4 Distribution of thrombocytopenia by severity among thrombocytopenic pregnant women ($n = 22$), St. Paul's Hospital Millennium Medical College Addis Ababa, Ethiopia, 2014

Severity	Number	Percentage (%)
Mild thrombocytopenia	20	90.91
Moderate thrombocytopenia	2	9.09
Severe thrombocytopenia	0	0
Total	22	100

in plasma volume is relatively greater than the increase in red cell mass, which results in a fall in maternal Hb and HCT. In late pregnancy, plasma volume increases slowly that lead to a slight rise in hemoglobin and hematocrit value, it may account for the slight rise in Hb and HCT in the third trimester [5, 19].

Our study also reported a gradual reduction in PLT count as pregnancy advanced but the mean difference between the three trimesters was not statically significant. Our finding is similar with study conducted by Ajibola et al. [22], Akinbami et al. [19] and James et al. [21]. The reduction of platelet count as pregnancy advanced may be due to an increase in blood volume, increased platelet activation, and decreased life span in the uteroplacental circulation [5–7]. The present study also found an increment of mean platelet volume as the pregnancy advanced. This result is in agreement with a study conducted in Port Harcourt, Nigeria [23].

The finding of 11.62% anemia in this study is comparable to studies conducted in Iranian pregnant women (13.6%), Nakhonsawan, Thailand (14.1%), Sudaneese (10%), and Ethiopian women from Hawassa (15.1%), Gondar (16.6%), and Debre Berhan (9.7%) [24–29].

The result of the present study is much lower than studies conducted in Karantaka India (82.9%), highlands of Tibet (ranges 41.3–77.9%), Nepal (41.02%), Uyo Nigeria (54.5%), Jamaica (34.8%), west Algeria (40.08%), Uganda (63.1%), Eastern Ethiopia (56.8%), south west Ethiopia (53.9%), and Arsi zone (Ethiopia) (36.6%) [30–39]. Our result is also lower than results reported by studies in Turkey (27.1%), Sokoto, Nigeria (21.3%), and two other studies from Ethiopia namely Azezo in Gondar (21.6%), and Tikur Anbessa Specialized Hospital in Addis Ababa (21.3%) [40–43].

The possible reason for the difference may be due to the differences in socio economic status, geographical variation and differences in dietary habits of the study participants. The lower result of our study may also be due to the Governments effort to achieve Sustainable Development Goals (SDGs).

The predominance of mild type of anemia in the current study fit well with studies conducted in Uyo Teaching Hospital Nigeria [33], Western Nepal [32], and studies conducted in different parts of Ethiopia: Tikur Anbessa Specialized Hospital [43], Debre Berhan Health Institutions [29], Southwest Ethiopia [38], and Gondar [28]. However, our result deviates from the findings from Karnataka India, west Algeria and Jimma (Ethiopia) which showed high rate of moderate Anemia [30, 35, 44].

The common morphological characteristic of anemia identified in our study, mainly microcytic hypochromic, and normocytic hypochromic, is deviated from studies conducted in Turkey [40], Northern Nigeria [45] and Gondar [28] which showed higher rate of normocytic normochromic type of anemia. Microcytic hypochromic and normocytic hypochromic blood picture are characteristic of iron deficiency anemia [33, 46], and our findings are in agreement with studies conducted in Sudan [47], Sokoto Nigeria [41], Uyo Nigeria [33], and New Delhi [46].

Thrombocytopenia is second to anemia as the most common hematologic abnormality encountered during pregnancy. The finding of 7.7% thrombocytopenia prevalence in the current study is similar to studies conducted in India (8.17%) and (8.8%), Iraq (8%), and Ahmedabad (7.67%) [48–51]. It also agrees with values indicated in a literature review conducted by Myers [15], which showed 8–10% rate of thrombocytopenia of all pregnancies. However, our result is lower than studies conducted in Ghana (15.3%) and Nigeria (13.5%) [22, 52].

The mildness of thrombocytopenia noted in the current study parallels findings from Iraq [51] Ghana, India, Nigeria, and Ahmedabad [22, 48, 49, 52]. The finding of predominantly mild thrombocytopeniamay be attributed to gestational thrombocytopenia (GT), which is of mild type and accounts for the majority of thrombocytopenias during pregnancy [7]. Though it is not associated with any adverse events for either the mother or baby and requires no specific treatment, other etiologies must be excluded (i.e. megaloblastic anemia, immune thrombocytopenia, eclampsia, and liver disorders) [6]. Especially, many features of GT are similar to mild immune thrombocytopenia and it can be difficult to distinguish between the two disorders [15].

The observed high prevalence of thrombocytopenia in the third trimester, which also agrees with other studies [22, 49, 51, 52], could be due to an increase in platelet

Table 5 Distribution of thrombocytopenia among pregnant women at different trimesters ($N = 284$), St. Paul's Hospital Millennium Medical College Addis Ababa, Ethiopia, 2014

Characteristics	Thrombocytopenia status		Total
	Thrombocytopenic (%)	Non-Thrombocytopenic (%)	
Trimester			
1st trimester	2 (4.2%)	46 (95.8%)	48
2nd trimester	4 (6.1%)	62 (93.9%)	66
3rd trimester	16 (9.4%)	154 (90.6%)	170

aggregation especially during last 8 weeks of gestation. It has been reported that significant fall in platelet count can occur from 32 weeks of gestation onwards [6]. In the third trimester, platelet count decreases due to hemodilution, increased platelet activation and consumption [5].

Conclusion

In conclusion, in this study WBC, Hb, HCT, RDW, lymphocyte and neutrophil counts showed statistically significant difference between trimesters ($P < 0.05$). The prevalence of anemia and thrombocytopenia, both predominantly of mild type, were 11.62 and 7.7%, respectively. Therefore, the pregnant women should be monitored and their hematological parameters properly interpreted to recognize and avoid pregnancy complications early. This will be of paramount importance in line with meeting the SDGs target related to maternal and child health.

Abbreviations

ANC: Antenatal care; EDTA: Ethylene DiamineTetra Acetic acid; GT: Gestational thrombocytopenia; Hb: Hemoglobin; HCT: Hematocrit; MCH: Mean cell hemoglobin; MCHC: Mean cell hemoglobin concentration; MCV: Mean cell volume; MPV: Mean platelet volume; PLT: Platelet; RBC: Red blood cell; RDW: Red cell distribution width; SDGs: Sustainable Development Goals; WBC: White blood cell; WHO: World health organization

Acknowledgements

We would like to thank Wollo University and Addis Ababa University for the financial and material support for this project. St. Paul's Hospital Millennium Medical College and ANC as well as hospital laboratory staffs are gratefully acknowledged for the support given to undertake this study in the hospital. Our special thanks and appreciation goes to all pregnant women who voluntarily participated in this study.

Funding

This study was funded by Addis Ababa University. The funder has no role in the design of the study and collection, analysis, and interpretation of data and in writing the manuscript.

Authors' contributions

AG, DB, and AT involved in proposal writing, designed the study and participated in all implementation stages of the project. AG and AT also analyzed the data and finalized the write up of the manuscript. AG, DB and AT were responsible for critically revising the proposal and the manuscript. All authors reviewed and approved the final manuscript.

Competing interests

The authors declare that they have no competing interests.

Author details

[1]Department of Medical Laboratory Science, College of Medicine and Health Science, Wollo University, Dessie, Ethiopia. [2]Department of Obstetrics and Gynecology, Saint Paul's Hospital Millennium Medical College, Addis Ababa, Ethiopia. [3]School of Medical Laboratory Science, College of Health science, Addis Ababa University, Addis Ababa, Ethiopia.

References

1. Carlin A, Zarko A. Physiological changes of pregnancy and monitoring. Best Pract Res Clin Obstet Gynaecol. 2008;22(5):801–23.
2. Datta S, Kodali BS, Segal S. Obstetric anesthesia handbook. 5th ed. Springer New York Dordrecht Heidelberg London; 2010.
3. Heidemann BH, McClure JH. Changes in maternal physiology during pregnancy. Br J Anaesth. 2003;3(3):65–8.
4. Pavord S, Hunt B. The obstetric hematology manual. New York: Cambridge University Press; 2010. 278 p
5. Chandra S, Tripathi AK, Mishra S, Amzaru M, Vaish AK. Physiological changes in hematological parameters during pregnancy. Indian J Hematol Blood Transfus. 2012;28(3):144–6.
6. Kaur S, Khan S, Nigam A. Hematological profile and pregnancy: a review. Int J Adv Med. 2014;1(2):68–70.
7. Townsley DM. Hematologic complications of pregnancy. Semin Hematol. 2013;50(3):222–31.
8. WHO. Haemoglobin concentrations for the diagnosis of anaemia and assessment of severity [Internet]. Vitamin and Mineral Nutrition Information System: Geneva, World Health Organization; 2011 [cited 2016 Jul 17]. Available from: http://www.who.int/vmnis/indicators/haemoglobin. pdf.
9. WHO. Worldwide prevalence of anaemia 1993–2005: WHO global database on Anaemia. In: World Health Organization; 2008.
10. McLean E, Mary C, Egli I, Wojdyla D, de BB. Worldwide prevalence of anemia, WHO vitamin and mineral nutrition information system, 1993–2005. Public Health Nutr. 2008:1–11.
11. Allen LH. Anemia and iron deficiency: effects on pregnancy outcome. Am Soc Clin Nutr. 71:1280S–4S.
12. Mohammed AA, Elnour MH, Mohammed EE, Ahmed SA, Abdelfattah AI. Maternal mortality in Kassala state - eastern Sudan: community-based study using reproductive age mortality survey (RAMOS). BMC Pregnancy Childbirth. 2011;11:102.
13. Rajasekhar A, Gernsheimer T, Stasi R, James AH. 2013 clinical practice guide on thrombocytopenia in pregnancy. American Society of Hematology; 2013.
14. Boehlen F. Thrombocytopenia during pregnancy Importance,diagnosis and management. Hamostaseologie. 2006;26:72–4.
15. Myers B. Thrombocytopenia in pregnancy. Obstet Gynaecol. 2009;11:177–83.
16. Das S, Char D, Sarkar S, Saha TK, Biswas S. Study of hematological parameters in pregnancy. IOSR J Dent Med Sci. 2013;12(1):42–4.
17. Osonuga I, Osonuga O, Onadeko A, Osonuga A, Osonuga A. Hematological profile of pregnant women in southwest of Nigeria. Asian Pac J Trop Dis. 2011:232–4.
18. Ifeanyi OE, Ndubuisi OT, Leticia EOB, Uche EC. Haematological profile of pregnant women in Umuahia, Abia state. Nigeria IntJCurrMicrobiolAppSci. 2014;3(1):713–8.
19. Akinbami AA, Ajibola SO, Rabiu KA, Adewunmi AA, Dosunmu AO, Adediran A, et al. Hematological profile of normal pregnant women in Lagos, Nigeria. Int J Women's Health. 2013;5:227–32.
20. Luppi P. How immune mechanisms are affected by pregnancy. Vaccine. 2003;21(24):3352–7.
21. James TR, Reid HL, Mullings AM. Are published standards for haematological indices in pregnancy applicable across populations: an evaluation in healthy pregnant Jamaican women. BMC Pregnancy Childbirth. 2008;8(8):1–4.
22. Ajibola SO, Akinbami A, Rabiu K, Adewunmi A, Dosunmu A, Adewumi A, et al. Gestational thrombocytopaenia among pregnant women in Lagos, Nigeria. Niger Med J. 2014;55(2):139–43.
23. Amah-Tariah F, Ojeka S, Dapper D. Haematological values in pregnant women in Port Harcourt, Nigeria II: serum iron and transferrin, total and unsaturated iron binding capacity and some red cell and platelet indices. Niger J Physiol Sci. 2011;26:173–8.
24. Barooti E, Rezazadehkermani M, Sadeghirad B, Motaghipisheh S, Tayeri S, Arabi M, et al. Prevalence of Iron deficiency Anemia among Iranian pregnant women; a systematic Reviewand meta-analysis. J Reprod Infertil. 2010;11(1):17–24.
25. Sukrat B, Suwathanapisate P, Siritawee S, Poungthong T, Phupongpankul K. The prevalence of iron deficiency anemia in pregnant women in Nakhonsawan. Thailand J Med Assoc Thai. 2010;93(7):765–70.
26. Abdelgader EA, Diab TA, Kordofani AA, Abdalla SE. Haemoglobnin level, RBCs indices, and iron status in pregnant females in Sudan. Basic Res J Med Clin Sci. 2014;3(2):8–13.
27. Gies S, Brabin B, Yassin M, Cuevas L. Comparison of screening methods for anemia in pregnant women in Awassa, Ethiopia. Tropical Med Int Health. 2003;8(4):301–9.

28. Melku M, Addis Z, Alem M, Enawgaw B. Prevalence and predictors of maternal Anemia during pregnancy in Gondar. Northwest Ethiopia: An Institutional Based Cross-Sectional Study Hindawi Publ Corp Anemia. 2014;2014:1–9.
29. Ayenew F, Abere Y, Timerga G. Pregnancy Anaemia prevalence and associated factors among women attending ante Natal Care in north Shoa zone. Ethiopia Reprod Syst Sex Disord. 2014;3(3)
30. Viveki RG, Halappanavar AB, Viveki PR, Halki SB, Maled VS, Deshpande PS. Prevalence of Anemia and its epidemiological determinants in pregnant women. Al Ameen J Med Sci. 2012;5(3):216–23.
31. Xing Y, Yan H, Dang S, Zhuoma B, Zhou X, Wang D. Hemoglobin levels and anemia evaluation during pregnancy in the highlands of Tibet: a hospital-based study. BMC Public Health. 2009;9(336)
32. Singh P, Khan S, Mittal R. Anemia during pregnancy in the women of western Nepal. Bali Med J. 2013;2(1):14–6.
33. Olatunbosun OA, Abasiattai AM, Bassey EA, James RS, Ibanga G, Morgan A. Prevalence of Anaemia among pregnant women at booking in the University of Uyo Teaching Hospital, Uyo, Nigeria. Hindawi Publ Corp BioMed Res Int. 2014;2014
34. Charles A, Campbell-Stennett D, Yatich N, Jolly P. Predictors of anemia among pregnant women in Westmoreland, Jamaica. Health Care Women Int. 2010;31(7):585–98.
35. Demmouche A, Khelil S, Moulessehoul S. Anemia among pregnant women in the Sidi Bel Abbes region (West Algeria) : an epidemiologic study. Blood Disord Transfus. 2011;2
36. Mbule M, Byaruhanga Y, Kabahenda M, Lubowa A. Determinants of anaemia among pregnant women in rural Uganda. Rural Remote Health. 2013;13:2259.
37. Alene KA, Dohe AM. Prevalence of Anemia and associated factors among pregnant women in an urban area of eastern Ethiopia. Anemia. 2014;2014
38. Getachew M, Yewhalaw D, Tafess K, Getachew Y, Zeynudin A. Anemia and associated risk factors among pregnant women in Gilgel gibe dam area,Southwest Ethiopia. Parasit Vectors. 2012;5(296)
39. Obse N, Mossie A, Gobena T. Magnitude of anemia and associated risk factors among pregnant women attending antenatal care in Shalla Woreda, west Arsi zone, Oromia region. Ethiopia Ethiop J Health Sci. 2013;23(2):165–73.
40. Karaoglu L, Pehlivan E, Egri M, Deprem C, Gunes G, Genc MF, et al. The prevalence of nutritional anemia in pregnancy in an east Anatolian province, Turkey. BMC Public Health. 2010;10:329.
41. Erhabor O, Isaac I, Isah A, Udomah F. Iron deficiency anemia among antenatal women in Sokoto, Nigeria. Br J Med Health Sci. 2013;1(4):47–57.
42. Alem M, Enawgaw B, Gelaw A, Kena T, Seid M, Olkeba Y. Prevalence of anemia and associated risk factors among pregnant women attending antenatal care in Azezo health center Gondar town, Northwest Ethiopia. J Interdiscipl Histopathol. 2013;1(3):137–44.
43. Jufar AH, Zewde T. Prevalence of Anemia among Pregnant Women Attending Antenatal Care at Tikur Anbessa Specialized Hospital, Addis Ababa Ethiopia. J Hematol Thromboembolic Dis. 2014;2(1)
44. Desalegn S. Prevalence of anemia in pregnancy in Jima town, southwestern Ethiopia. Ethiop Med J. 1993;31(4):251–8.
45. Nwizu E, Iliyasu Z, Ibrahim S, Galadanci H. Socio-Demographic and Maternal factors in Anaemia in pregnancy at booking in Kano, Northern Nigeria. Afr J Reprod Health. 2011;15(4):33–41.
46. Gautam V, Bansal Y, Taneja D, Saha R. Prevalence of anemia amongst pregnant women and its socio demographic associates in a rural area of Delhi. Indian J Community Med. 2002;XXVII(4):157–60.
47. Elgari M. Evaluation of hematological parameters of Sudanese pregnant women attending at Omdurman Al Saudi maternity hospital. Egypt Acad J Biol Sci. 2013;5(1):37–42.
48. Vyas R, Shah S, Yadav P, Patel U. Comparative study of mild versus moderate to severe thrombocytopenia in third trimester of pregnancy in a tertiary care hospital. NHL. J Med Sci. 2014;3(1):8–11.
49. Nisha S, Amita D, Pushplata S, Uma S, Tripathi AK. Prevalence and characterization of thrombocytopenia in pregnancy in Indian women. Indian J Hematol Blood Transfus. 2012;28(2):77–81.
50. Dwivedi P, Puri M, Nigam A, Agarwal K. Fetomaternal outcome in pregnancy with severe thrombocytopenia. Eur Rev Med Pharmacol Sci. 2012;16:1563–6.
51. Shamoon RP, Muhammed NS, Jaff MS. Prevalence and etiological classification of thrombocytopenia among a group of pregnant women in Erbil City. Iraq Turk J Hematol. 2009;26:123–8.
52. Olayemi E, Akuffo FW. Gestational thrombocytopenia among pregnant Ghanaian women. Pan Afr Med J. 2012;12(34)

Prevalence of anemia and its associated factors in human immuno deficiency virus infected adult individuals in Ethiopia. A systematic review and meta-analysis

Ayenew Negesse[1*], Temesgen Getaneh[2], Habtamu Temesgen[1], Tesfahun Taddege[3], Dube Jara[4,5] and Zeleke Abebaw[6]

Abstract

Background: Anemia is a common hematologic disorder among human Immunodeficiency virus (HIV) infected adult Individuals. However, there is no concrete scientific evidence established at national level in Ethiopia. Hence, this review gave special emphasis on Ethiopian HIV infected adult individuals to estimate pooled prevalence of anemia and its associated factors at national level.

Methods: Studies were retrieved through search engines in PUBMED/Medline, Cochrane Library, and the web of science, Google and Google scholar following the Preferred Reporting Items for Systematic Review and Meta-Analysis Protocols (PRISMA-P). Joanna Briggs Institute Meta-Analysis of Statistical Assessment and Review Instrument (JBI-MAStARI) was used for critical appraisal of the included studies. Random effects meta-analysis was used to estimate the pooled prevalence of anemia and associated factors at 95% Confidence interval with its respective odds ratio (OR). Meta regression was also carried out to identify the factors. Moreover, Sub-group analysis, begs and egger test followed by trim-and-fill analysis were employed to assess heterogeneity and publication bias respectively.

Result: A total of 532 articles were identified through searching of which 20 studies were included in the final review with a total sample size of 8079 HIV infected adult individuals. The pooled prevalence of anemia was 31.00% (95% CI: 23.94, 38.02). Cluster of Differentiation 4 (CD4) count <= 200 cells/μl with OR = 3.01 (95% CI: 1.87, 4.84), World Health Organization (WHO) clinical stage III&IV with OR = 2.5 (95% CI: 1.29, 4.84), opportunistic infections (OIs) with OR = 1.76 (95% CI: 1.07, 2.89) and body mass index (BMI) < 18.5 kg/M^2 with OR = 1.55 ((95% CI: 1. 28, 1.88) were the associated factors.

Conclusion: This review demonstrates high prevalence of anemia among HIV infected adults. Low CD4 count, WHO clinical stage III&IV, OIs and low level of BMI were found to have significant association with the occurrence of anemia. Therefore, the responsible stockholders including anti retro viral treatment (ART) clinics should strengthen the system and procedures for the early diagnosis of opportunistic infection and screening of underlying problems. There should be also early screening for OIs and under nutrition with strict and frequent monitoring of HIV infected individuals CD4 count.

Keywords: Anemia, Adult individuals, Pooled prevalence, Ethiopia, HIV/AIDS

* Correspondence: ayenewnegesse@gmail.com
[1]Department of Human Nutrition and Food Sciences, College of Health Science, Debre Markos University, P.O. Box 269, Debre Markos, Ethiopia
Full list of author information is available at the end of the article

Background

Anemia is occurs when the number of red blood cells or their oxygen carrying capacity becomes insufficient to meet the physiologic condition [1]. Anemia is also common hematologic disorder among HIV infected individuals [2] with impact on quality of life and clinical outcomes among these individuals [3].

This hematologic disorder may be attributed by HIV infection itself (the incidence is increased from asymptomatic to final Acquired Immuno Deficiency Syndrome (AIDS) stage) [4],OIs, gastrointestinal bleeding, nutritional deficiencies and erythropoietin depletion [5–7]. The complex interplay of all those factors cause life threatening symptoms, which also increases the hazard of mortality among HIV infected individuals [5, 8].

A compressive global estimate of anemia in the year from 1990 to 2010 was 32.9%, resulting in 68.4 million years lived with disability (YLD) [9]. Another systematic analysis of global anemia in the year 1990–2013 also reported the high burden of anemia in which developing countries account nearly 90 % of all anemia-related disability [10].

The prevalence of anemia among HIV infected adult individuals ranges from 20 to 80% and associated with high burden of morbidity and mortality [11]. Anemia among HIV infected individuals is a well-documented phenomenon and need to be the focus area of research to determine the prevalence and its predictors in a specific country [11, 12].

Based on this recommendation, a number of researches were done and reported that the prevalence of anemia among HIV infected adult individuals was:11.2% at northwest parts of Ethiopia in 2014 [3], 11.4% at Addis Ababa in 2018 [13],11.5% at northwest parts of Ethiopia in 2014 [14], 12% at southern parts of Ethiopia in 2005–2010 [15],14.3% at Addis Ababa in 2011/2012 [16], 22.6 at southern parts of Ethiopia in 2016 [17], 23%at northwest parts of Ethiopia in 2015 [18], 23.1% at Southwest parts of Ethiopia in 2012 [19], 25% at Northwest parts of Ethiopia in 2016 [20], 32.48% at Addis Ababa in 2011/2012 [21], 33% at Addis Ababa in 2008–2012 [22], 34.4% at northeast parts of Ethiopia in 2010–2013 [23], 35% at northwest Ethiopia in 2011/2012 [24], 41.2% at Eastern parts of Ethiopia in 2014 [25], 43% at northwest parts of Ethiopia in 2012/2013 [26], 51.74% at Gambella region in Southwest parts of Ethiopia in 2014 [27], 53.3% in Southern parts of Ethiopia in 2016–2013 [3] and 70.1% at northwest parts of Ethiopia in 2011/2012 [28].

The above individual studies revealed that the findings pertaining to the prevalence of anemia are inconsistent across regions and had variations over time. Similar to the prevalence of anemia, predictor variables were also inconsistent among the aforementioned studies. In addition to this gap, lack of documented data on pooled prevalence of anemia and its associated factors among HIV infected adult individuals at national level hinders program managers to design and implement effective strategies.

With the existing meager evidence in developing countries, we set out to explore the evidence on national pooled prevalence of anemia, and to our knowledge, found no published systematic review and meta-analysis so far on this topic to help guide decision-making. Therefore, this review would summarize the available evidence on the pooled prevalence of anemia among HIV infected adult individuals and associated factors.

Methods

Search strategy

Initially databases were searched for same systematic review and meta-analysis to avoid duplications. First DARE database (http://www.library.UCSF.edu) was explored in an attempt to confirm whether systematic review or meta-analysis exists and for availability of ongoing projects related to the topic. We also searched the three Trials Registries: ICTRP, Clinical Trials.gov and PROSPERO (searched January 2018). By using this method, it was confirmed that there was no any review and meta-analysis was conducted in similar to with this topic.

We systematically reviewed and analyzed published research articles to determine the pooled prevalence of anemia and its associated factors among HIV infected adult individuals in Ethiopia. To identify published articles, major databases such as PUBMED/MEDLINE, WHOLIS, Cochrane library, web of science, Google and Google Scholar were used accordingly. In addition, reference lists of relevant studies were identified and the full-text articles reviewed for inclusion. The key term used for PubMed search were "Prevalence" OR "incidence" AND "Anemia" AND "HIV" OR "AIDS" AND "Ethiopia". The Search terms were pre-defined to allow a comprehensive search strategy that included all fields within records and Medical Subject Headings (MeSH terms) was used to help expand the search in advanced PubMed search. This study also used Boolean operator (within each axis we combined keywords with the "OR" operator and we then linked the search strategies for the two axes with the "AND" operator). We followed the Preferred Reporting Items for Systematic Reviews and Meta-Analyses (PRISMA) guideline during the systematic review [29].

Eligibility criteria

We reviewed abstracts from initial search using defined inclusion and exclusion criteria.

Inclusion criteria

Study scope

All studies which determine the prevalence of anemia and which identify the associated factors of it among

HIV infected adult individuals were included under this systematic review and meta-analysis.

Study design

Both cross sectional and cohort study designs were included.

Study setting

Both community and health institution level studies.

Language

All articles published in English language were included.

Population

All HIV infected adult individuals in Ethiopia.

Exclusion criteria

Based on the eligibility criteria, we read their titles and abstracts. If studies are relevant for our review, we examined the full texts. Those papers which didn't fully accessed at the time of our search process were excluded from this review after contact was attempted with the principal investigator through email at least two times. After reading the abstracts, if the studies are relevant to our review, we examined the full texts. The reason for the exclusion of these articles is that we are unable to assess the quality of each article in the absence of their full texts. Studies which didn't report specific outcomes for anemia and associated factors quantitatively were also excluded from this systematic review and meta-analysis. Moreover, studies with poor quality as per settled criteria and review articles were also excluded from the review.

Data abstraction

The Database search results were combined and duplicate articles were removed manually using Endnote (version X8). Data were extracted by two authors using a standardized data extraction spread sheet. The data extraction spreadsheet was piloted on 7 randomly selected papers and modified accordingly. Data extraction sheet included study characteristics such as: (1) Authors' name, year, region, study or publication year, study design, study setting and study population; (2) incidence or prevalence of anemia (3) data extracted on sex, OIs, CD4 counts, WHO clinical stages, residence, their nutritional status, residence and their history of malaria infestation; (4) studies' quality score, sampling technique, study area, estimating technique of anemia using Hemoglobin measurement and their mean age of the study participants were also extracted from each individual studies.

Quality assessment (appraisal) of the individual studies

The Database search results were combined and duplicate articles were removed manually using Endnote (version X8). Joanna Briggs Institute Meta-Analysis of Statistics Assessment and Review Instrument (JBI-MAStARI) adapted for both cross sectional and follow up study design was used [30]. Three independent reviewers critically appraised each individual paper. Disagreements between those reviewers were solved by discussion. If not third reviewer was involved to resolve inconsistencies in between the two independent reviewers. Studies which score five and above were included in the final systematic review and meta-analysis.

Outcome measurements

This review has two main outcomes. The primary outcome was prevalence of anemia among HIV infected adult individuals which was calculated as number of adult HIV infected individuals who experienced anemia divided by total adult HIV infected individuals who were at risk of developing anemia and multiplied by 100%. The second aim of this review was to identify predictors of anemia among adult HIV infected individuals in Ethiopia.

Data analysis and synthesis

The extracted data were entered into computer using excel sheet and imported to STATA 14 for analysis. Evidence of publication bias was assessed using both egger's test and begg's test with *p*-value of less than 0.05 as a cut of point to declare the presence of publication bias [31, 32]. Heterogeneity across studies was checked using the inverse variance (I^2) with Cochran Q statistic at 25, 50 and 75% as low, moderate and sever heterogeneity respectively [33]. Forest plot was also used to visualize the presence of heterogeneity. *P* value less than 0.05 was also used to declare the presence of heterogeneity across studies. Potential differences between studies were explored by sub-group analyses and Meta regression. The impact of heterogeneity across studies on the meta-analysis was quantified by I-square statistic (TAU) and a cutoff point of 50% was used to declare substantial heterogeneity. The effect size of categorical data was expressed using odds ratio.

Measures of effect and reporting

PRISMA flow diagrams used to summarize the study selection process. Random effects (DerSimonian and laird) model was used during analysis and Odds Ratios with their 95% CI were used to present the pooled effect sizes.

Results

Selection of studies

A total of 532 articles searched through the electronic (526) and supplementary (6) searches of which 78 duplicated articles were excluded. From the remaining 454 articles, 429 articles were excluded after reading of titles and abstracts based on the pre-defined inclusion criteria's. Finally, 25 full text articles were accessed and assessed for eligibility criteria. Based on the pre-defined criteria and after critical appraisal, only 20 articles were included for the final analysis (Fig. 1).

Characteristics of included studies

A total of twenty articles met the inclusion criteria. All the included studies were published between 2005 and 2017. Both cross sectional and cohort studies were included accordingly using an estimated sample size range from 172 [27] up to 1061 [16] adult HIV infected individual samples who were taken at Southwest parts of Ethiopia in the year 2014 and Addis Ababa city in the year 2011/2012 respectively. About 3139 men and 4920 women with a total sample of 8, 059 adult HIV infected individuals were included to estimate the pooled prevalence of anemia and its associated factors among adult HIV infected individuals (Table 1).

Of the total 20 articles, more than one third of studies were conducted in Amhara regional state health institutions [2, 14, 18, 20, 23, 24, 26, 28]; four studies in Addis Ababa health institutions [13, 16, 21, 22]; four studies at South Nations Nationalities and peoples of Ethiopia national regional state (SNNP) [3, 15, 17, 34]; one study at Oromia national regional state [19], one study at Gambella national regional state [27], one study at Tigray regional national state [35] and one study at Dire Dawa town administration of Ethiopia [25].

Regarding the study designs, 13 studies [3, 13, 15, 17–20, 25–28, 34, 35] and the remaining seven were cross sectional and cohort studies respectively. After critical appraisal of each articles based on JBI-MAStARI, both in peer and independently, they scored in the range of 5-up to 8 out of 9 values (see Table 1).

Prevalence of anemia among adult HIV infected individuals in Ethiopia (Meta-analysis)

As shown in the forest plot below, the pooled prevalence of anemia among adult HIV infected individuals in Ethiopia was 31.00% (95% CI: 23.94, 38.02) (Fig. 2). Substantial level of statistically significant heterogeneity was detected (I^2 = 98%; $p < 0.001$) suggesting that the use of random effects model in estimating the pooled estimates is appropriate. The substantial magnitude of the heterogeneity also suggests the need to conduct subgroup analysis which demands identifying the sources of heterogeneity (Fig 2).

Subgroup analysis

Since this review is exhibited with substantial heterogeneity, subgroup analysis based on study year, type of study design, study year, mean age in years, gender distribution, sample size and sampling technique they used were considered to identify the possible source of heterogeneity across studies (Table 2). However the subgroup analysis result indicated that the source of heterogeneity was not due to type of study design, study year, mean age in years, gender distribution, sample size and sampling technique they used.

Publication bias was observed using both begg's and egger's test [36, 37] and the value was found to be significant at p value of 0.002 and 0.004 respectively. So that trim and fill meta-analysis [38] has been done to

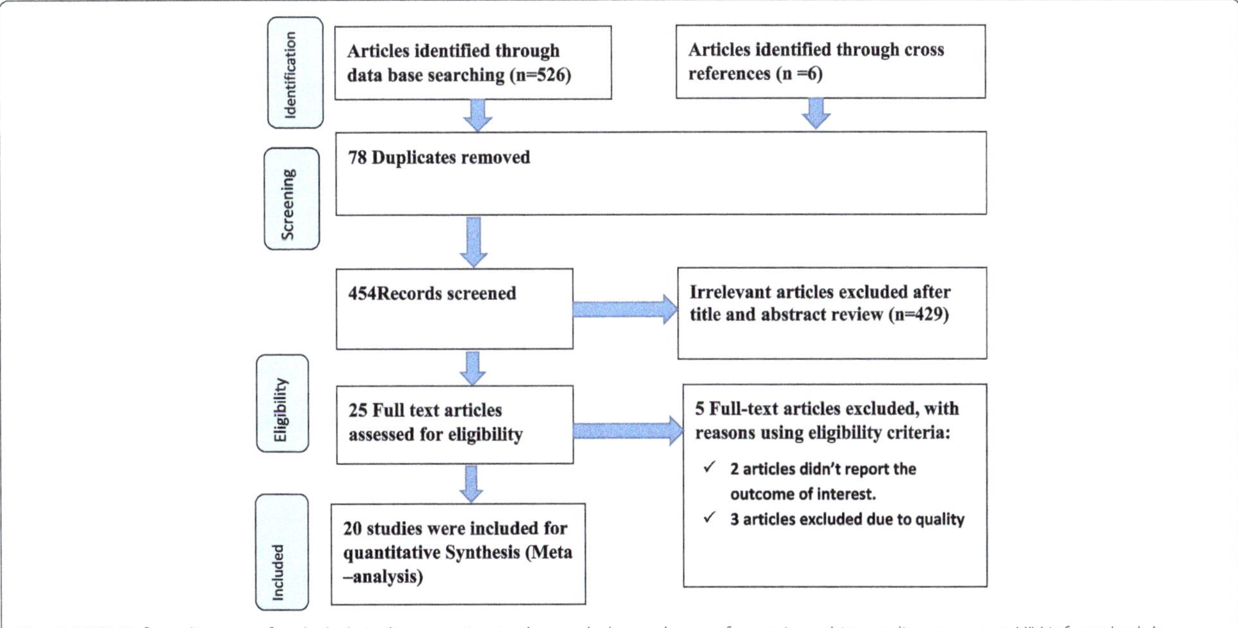

Fig. 1 PRISMA flow diagram of included studies to estimate the pooled prevalence of anemia and its predictors among HIV infected adult individuals in Ethiopia from 2005 up to 2017

Table 1 characteristics of included studies to estimate the pooled prevalence of anemia and its predictors among adult HIV infected individuals in Ethiopia from 2005 up to 2017

ID	Region	Author	Study year	Publication year	Study design	Sampling method	Sample size	Gender distribution		Mean age In years	Measurement of anemia	Quality score
								Male	Female			
1	Addis Ababa	Tamir Z et al. [21]	2011/2012	2018	Cohort	_	394	142	252	_	Hemoglobin level	7
2	SNNP	Alamdo A et al. [3]	2006–2012	2015	Cross sectional	_	411	216	195	33.9	Hemoglobin level	6
3	Addis Ababa	Woldeamanuel G et al. [13]	2017	2018	Cross sectional	Simple random	255	148	107	40.6	Hemoglobin level	8
4	Amhara	Beyene H et al. [26]	2012/2013	2017	Cross sectional	_	528	278	250	33.69	Hemoglobin level	8
5	Amhara	Melese H et al. [18]	2015	2017	Cross sectional	Simple random	377	234	143	35.21	Hemoglobin level	8
6	Amhara	Alem M et al. [28]	2011/2012	2013	Cross sectional	Simple random	384	233	151	37	Hemoglobin level	8
7	Amhara	Deressa et al. [20]	2016	2018	Cross sectional	Systematic	320	203	117	_	Hemoglobin level	6
8	Amhara	Fiseha T et al. [23]	2010–2013	2013	Cohort	Simple random	373	233	140	34.6	Hemoglobin level	8
9	Amhara	Tesfaye Z et al. [14]	2014	2014	Cohort	_	349	218	131	34.6	Hemoglobin level	8
10	Oromia	Gedefaw L et al. [19]	2012	2013	Cross sectional	_	234	145	89	32.09	Hemoglobin level	6
11	Addis Ababa	Wolde H et al. [22]	2008–2012	2014	Cohort	Simple random	616	401	215	_	Hemoglobin level	5
12	Addis Ababa	Assefa M et al. [16]	2011/2012	2015	Cohort	Simple random	1061	632	429	_	Hemoglobin level	8
13	Amhara	Bamlaku E et al. [2]	2012/2013	2014	Cohort	_	319	202	117	_	Hemoglobin level	5
14	SNNP	Daka D et al. [15]	2005–2010	2013	Cross sectional	_	384	254	130	33.64	Hemoglobin level	7
15	Amhara	Ferede G et al. [24]	2011/2012	2013	Cohort	_	400	278	122	_	Hemoglobin level	5
16	Dire Dawa	Geleta D et al. [25]	2014	2016	Cross sectional	Simple random	425	275	150	34	Hemoglobin level	8
17	Gambella	Sahle T et al. [27]	2014	2017	Cross sectional	Systematic	172	68	104	31.95	Hemoglobin level	8
18	SNNP	Muluken W et al. [17]	2016	2018	Cross sectional	Simple random	376	195	181	_	Hemoglobin level	5
19	SNNP	Gedel G et al. (2015) [34]	2013/2014	2015	Cross sectional	Systematic	305	189	116	39.5	Hemoglobin level	8
20	Tigray	Hadgu T et al. (2013) [35]	2012	2013	Cross sectional	Systematic	376	376	_	32.5	Hemoglobin level	8

account for the publication bias. Based on this analysis, the prevalence of anemia among HIV infected individuals was 31% (95% CI: 23.97, 38.02) and no significant change was exhibited as compared with the main meta-analysis.

Meta regression

In addition to subgroup analysis and publication bias, Meta regression was also undertaken by considering both continuous and categorical data to identify associated factors with the pooled prevalence of anemia. Sample size, study year, publication year, study design, Gender distribution, sampling technique and mean age in years for each individual studies were considered in the meta-regression. But the meta regression showed that the pooled prevalence of anemia among HIV infected adult individuals was not associated with sample size, study year, publication year, study design, Gender

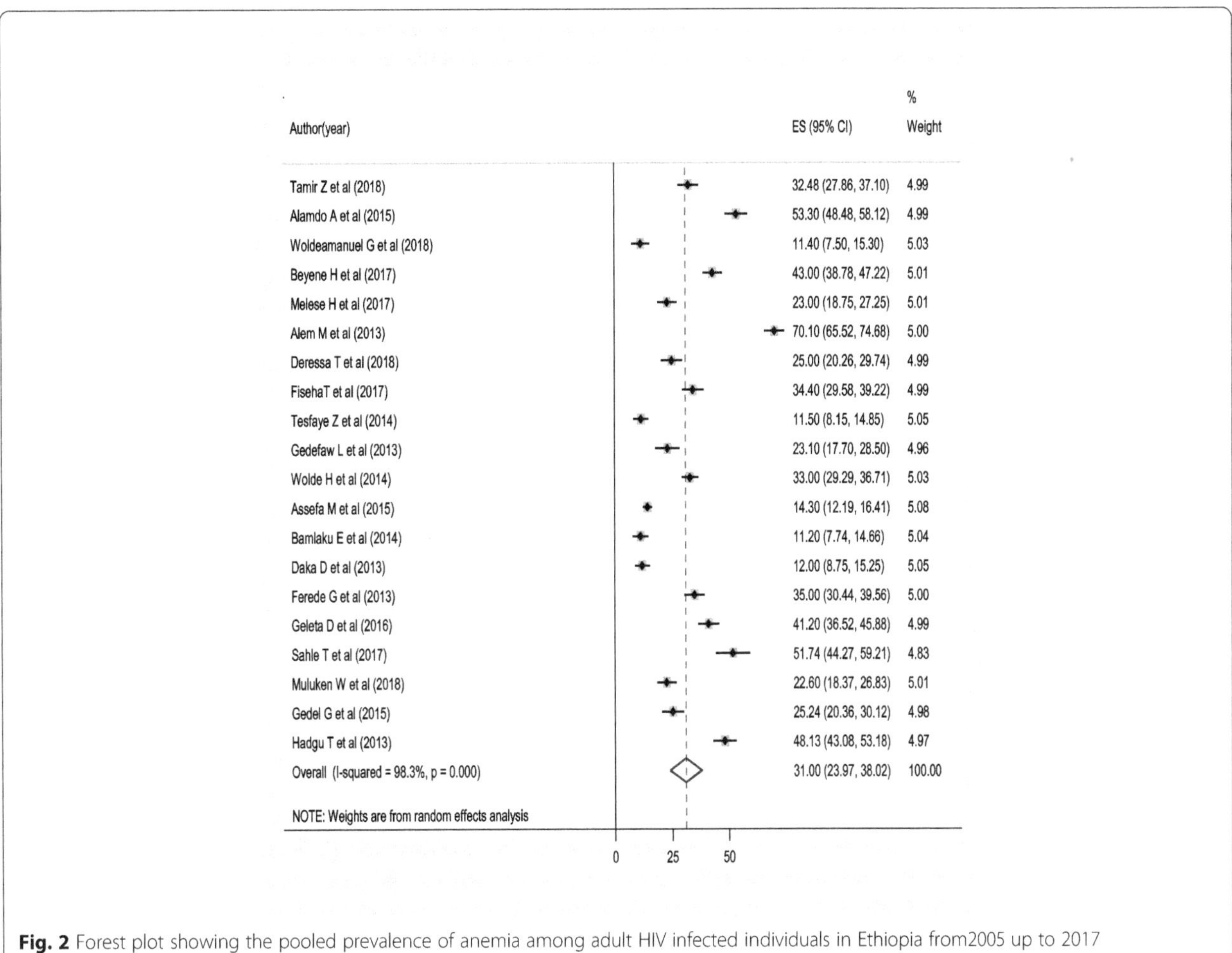

Fig. 2 Forest plot showing the pooled prevalence of anemia among adult HIV infected individuals in Ethiopia from2005 up to 2017

Table 2 Sub group analysis which describes pooled prevalence of anemia and its predictors among adult HIV infected individuals in Ethiopia

Sub group		Number of included studies	Prevalence (95% CI)	Heterogeneity statistics	*P* value	I^2
By study design	Cross sectional	13	34.54 (24.54, 44.55)	761.77	< 0.001	98.4
	Cohort	7	24.44 (16.18, 32.70)	228.57	< 0.001	97.4
Time of study year	Before 2015	16	33.65 (25.13, 42.16)	1077.02	< 0.001	98.6
	2015 and above	4	20.43 (14.12, 26.74)	26.29	< 0.001	88.6
Gender distribution	Male	12	41.21 (27.07,55.36)	774.85	< 0.001	98.6
	Female	12	34.52(24.27,44.77)	309.79	< 0.001	96.4
sampling method	Simple random	8	31.20 (18.86, 43.54)	598.36	< 0.001	98.8
	Systematic	4	37.37 (23.72, 51.02)	77.69	< 0.001	96.1
	Un-defined	8	27.64 (16.62, 38.66)	413.30	< 0.001	98.3
Mean age in years	<= 35	8	34.31 (21.75, 46.88)	432.49	< 0.001	98.4
	> 35	5	34.54 (14.59, 54.49)	422.51	< 0.001	99.1
	No report of mean age	7	24.71(17.28, 32.14)	172.93	< 0.001	96.5
Sample size	< 384	11	25.91 (18.63, 33.19)	296.43	< 0.001	98.3
	> = 384	9	37.1 (24.68,49.51)	1141.04	< 0.001	99.0

distribution, sampling technique and mean age in years (Table 3).

Associated factors of anemia among HIV infected adult individuals in Ethiopia

Low CD4 count, WHO clinical stage III&IV, OIs and low level of BMI were found to have significant association with the occurrence of anemia among HIV infected adult Individuals.

The odds of developing anemia were 3 times higher among HIV infected individuals with CD4 count of < 200 cell/ul compared with HIV infected individuals with CD4 count is > = 200/ul [(OR = 3.01 (95% CI: 1.87, 4.84))] (Fig. 3a). The odds of developing anemia were 2.5 times higher among HIV infected Individuals with WHO clinical stage III &IV compared with individuals with WHO clinical stage I&II [OR = 2.5 (95% CI: 1.29, 4.84)] (Fig. 3b). The odds of developing anemia were 1.8 times higher among HIV infected Individuals with opportunistic infection had compared with individuals free of opportunistic infections [OR = 1.76 (95% CI: 1.07, 2.89)] (Fig. 3c). The odds of developing anemia were 1.6 times higher among HIV infected Individuals whose body mass index (BMI) < 18.5 kg/m^2 had compared with those whose BMI was > = 18.5 kg/M^2[OR = 1.55 ((95% CI: 1. 28, 1.88)](Fig. 3d).

Discussion

This systematic review and meta-analysis was established out to estimate the pooled prevalence of anemia and its associated factors among HIV infected adult individuals in Ethiopia from 2005 [15] up 2017 [13].

According to this review, one third of HIV infected adult individuals were found to be anemic in Ethiopia. The prevalence of anemia in the current systematic review is higher than the finding of the study conducted in Tanzania [39] which estimated only severe form of anemia. The finding is also lower than the finding of the study conducted in European countries [40] and south India [41].

This variation may be due to variation in hemoglobin cut off point to define anemia across those regions. In Ethiopian studies anemia was defined if hemoglobin level was less than 11 g/dl for both men and women according to WHO definition criteria for anemia. However, in the studies conducted in European countries anemia was considered as less than or equal to 14 g/dl for men and less than or equal to 12 g/dl for women. On the other hand, anemia was considered as less than 13 g/dl for men as and less than 12 g/dl for women in the South Indian stud.

Another explanation for the difference in magnitude may be attributed to the geographic location variation where altitude difference across Ethiopia, Tanzania and European countries may change the level of hemoglobin concentration. The meta analysis results also indicated that CD4 count of HIV infected individual was found to have statistically significant association with anemia. Decrease in CD4 count of HIV infected individual leads to the increase progression to [42]. This finding is consistent with the findings reported in the study conducted in the Kathmandu [43], the united states [4], in south Africa [44], in Tanzania [39], in China [45] and Central region of Ghana [46]. This is due to patients with low Cd4 count may exposed with different opportunistic infections that in turn exposed to anemia. Hence rate of falling hemoglobin level also indicates falling of CD4 count, which is a gold standard for monitoring HIV progression [47].

Table 3 Meta regression for the included studies to identify source of heterogeneity for the prevalence of anemia among HIV infected adult individuals in Ethiopia from 2005 up to 2017

Variables	Characteristics	Coefficients	P-value
Year	Publication year	−.8434435	0.672
Study year	Before 2015	Reference	Reference
	2015 and above	−13.14142	0.156
Sample	Sample size of each articles	−.0092616	0.665
Study design	Cohort	−10.0263	0.199
	Cross sectional	Reference	Reference
Gender distribution	Male	.0071367	0.883
	Female	Reference	Reference
Sampling technique	Simple random	3.11105	0.747
	Systematic	15.15263	0.385
	Undefined	Reference	Reference
Mean age in years	<=35	9.531214	0.282
	> 35	9.762604	0.328
	No report of mean age	Reference	Reference

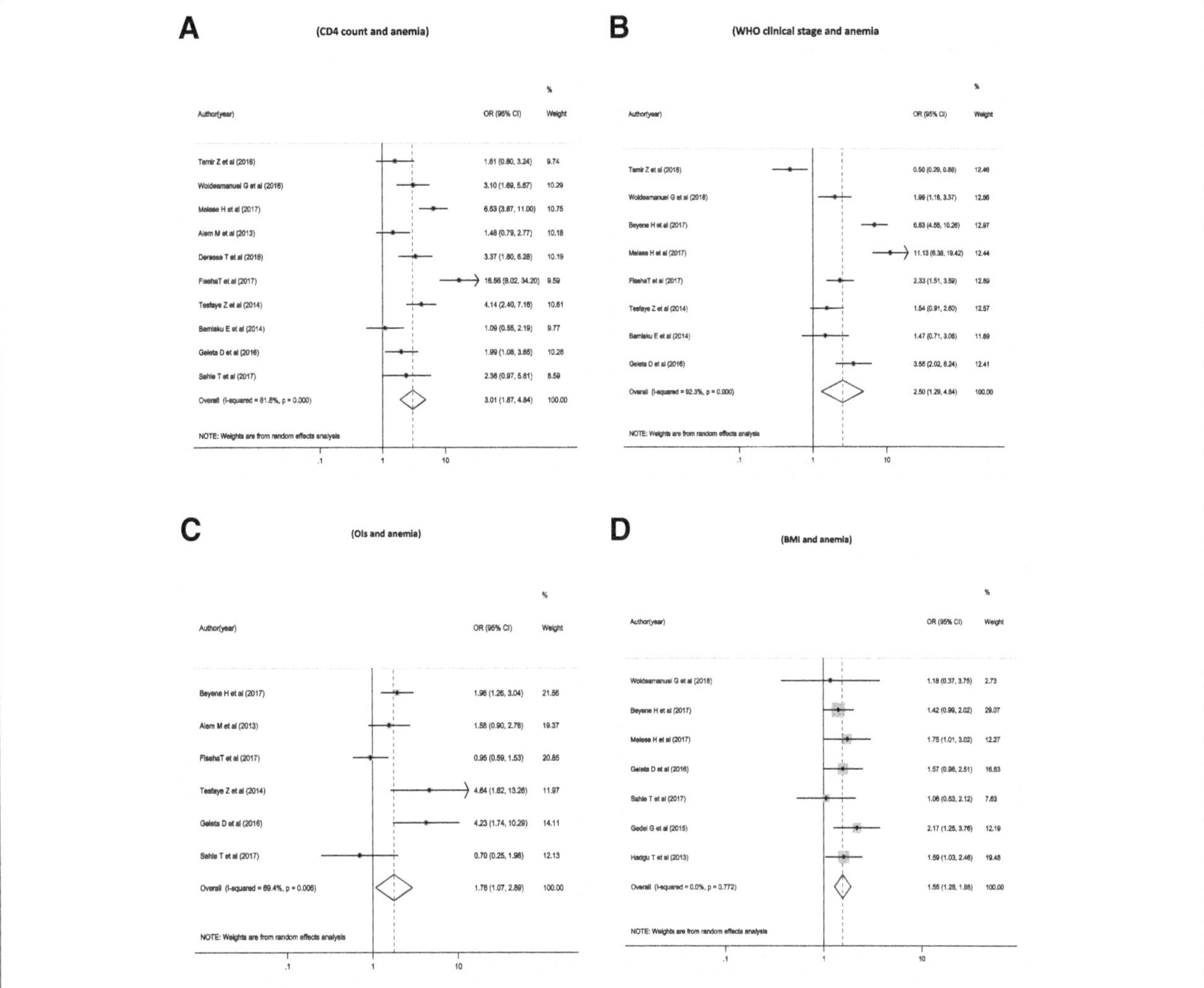

Fig. 3 Forest plots which describe associated factors of anemia among HIV infected adult individuals in Ethiopia. **a** Forest plot which describe the association between anemia and CD4 count response among HIV infected adult individuals in Ethiopia. **b** Forest plot which describe the association between anemia and WHO clinical stage among HIV infected adult individuals in Ethiopia. **c** Forest plot which describe the association between anemia and OIs among HIV infected adult individuals in Ethiopia. **d** Forest plot which describe the association between anemia and BMI among HIV infected adult individuals in Ethiopia

The finding of current review is also consistent with the findings of studies conducted in South Africa [44], south India [41], Tanzania [39] in which WHO clinical stage III/IV of HIV, low level of body mass index (< 18.5 kg/m^2) and different forms of opportunistic infections were an independent predictors of anemia among HIV infected individuals.

In addition, evidences also documented that individuals with advanced stage of HIV exposed to OIs [48]. These OIs also may cause dietary problems which would led to nutritional deficiencies and problems of absorbing nutrients which in turn would lead to anemia and malnutrition [49].

Theoretical and practical implications

HIV infected adult individuals are more prone to develop concomitant infections demanding comprehensive package of health services including ART. This review evidence also indicated that those anemic HIV infected individuals deserve more attention where integrated service provision is critical to identify and manage underlying causes for anemia at early stages. Hence, specific considerations tailored to anemia screening and management needs to be taken into account during ART program design and implementation across the health system. Despite the vast investment of resources in tackling the occurrence of anemia in low and middle income countries few studies, are available to inform policy and decision making. Therefore, further studies are also recommended to generate pooled evidence at global level in general and in developing countries in particular.

Strengths and limitations

The main strength of the current review lies in our adherence to international standardized guidelines on the conduct and reporting of systematic reviews. We included studies only from peer-reviewed English-language journals, which may have restricted our findings. Though searching was done for unpublished papers, only published studies were included.

Conclusion

This systematic review and meta-analysis showed a high prevalence of anemia among HIV infected adult individuals in Ethiopian in which in 1/3 of HIV infected adult individuals were anemic. The review found that low CD4 count; advanced stage of the disease (WHO clinical stage III &IV), opportunistic infection and low level of BMI were found to have positive significant association with the development of anemia. Therefore, the responsible stockholders including ART clinics should strengthen the system and procedures for the early diagnosis of opportunistic infection and screening of underlying problems like under nutrition. The system should focus on technical update training on opportunistic infection diagnosis and treatment guidelines, on nutritional assessment, counseling and support (NACs), strengthening of laboratory facilities which can detect opportunistic infections early in infection. Moreover linkage of case managers, mother groups and HIV/AIDs union with ART clinic should also be strengthened for better referral linkage which can indirectly help for early screening of opportunistic infection and undernutrition. There should also be strict and frequent monitoring of HIV infected individuals CD4 count than previous in order to minimize anemia and related burdens.

Abbreviations

BMI: Body mass index; CD4: Cluster of differentiation 4; CI: Confidence Interval; HIV: Human immuno virus; OIs: Opportunistic Infections; SNNP: South Nations Nationalities and peoples of Ethiopia

Funding

Not applicable.

Acknowledgments

We would like to thank all authors of studies included in this systematic review and meta-analysis.

Authors' contributions

AN and TG developed the protocol and involved in the design, selection of study, data extraction, statistical analysis and developing the initial drafts of the manuscript. ZA, TT, DJ and HT involved in quality assessment. AN, TG and DJ prepared and revising subsequent drafts. AN, ZA and TT prepared the final draft of the manuscript. All authors read and approved the final draft of the manuscript.

Competing interests

The authors declare that they have no competing interests.

Author details

[1]Department of Human Nutrition and Food Sciences, College of Health Science, Debre Markos University, P.O. Box 269, Debre Markos, Ethiopia. [2]Department of Midwifery, College of Health Science, Debre Markos University, P.O. Box 269, Debre Markos, Ethiopia. [3]Ethiopia Field Epidemiology and Laboratory Training Program (EFELTP) Resident, University of Gondar, P.O. Box 196, Gondar, Ethiopia. [4]Department of Public Health, College of Health Science Debre Markos University, P.O. Box 269, Debre Markos, Ethiopia. [5]School of Public Health, College of Health Science, Addis Ababa University, Addis Ababa, Ethiopia. [6]Department of Health Informatics, University of Gondar, P.O. Box 196, Gondar, Ethiopia.

References

1. World Health Orgnanization: health topics on Anemia which is available at http://www.who.int/topics/anaemia/en/.
2. Enawgaw B, Tadele A, Melku M, et al. Prevalence of zidovudine induced megaloblastic anemia among human immunodeficiency virus positive patients attending University of Gondar hospital antiretroviral therapy clinic, Northwest Ethiopia. HIV Advance Res Dev. 2014;1(1):105.
3. Gizaw AA, Temesgen F, Amanuel T, et al. Anemia and its associated risk factors at the time of antiretroviral therapy initiation in public health facilities of Arba Minch Town, Southern Ethiopia. Health. 2015;7(12):1657.
4. Sullivan Patrick S, Hanson Debra L, Chu Susan Y. Epidemiology of anemia in human immunodeficiency virus (HIV)-infected persons: results from the multistate adult and adolescent spectrum of HIV disease surveillance project. Blood. 1998;91(1):301–8.
5. Sudhir M, Srinivasa J, Dinesh G. Hematologic manifestations of HIV/AIDS. Medicine. 2011;9:484–90.
6. Richman Douglas D, Fischl Margaret A, Grieco MH. The toxicity of azidothymidine (AZT) in the treatment of patients with AIDS and AIDS-related complex. N Engl J Med. 1987;317(4):192–7.
7. Camacho J, Poveda F, Zamorano AF, et al. Serum erythropoietin levels in anaemic patients with advanced human immunodeficiency virus infection. Br J Haematol. 1992;82(3):608–14.
8. Volberding Paul A, Bake Kelty R, Levine Alexandra M. Human immunodeficiency virus hematology. ASH Educ Program Book. 2003;2003(1): 294–313.
9. Kassebaum Nicholas J, Rashmi J, Mohsen N, et al. A systematic analysis of global anemia burden from 1990 to 2010. Blood. 2014;123(5):615–24.
10. Kassebaum Nicholas J, Yousef K. The global burden of Anemia. 2016;30.
11. Belperio Pamela S, Rhew David C. Prevalence and outcomes of anemia in individuals with human immunodeficiency virus: a systematic review of the literature. Am J Med. 2004;116(7):27–43.
12. Rawat Rahul MCSI, Suneetha AK. Poor diet quality is associated with low CD4 count and anemia and predicts mortality among antiretroviral therapy–naive HIV-positive adults in Uganda. J. Acquir. Immune Defic. Syndr. 2013;62(2):246–53.
13. Garedew WG, Haile WD. Prevalence of anemia before and after initiation of antiretroviral therapy among HIV infected patients at black lion specialized hospital, Addis Ababa, Ethiopia: a cross sectional study. BMC Hematology. 2018;18(1):7.
14. Zelalem T, Bamlaku E. Prevalence of anemia before and after initiation of highly active antiretroviral therapy among HIV positive patients in Northwest Ethiopia: a retrospective study. BMC. Res. Notes. 2014;7(1):745.
15. Deresse D, Dereje L, Aderajew A, et al. Prevalence of anaemia before and after the initiation of antiretroviral therapy at ART centre of Hawassa University Referral Hospital, Hawassa, South Ethiopia. Sch J Med. 2013;3(1):1–6.
16. Muluken A, Erku AW, Aster S, et al. Prevalence and correlates of anemia among HIV infected patients on highly active anti-retroviral therapy at Zewditu memorial hospital, Ethiopia. BMC Hematology. 2015;15(1):6.

17. Wubetu M, Mebratu E. Assessment of the prevalence of zidovudine induced Anemia among adult HIV/AIDS patients on HAART in an Ethiopian Hospita. Occupational Medicine & Health Affairs. 2018;6:271.
18. Hermela M, Mesele WM, Haile W, et al. Anemia among adult HIV patients in Ethiopia: a hospital-based cross-sectional study. HIV/AIDS (Auckland, NZ). 2017;9:25.
19. Lealem G, Tilahun Y, Zewdineh S, et al. Anemia and risk factors in HAART naive and HAART experienced HIV positive persons in south West Ethiopia: a comparative study. PLoS One. 2013;8(8):e72202.
20. Tekalign D, Debasu D, Meseret W, et al. Anemia and thrombocytopenia in the cohort of HIV-infected adults in Northwest Ethiopia: a facility-based cross-sectional study. EJIFCC. 2018;29(1):36.
21. Zemenu T, Jemal A, Aster T. Anemia among HIV infected individuals taking art with and without zidovudine at Addis Ababa, Ethiopia. Ethiopian J Health Sci. 2018;28(1):73–82.
22. Milkias WH, Lerebo WT, Melaku YA, et al. Incidence and risk factors of Anemia among HIV/AIDS patients taking anti-retroviral erapy at tertiary hospitals in Addis Ababa, Ethiopia: a retrospective cohort study. J HIV AIDS Infect Dis2. 2014:1–06.
23. Temesgen F, Zemenu T, Abdurahaman S, et al. Prevalence of anemia in renal insufficiency among HIV infected patients initiating ART at a hospital in Northeast Ethiopia. BMC Hematology. 2017;17(1):1.
24. Getachew F, Yitayih W. Prevalence and related factors of anemia in HAART-naive HIV positive patients at Gondar University hospital, Northwest Ethiopia. BMC Blood Disorders. 2013;13(1):8.
25. Dessalegn G, Bayissa DD, Birhanu S, et al. Prevalence of Anemia and associated factors among PHIVs attendants antiretroviral therapy clinics in public health institutions in Dire Dawa town, East Ethiopia. J Med, Physiol and Biophys. 2016;22.
26. Bedimo BH, Mulualem T, Disass H. Concurrent Plasmodium infection, anemia and their correlates among newly diagnosed people living with HIV/AIDS in northern Ethiopia. Acta Trop. 2017;169:8–13.
27. Tsion S, Tilahun Y, Lealem G. Effect of malaria infection on hematological profiles of people living with human immunodeficiency virus in Gambella, southwest Ethiopia. BMC Hematology. 2017;17(1):2.
28. Meseret A, Tigist K, Negash B, et al. Prevalence of anemia and associated risk factors among adult HIV patients at the anti-retroviral therapy clinic at the University of Gondar Hospital, Gondar, Northwest Ethiopia. Scientific Reports. 2013;2:article 3.
29. David M, Alessandro L, Jennifer T, et al. Preferred reporting items for systematic reviews and meta-analyses: the PRISMA statement. Phys Ther. 2009;89(9):873–80.
30. Institute Jonna Briggs. Meta-analysis of statistics: assessment and review instrument (JBI Mastari). Adelaide: Joanna Briggs Institute; 2006. p. 20032.
31. Begg Colin B, Madhuchhanda M. Operating characteristics of a rank correlation test for publication bias. Biometrics. 1994:1088–101.
32. Matthias E, Davey SG, Martin S, et al. Bias in meta-analysis detected by a simple, graphical test. BMJ. 1997;315(7109):629–34.
33. Higgins Julian PT, Thompson Simon G, Deeks Jonathan J, et al. Measuring inconsistency in meta-analyses. BMJ: British Medical Journal. 2003;327(7414):557.
34. Dereje G, Baye G, Dagnachew M, et al. Prevalence of malnutrition and its associated factors among adult people living with HIV/AIDS receiving anti-retroviral therapy at Butajira Hospital, Southern Ethiopia. BMC Nutrition. 2015;1(1):5.
35. Hailu HT, Walelegn W, Desalegn T, et al. Undernutrition among HIV positive women in Humera hospital, Tigray, Ethiopia, 2013: antiretroviral therapy alone is not enough, cross sectional study. BMC Public Health. 2013;13(1):943.
36. Begg CB, Mazumdar M. Operating characteristics of a rank correlation test for publication bias. Biometrics. 1994:1088–101.
37. Egger M, Smith GD, Schneider M, Minder C. Bias in meta-analysis detected by a simple, graphical test. BMJ. 1997;315(7109):629–34.
38. Duval S, aT R. Trim and fll: a simple funnel-plot–based method of testing and adjusting for publication bias in meta-analysis. Biometrics. 2000;56(2):455–63.
39. Abel M, James O, Donna S, et al. Burden and determinants of severe anemia among HIV-infected adults: results from a large urban HIV program in Tanzania, East Africa. J Int Assoc Providers of AIDS Care (JIAPAC). 2015; 14(2):148–55.
40. Amanda M, Ole K, Barton Simon E, et al. Anaemia is an independent predictive marker for clinical prognosis in HIV-infected patients from across Europe. Aids. 1999;13(8):943–50.
41. Ramnath S. Anemia among HIV-infected individuals in South India; 2007.
42. Spivak Jerry L. Serum Immunoreactive erythropoietin. Jama. 1989;261:3104–7.
43. Raj BK, Surya D, Midhan S, et al. Profile of Anaemia in HIV positive patients. J College of Med Sci-Nepal. 2016;12(2):70–3.
44. Simbarashe T, Mhairi M, Brennan Alana T, et al. Anemia among HIV-infected patients initiating antiretroviral therapy in South Africa: improvement in hemoglobin regardless of degree of immunosuppression and the initiating ART regimen. J Tropical Medicine. 2013;2013:6.
45. Yinzhong S, Zhenyan W, Hongzhou L, et al. Prevalence of anemia among adults with newly diagnosed HIV/AIDS in China. PLoS One. 2013;8(9):e73807.
46. Christian O, Yeboah Francis A, et al. Blood haemoglobin measurement as a predictive indicator for the progression of HIV/AIDS in resource-limited setting. J Biomed Sci. 2009;16(1):102.
47. Langford Simone E, Jintanat A, Cooper David A. Predictors of disease progression in HIV infection: a review. AIDS Res Ther. 2007;4(1):11.
48. Center for Disease prevention and control (CDC): Opportunistic infection among HIV infected indviduals last updated may 30/2017: available at https://www.cdc.gov/hiv/basics/livingwithhiv/opportunisticinfections.html.
49. Porter C. A report on HIV/AIDS and malnutrition locked in vicious cycle. Washington File, 16 October 2006: available at http://aids.immunodefence.com/2006/10/hivaids-and-malnutrition-locke.html.

Prevalence of cytopenias in both HAART and HAART naïve HIV infected adult patients in Ethiopia: a cross sectional study

Tamirat Edie Fekene[1*], Leja Hamza Juhar[1], Chernet Hailu Mengesha[2] and Dawit Kibru Worku[3]

Abstract

Background: In individuals infected with HIV, hematological abnormalities are common and are associated with increased risk of disease progression and death. However, the profile of hematological abnormalities in HIV infected adult patients is not known in Ethiopia. Thus, the aim of this study was to assess the hematological manifestations of HIV infection and to identify the factors associated with cytopenias in both HAART and HAART naïve HIV infected adult patients in Ethiopia.

Method: We conducted a cross-sectional quantitative study of HIV-infected adult patients attending the ART follow-up clinic of Jimma University Specialized Hospital in Jimma, Ethiopia, from July 2012 to September 2012. We used a structured questionnaire to collect socio-demographic and clinical information. After interviewing, 4 ml of venous blood was drawn from each study subject for hematologic and immunologic parameters.

Result: The prevalence of anemia, leucopenia, thrombocytopenia and lymphopenia among the study individuals were 51.5%, 13%, 11.1% and 5% respectively. Presence of opportunistic infection ($p = 0.001$), use of CPT ($p = 0.04$) and CD4 count < 200 cells/μl ($p = 0.002$) were associated with an increased risk of anemia.

Conclusion: Hematologic abnormalities were common in HIV infected adult patients. Of the cytopenias anemia was the most common. Use of CPT was independently associated with increased risk of anemia and leucopenia. Therefore, large scale and longitudinal studies, giving emphasis on the association of CPT and cytopenia, are recommended to strengthen and explore the problem in depth.

Keywords: Anemia, Leucopenia, Lymphopenia, Thrombocytopenia, HIV, HAART, CPT

Background

In 2008, an estimated 33.4 million people were living with HIV/AIDS worldwide; nearly 70% of these were found in sub-Saharan Africa. Since the beginning of the epidemic, almost 60 million people have been infected with HIV and 25 million people have died of HIV-related causes. [1].

Altered hematopoiesis (blood cell production) occurs in patients with HIV infection. This change affects all three cell lines (red blood cells, white blood cells, and platelets) and consequently, HIV-infected patients may suffer from anemia, leucopenia, thrombocytopenia, or any combination of these three. They are common throughout the course of HIV infection and may be the direct result of HIV; at the stem cell level or the mature blood cell level; manifestations of secondary infections and neoplasms, or side effects of therapy. The use of cART could positively or negatively affect these parameters, depending on the choice of combination used. But generally, it will reverse most of the complications that are the direct result of HIV infection [2–4].

Anemia is the most commonly encountered hematologic abnormality, occurring in approximately 30% of patients with asymptomatic HIV and in as many as 75% to 80% of those with clinical AIDS; making it more common than thrombocytopenia or leucopenia in patients with AIDS [5, 6]. Its prevalence is significantly higher among HAART naive patients than those on HAART [7]. Anemia is

* Correspondence: tamiratemn1@yahoo.com
[1]Department of internal medicine, College of Public Health and Medical Sciences, Jimma University, P.O. Box376, Jimma, Ethiopia
Full list of author information is available at the end of the article

associated with progression to AIDS [8], shorter survival times [9],and it is a predictor of poorer prognosis for HIV infected patients independent of the CD4 count [10].

Leucopenia and neutropenia and/or lymphopenia often accompany HIV, and their prevalence increases from asymptomatic HIV-infected individuals to individuals with AIDS. Severe uncommon infections such as spontaneous bacterial infections, and rare fungal infections like aspergillosis or mucormycosis may occur in the course of HIV infection due to neutropenia, which may be seen in half of HIV-infected patients. The commonest cause of neutropenia is the result of drugs such as Zidovudine (AZT), the anti-CMV drug ganciclovir, or drugs used to treat cancers and tumors. [11, 12].

Thrombocytopenia is a common finding in individuals infected with HIV, occurring in about 40% of HIV-infected patients and the degree is generally mild to moderate; however, severe reduction of platelet count below 50,000/μL also occurs. With the advent of HAART, thrombocytopenia is more commonly seen in the setting of uncontrolled HIV infection and Hepatitis C co-infection. Thrombocytopenia in HIV infection can be due to either primary HIV-associated thrombocytopenia or secondary thrombocytopenia. Of which PHAT is the most common cause; clinically it resembles classic ITP. [13–15].

Despite the fact that hematologic manifestations of HIV infection are a well-recognized complication of the disease and it increases progression to AIDS; there are no studies done on its magnitude in Ethiopia. Hence this research aims to determine the magnitude and possible associated factors of hematological abnormalities among HIV-infected adult patients in the ART follow-up clinic of Jimma University Specialized Hospital, Jimma, Ethiopia.

Methods

Study design

A quantitative cross-sectional study was conducted from July 2012 to September 2012, at Jimma University Specialized Hospital, Jimma, Ethiopia; one of the teaching and referral Hospital in the country.

Sample size determination, sampling procedure and study subjects

All adult patients diagnosed with HIV and attending the ART follow-up clinic of Jimma University Specialized Hospital were the source population.

The sample size was calculated based on single population formula using a confidence interval (CI) of 95% and previous prevalence of cytopenias being 50% (unknown) among HAART and HAART naïve HIV-infected adult patients. A sample size of 361 was calculated and Quota sampling technique was used to recruit 130 HAART and 231 HAART naïve patients.

The study population was all adult HIV- infected patients who were on follow-up care at Jimma University Specialized Hospital during July 2012 to September 2012. Those adult patients, who have received chemotherapeutic agents (for any malignancy) within 6 months prior to the study, and blood transfusion within 3 months prior to the study, were excluded. Pregnant women and patients unable to give consent were also excluded from the study.

Data collection instrument and procedures

Structured questionnaires in English were used to collect the data. The questionnaires were constructed with socio-demographic characteristics, clinical data (duration of HIV infection, WHO clinical stage, opportunistic infection, malignancy and other co morbidity status) and medication data (ART status, ART regimen, ART duration and use of CPS).

A total of six health professionals, four ART nurses and an intern as data collectors, and the principal investigator as supervisor were involved in the data collection process of the study.

The study population was separated into HAART and HAART naïve groups. Each client who visited the clinic during the study period was evaluated for eligibility to be included in the study. Those eligible were included in the study consecutively for either of the two groups. The selection and inclusion of patients was continued until the specific number of patients (quota) was obtained for each category.

After patient interview and a detailed review of the medical record, about 4 ml of venous blood was collected by experienced laboratory technologist from each subject for immunologic (CD4 count) and hematologic parameters (CBC) analysis.

Data quality control

Pretesting of the questionnaires was done in a sample of 20 HIV-infected adult patients attending ALERT Hospital, located in the capital Addis Ababa, Ethiopia, before the actual study begun. The collected data was checked for completeness and internal consistency. Necessary correction of questionnaire was made accordingly after the pretest. These subjects were not included in the actual study result. Training was given to recruited data collectors. During data collection, the principal investigator ensured quality data collection by supervision, on spot corrective action and recollecting data on 5% of the study population. Each day the principal investigator reviewed all collected data, he checked for completeness and internal consistency and took immediate remedial action accordingly. Each sampled blood was analyzed within two hours using the Cell-Dyn 1800 auto analyzer machine for CBC and the Becton Dickenson(BD) FACS caliber for CD4 count. The performance of these machines was controlled by running quality control samples alongside the study subjects' sample.

Operational definitions

The 2011 World Health Organization (WHO) report on Hb concentration level to diagnose anemia was used to define and grade anemia [16]. Accordingly, for males Hb concentration of 13 g/dL or higher was considered non-Anemia(normal) and **anemia** was defined as Hb concentration < 13 g/dL (11.0–12.9 g/dL = mild; 8.0– 10.9 g/ dL moderate, and < 8.0 g/dL = severe), whereas for females Hb concentration of 12 g/dL or higher was considered non-Anemia(normal) and **anemia** was defined as Hb < 12. 0 (11.0–11.9 g/ dL = mild, 8.0–10.9 g/ dL = moderate, and < 8.0 g/dL = severe).

Patterns of anemia were classified as **normocytic** (MCV 80 -100 fL), **microcytic** (MCV < 80 fL), **macrocytic** (MCV > 100 fL), **normochromic** (MCH ≥27 pg) and **hypo chromic** (MCH < 27 pg). **MCHC** of < 32.3 g/dl, 32.3-35.9 g/dl and ≥ 36 g/dl were considered low, normal and high respectively.

Leucocyte count of 4-11 × 10^3/μl was considered normal and **leucopenia** was defined as total WBC count < 4 × 10^3 /μl. Neutrophils constitute 40-70% of the total WBC count and **neutropenia** was defined as absolute neutrophil count < 1000 cells/μl. Lymphocytes constitute 20-50% of the total WBC count and **lymphopenia** was considered when absolute lymphocyte count is < 800 cells/μl. **Platelet** count of 150-450× 10^3/μl was considered normal and **Thrombocytopenia** was defined as total platelet count < 150 × 10^3/μl [17].

Isolated cytopenia- presence of anemia, thrombocytopenia, or leucopenia.

Bicytopenia- presence of any 2 of the following 3: anemia, thrombocytopenia and leucopenia.

Pancytopenia- presence of anemia, thrombocytopenia, and leucopenia all together.

A normal **CD4** count in adults ranges from 500 to 1200 cells/mm^3.

Subjects were classified in to **stage1**, **stage 2**, **stage 3** and **stage 4**, based on WHO clinical staging of HIV disease in adults and adolescents [18].

HAART use was defined as receipt of two nucleoside reverse transcriptase inhibitors (NRTI) and one non-nucleoside reverse transcriptase inhibitor (NNRTI) or one protease inhibitor (PI).

Data processing and analysis

The collected data were categorized, coded, entered onto a computer, cleaned (verified) and analyzed using SPSS Windows version 20.0 software packages for statistical analysis. Descriptive analysis was done to determine the prevalence of anemia, leucopenia, neutropenia, lymphopenia, and thrombocytopenia; and patterns of anemia; and was presented using tables, diagrams and summary measures as appropriate. Before analysis, continuous variables were checked on whether they were normally distributed or not using normal graph curves. Normally distributed Continuous variables were compared with dependent variables using T- test and ANOVA; when ANOVA revealed significant difference further post hoc-multivariate comparison were done. Categorical variables were compared with dependent variables using chi- square test and fisher exact test when appropriate. When association was found the odds ratio was used to measure the strength of association. Finally, for variables which had statistically significant association with dependent variable multiple logistic regression analysis were done to come up with the independent predictors of outcome variables (dependent variable). All tests were two tailed and statistical significance was considered at $p < 0.05$ with 95%CI.

Results

Socio-demographic characteristics

Three hundred sixty-one HIV infected individuals were involved in this study, made up of 149(41.3%) males and 212(58.7%) females (Table 1). The overall mean age for the study population was 34.7 ± 10.1 years (range 16-70). The mean age of 32.1 ± 9.37 and 38.4 ± 10.04 years was obtained for females and males, respectively, with a minimum of 16 and 17, and a maximum of 70 and 68 years for females and males, respectively (Table 2). Majority of the study subjects (87.8%) were living in urban areas and more than three fourth (77.5%, $n = 280$) of the subjects had at least primary school education or more. Nearly half (49.6%, $n = 179$) of the participants were married, 18.8% single, 21.6% divorced and 10% were widows or widowers. 22.7% of the individuals were dependent and 54% earned monthly personal income below 500 birr ($ 27.78) (Table 1).

Base line clinical profile

The mean duration since the diagnosis of HIV for the study subjects was 30.3 ± 26.3 months (range 1-117). The mean duration for females and males was 31 ± 27.6 and 29 ± 24.3 months, respectively, with a minimum of 1 month for both and a maximum of 117 and 96 months for females and males, respectively (Table 2). According to WHO clinical staging, about two third (64%, $n = 231$) of the study subjects were in stage I and II, while 36% ($n = 130$) of the individuals had advanced clinical stage (stage III and IV) (Table 3).

13.3% ($n = 48$) of the individuals had history of opportunistic infection (OI) at the time of the study, the commonest being tuberculosis (TB) seen in 54.2% ($n = 26$) of cases, followed by chronic GE, pneumonia and candidiasis

Table 1 Distribution of socio-demographic characteristics of the study subjects, at JUSH from July-September 2012

Variables	On HAART N (%)	HAART naive N (%)	Total N (%)
Age in years			
16-26	17(13.1)	61(26.4)	78(21.6)
27-37	56(43.1)	107(46.3)	163(45.2)
38-48	40(30.8)	46(19.9)	86(23.8)
49-59	15(11.5)	7(3.0)	22(6.1)
60-70	2(1.5)	10(4.3)	12(3.3)
Total	130(100)	231(100)	361(100)
Mean age ± SD	33.5 ± 10.3	36.8 ± 9.5	
Sex			
Male	50(38.5)	99(42.9)	149(41.3)
Female	80(61.5)	132(57.1)	212(58.7)
Marital status			
Married	57(43.8)	122(52.8)	179(49.6)
Single	17(13.1)	51(22.1)	68(18.8)
Divorced	34(26.2)	44(19.0)	78(21.6)
Widowed	22(16.9)	14(6.1)	36(10.0)
Monthly personal income (Birr)			
< 500	84(64.6)	111(48.1)	195(54.0)
500-1000	21(16.2)	91(39.4)	112(31.0)
1001-1500	13(10.0)	24(10.4)	37(10.2)
> 1500	12(9.2)	5(2.2)	17(4.7)
Total	130(100)	231(100)	361(100)

(oral± esophageal) seen in 25% (n = 12), 10.4% (n = 5) and 10.4% (n = 5) of cases, respectively (Table 3).

The mean CD4 lymphocyte count for the study population was 380 ± 221 (range 5-1421). Mean CD4 count of 406 ± 232.6 and 343 ± 199 cells/μl was obtained for females and males, respectively, with a minimum of 5 and 36 and a maximum of 1377 and 1421 cells/μl for females and males respectively (Table 2). The majority of the study subjects (60.9%) had a CD4 count of 200-499 cells/μl; whereas 21. 1% and 18% of the subjects had CD4 lymphocyte count of ≥500 cells/μl and < 200 cells/μl, respectively (Table 3).

Of the 361 individuals about two third (64%, n = 231) were HAART naive and 36% (n = 130) were taking

Table 3 Clinical and immunological characteristics of the study subjects, at JUSH from July-September 2012

Variables	Females N (%)	Males N (%)	Total N (%)
WHO clinical stage			
Stage I	56(62.2)	34(37.8)	90(24.9)
Stage II	80(56.7)	61(43.3)	141(39.1)
Stage III	66(64.7)	36(35.3)	102(28.3)
Stage IV	10(35.7)	18(64.3)	28(7.8)
Opportunistic infections			
TB	12(46.2)	14(53.8)	26(7.2)
Chronic GE	6(50)	6(50)	12(3.3)
Pneumonia	1(20)	4(80)	5(1.4)
Candidiasis	4(80)	1(20)	5(1.4)
No	189(60.4)	124(39.6)	313(86.7)
Total	212(58.7)	149(41.3)	361(100)
Co- morbidities			
HTN	2(100)	0(0)	2(0.5)
DM	0(0)	2(100)	2(0.5)
CLD	2(100)	0(0)	2(0.5)
No	208(58.6)	147(41.4)	355(98.3)
Total	212(58.7)	149(41.3)	361(100)
Immunologic stage			
CD4 ≥ 500	53(69.7)	23(30.3)	76(21.1)
CD4 200-499	127(57.7)	93(42.3)	220(60.9)
CD4 < 200	32(49.2)	33(50.8)	65(18.0)

Table 2 Clinical and hematological parameter distribution of the study subjects, at JUSH from July-September 2012

Variables	Female		Male		HAART patients		HAART naïve		Total	
	Min-Max	Mean ± SD	MIn-Max	Mean ± SD	Min-Max	Mean ± SD	Min-Max	Mean ± SD	Min-Max	Mean ± SD
Age	16-70	32.1 ± 9.38	17-68	38.4 ± 10.04	20-67	36.9 ± 9.5	16-70	33.5 ± 10.3	16-70	34.7 ± 10
HIV dur. (months)	1-117	31 ± 27.6	1-96	29 ± 24.3	1-117	50.6 ± 25.7	1-90	18.9 ± 18.7	1-117	30 ± 26.3
ART dur. (months)	1-96	41 ± 25.8	1-76	36 ± 21.9	1-96	39 ± 24.5	–	–	1-96	39.11 ± 24.46
CD4 count	5-1377	406 ± 232.6	36-1421	343 ± 199.07	5-1314	429.2 ± 337.5	7.6-16.9	352 ± 207	5-1421	380 ± 221
Hemoglobin	4.3-15.6	11.9 ± 1.65	7.8-18.6	12.6 ± 2.1	4.3-18.6	12.6 ± 1.85	2.4-13	11.9 ± 1.8	4.3-18.6	12.2 ± 1.9
WBC × 10^3	1.8-13.0	6.007 ± 1.92	2.3-11.6	6.069 ± 1.78	1.8-12.5	6.28 ± 2	1.2-9.88	5.89 ± 1.76	1.8-13	6.03 ± 1.86
ANC × 10^3	1.062-9.88	3.549 ± 1.56	.920-8.424	3.530 ± 1.39	0.92-9.5	3.76 ± 1.7	0.35-5.05	3.42 ± 1.3	0.92-9.88	3.54 ± 1.48
TLC × 10^3	0.349-5.05	1.854 ± 0.76	.543-4.325	1.854 ± 0.706	0.57-4.3	1.9 ± 0.7	13-987	1.82 ± 0.75	0.349-5.05	1.85 ± 0.74
Platelet count × 10^3	62.0-987.0	296.769 ± 135.22	13-890	276.953 ± 149.89	73-750	290.3 ± 111.5	21-1421	287.6 ± 156.2	13-987	288.59 ± 141.59

HAART. 37.7% ($n = 80$) of female and 33.6% ($n = 50$) of male study subjects were on HAART (Table 3). Mean age of 33.5 ± 10.3 and 36.8 ± 9.5 years was obtained for HAART naïve and HAART patients respectively ($p = 0.002$) (Table 2). The mean CD4 count of HAART patients (429 ± 237) was 1.2 times higher than that of their HAART naïve counterparts (352 ± 207) ($p = 0.01$). 40% of HAART patients ($n = 52$) were taking TDF based first line regimen, while 39. 2% ($n = 51$) and 20% ($n = 26$) of individuals were taking AZT based and D4T based first line regimen, respectively, whereas only one individual (0.8%) was taking TDF based second line regimen. The overall mean duration since the initiation of HAART was 39 ± 24.5 months (range 1-96 months), it was 41 ± 25.8 and 36 ± 21.9 months for females and males respectively (Table 2).

60.9%($n = 220$) of the study subjects were taking co-trimoxazole prophylaxis therapy, 7.5%($n = 27$) were taking INH prophylaxis, 7.2%(n = 26) were taking anti TB treatment and another 7.5%(n = 27) were taking different drugs including fluconazole, antibiotics and vitamins.

Mean cell count values and prevalence of cytopenias

Hemoglobin concentration and anemia prevalence, severity and pattern

Anemia was the most common cytopenia in this study; seen in 186 (51.5%) cases (Table 4). The prevalence of anemia was 47.2% (100/212) in female patients and 57. 7% (86/149) in male patients ($p = 0.062$) (Table 4), it was 56.3%(130/231) and 43.1%(56/130) for HAART naïve and HAART patients, respectively, ($p = 0.021$) (Table 5). Anemia prevalence was 88.9% for patients with CD4 count < 50 cells/μl and 85.7% for CD4 count 50-99 cells/μl, 81% for CD4 count 100-199 cells/μl, 65.3% for CD4 count 200-349 cells/μl, 32.7% for CD4 count 350-500 cells/μl and 28.6% for CD4 count > 500 cells/μl ($p = 0.000$) (Table 6). We found 71.4% prevalence of anemia for WHO clinical stage IV patients and 62.7% for stage III, 57.4% for stage II and 23.3% for stage I patients ($p = 0.000$) (Table 7). There was no difference between the prevalence of anemia in relation to ART regimen (AZT vs non-AZT based) ($p = .0.58$) (data not shown).

Most of the anemic patients, 79.6%($n = 148$), had mild degree of anemia (Hb ≥ 11 g/dl), while 19.3%($n = 36$) had moderately severe anemia (Hb 8-10.9 g/dl) and two individuals (1.1%) had severe anemia (Hb < 8 g/dl) (Table 5). Moderately severe anemia was seen in 35.2% and 13.6% of patients with CD4 count < 200cells /μl and CD4 count ≥200cells /μl, respectively, ($p = 0.001$); in 9.5%, 12. 3%, 28.1% and 35% of patients with WHO clinical stage I, II, III and IV, respectively, ($p = 0.007$) (data not shown); in 7.1% and 24.6% of HAART and HAART naïve patients, respectively ($p = 0.017$) (Table 5). Whereas, there was no difference between the severity of anemia in relation to gender.

The most common pattern of anemia was normocytic normochromic in 98 (52.7%) cases followed by macrocytic anemia in 60 (32.2%) cases, normocytic hypo chromic anemia in 17 (9.1%) cases and microcytic hypo chromic anemia in 11(5.9%) cases (Fig. 1). Normocytic normochromic, normocytic hypo chromic, microcytic

Table 4 Frequency distribution of cytopenia in the study subjects, at JUSH from July-September 2012 ($n = 361$)

Cytopenia	Female ($n = 212$) N (%)	Male ($n = 149$) N (%)	Total (361) N (%)
Anemia	100(53.8)	86(57.7)	186(51.5)
Leucopenia	28(13.2)	19(12.8)	47(13)
Thrombocytopenia	18(8.5)	22(14.80	40(11.1)
Lymphopenia	13(6.1)	5(3.4)	18(5)
Neutropenia	0(0)	1(0.7)	1(0.3)
Isolated cytopenia	100(47.2)	83(55.7)	183(50.7)
Bicytopenia	9(4.2)	13(8.70	22(6.1)

Table 5 Distribution of categories of hematologic values of the study subjects, at JUSH from July-September 2012

Variables	On HAART N (%)	HAART naïve N (%)	Total N (%)	*P*-value
Hemoglobin (g/dl)				
Not anemic	74(56.9)	101(43.7)	175(48.5)	0.021
Anemic	56(43.1)	130(56.3)	186(51.5)	
Total	130(100)	231(100)	361(100)	
Anemia severity				
Grade 1	50(89.3)	98(75.4)	148(79.6)	
Grade 2	4(7.1)	32(24.6)	36(19.3)	
Grade 3	2(3.6)	0(0.0)	2(1.1)	
Total	56(100)	130(100)	186(100)	
WBC (cells/μl)				
≥4000	114(87.7)	200(86.6)	314(87.0)	0.890
< 4000	16(12.3)	31(13.4)	47(13.0)	
Total	130(100)	231(100)	361(100)	
ANC (cells/μl)				
≥1000	129(99.2)	231(100.0)	360(99.7)	
< 1000	1(0.8)	0(0.0)	1(0.3)	
Total	130(100)	231(100)	361(100)	
TLC (cells/μl)				
≥800	126(96.9)	217(93.9)	343(95.0)	0.318
< 800	4(3.1)	14(6.1)	18(5.0)	
Total	130(100)	231(100)	361(100)	
Platelet count (cells/μl)				
$\geq 150 \times 10^3$	121(93.1)	200(86.6)	321(88.9)	0.087
$< 150 \times 10^3$	9(6.9)	31(13.4)	40(11.1)	
Total	130(100)	231(100)	360(100)	

Table 6 Association of immunologic stages with cytopenias in the study subjects, at JUSH from July-September 2012

Immunologic stage	Total N (%)	Anemia N (%)	P-value	Leucopenia N (%)	*P*-value	Thrombocytopenia N (%)	P-value	Lymphopenia N (%)	*P*-value
> 500	77 (21.3)	22(28.6)	0.000	3(3.9)	0.000	5(6.5)	0.261	0(0)	0.000
350-500	101 (28)	33(32.7)		6(5.9)		10(9.9)		0(0)	
200-349	118 (32.7)	77(65.3)		16(13.6)		13(11)		5(4.20	
100-199	42 (11.6)	34(81.00		14(33.3)		9(21.4)		5(11.9)	
50-99	14 (3.9)	12(85.7)		4(28.6)		2(14.3)		6(42.9)	
< 50	9 (2.5)	8(88.9)		4(44.4)		1(11.1)		2(22.2)	
Total	361(100)	186(51.5)		47(13)		40(11.1)		18(5)	

hypo chromic and macrocytic anemia were seen in 60. 8%, 12.3%, 8.5% and 18.5% and 33.9%, 1.8%, 0% and 64. 3% of HAART naïve and HAART patients, respectively, ($p = 0.000$). Whereas there was no difference between the pattern of anemia in relation to gender, WHO clinical stage and immunologic stage (data not shown).

The mean ± standard deviation (SD) hemoglobin concentration for the study population was 12.2 ± 1.86 (range 4.3-18.6) (Table 2), it was 11.9 ± 1.65 g/dl and 12. 6 ± 1.65 g/dl for female and male patients respectively ($p = 0.000$) (Table 2), 10.9 ± 1.9 g/dl and 12.47 ± 1.7 g/dl for CD4 count < 200 cells/μl and ≥ 200 cells/μl, respectively (p = 0.000) (data not shown), 12.6 ± 1.84 and 11.9 ± 1. 83 for HAART and HAART naïve patients, respectively (Table 2) ($p = 0.002$) and it was 12.5 ± 1.77 and 11.6 ± 1.87 for patients with early and advanced WHO clinical stages, respectively ($p = 0.000$). There was no difference between the mean hemoglobin concentration in relation to ART regimen (data not shown).

Mean WBC count and prevalence of leucopenia

Leucopenia (WBC < 4000/μL) was found in13%($n = 47$) of the participants, the prevalence was 13.2% (28) in female patients and 12.8% (19) in male patients (Table 4), ($p = 1.000$). Leucopenia was found in 3.9%, 5.9%, 13.6%, 33.3%, 28.6% and 44.4% of patients with CD4 count> 500 cells/μl, 350-500 cells/μl, 200-349 cells/μl, 100-199 cells/μl, 50-99 cells/μl and < 50 cells/μl respectively ($p = 0.000$) (Table 6). Whereas there was no difference between the prevalence of leucopenia in relation to WHO clinical stages (Table 7), ART status (Table 5) and ART regimen (data not shown).

The mean ± standard deviation (SD) WBC count for the study population was $6.03 \pm 1.86 \times 10^3$ (range 1.8-13) (Table 2), it was 5.11 ± 1.88 and $6.24 \pm 1.8 \times 10^3$ for patients in the CD4 count group < 200 and ≥ 200/μl, respectively, ($p = 0.000$) (data not shown). Otherwise there was no difference between the mean WBC count in relation to gender, WHO clinical stages, ART status and ART regimen (data not shown).

Mean platelet count and prevalence of thrombocytopenia

Thrombocytopenia (platelet< 150,000/μL) was found in 11.1%($n = 40$) of the study subjects, the prevalence was 8. 5%(18/212) and 14.8%(22/149) for female and male patients respectively (Table 4), ($p = 0.089$); 2%(1/51) and 10. 1%(8/79) for AZT and non AZT based HAART patients, respectively, ($p = 0.579$) (data not shown).There was no difference between the prevalence of thrombocytopenia in relation to immunologic stage (CD4 category) (Table 6), WHO clinical stages (Table 7) and ART status (Table 5).

The mean ± standard deviation (SD) platelet count for the study population was $288.6 \pm 141.6 \times 10^3$ (range 13-987) (Table 2), it was 255.3 ± 135.7 and $295.9 \pm 142.02 \times 10^3$ for patients in the CD4 count group < 200 and ≥ 200/μl, respectively, ($p = 0.036$); 303.7 ± 119.2 and 281.7 ± 106. 2×10^3 for AZT and non-AZT based HAART, respectively, ($p = 0.273$). There was no difference between the mean platelet count in relation to gender, WHO clinical stages, ART status and ART regimen (data not shown).

Mean TLC and prevalence of lymphopenia

Lymphopenia (TLC < 800/μL) was found in 5%($n = 18$) of the participants, the prevalence was 6.1%(13/212) and

Table 7 Association of clinical stage with cytopenia in the study subjects, at JUSH from July-September 2012

Clinical stage	Total N (%)	Anemia N (%)	P-value	Leucopenia N (%)	P-value	Thrombocytopenia N (%)	*P*-value	Lymphopenia N (%)	*P*-value
Stage I	90(24.9)	21(23.3)	0.000	9(10)	0.132	9(10)	0.982	2(2.2)	0.138
Stage II	141(39.1)	81(57.4)		15(10.6)		16(11.3)		5(3.5)	
Stage III	102(28.3)	64(62.7)		16(15.7)		12(11.8)		9(8.8)	
Stage IV	28(7.8)	20(71.4)		7(25)		3(10.7)		2(7.1)	
Total	361(100)	186(51.5)		47(13)		40(11.1)		18(5)	

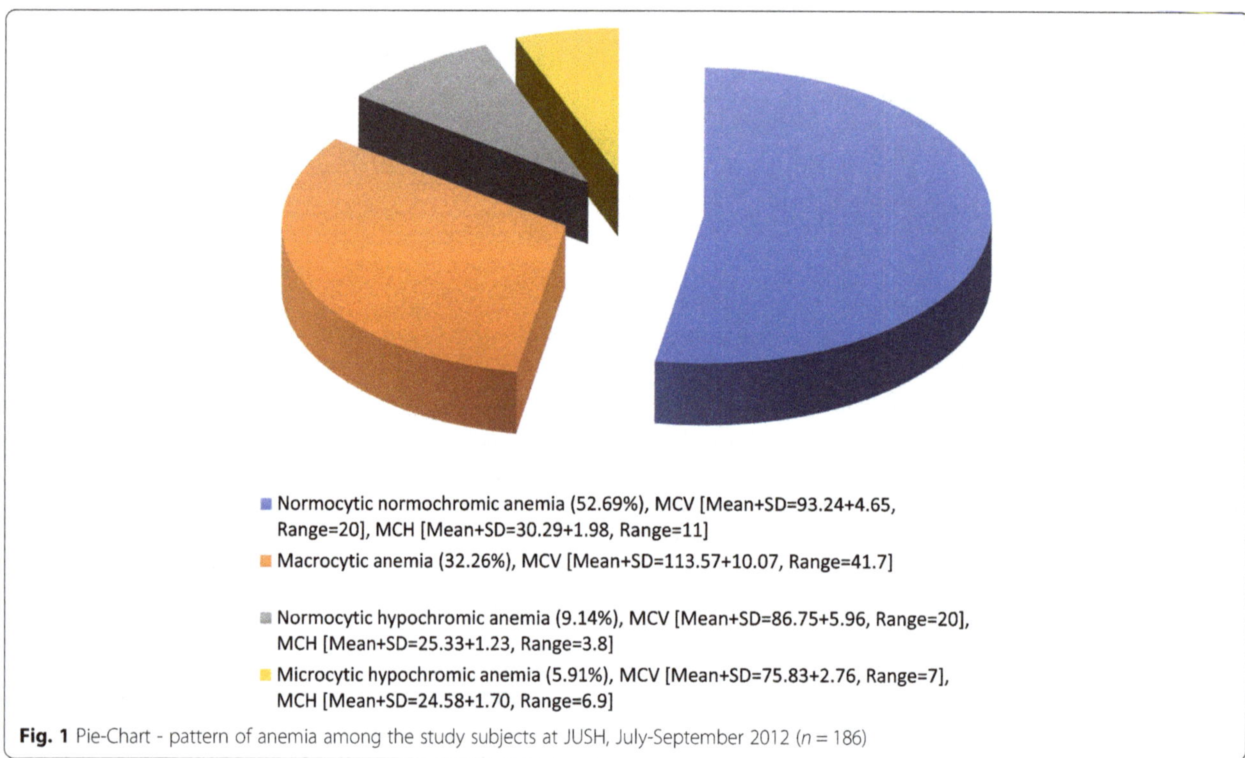

Fig. 1 Pie-Chart - pattern of anemia among the study subjects at JUSH, July-September 2012 ($n = 186$)

3.4%(5/149) for female and male patients, respectively (Table 4), ($p = 0.343$). The prevalence of lymphopenia was 0%, 0%, 4.2%, 11.9%, 42.9% and 22.2% for patients with CD4 count > 500, 350-500, 200-349, 100-199, 50-99 and < 50 cells/μl, respectively, ($p = 0.000$) (Table 6). Otherwise there was no difference between the prevalence of lymphopenia in relation to WHO clinical stages (Table 7), ART status (Table 5) and ART regimens (data not shown).

The mean ± standard deviation (SD) TLC for the study population was $1.85 \pm 0.735 \times 10^3$ (range 0.349-5.05) (Table 2), it was 1.39 ± 0.66 and $1.96 \pm 0.7 \times 10^3$ for patients in the CD4 count group < 200 and ≥ 200/μl, respectively, ($p = 0.000$); whereas there was no difference between the mean TLC in relation to gender, WHO clinical stages, ART status and ART regimens (data not shown).

Mean ANC and prevalence of neutropenia, isolated cytopenia and bicytopenia

Neutropenia (ANC < 1000/μL) was present in only one individual (0.3%) and isolated cytopenia and bicytopenia were found in 50.7%($n = 183$) and 6.1%($n = 22$) of the participants respectively, and there was no one with Pancytopenia (Table 4).

The mean ± standard deviation (SD) ANC for the study population was $3.54 \pm 1.49 \times 10^3$ (range 0.92-9.88) (Table 2) , it was 3.42 ± 1.3 and $3.76 \pm 1.74 \times 10^3$ for HAART naïve and HAART patients (Table 2), respectively, ($p = 0.037$) and 3.2 ± 1.46 and $3.6 \pm 1.5 \times 10^3$ for patients in the CD4 count group < 200 and ≥ 200/μl, respectively, ($p = 0.031$) (data not shown); whereas there was no difference between the mean ANC in relation to gender, WHO clinical stages and ART regimens (data not shown).

Risk factors for cytopenias

A univariate analysis showed that many risk factors were associated with prevalent anemia. Risk factors associated with increased risk of anemia were: Advanced WHO clinical stage OR 2.3(IC 95% 1.48-3.59; $p = 0.000$), presence of opportunistic infection OR 10.2(IC 95% 3.94-26.5; $p = 0.000$), lack of HAART OR 1.7(IC 95% 1.1-2.6; $p = 0.021$), use of co-trimoxazole prophylaxis therapy OR 1.99(IC 95% 1.29-3. 05; $p = 0.002$), CD4 count < 200 cells/μl OR 6.1(IC 95% 3.1-12.1; $p = 0.000$), WBC count < 4000/μl OR 2.78(IC 95% 1. 41-5.48; $p = 0.004$) and TLC < 800 cells/μl OR 17.5(IC 95% 2.3-132.98; $p = 0.000$). Presence of opportunistic infection, use of co-trimoxazole prophylaxis therapy and CD4 count < 200 cells/μl were associated with an increased risk of anemia in the multivariate analysis with OR 5.72(IC 95% 2. 05-15.97; $p = 0.001$), OR 1.65(IC 95% 1.02-2.67; $p = 0.040$) and OR 3.34(IC 95% 1.57-7.1; $p = 0.002$) respectively (Table 8).

A univariate analysis showed that use of co-trimoxazole prophylaxis therapy, CD4 count < 200cells /μl, presence of anemia and presence of lymphopenia were associated with increased risk of leucopenia with OR 3.06(IC 95% 1.43-6. 55; $p = 0.005$), OR 5.54(IC 95% 2.87-10.7; $p = 0.000$), OR 2.

Table 8 Factors associated with anemia in the study subjects, at JUSH from July-September 2012

Variables	Anemia present $n = 186$ N (%)	No anemia $n = 175$ N (%)	COR (95% CI) *p*-value	AOR (95% CI) *p*-value
Clinical stage				
Advanced (stage III and IV)	84(45.2)	46(26.3)	2.3(1.48-3.6) 0.000	1.59(0.93-2.72) 0.089
Early (stage I and II)	102(54.8)	129(73.7)		
Opportunistic infection				
Present	43(23.1)	5(2.9)	10.2(3.94-26.5) 0.000	5.72(2.05-15.92) 0.001
Absent	143(76.9)	170(97.1)		
HAART status				
HAART naïve	130(69.9)	101(57.7)	1.7(1.1-2.6) 0.021	1.53(0.91-2.56) 0.109
On HAART	56(30.1)	74(42.3)		
Use of CPT				
On CPT	128(68.8)	92(52.6)	1.99(1.29-3.05) 0.002	1.65(1.02-2.67) 0.04
Not on CPT	58(31.2)	83(47.4)		
CD4 count				
1 < 200	54(29)	11(6.3)	6.1(3.1-12.1) 0.000	3.34(1.57-7.1) 0.002
≥200	132(71)	164(93.7)		
WBC count				
< 4000	34(18.3)	13(7.4)	2.78(1.41-5.48) 0.004	1.44(0.66-3.14) 0.356
≥4000	152(81.7)	162(92.6)		
TLC				
< 800	17(9.1)	1(0.6)	17.5(2.3-132.98) 0.000	7.26(0.867-60.74)
≥800	169(90.9)	174(99.4)		

78(IC 95% 1.41-5.48; $p = 0.004$) and OR 6.23(IC 95% 2.32-16.74; $p = 0.000$), respectively. In the multivariate analysis only CD4 count < 200 cells/μl and use of co-trimoxazole prophylaxis therapy were associated with increased risk of leucopenia with OR 3.34(IC 95% 1.59-7.02; $p = 0.001$) and OR 2.34(IC 95% 1.05-5.19; $p = 0.036$) respectively (Table 9).

In a univariate analysis, there wasn't any risk factor associated with prevalence of thrombocytopenia. It was found in 6.5%, 9.9%, 11%, 21.4%, 14.3% and 11. 1% of patients with CD4 count > 500 cells/μl, 350-500 cells/μl, 200-349 cells/μl, 100-199 cells/μl, 50-99 cells/μl and < 50 cells/μl respectively ($p = 0.261$) (Table 6). Although statistically not significant HAART naïve patients were more than 2 times at risk of having thrombocytopenia compared to those on HAART ($p = 0.087$) (Table 5). Patients on non-AZT based HAART were more than 5 times at risk of having thrombocytopenia compared to those on AZT based HAART, however it wasn't statistically significant ($p = 0.151$) (data not shown).

Table 9 Factors associated with prevalent leucopenia in the study subjects, at JUSH from July-September 2012

Variables	Leucopenia present $n = 47$ N (%)	No leucopenia $n = 314$ N (%)	COR (95% CI) *p*-value	AOR (95% CI) *p*-value
Use of CPT				
On CPT	38(80.9)	182(58)	3.06(1.43-6.55) 0.005	2.34(1.05-5.19) 0.036
Not on CPT	9(19.1)	132(42)		
CD4 count				
< 200	22(46.8)	43(13.7)	5.54(2.87-10.7) 0.000	3.34(1.59-7.02) 0.001
≥200	25(53.2)	271(86.3)		
Anemia status				
Present	34(72.3)	152(48.4)	2.78(1.41-5.48) 0.004	1.6(0.76-3.34) 0.211
Absent	13(27.7)	162(51.6)		
TLC				
< 800	8(17)	10(3.2)	6.23(2.32-16.74	2.78(0.908-8.54) 0.073
≥800	39(83)	304(96.8)		

A univariate analysis showed that many risk factors were associated with prevalence of lymphopenia. Risk factors associated with increased risk of lymphopenia were: duration since the diagnosis of HIV ≤ 6 months OR 12.3(IC 95% 3.9-38.4; $p = 0.000$), duration since the initiation of HAART ≤ 6 months OR 26.07(IC 95% 2.52-269.3; $p = 0.006$), CD4 count < 200 cells/µl OR 14.5(IC 95% 4.97-42.53), presence of anemia OR 17.5(IC 95% 2. 3-132.98; p = 0.000), presence of leucopenia OR 6.23(IC 95% 2.32-16.74; p = 0.000) and presence of opportunistic infection OR 3.58(IC 95% 1.27-10.05; $p = 0.021$). In the multivariate analysis, none of them were associated with increased risk of lymphopenia (data not shown).

Discussion

Our study revealed that 51.5% of the study population was anemic, a value that agrees with the Benin city and India studies [7, 19]. In contrast to other studies, there were no gender difference in the prevalence of anemia in this study, women (47.2%) and men (57.7%) ($p = 0.062$) [20]. Also, we did not observe any difference in the prevalence of microcytic anemia among women (6%) and men (5.8%) ($p = 0.918$). These indicate that iron deficiency was not the main cause of anemia in the study population.

This study confirms that anemia is directly related with the degree of immunosuppression, a finding that agrees with those found by others [20–22]; the lower the CD4 count the higher the prevalence of anemia.

We also proved that anemia is associated with advanced WHO clinical stage, a finding that is in accordance with the literature [18, 20, 22]; the advanced the clinical stage the higher the prevalence of anemia.

In accordance with the Benin city and Rwanda studies [7, 22], we did find a higher prevalence of anemia in HAART naïve patients compared to patients on HAART. We did not observe any significant difference between the hemoglobin level in relation to ART regimens (AZT based HAART vs non-AZT based HAART); a finding that differs from those observed by others who have observed a higher prevalence of anemia in patients taking AZT based HAART [20]. The possible explanation could be that, in contrast to the pre-HAART era, the risk of anemia with AZT therapy has been reduced with the advent of HAART [23].

Our study revealed that use of co-trimoxazole prophylaxis therapy is positively associated with prevalence of anemia, a finding in sharp contrast with that found by others, who have found a negative association between use of CPT and prevalence of anemia [20]. One possible explanation could be that trimethoprim is a weak inhibitor of dihydrofolate reductase and in high doses, it has been implicated in Megaloblastic Pancytopenia, particularly in patients who are not on folate supplementation like our patients [24]. However, the usage of co trimoxazole therapy wasn't different between macrocytic (73.3%) and other patterns of anemia (66.6%) ($p = 0.816$).

Moreover, this study found that, presence of an opportunistic infection at the time of the study was associated with an increased prevalence of anemia, irrespective of clinical stage and degree of immunosuppression, which could perhaps be explained by anemia related to secondary infections.

The study found normocytic normochromic anemia as the most common pattern of anemia (52.7%); a finding that is in agreement with the literature [25, 26]. Macrocytic RBC morphology was seen in 32.2% of the anemic subjects, a finding with a value higher than others (9%) [25]. Possible explanation for this could be higher rate of co trimoxazole usage in our patients, which as already mentioned above is associated with Megaloblastic anemia in patients who lack folate supplementation.

The prevalence of leucopenia in our patients, defined as WBC count less than 4000/µl, was 13%, a value somewhat lower than those found by other studies, which were done on HAART naive patients [21, 25]. The possible explanation for this could be the presence of HAART patients in our study which, to a certain degree, lowered the prevalence.

The study confirmed that leucopenia is directly related with the degree of immunosuppression, a finding that agrees with the literature [21]. Our study also revealed that use of co-trimoxazole prophylaxis therapy is positively associated with prevalence of leucopenia, a finding not addressed by others. This could be due to the megaloblastic side effect of co trimoxazole therapy in the absence of folate supplementation.

The prevalence of thrombocytopenia (platelet count less than 150×10^3) in our patients was 11.1%, a value somewhat similar to that found by others [19]. This study confirmed that prevalence of thrombocytopenia is not associated with neither the degree of immunosuppression nor with the clinical stage of HIV, a finding that is in accordance with the literature [18, 21]. Most importantly, this study also showed a higher prevalence of thrombocytopenia among patients on non-AZT based HAART regimen as compared to those on AZT based HAART regimen. The possible explanation could be that AZT can rapidly increase platelet count in patients with HIV related thrombocytopenia [27, 28].

The prevalence of lymphopenia in our patients, defined as TLC less than 800 cells/µl, was 5%, a value lower than those found by a study undertaken on HAART naive patients [29]. This could be due to the presence of HAART patients in our study which, to a certain degree, lowered the prevalence. As expected, we found that patients with CD4 count less than 200cells/µl presented with a significantly increased prevalence of lymphopenia. Our study revealed that lymphopenia is inversely related with the duration of HIV infection, higher prevalence observed in a group of patients diagnosed in the prior 6 months. This might be due to the rapid viral replication and associated lymphocyte cell death occurring in the acute phase of HIV infection. The study also revealed that prevalence of lymphopenia is inversely related with the duration of HAART treatment, lower prevalence observed in a group of patients with HAART duration greater than 6 months. This could be due to the hematologic recovery that occurs after 6 months of HAART treatment [29].

Neutropenia, defined as ANC less than 1000/μl, was found only in one individual, a finding that agrees with the Indian study which found no patient with neutropenia [26]. The mean Neutrophil count was lower in HAART naïve and immunologic AIDS patients, a finding that is in accordance with the literature [27, 28, 30].

In summary, the hematologic abnormalities that we have observed in our patients could be the direct result of the HIV infection itself; nutritional deficiencies; manifestations of secondary infections and neoplasms, or side effects of therapy. Cytopenias, particularly anemia, could be associated with progression to AIDS, shorter survival times, and a predictor of poorer prognosis in our patients.

Conclusion and recommendation

Conclusion

In conclusion in this study anemia, leucopenia, thrombocytopenia and lymphopenia were common among the study subjects in both HAART naïve and HAART patients. Of the cytopenias, anemia was the most common manifestation and the most frequent patterns were normocytic normochromic and macrocytic forms, whereas neutropenia was rare.

Prevalence of anemia, leucopenia and lymphopenia correlates with disease progression. Thrombocytopenia occurs independent of disease progression. The present study also showed that use of co-trimoxazole prophylaxis therapy was independently associated with an increased risk of anemia and leucopenia; a finding that needs to be strengthened by further study.

Recommendation

Based on these findings it is recommended that physicians giving care for HIV infected adults should routinely investigate and treat hematologic abnormalities in both HAART and HAART naïve patients to reduce the morbidity and mortality of the patients.

Additionally, co trimoxazole prophylaxis therapy should be avoided in HIV-infected adult patients who have folic acid deficiency or who are pregnant, and instead the other alternatives for PCP prophylaxis can be used. And in the rest group of HIV patients co trimoxazole prophylaxis therapy should only be used if the potential benefit outweighs the possible hematologic risk (patients with CD4 count< 200 cells/μl, prior bout of PCP).

However, large scale and longitudinal studies, giving emphasis on the association of co trimoxazole prophylaxis therapy and cytopenia, are recommended to strengthen and explore the problem in depth.

Abbreviation

AIDS: Acquired Immuno deficiency syndrome; ANC: Absolute Neutrophil count; ANOVA: One-way analysis of variance; ART: Anti-retroviral therapy; AZT: Zidovudine; CART: Combined Anti-retroviral therapy; CBC: Complete blood count; CDC: Center for disease control; CMV: Cytomegalovirus; CPT: Cotrimoxazole prophylaxis therapy; Fl: Femto liter; GCSF: Granulocyte colony stimulating factor; HAART: Highly active antiretroviral therapy; Hb: Hemoglobin; HIV: Human immunodeficiency virus; ITP: Idiopathic thrombocytopenic purpura; JUSH: Jimma university specialized hospital; MCH: Mean Corpuscular hemoglobin; MCHC: Mean cell hemoglobin concentration; MCV: Mean Corpuscular Volume; NNRTI: Non- Nucleoside reverse transcriptase inhibitor; NRTI: Nucleoside reverse transcriptase inhibitor; PCV: Packed cell volume; Pg: Pico gram; PHAT: Primary HIV associated thrombocytopenia; PI: Protease inhibitor; PLWHA: Patient living with HIV/AIDS; RBC: Red blood cell; SPSS: Statistical Package for Social Science; TB: Tuberculosis; TLC: Total lymphocyte count; TTP-HUS: Thrombotic thrombocytopenic purpura- hemolytic uremic syndrome; WBC: White blood cell count; WHO: World Health Organization

Acknowledgments

The authors thank all nurses, interns and laboratory staffs who participated during data collection and laboratory analysis activities. The authors are also grateful to thank the study subjects for their voluntary participation in the study. Our special thanks to Kurt McCray and Kerry Boyd, Ekg quality assurance specialists at Medi-lynx for their major contribution in editing the manuscript. Lastly, we would like to thank Jimma University and Jimma Specialized Hospital for logistic support.

Funding

The research was 100% funded by the primary author.

Authors' contributions

TEF conceived and designed the study, collected the data, performed the statistical analysis and drafted the manuscript. LH, CH and DKW participated in its design and coordination and helped to draft the manuscript. All authors read and approved the final manuscript.

Competing interests

The authors declare that they have no competing interests.

Author details

[1]Department of internal medicine, College of Public Health and Medical Sciences, Jimma University, P.O. Box376, Jimma, Ethiopia. [2]Department of Epidemiology, Jimma University, P.O. Box 376, Jimma, Ethiopia. [3]Department of Internal Medicine, Bahir Dar University, -79 Bahir Dar, Ethiopia.

References

1. UNAIDS – Joint United Nations Program on HIV/ADIS. Annual report. 2009. http://data.unaids.org/pub/report/2010/2009_annual_report_en.pdf Accessed 15 June 2010.?
2. Longo DL, Fauci AS. Human immunodeficiency virus disease: AIDS and related disorders. In: Fauci A, Braunwald E, Kasper D, Hauser S, Longo D, editors. Harrison's principles of internal medicine. 18th ed. New York City: McGraw-Hill Companies; 2011. p. 1500–85.
3. Coyle TE. Hematologic complications of human immunodeficiency virus infection and the acquired immunodeficiency syndrome. Med Clin North Am. 1997;81:449–70.
4. RD KJC, Chaisson RE. Anemia and survival in HIV infection. J Acquire Immune Defic Syndr Hum Retrovirol. 1998;19:29–33.
5. Volberding P. The impact of anemia on quality of life in human immunodeficiency virus infected patients. J Infect Dis. 2002;185(2):110–4.
6. Levine AM. Anemia, neutropenia, and thrombocytopenia: pathogenesis and evolving treatment options in HIV-infected patients. Medscape HIV Clinical · Management Series. 1999;10:1–27. https://www.medscape.org/viewarticle/420904_6. Accessed 29 June 2010
7. Omoregie R, Omokaro EU, Palmer O, Ogefere HO, Egbeobauwaye A, Adeghe JE, Osakue SI, Ihemeje V. Prevalence of anemia among HIV-infected patients in Benin City, Nigeria. Tanzan J Health Res. 2009;11(1):1–4.
8. Morfeldt-Månson L, Böttiger B, Nilsson B, von Stedingk LV. Clinical signs and laboratory markers in predicting progression to AIDS in HIV-1 infected patients. Scand J Infect Dis. 1991;23:443–9.
9. Ellaurie M, Burns ER, Rubinstein A. Hematologic manifestations in pediatric HIV infection: severe anemia as a prognostic factor. Am J Pediatric Hematol Oncol. 1990;12:449–53.
10. Mocroft A, Kirk O, Barton SE, Dietrich M, Proenca R, Colebunders R, Pradier C, Darminio Monforte A, Ledergerber B, Lundgren JD. Anemia is an independent predictive marker for clinical prognosis in HIV infected patients from across Europe. AIDS. 1999;13:943–50.
11. Murphy MF, Metcalfe P, Waters AH, Carne CA, Weller IV, Linch DC, Smith A. Incidence and mechanism of neutropenia and thrombocytopenia in patients with HIV infection. Br J Hem. 1987;66:337–40.
12. Rossi G, Gloria R, Stellini R, Franceschini F, Bettinzioli M, Cadeo G, Sueri L, Cattaneo R, Marinone G. Prevalence, clinical and laboratory features of thrombocytopenia among HIV-infected individuals. AIDS Res Hum Retrovir. 1990;6:261–9.
13. Sioand EM, Klein HG, Banks SM, Vareldziz B, Merritt S, Pierce P. Epidemiology of thrombocytopenia in HIV infection. Eur J Hematol. 1992;48:168–72.
14. The Swiss Group for Clinical Studies on the Acquired Immunodeficiency Syndrome (AIDS). Zidovudine for the Treatment of Thrombocytopenia Associated with Human Immunodeficiency Virus (HIV): A Prospective Study. Ann Intern Med. 1988;109(9):718–21.
15. Jackson GG, Paul DA, Falk LA, Rubenis M, Despotes JC, Mack D, Knigge M, Emeson EE. Human immunodeficiency virus antigenemia in the acquired immunodeficiency syndrome and the effect of treatment with zidovudine. Ann Intern Med. 1988;108:175–80.
16. World Health Organization. Hemoglobin Concentration for the Diagnosis of Anemia and Assessment of Severity. In: Vitamin and Mineral Nutrition Information System. 2011. http://apps.who.int/iris/bitstream/handle/10665/85839/WHO_NMH_NHD_MNM_11.1_eng.pdf;jsessionid=BD9F9FB066817BF287AD4BD8B057B0ED?sequence=3. Accessed 15 Sep 2011.
17. Henry PH, Longo DL. Disorders of granulocytes and monocytes. In: Kasper DL, Braunwald E, Hauser S, Longo D, Larry Jameson J, Fauci AS, editors. Harrison's principles of internal medicine (16th edition). New York City: McGraw-Hill Companies; 2005. p. 1137–203.
18. Adewuyi JO, Coutts AM, Latif AS, Smith H, Abayomi AE, Moyo AA. Haematologic features of the human immunodeficiency virus (HIV) infection in adult Zimbabweans. Cent Afr J Med. 1999;45:26–30.
19. Dikshit B, Wanchu A, Sachdeva RK, Sharma A, Das R. Profile of hematological abnormalities of Indian HIV infected individuals. BMC Blood Disord. 2009;9:5.
20. Sullivan PS, Hanson DL, Chu SY, Jones JL, John W. Ward, and group. Epidemiology of Anemia in human immunodeficiency virus (HIV)-infected persons: results from the multistate adult and adolescent Spectrum of HIV disease surveillance project. Blood. 1998;91:301–8.
21. Akinbami A, Oshinaike O, Adeyemo T, Adediran A, Owolabi D, Dada M, Durojaiye I, Adebola A, Vincent O. Hematologic abnormalities in treatment-Naïve HIV patients infectious diseases. Research and Treatment. 2010;3:45–9.
22. Masaisa F, Gahutu JB, Mukiibi J, Delanghe J, Philippé J. Anemia in human immunodeficiency virus–infected and uninfected women in Rwanda. Am J Trop Med Hyg. 2011;4:456–60.
23. Semba RD, Shah N, Klein RS, Mayer KH, Schuman P, Vlahov D. Prevalence and cumulative incidence of and risk factors for anemia in a multicenter cohort study of human immunodeficiency virus-infected and uninfected women. Clin Infect Dis. 2002;34:260–6.
24. Pattishall KH, Acar J, Burchall JJ, et al. Two distinct types of trimethoprim-resistant dihydrofolate reductase specified by R-plasmids of different compatibility groups. J Biol Chem. 1977;252:2319.
25. Pande A, Bhattacharyya M, Pain S, Ghosh B, Saha S, Ghosh A, Banerjee A. Anemia in antiretroviral Naïve HIV/AIDS patients: a study from eastern India. Online J Health Allied Scs. 2011;10:4.
26. Erhabor O, Ejele OA, Nwauche CA, Buseri FI. Some hematological parameters in human immunodeficiency virus (HIV) infected Africans: the Nigerian perspective. Niger J Med. 2005;14:33–8.
27. Zon LI, Arkin C, Groopman JE. Hematologic manifestations of the human immunodeficiency virus (HIV). Br J Hematol. 1987;66:251.
28. Murphy PM, Lane HC, Fauci AS, Gallin JI. Impairment of neutrophil bactericidal capacity in patients with AIDS. J Infect Dis. 1988;158:627–30.
29. Choi SY, Kim I, Kim NJ, Lee S-A, Choi Y-A, Bae J-Y, Kwon JH, Choe PG, Park WB, Yoon S-S, Park S, Kim BK, Oh M-D. Hematological manifestations of human immunodeficiency virus infection and the effect of highly active anti-retroviral therapy on cytopoenia. Korean J Hematol. 2011;46:253–7.
30. Zon LI, JE. Groopman hematologic manifestations of the human immune deficiency virus (HIV). Semin Hematol. 1988;25:208–18.

An outline of anemia among adolescent girls in Bangladesh: findings from a cross-sectional study

Sabuj Kanti Mistry[1*], Fatema Tuz Jhohura[1], Fouzia Khanam[1], Fahmida Akter[1], Safayet Khan[1], Fakir Md Yunus[3], Md Belal Hossain[1], Kaosar Afsana[2], Md Raisul Haque[2] and Mahfuzar Rahman[1]

Abstract

Background: Anemia is a significant wide spread public health threat especially among the adolescent girls who are more vulnerable towards low level of hemoglobin particularly of low and middle income countries (LMICs). We investigated the prevalence of anemia among the adolescent girls (10–19 years) in Bangladesh and its socio-demographics distribution.

Methods: We collected data digitally in ODK platform from a sub-sample of a nationwide cross-sectional survey of 1314 adolescent girls in 2015. Capillary blood hemoglobin level was estimated using HemoCue®; anthropometric measurements through standardized procedure and details socio-demographic information were captured and analyzed. Malnutrition was defined as BMI-for-age Z-score below -2SD (BAZ < −2SD), measured in WHO-AnthroPlus. Univariate analysis followed by multiple logistic regression were performed to examine the association between socio-demographic variables and anemia, while controlling the effect of potential confounding variables.

Results: Overall, 51.6% girls were suffering from any form of anemia (non-pregnant-Hb < 12 g/dl; pregnant-Hb < 11 g/dl) while 46% were mildly (non-pregnant-Hb: 10–11.9 g/dl; pregnant-Hb: 10–10.9 g/dl) and 5.4% were moderately (Hb: 7–9.9 g/dl) anemic while only 0.2% were severely anemic. After controlling for relevant covariates in multiple logistic regression model, malnutrition (AOR: 1.42, 95% CI = 1.0–2.10, p-value = 0.083), non-pregnancy (AOR: 6.10, 95% CI = 2.70–13.78, p-value < 0.001), and households with bottom wealth quintile (AOR: 1.54, 95% CI = 1.03–2.30, p-value = 0.037) were identified as significant risk factors of anemia among adolescent girls of Bangladesh.

Conclusions: Higher number of adolescent girls are still suffering from anemia in Bangladesh and non-pregnant adolescent girls contributed the most. Immediate, long term and sustainable public health intervention would require to combat the situation.

Keywords: Adolescent anemia, Malnutrition, Hemoglobin, Socio-demographic factors

Background

Anemia is a major public health problem affecting around 1.62 billion people globally [1, 2]. It is defined as a common blood disorders in which number of red blood cells, or the hemoglobin (Hb) concentration, falls below an established cut-off value, consequently impairing the capacity of the blood to transport oxygen around the body [3]. Anemia may develop at any stage of the life cycle [1] but children, adolescent girls and women of reproductive age are high risk groups for developing anemia [4, 5]. Anemia is a particular concern for adolescent girls i.e., aged 10–19 years [6], as this is a period of intense growth with higher iron requirement. This compounded with frequent menstrual blood losses and inadequate dietary iron intake in this period results in anemia [7]. Though anemia has multifaceted etiology, it primarily results from iron deficiency [3, 7, 8]. Worldwide, about 50% cases of anemia is caused by iron

* Correspondence: sabuj.km@brac.net
[1]Research and Evaluation Division, BRAC, BRAC Centre, 75 Mohakhali, Dhaka 1212, Bangladesh
Full list of author information is available at the end of the article

deficiency [9], but based on local conditions, this proportion may vary among population groups and areas [9, 10]. Some other haemopoietic micronutrient deficiencies like folate, riboflavin, Vitamins A and B_{12} may increase risk for anemia [7]. Infectious diseases such as malaria, tuberculosis and HIV/AIDS can also contribute to anemia, particularly prevalent in Africa and sub- Saharan Africa [4, 7]. Excessive blood loss resulting from hookworm infection and schistosomiasis can also lead to anemia [7, 11]. Some genetic or inherited hemoglobin disorders caused by inherited mutations of the globin genes leading to qualitative and quantitative abnormalities of globin synthesis (sickle-cell disease and thalassemia) also increases the risk for anemia, mainly in Mediterranean and Southeast Asian countries [4, 7, 12]. In Bangladesh more than 7000 children born each year with thalassemia and WHO report estimates that there are about 3% beta-thalassemia carrier and about 4% HB E/beta-thalassemia carrier in Bangladesh [13].

Anemia has serious consequences in adolescence with growth retardation [14] as well as impaired physical and cognitive performance [15]. Iron is also an essential nutrients for the functioning of neurotransmitter having a role in cognition, and in scarcity of hemoglobin, hypoxia develops with decreased cardiac output [16]. Several studies reported that iron supplementation among anemic adolescents and women had a role in cognition [17]. Higher behavioral disturbances along with reduced learning capacities and suboptimal school performance have also been documented among anemic school children [18]. Moreover, adolescent girls with anemia tend to commence their pregnancy with increased risk of morbidities and mortality for both mother and child [10].

Adolescent anemia is mostly prevalent in developing countries [4, 7, 19], and girls are more vulnerable than boys [20]. Studies identified that a large number of adolescent girls of South Asian region including Bangladesh are suffering from anemia along with other forms of malnutrition [21, 22]. Prevalence of anemia ranged from 31.6% to 99.9% among adolescent girls in India [2, 5] while in Nepal, the prevalence was as high as 68.8% [23]. Meanwhile, as of 2000, a study carried out in peri-urban areas of Bangladesh reported that the prevalence of anemia to be 27% among adolescent girls [24]. Recent study reported in 2016 that national prevalence of iron deficiency (serum ferritin level < 15.0 ng/ml) among non-pregnant non lactating women and children aged 12–14 years was 7.1% and 9.5% respectively in Bangladesh. It was found much higher (10%) among the children (12–14 years) in the rural Bangladesh. Furthermore, the study estimated that iron deficiency anemia could be much lower than anticipated among the Bangladeshi population of non-pregnant no lactating women (4.8%) and children aged 12–14 years (1.8%) [25]. However, there are still limited information till date in Bangladesh on the prevalence of anemia among adolescent girls (10–19 years) and its distribution. Other studies revealed the causal factors of anemia such consumption of traditional carbohydrate based diet lacking iron rich animal products, irregular eating habits [2], parent's education [26], father's occupation [27], age [19, 28], malaria [28], body mass index [19], menstruation 'when marked as heavy' [28], helminthes infestation [19, 28] and post-meal tea consumption [26]. However, all of these studies were carried out outside Bangladesh. This study will shed light on not only the number of adolescents suffering from low blood hemoglobin level but will also provide information on the factors associated with it.

Methods

Study site and participants

The data used for this study was collected as a part of a large scale multistage cluster sampled nationally representative cross-sectional survey. The base survey was conducted among the 11,428 mothers of children aged less than 5 years between October 2015 to January 2016 by BRAC Research and Evaluation Division in collaboration with the BRAC's Health, Nutrition and Population Programme. In the base survey, the sample was drawn from 21 equally divided clusters encompassing the entire country, of which 7 clusters were randomly selected for the present study. Thus, we opt to select all the adolescent girls (1467) from the selected households of 7 clusters as participants of the present study. However, we were unable to reach 10% of them due to unavailability and 1314 adolescent girls were finally selected. Inclusion criteria included was aged between 10 and 19 years, female and member of the surveyed households. The entire sampling strategy is summarized in Fig. 1.

Data collection tools and techniques

Household level socio-economic and demographic information was collected through face-to-face interview of the targeted mothers, while other specific information pertaining to the adolescent girls were gathered by directly interviewing/measuring the girls. The entire data was collected electronically using ODK (Open Data Kit version 2.0), an android based open-source mobile platform software. ODK has easy interface that can be used in low-resource settings to support frontline health workers who has minimum education to collect data electronically. This easily customizable mobile app can work both online and offline, and has features like short message service (SMS) and GPS tracker which enable the real-time data collection monitoring. A total of 28 skilled female interviewers (having survey experience) were recruited for data collection. A fifteen-day intensive training were organized which included lectures, mock interviews, role play and field practice at the community level. A training manual was

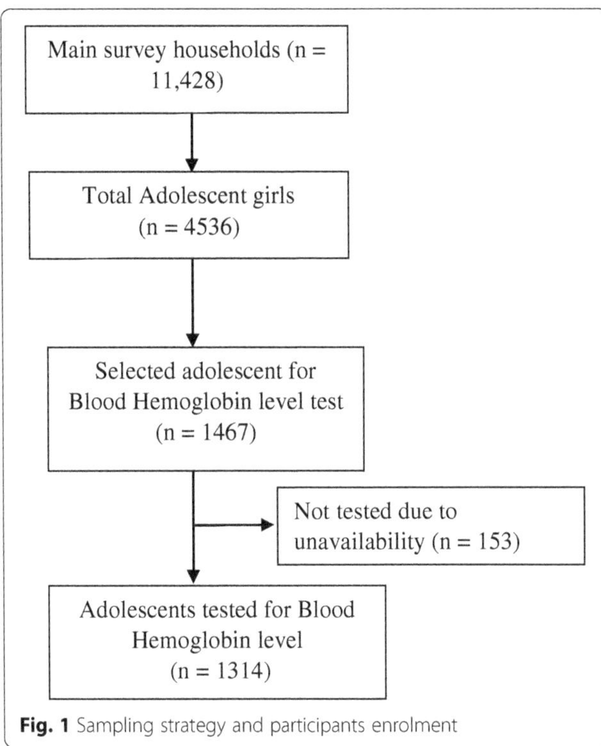

Fig. 1 Sampling strategy and participants enrolment

developed to guide the interviewers in the field. Several extensively trained teams of enumerators were formed for data collection each consisting of one supervisor and interviewers. The ODK was used in offline during the data collection and the questionnaires were uploaded every evening. The ODK server was hosted at the Head Office and was maintained by an experienced ICT person.

To ensure accuracy of information of such a large dataset, a number of quality control measures were undertaken at different stages of the data collection procedure. For example, a researcher statistician was position at the head office to check the live data and to provide feedback thereby. Considering the fact that our main respondents were women, we recruited experienced female field enumerators for data collection to minimize bias [29]. We established a multilayered monitoring system to validate, standardize and maintain data quality and performed tasks such as spot checking, thorough checking of the filled questionnaire in tablet, back checking and provided necessary feedback. Seven teams were working throughout the country headed by an experienced monitor for each, and researchers from headquarter also visited the survey areas frequently with the main task of supervision of data collection process.

Variables assessed/measured

Wealth index

Construction of the wealth index was based on principal component analysis (PCA) of key socioeconomic variables. Each variable was given a weight based on its loading in the first general factor identified in the PCA. The resulting score for each household was then standardized with mean '0' and standard deviation '1' [30]. Households were then ranked and assigned a score ranging from 1 to 5 with 5 identifying the wealthiest households.

Hematological assessment

Capillary blood was collected from all participants through pricking the fingertips by lancet, while strict aseptic environment was maintained throughout the entire process. A separate lancet was used for each individual and hemoglobin (the oxygen carrying part of the blood cell) concentration was determined using the Hemocue portable hemoglobinometer (B-Hemoglobin Photometer, HemoCue AB, Angelhom, Sweden). A total of 7 machines were used and the enumerators were trained by a physician on the procedure and aseptic techniques. Researchers frequently visited the field and rechecked a number of adolescent girls for their Hb concentration to validate the enumerators' activities. WHO cut-off point was used for classifying severity of anemia. Non pregnant adolescent girls with Hb level < 12 g/dl considered suffering from any form of anemia; 10.0–11.9 g/dl mildly anemic, 7.0–9.9 g/dl moderately anemic and <7.0 g/dl were considered severely anemic. For pregnant adolescent girls, the cut off value of any form of anemia was < 11.0 g/dl; mild anemia 10.0–10.9 g/dl, moderate anemia 7–9.9 g/dl and girls with Hb level < 7 g/dl were considered severely anemic [31].

Anthropometric measurement and calculation of BMI

Height was measured to the nearest 0.1 cm by using a board with an upright wooden base and a movable headpiece, on a flat surface. Weight was measured with an electronic scale at 0.1 kg precision. Body mass index (BMI), defined as weight in kg/(height in meter)^2 is the preferred method to classify nutritional status of adults. However, since adolescence is a period of intense growth, both height and weight changes rapidly during this period. Thus, BMI-for-age Z-score (BAZ) is the recommended indicator for assessing nutritional status among adolescent girls aged 10–19 years [32]. The nutritional status of the selected adolescent girls was measured using BAZ through WHO Anthro Plus software. Malnourished (< −2SD), Well nourished (− 2SD to +1SD), and Over nourished (> +1SD) were estimated.

Statistical analysis

Statistical analysis was conducted using STATA software (version 12.0). We used Chi-square test to assess the association between anemia and associated factors in contingency tables with a statistical significance level ≤ 0.05.

Simple logistic regression (also called single covariate logistic regression) model was employed to analyze the potential risk factors for anemia among adolescent girls and crude odds ratio (COR) with 95% confidence interval (CI) were calculated. We followed the model building strategy as described by Akaike (1973) where the multiple logistic regression model with smallest Akaike Information Criteria (AIC) value considered as the best model [33].

Results

Background characteristics of the respondents

Table 1 presents detailed socio-demographics of the study participants. It was found that, nearly half of the respondents (47.9%) were aged between 10 and 14 years. Among them, around 18.9% and 17.5% of the adolescent girls belonged to the wealthiest and poorest households respectively. Majority (80.8%) of them were literate and mostly (85.5%) from rural areas. Nearly 60% of the girls were single and over one third (38.3%) were married before they reached 19 years, while 3.4% ware pregnant at the time of survey. Moreover, 20 of the 45 currently pregnant women were consuming Iron and Folic Acid (IFA) supplement tablets.

Table 1 Demographic and socioeconomic characteristics of adolescent girls

Characteristics	Frequency (Total N = 1314)	Percentage (%)
Age category		
10–14 years	629	47.9
15–19 years	685	52.1
Wealth index		
Lowest	230	17.5
Second	265	20.2
Middle	276	21.0
Fourth	295	22.4
Highest	248	18.9
Literacy		
Literate	1061	80.8
Illiterate	253	19.2
Region		
Rural	1123	85.5
Urban	191	14.5
Marital status		
Single	811	61.7
Married	503	38.3
Currently pregnant		
Yes	45	3.4
No	1269	96.6

Prevalence of anemia

Overall, 51.6% of the surveyed adolescent girls were found sufferings from any form of anemia. Most of them (46%) were suffering from mild form of anemia, followed by moderate anemia prevalence of 5.4%, and only a few of them (0.2%) were severely anemic. Mild anemia was comparatively higher among younger girls of age 10–14 years than older girls aged 15–19 years (48.3% versus 43.8%). However, moderate anemia prevalence was higher among older group (6.1%) than those of younger age (4.6%) (Data not shown).

Socio-demographic distribution of anemia

Socio-demographic distribution of anemia is summarized in Table 2. Higher proportion (54.4%) of adolescent girls from lowest wealth quintile were suffering from anemia compare to those of the richest (47.2%). Not much difference was observed in anemia prevalence between single and married adolescent girls, roughly

Table 2 Socio-demographic characteristics and anemia status among adolescent girls

Socio-demographic characteristics	Anemic % (n)	Total n	Chi-square	p-value
Total	51.6 (678)	1314		
Age				
10–14 years	53.3 (335)	629	1.333	0.248
15–19 years	50.1 (343)	685		
Household wealth quintile				
Lowest quintile (Poorest)	54.4 (125)	230	3.519	0.475
Second lowest quintile	54.3 (144)	265		
Middle quintile	50.7 (140)	276		
Second highest quintile	51.5 (152)	295		
Highest quintile (Richest)	47.2 (117)	248		
Region				
Rural	51.3 (576)	1123	0.292	0.589
Urban	53.4 (102)	191		
Marital status				
Currently single	52.7 (427)	811	0.94	0.332
Currently married	49.9 (251)	503		
Household food security				
Unsecured	51.8 (199)	384	0.0492	0.824
Secured	51.5 (479)	930		
Currently pregnant				
No	52.9 (671)	1269	24.237	<0.001***
Yes	15.6 (7)	45		
BMI for age				
Well nourished	50.8 (607)	1196	3.8137	0.05 1*
Malnourished	60.2 (71)	118		

***$p \leq 0.01$, *$p \leq 0.10$

around 50% among both groups. Similar result was also noticed in terms of household food security and anemia status, prevalence varies around 51% among secured and unsecured households. Anemia prevalence was slightly higher among adolescent girls from urban slums compared to those from rural (53% versus 51%, p-vale = 0.589). Pregnancy status identified as a significant factor associated with anemia among adolescent girls. Nearly 16% of the pregnant adolescents were anemic while 47% of non-pregnant adolescents were anemic (p-value < 0.001). Also, among the malnourished adolescent girls (BMI-for-age Z-score < –2SD) 60% were anemic compared to around 50% of well-nourished girls (p-value = 0.051). Meanwhile, mean height and weight was 144.1 ± 16.1 cm and 39.5 ± 11.1 kg respectively and higher among non-anemic girls compared to anemic. It was also noted that mean hemoglobin level was 11.82 ± 1.15 g/dl, while it was 10.99 ± 0.9 g/dl and 12.7 ± 0. 61 g/dl respectively among anemic and non-anemic adolescent girls with a p-value <0.001 (Data not shown).

Risk factors of anemia

In simple logistic regression analyses, malnutrition and pregnancy status were significantly associated with anemia among adolescent girls (Table 3). The crude odds ratio (COR) for malnutrition status with anemia is found as 1.5 with p-value 0.052 where the 95% confidence interval was found as (1.0, 2.2). Likewise, the COR for non-pregnancy compared to pregnancy status with anemia was found 0.2 with p-value < 0.001 where the 95% confidence interval was (0.1–0.4).

However, after adjusting for potential covariates such as age, wealth index, marital status, regional effect and food security in multiple logistic model, malnutrition remained as an independent risk factors for anemia. Indeed, a malnourished adolescent girl had 40% more chance of anemia than a non-malnourished girl. It was also found that a pregnant adolescent girl had 5 times less chance of anemia compare to a pregnant girl. On the other hand, adolescent girls hailing from poorest or second poorest households were 50% more prone to become anemic compared to those from richest households. Besides, other covariates such as marital status, region and household food security status did not show any significant association with anemia status among adolescent girls.

Discussion

Our study reports the prevalence of anemia and distribution of severity of anemia in different socio-demographic strata among adolescent girls of the age bracket of 10–19 years in Bangladesh. The study further examines the risk factors of anemia among them. While, the prevalence of all form of anemia were found 51.6%, most of them (46%) were mildly anemic and few (5.4%) were moderate with only 0.23% severely anemic. Our study also found that malnutrition, pregnancy status and wealth quintile are significant risk factors of anemia among adolescent girls in Bangladesh.

Prevalence of anemia reported in our study was similarly high to the most recent Bangladesh Demographic and Health Survey (BDHS) where the prevalence of any form anemia were 48.6%, while mild, moderate and severe anemia were 39.2%, 9.4% and 0.0% respectively among adolescent girls of 15–19 years [22]. Though the participants of that survey were married adolescent girls, the findings are comparable as very little difference was observed in terms of anemia status between married and unmarried adolescent girls in our study. Our study is unique in that sense as it covered nationally representative sample of adolescent girls regardless their all socio-demographic variables including marital status, and habitat. Several other similar studies [27, 34, 35] conducted in India also found that girls were mostly suffering from mild to moderate anemia.

Few other studies [24, 36–39] were carried out till date examining the prevalence and risk factors of anemia among adolescent girls in Bangladesh. Most of the studies were outdated and conducted in school setting, while a few were carried out at community level. A study [37] conducted among adolescent girls aged 11–16 years in rural community found that 43.0% of the girls were anemic, which indicates that the situation is as worse as it was previously. School based studies were carried out in urban [38] or per-urban [24] areas and anemia prevalence was ranged from 22 to 27%. Studies [16, 27, 40] conducted in community setting of India also found a very high prevalence of anemia among adolescent girls and it ranged between 48 and 85%. The prevalence was 30.9% in Afghanistan and 58.1% in Sri Lanka [41] and 23% in Iran [42]. Several other studies conducted in sub-Saharan Africa also found high prevalence of anemia among adolescent girls [43].

Several socioeconomic and physiological factors such as literacy [44], father's occupation [27], lower socio-economic status [35], traditional and irregular feeding habit [2] and lower BMI [45] are reported as the most important factors associated with anemia among adolescent girls. Nutritional deprivation has long been identified as one of the most important causes of anemia, particularly among adolescent girls from underdeveloped countries [28]. Our study identified that malnutrition (BMI-for-age Z-score < –2SD) is a significant risk factor of anemia among adolescent girls. Studies conducted in similar setting also found that lower BMI is associated with higher rate of anemia among adolescent girls [23, 27]. However, contradictory to this, BMI had not significantly been

Table 3 Association of socio-demographic variables with anemia status

Characteristics	Crude			Adjusted		
	OR	*p*-value	95% CI	OR[a]	*p*-value	95% CI
Household wealth quintile						
Highest quintile (Richest)	1.0			1.0		
Second highest quintile	1.2	0.313	0.9–1.7	1.3	0.187	0.9–1.8
Middle quintile	1.2	0.417	0.8–1.6	1.3	0.154	0.9–1.9
Second lowest quintile	1.3	0.105	0.9–1.9	1.5	0.043**	1.0–2.2
Lowest quintile (Poorest)	1.3	0.118	0.9–1.9	1.5	0.041**	1.0–2.3
Region						
Rural	1.0			1.0		
Urban	1.1	0.589	0.8–1.5	1.3	0.119	0.9–1.9
Household food security						
Unsecured	1.0			1.0		
Secured	1.0	0.917	0.8–1.3	1.1	0.547	0.8–1.4
Marital status						
Single	1.0			1.0		
Married	1.1	0.332	0.7–1.1	0.9	0.650	0.7–1.3
Currently pregnant						
No	1.0			1.0		
Yes	0.2	<0.001***	0.1–0.4	0.2	<0.001***	0.1–0.4
BMI for age						
Well nourished	1.0			1.0		
Malnourished	1.5	0.052*	1.0–2.2	1.4	0.093*	1.0–2.1

[a]OR adjusted with girls age, $^{***}p \leq 0.01$, $^{**}p \leq 0.05$, $^{*}p \leq 0.10$

associated with anemia among adolescent girls from rural India [40].

A number of studies affirmed the association between low socio-economic status and anemia among adolescent girls from low and middle income countries [35]. Studies conducted in Bangladesh also clearly demonstrated the influence of poor socio-economic status on higher anemia prevalence and reported that around half of the anemic girls belong to the low socioeconomic status group [36]. Present study pointed that girls from the poorest wealth quintile were more prone to become anemic compared to those from the richest wealth quintile. Adolescent girls of poor socioeconomic condition tends to consume less diversified diet [46] with lesser micronutrient content which might have resulted in lower BMI with concomitant higher prevalence of anemia.

In Bangladesh, adolescent pregnancy is a major social and health concern as 31% of adolescents aged 15–19 was childbearing mother [47]. We also found than non-pregnant adolescent girls were more prone to become anemic compared to that of the pregnant girls. This may mean that non-pregnant adolescent girls would require more attention from different stakeholders, however, prevalence of anemic among pregnant adolescent was still high.

Our study has several strengths over other studies of that kind. It followed a multistage cluster sampling procedure covering a wide region of both rural and urban areas and is generable to the entire population. The biochemical procedure of testing blood hemoglobin level to ascertain anemia is one of the most effective methods of measuring anemia at community setting compared to other methods such as clinical examination. Another advantage is as it is a community based study it provides a population level assessment of anemia prevalence especially severe anemia, which is unlikely to be detected through school-based studies where only school going adolescent are available [27].

However, the study was subjected to certain limitations. Although, the study identified prevalence of anemia it cannot be confirmed whether the anemia is resulting from iron deficiency, as we have no data on dietary iron intake or serum ferritin level. Also, the study was unable to confirm the types and causes of anemia without the data on RBC indices (MCV, MCH, MCHC) and blood plates, which can be measured using Hematology analyzers. Furthermore, as the data was cross-sectional in nature, temporal relationship between the socio-demographics and anemia should be interpreted with caution. However, it is estimated that at least half of anemia worldwide is due to nutritional iron deficiency anemia [10] and 32% anemia in Bangladesh is iron deficiency anemia [24]. However, other research reported a low prevalence of iron deficiency anemia among Bangladeshi women, most of them above the age of adolescence [8]. And although, Bangladesh has a nationwide program to distribute iron and folic acid for pregnant women, no such program exists for adolescent girls. We also did not assess energy, protein or other macro or micronutrient intakes. Studies identified that hookworm infestation is significantly associated with anemia in adolescent girls [19, 40]. But this study did not collect information regarding hookworm infestation. Further studies regarding these issues would enhance our understanding and therefore more work is needed to determine the cause of anemia in these adolescent girls to determine what effective interventions are warranted.

Conclusions

Our study reaffirm the fact that anemia is a major problem for adolescent girls in Bangladesh which need to be given highest priority. Malnourished girls are highly vulnerable to anemia, most of which belong to the poor socioeconomic class. Currently there is actually no large scale intervention focusing on to control anemia among adolescent girls of the country. Thus, it is essential to initiate interventions to improve dietary iron intake along with measures to control infections and infestations which involves unusual blood loss resulting anemia.

Abbreviations

AIDS: Acquired immune deficiency syndrome; AOR: Adjusted odds ratio; BMI: Body mass index; COR: Crude odds ratio; HIV: Human immunodeficiency virus; ODK: Open data kit; PCA: Principal component analysis; WHO: World Health Organization

Acknowledgements

The authors thank Dr. Sujay Kakarmath, Harvard University for initial review of the manuscript.

Funding

This research was funded by the Strategic Partnership Arrangement (SPA) between BRAC, the UK Department for International Development (DFID), and the Australian Department of Foreign Affairs and Trade (DFAT).

Authors' contributions

SKM, MR and KA conceived and designed the study. FK, FA and FTJ contributed to the data collection. MBH and FTJ conducted the data analysis and participated in the result interpretation. SKM, FK and FA wrote the manuscript. FMY, MRH and SK commented on the manuscript draft. All authors read and approved the final manuscript.

Competing interests

The authors declare that they have no competing interests.

Author details

[1]Research and Evaluation Division, BRAC, BRAC Centre, 75 Mohakhali, Dhaka 1212, Bangladesh. [2]Health, Nutrition and Population Programme, BRAC, BRAC Centre, 75 Mohakhali, Dhaka 1212, Bangladesh. [3]College of Pharmacy and Nutrition, The University of Saskatchewan, 104 Clinic Place, Saskatoon, SK S7N 2Z4, Canada.

References

1. McLean E, Cogswell M, Egli I, Wojdyla D, de Benoist B. Worldwide prevalence of anaemia, WHO Vitamin and Mineral Nutrition Information System, 1993-2005. Public Health Nutr. 2009;12:444–54.
2. Işık Balcı Y, Karabulut A, Gürses D, Ethem Çövüt I. Prevalence and Risk Factors of Anemia among Adolescents in Denizli, Turkey. Iran J Pediatr. 2012;22:77–81.
3. WHO. Global nutrition targets 2025: anaemia policy brief(WHO/NMH/NHD/14.4). Geneva: World Health Organization; 2014.
4. Balarajan Y, Ramakrishnan U, Özaltin E, Shankar AH, Subramanian S. Anaemia in low-income and middle-income countries. Lancet. 2012;378:2123–35.
5. Bharati P, Shome S, Chakrabarty S, Bharati S, Pal M. Burden of anemia and its socioeconomic determinants among adolescent girls in India. Food Nutr Bull. 2009;30:217–26.
6. Anthony D. The state of the world's children 2011-adolescence: an age of opportunity. New York: United Nations Children's Fund (UNICEF); 2011.
7. Tolentino K, Friedman JF. An update on anemia in less developed countries. Am J Trop Med Hyg. 2007;77:44–51.
8. Merrill RD, Ahmed Shamim A, Ali H, Labrique AB, Schulze K, Christian P, West KP Jr. High prevalence of anemia with lack of iron deficiency among women in rural Bangladesh: a role for thalassemia and iron in groundwater. Asia Pac J Clin Nutr. 2012;21:416.
9. Stevens GA, Finucane MM, De-Regil LM, Paciorek CJ, Flaxman SR, Branca F, Peña-Rosas JP, Bhutta ZA, Ezzati M, Group NIMS. Global, regional, and national trends in haemoglobin concentration and prevalence of total and severe anaemia in children and pregnant and non-pregnant women for 1995-2011: a systematic analysis of population-representative data. Lancet Glob Health. 2013;1:e16–25.
10. ML SRJ, Black RE. Iron deficiency anaemia. Geneva: World Health Organization; 2004.
11. Smith JL, Brooker S. Impact of hookworm infection and deworming on anaemia in non-pregnant populations: a systematic review. Tropical Med Int Health. 2010;15:776–95.
12. Weatherall DJ. The inherited diseases of hemoglobin are an emerging global health burden. Blood. 2010;115:4331–6.
13. Palit S, Bhuiyan RH, Aklima J, Emran TB, Dash R. A study of the prevalence of thalassemia and its correlation with liver function test in different age and sex group in the Chittagong district of Bangladesh. J Basic Clinical Pharm. 2012;3:352.
14. Bandhu R, Shankar N, Tandon O. Effect of iron on growth in iron deficient anemic school going children. Indian J Physiol Pharmacol. 2003;47:59–66.
15. Grantham-McGregor S, Ani C. A review of studies on the effect of iron deficiency on cognitive development in children. J Nutr. 2001;131:649S–68S.
16. Sen A, Kanani SJ. Deleterious functional impact of anemia on young adolescent school girls. Indian Pediatr. 2006;43:219–26.
17. Falkingham M, Abdelhamid A, Curtis P, Fairweather-Tait S, Dye L, Hooper L. The effects of oral iron supplementation on cognition in older children and adults: a systematic review and meta-analysis. Nutr J. 2010;9:4.

18. Soemantri AG, Pollitt E, Kim I. Iron deficiency anemia and educational achievement. Am J Clin Nutr. 1985;42:1221–8.
19. Ramzi M, Haghpanah S, Malekmakan L, Cohan N, Baseri A, Alamdari A, Zare N. Anemia and iron deficiency in adolescent school girls in kavar urban area, southern iran. Iran Red Crescent Med J. 2011;13:128–33.
20. Akramipour R, Rezaei M, Rahimi Z. Prevalence of iron deficiency anemia among adolescent schoolgirls from Kermanshah, Western Iran. Hematology. 2008;13:352–5.
21. WHO. Adolescent nutrition: a review of the situation in selected South-East Asian countries (SEA/NUT/163). In: Regional Office for South East Asia. New Delhi: World Health Organization; 2006.
22. research NIop, training (NIPORT), Mitra and Associates all. Bangladesh Demographic and Health Survey, 2011. Dhaka and Calverton: NIPORT, Mitra and Associates, and ICF International; 2013.
23. Shah BK, Gupta P. Weekly vs daily iron and folic acid supplementation in adolescent Nepalese girls. Arch Pediatr Adolesc Med. 2002;156:131–5.
24. Ahmed F, Khan MR, Islam M, Kabir I, Fuchs GJ. Anaemia and iron deficiency among adolescent schoolgirls in peri-urban Bangladesh. Eur J Clin Nutr. 2000;54:678–83.
25. Rahman S, Ahmed T, Rahman AS, Alam N, Ahmed AS, Ireen S, Chowdhury IA, Chowdhury FP, Rahman SM. Determinants of iron status and Hb in the Bangladesh population: the role of groundwater iron. Public Health Nutr. 2016;19:1862–74.
26. Tayel DI, Ezzat S. Anemia and Its Associated Factors among Adolescents in Alexandria, Egypt. Int J Health Sci Res (IJHSR). 2015;5:260–71.
27. Verma A, Rawal V, Kedia G, Kumar D, Chauhan J. Factors influencing anaemia among girls of school going age (6-18 years) from the slums of Ahmedabad city. Indian J Community Med. 2004;29:25.
28. Leenstra T, Kariuki SK, Kurtis JD, Oloo AJ, Kager PA, ter Kuile FO. Prevalence and severity of anemia and iron deficiency: cross-sectional studies in adolescent schoolgirls in western Kenya. Eur J Clin Nutr. 2004;58:681–91.
29. Davis RE, Couper MP, Janz NK, Caldwell CH, Resnicow K. Interviewer effects in public health surveys. Health Educ Res. 2010;25:14–26.
30. Gwatkin D, Rutstein S, Johnson S, Pande R, Wagstaff A. Differences in health, nutrition, and population in Bangladesh 1996/1997, 1999/2000, 2004. Washington: World Bank; 2007. *Human Development Network*
31. WHO. Haemoglobin concentrations for the diagnosis of anaemia and assessment of severity. Geneva: World Health Organization; 2011.
32. Lourenço BH, Villamor E, Augusto RA, Cardoso MA. Influence of early life factors on body mass index trajectory during childhood: a population-based longitudinal analysis in the Western Brazilian Amazon. Maternal & child nutrition. 2015;11:240–52.
33. Akaike H. Theory and an extension of the maximum likelihood principal. In: International symposium on information theory Budapest. Akademiai Kaiado: Hungary; 1973.
34. Gupta A, Parashar A, Thakur A, Sharma D. Anemia among adolescent girls in Shimla Hills of north India: does BMI and onset of menarche have a role? Indian J Med Sci. 2012;66:126–30.
35. Deshpande NS, Karva D, Agarkhedkar S, Deshpande S. Prevalence of anemia in adolescent girls and its co-relation with demographic factors. Int J Med Public Health. 2013;3:235.
36. Ahmed F, Khan MR, Banu CP, Qazi MR, Akhtaruzzaman M. The coexistence of other micronutrient deficiencies in anaemic adolescent schoolgirls in rural Bangladesh. Eur J Clin Nutr. 2008;62:365–72.
37. IPHN H. Iron deficiency anemia throughout the lifecycle in rural Bangladesh. National Vitamin A Survey, 1997–98. Dhaka: Helen Keller International; 1999.
38. Ahmed F, Khan MR, Karim R, Taj S, Hyderi T, Faruque MO, Margetts BM, Jackson AA. Serum retinol and biochemical measures of iron status in adolescent schoolgirls in urban Bangladesh. Eur J Clin Nutr. 1996;50:346–51.
39. Ahmed F, Hasan N, Kabir Y. Vitamin A deficiency among adolescent female garment factory workers in Bangladesh. Eur J Clin Nutr. 1997;51:698–702.
40. Kaur S, Deshmukh P, Garg B. Epidemiological correlates of nutritional anemia in adolescent girls of rural Wardha. Indian J Community Med. 2006;31:255–8.
41. Hettiarachchi M, Liyanage C, Wickremasinghe R, Hilmers DC, Abrahams SA. Prevalence and severity of micronutrient deficiency: a cross-sectional study among adolescents in Sri Lanka. Asia Pac J Clin Nutr. 2006;15:56–63.
42. Sarraf Z, Goldberg D, Shahbazi M, Arbuckle K, Salehi M. Nutritional status of schoolchildren in rural Iran. Br J Nutr. 2005;94:390–6.
43. Hall A, Bobrow E, Brooker S, Jukes M, Nokes K, Lambo J, Guyatt H, Bundy D, Adjei S, Wen ST, et al. Anaemia in schoolchildren in eight countries in Africa and Asia. Public Health Nutr. 2001;4:749–56.
44. Naidu C, Venela P, Ammika P, Kattula SR, Kokkiligadda SV, Deshmukh H. Factors Influencing Anaemia among Adolescent Girls from Urban Slums of Hyderabad-A Cross Sectional Cohort Study. Indian J Public Health Res Dev. 2014;5:16–21.
45. Kanani SJ, Poojara RH. Supplementation with iron and folic acid enhances growth in adolescent Indian girls. J Nutr. 2000;130:452S–5S.
46. JPGSPH Ha. State of food security and nutrition in Bangladesh:2013. Dhaka: Helen kellar International (HKI) and James P. Grant School of Public Health (JPGSPH); 2014.
47. International NMaAal. Bangladesh Demographic and Health Survey 2014: Key Indicators. Dhaka and Rockville: NIPORT, Mitra and Associates, and ICF International; 2015.

28

Storage related haematological and biochemical changes in *Plasmodium falciparum* infected and sickle cell trait donor blood

Enoch Aninagyei[1*], Emmanuel Tetteh Doku[2], Patrick Adu[3], Alexander Egyir-Yawson[1] and Desmond Omane Acheampong[1*]

Abstract

Background: In sub-Saharan Africa where sickle cell trait (SCT) and malaria is prevalent, significant proportions of blood donors may be affected by one or more of these abnormalities. The haemato-biochemical properties of SCT and asymptomatic malaria in donor blood have not been evaluated. This study evaluated the haemato-biochemical impact of SCT and asymptomatic malaria infections in citrate-phosphate-dextrose-adenine (CPDA-1) stored donor blood units.

Methods: Fifty-milliliters of sterile CPDA-1 anti-coagulated blood were drained into the sample pouch attached to the main blood bag. Ten units each of sickle cell/malaria negative, sickle cell and malaria positive blood were analyzed. Baseline and weekly haematological profiling and week 1, 3 and 5 concentrations of plasma haemoglobin, % haemolysis, sodium, potassium and chloride and lactate dehydrogenase (LDH) were assayed. Differences between baseline and weekly data were determined using one-way analysis of variance (ANOVA) and Kruskal-Wallis test, whereas differences between baseline parameters and week 1–3 data pairs were determined using paired t-test. *P*-value < 0.05 was considered statistically significant.

Results: Storage of SCT and malaria infected blood affected all haematological cell lines. In the SCT donors, red blood cells (RBC) ($4.75 \times 10^{12}/L \pm 1.43^{baseline}$ to $3.49 \times 10^{12}/L \pm 1.09^{week\text{-}5}$), haemoglobin ($14.45\ g/dl \pm 1.63^{baseline}$ to $11.43\ g/dl \pm 1.69^{week\text{-}5}$) and haematocrit ($39.96\% \pm 3.18^{baseline}$ to $33.22\% \pm 4.12^{week\text{-}5}$) were reduced. In the asymptomatic malaria group, reductions were observed in RBC ($5.00 \times 10^{12}/L \pm 0.75^{baseline}$ to $3.72 \times 10^{12}/L \pm 0.71^{week\text{-}5}$), haemoglobin ($14.73\ g/dl \pm 1.67^{baseline}$ to $11.53\ g/dl \pm 1.62^{week\text{-}5}$), haematocrit ($42.72\% \pm 5.16^{baseline}$ to $33.38\% \pm 5.80^{week\text{-}5}$), mean cell haemoglobin concentration ($35.48\ g/dl \pm 1.84^{baseline}$ to $35.01\ g/dl \pm 0.64^{week\text{-}5}$) and red cell distribution width coefficient of variation ($14.81\% \pm 1.54^{baseline}$ to $16.26\% \pm 1.37^{week\text{-}5}$). Biochemically, whereas plasma LDH levels significantly increased in asymptomatic malaria blood donors (319% increase at week 5 compared to baseline), SCT blood donors had the most significant increase in plasma potassium levels at week 5 (382% increase). Sodium ions significantly reduced in SCT/malaria negative and sickle cell trait blood at an average rate of 0.21 mmol/L per day. Moreover, elevations in lymphocytes-to-eosinophils and lymphocytes-to-neutrophils ratios were associated with SCT and malaria positive blood whilst elevation lymphocytes-to-basophils ratio was exclusive to malaria positive blood.

Conclusion: Severe storage lesions were significant in SCT or malaria positive donor blood units. Proper clinical evaluation must be done in prospective blood donors to ensure deferral of such donors.

Keywords: Sickle cell trait donor, Asymptomatic malaria donor, % haemolysis, Storage lesions, Plasma haemoglobin, Biochemical changes, Blood transfusion

* Correspondence: enochaninagyei@yahoo.com; dacheampong@ucc.edu.gh
[1]Department of Biomedical Sciences, School of Allied Health Sciences, University of Cape Coast, Cape Coast, Ghana
Full list of author information is available at the end of the article

Background

There are two major outcomes of *Plasmodium* infections, thus symptomatic and asymptomatic infections. Symptomatic infections occur in patients with compromised anti-disease immunity [1] and asymptomatic infections occur in individuals with competent malaria immunity [2]. Despite being asymptomatic, parasites may be present in red blood cells, but at low density and can persist for many months [3]. Prevalence of asymptomatic *Plasmodium* infections differs from one geographical region to another. In Brazil, Solomon Islands and Cambodia, asymptomatic malaria has been found to be 37.5, 82.2 and 92% respectively [4–6]. In Africa, the prevalence of asymptomatic malaria in blood donors in Ghana has been found to be 10.0% [7]. In Cameroon, Senegal, Benin and Nigeria, asymptomatic malaria parasitaemia in blood donors have been found to be 27.54% [8], 65.3% [9], > 30% [10] and 40% [11] respectively.

Sickle cell haemoglobin result when valine substitutes for glutamic acid at position 6 of the β-globin chain. This mutation consequently changes the physico-chemical properties of the haemoglobin molecule [12]. A person who inherits haemoglobin S from one parent and haemoglobin A (normal gene) from the other has a sickle cell trait (SCT) or is said to be a carrier of sickle cell disease [13]. The prevalence of sickle cell trait (SCT) is highest in Africans and people of African descent. In Africa, Nigeria probably has the highest number of people with SCT as close to 30% of the population carry haemoglobin S gene [14]. Liberia, Ghana and Uganda have 10–15% of their population being carriers of haemoglobin S gene [13, 15, 16]. Cameroon and Gabon have haemoglobin S gene prevalence of 19 and 22%, respectively [17, 18]. SCT individuals are clinically healthy to donate blood [19]. Populations with high prevalence of sickle cell trait and asymptomatic *Plasmodium falciparum* infections can result in high number of healthy blood donors with sickle cell trait and/or asymptomatic *Plasmodium* infections. In Kenya and Nigeria, proportion of their blood donor population who were sickle cell carriers were 3.9 and 27.1% respectively [20, 21]. In Ghana, studies done in Brong Ahafo and Greater Accra regions reported prevalence of SCT in blood donors to be 12.5 and 11.3% respectively [12, 22].

Majority of the blood banks in SSA still practice whole blood banking [23, 24]. Although donated blood units are stored in anticoagulants supplemented with phosphate, dextrose, and/or adenine to assure long-term viability, storage lesions are inevitable when blood is stored for long periods [25]. RBC storage lesions include decreased RBC stability, alterations in various metabolites and the metabolic status of the cell, including decrease of intracellular adenosine triphosphate (ATP) and 2,3-biphosphoglycerate (2,3 BPG) [26–28]. These changes in RBC during storage have been known for years but the exact changes conferred on blood collected from SCT donors and those infected with *Plasmodium* parasites are unknown. The aim of this study therefore was to evaluate, for the first time, the haematological and biochemical variations in sickle cell trait blood and blood infected with *Plasmodium falciparum* stored in CPDA-1 anticoagulant up to 35 days.

Methods

Study design

This cross-sectional laboratory based experimental study was done in sterile blood units. Donors were selected according to Medical History Guide for Donor Selection [29].

Donor selection, phlebotomy and specimen collection

The selections of the healthy blood donors were double-blinded as researchers and National Blood Service Ghana staff could not link the study specimens to any donor. Participant consent form was signed by all participated donors. Blood was collected from each of the donors following a modification of the technique described by Cheesbrough [25]. For the purpose of the study, 7 ml of the CDPA-1 anticoagulant was allowed into the sample pouch attached to the main blood bag, which was filled with the initial 50 ml of whole blood. The rest of the whole blood was directed into the main blood bag.

Inclusion criteria

Donor blood included in the study were TTIs-negative blood with baseline biochemical parameters that fell within these ranges; haemoglobin 12.5–18.00 g/dl, plasma haemoglobin-0 g/dl, percentage haemolysis-0.0%, plasma sodium, potassium, chloride and LDH that fell within these respective ranges 135-145mmo/l, 3.0–5.2 mmol/l, 95-108 mmol/l and 100-250 U/L.

Laboratory procedures

Post-phlebotomy laboratory procedures were done as follows: 5 ml of well mixed whole blood was aspirated into plain glass vacutainer tubes (All-Pro, Dusseldorf, Germany). Portion of the blood was used to screen for transfusion-transmitted infections (TTIs) using fourth generation enzyme immuno-assay (Abnova, Taiwan). The ELISA microtitre plate wells were pre-coated with hepatitis B surface monoclonal antibodies, gp36/gp41, hepatitis C antigens (core, NS3 and NS5) and *Treponema pallidum* antigens for qualitative detection of hepatitis B virus, HIV I&II, hepatitis C virus and *Treponema pallidum* respectively. Donor screening of sickle cells was done as described by Antwi-Baffour [13] whilst phenotyping was done in alkaline medium (pH = 8.6). Separation of haemolysate was done on cellulose acetate paper using 250 V voltage and 50 mA current for

30 min. The separated haemoglobin molecules were interpreted against pooled haemoglobin AFSC controls. Screening of malaria was done with PfHRP-2/Pf-LDH SD Bioline rapid diagnostic test kit (Gyeonggi-do, Republic of Korea). The kit detected *Plasmodium falciparum* specific HRP-2 proteins and lactate dehydrogenase enzymes. Five microliters of whole blood were dropped on the sample column of the rapid test kit. Four drops of assay diluent (PfHRP-2/Pf-LDH SD Bioline, Korea) were added to the buffer window of the kit. Results were read after 15 min. Baseline haematological parameters using 5-part differential Urit-5160 (Guangxi, China), plasma electrolytes (sodium, potassium and chloride) measured by FT-320 electrolyte analyzer (China), lactate dehydrogenase (measured by PKL-125 Italia fully automated chemistry analyzer using ELItech LDH kinetic reagent, France), plasma haemoglobin (Urit-5160, China) and percentage haemolysis calculated by using formulae used by Sawant et al. [30] was done on same day of blood collection (baseline). The donor whole blood study samples were stored in the blood bank refrigerator (Fiocchetti Scientific Refrigerator, Italy) for 5 weeks. Internal storage temperature was taken twice daily. Haematological parameters were determined weekly for 5 weeks whilst plasma haemoglobin, % haemolysis, plasma electrolytes and LDH were measured at the end of week 1, week 3 and week 5.

Data processing and statistical analysis

Baseline and weekly data was entered into Microsoft Excel 2010. Statistical analysis was done by SPSS Version 24 (Chicago, IL, USA). Based on SCT status and/or asymptomatic malaria infection status, participants were grouped into three: SCT blood donors, asymptomatic malaria blood donors and no SCT/asymptomatic malaria blood donors for subsequent analysis. Differences between baseline and the 5 weeks haematological profile and biochemical data set were determined by one-way analysis of variance (ANOVA) and Kruskal-Wallis test statistical models. Differences between baseline haematological parameters and week 1 to 3 data pair were determined by paired student T-test. *P*-value of < 0.05 was considered statistically significant.

Results

Storage related changes in TWBC and WBC differential counts

The study recorded significant changes in total white blood cells (TWBC) and WBC differential in all the three donor groups (Table 1). There were consecutive reductions in TWBC and neutrophil proportion in all donor groups. Whereas the largest significant TWBC reduction occurred in the sickle cell/malaria negative group (62.3% reduction in week 5), the largest significant reduction in neutrophil% occurred in the SCT donors (53.9% reduction in week 5). However, there were successive increases in %lymphocytes, basophils and monocytes in all donor groups when weekly estimates were compared to baseline values. Whereas the highest increase in %lymphocytes occurred in the sickle cell/malaria negative donors (84.3% increase compared to baseline), the highest %monocyte increase occurred in the SCT donor group (75.6% increase compared to baseline). Additionally, although there was a consecutive reduction in %eosinophil count in the SCT group, the changes in %eosinophil count fluctuated in the sickle cell/malaria negative, and the asymptomatic malaria donor groups.

Storage related changes in RBC and RBC indices

This study also found significant changes in RBC count and RBC indices in all the three donor groups (Table 2). In all donor groups, there were consecutive reductions of RBC count, haemoglobin level, and HCT in all successive weekly estimations compared to baseline values. Whereas the most significant reduction in RBC count occurred in the SCT blood donor group, (26.5% decrease compared to baseline), the highest reductions in haemoglobin and HCT occurred in the sickle cell/malaria negative blood donor group [26.5% (Hb), and 25.2% (HCT) reductions compared to baseline]. Also, RDW-CV% values consecutively increased in all donor groups with respect to successive weekly measurement. However, whereas weekly MCV and MCH values consistently decreased in asymptomatic malaria donor group, these values fluctuated in SCT or sickle cell/malaria negative donor groups.

Storage related changes in platelets and platelet indices

Changes in platelet count and related platelet indices were also observed in the donor population (Table 3). Consecutively, weekly platelet count estimates successively decreased in all blood donor groups; the highest significant reduction occurring in asymptomatic malaria blood donor group (49.9% decrease compared to baseline). Also, whereas weekly MPV and P_LCR successively increased in sickle cell/malaria negative and asymptomatic malaria donor group, the levels of these measurements fluctuated in the SCT blood donor group.

Storage related changes in leukocyte ratios

There was progressive increase in lymphocyte-to-eosinophils ratio (LER) in the three blood donor groups but the differences in the SCT/malaria negative group were not significant (%Δ 4.0–20.7%, $F = 2.363$, $p = 0.052$) whilst significant differences were seen in the SCT (%Δ 55.9–178%, $F = 5.16$, $p = < 0.05$) and the malaria positive donor group (%Δ 35.5–514.7%, $F = 4.46$, $p = < 0.05$). In addition to LER,

Table 1 Leukocytes and percentage differential storage changes in donor blood

TWBC and differentials	Baseline Mean	Week 1 Mean (%Δ)	Week 2 Mean (%Δ)	Week 3 Mean (%Δ)	Week 4 Mean (%Δ)	Week 5 Mean (%Δ)	*P*-value
Sickle cell/malaria negative donor blood							
TWBCx10^9/L	5.63	3.89(−30.9)	2.90(−48.4)	2.49(−55.7)	2.27(− 59.6)	2.09(−62.3)	0.001[*,a]
Neut %	66.18	60.09(− 9.2)	52.77(−20.2)	49.49(− 25.2)	44.21(− 33.2)	40.88(− 38.2)	0.054[b]
Lymp %	27.28	33.42(22.5)	39.83(46.0)	41.92(53.6)	46.94(72.0)	50.28(84.3)	0.092[b]
Eos %	3.03	2.73(−9.9)	2.42(−20.1)	3.32(9.5)	3.00(−0.9)	3.49(15.2)	0.845[a]
Mon %	3.27	3.52(7.6)	4.64(41.9)	4.94(51.1)	5.50(68.2)	4.96(51.6)	0.009[b]
Bas %	0.24	0.25(4.1)	0.35(45.8)	0.33(37.5)	0.35(45.8)	0.39(62.5)	0.033[b]
Sickle cell trait donor blood							
TWBCx10^9/L	6.36	5.08 (−20.1)	4.42 (−30.5)	4.24 (−33.3)	3.74 (−41.2)	3.57 (−43.8)	0.001[*,b]
Neut %	56.26	50.91 (−9.5)	39.58(−29.6)	32.64 (−41.9)	31.99 (− 43.1)	25.90 (− 53.9)	0.001[*,b]
Lymp %	37.50	43.06 (14.8)	51.48 (37.3)	61.46 (63.9)	62.79 (67.4)	66.28 (76.7)	0.001[*,1]
Eos %	3.34	2.45 (−26.6)	2.50 (− 25.1)	1.56 (−53.3)	1.69 (−49.4)	2.77 (−17.0)	0.020[a]
Mon %	2.71	3.59 (32.4)	3.94 (45.4)	4.02 (48.3)	3.24 (19.5)	4.76 (75.6)	0.179[b]
Bas %	0.20	0.20 (0.0)	0.38 (90.0)	0.32 (60.0)	0.30 (50.0)	0.29 (45.0)	0.069[b]
Asymptomatic malaria donor blood							
TWBCx10^9/L	6.08	4.49 (−26.1)	4.13 (−32.1)	3.77 (−37.9)	3.54 (−41.7)	3.21 (−47.2)	0.001[a]
Neut %	72.09	60.89 (−15.5)	47.78 (−33.7)	39.79 (−44.8)	42.91 (−40.4)	36.07 (− 49.9)	0.001[*,b]
Lymp %	31.67	32.53 (2.7)	45.65 (44.1)	52.53 (65.8)	49.52 (56.3)	55.63 (75.6)	0.001[*,b]
Eos %	2.38	2.50 (5.0)	2.01 (−15.5)	2.26 (−5.0)	2.39 (0.4)	2.69 (13.0)	0.265[a]
Mon %	3.56	3.72 (4.5)	4.68 (31.4)	5.08 (42.6)	4.57 (28.4)	5.29 (48.6)	0.095[b]
Bas %	0.30	0.36 (20.0)	0.33 (10.0)	0.34 (13.3)	0.31 (3.3)	0.32 (6.6)	0.804[a]

Abbreviations: *TWBC* = total white blood cells, *Neut* = Neutrophils, *Lymp* = Lymphocytes, *Eos* = Eosinophils, *Mon* = Monocytes, *Bas* = Basophils, % = Percent, *L* = Liter, *ANOVA* = Analysis of variance, *SD* = Standard deviation

[*]*p* values less than 0.001, [a]*p*-value determined by Kruskal-Wallis H test, [b]*p*-value determined by one-way ANOVA

significant increase in lymphocyte-to-basophils ratio (LBR) was observed in malaria positive donor group (%Δ 25.3–151.9%, F = 5.11, $p = < 0.05$) but not in SCT group (F = 0.73, $p = 0.602$) and SCT/malaria negative group (F = 0.34, $p = 0.882$). There were gradual increases in lymphocytes-to-monocytes ratio (LMR) in both the SCT and the malaria positive group but the differences between the values were not significant. Lymphocyte-to-neutrophil ratio (LNR) increased in the three groups but significant increases were seen in SCT (29.1–308.8%, F = 4.53, $p = 0.001$) and malaria positive blood (75–437.5%, F = 10.9, $p < 0.05$) (Table 4).

Moreover, when the weekly estimates in haematological parameters were compared to baseline using paired t-test analyses, most of the significant changes occurred in the SCT blood donors or the asymptomatic malaria positive blood donors (Additional file 1: Table S1).

Effect of storage on haemolytic and biochemical parameters in donor blood

The storage lesions related to haemolytic and biochemical parameters presented in Table 5. The plasma haemoglobin and %haemolysis consecutively increased with the successive weekly estimations in all blood donor groups. Additionally, weekly LDH and plasma potassium levels consecutively increased in weekly estimates compared to baseline in all blood donor groups. Whereas the most significant increase in LDH occurred in asymptomatic malaria blood donor group (319% increase over baseline), the most significant increase in plasma potassium levels occurred in SCT blood donor group (382% increase over baseline levels). However, weekly plasma sodium and chloride levels successively decreased in all blood donor group; the highest significant reductions occurring in asymptomatic malaria blood donor group [10.0% (sodium) and 21.3% (chloride) decreases compared to baseline].

Comparison of haemolytic and biochemical parameters across blood donor groups

The storage lesions in donor blood were quantitatively compared across the groups with respect to the weeks in storage (Table 6). Plasma haemoglobin and %haemolysis were significantly higher in SCT blood donors with respective weekly measurements compared to the other blood donor groups. However, respective weekly plasma

Table 2 RBC and RBC indices storage changes in donor blood

RBC and RBC indices	Baseline Mean	Week 1 Mean (%Δ)	Week 2 Mean (%Δ)	Week 3 Mean (%Δ)	Week 4 Mean (%Δ)	Week 5 Mean (%Δ)	*P*-values
Sickle cell and malaria negative donor blood							
RBC ($\times10^{12}$/L)	4.72	4.27 (−9.5)	4.08 (− 13.5)	4.03 (− 14.6)	3.98(−15.6)	4.04 (− 14.4)	0.147[a]
Hb (g/dl)	13.17	11.35 (−13.8)	10.49 (− 20.3)	9.97 (− 24.3)	10.06 (−23.6)	9.74 (−26.0)	0.022[a]
HCT (%)	37.54	33.52 (−10.7)	28.83 (− 23.2)	28.52 (−24.0)	28.48(− 24.1)	28.06(− 25.2)	0.013[a]
MCV (fL)	75.88	76.99 (1.5)	75.34 (−0.7)	74.37 (−1.9)	74.67 (−1.6)	75.22 (− 0.9)	0.952[a]
MCH (pg)	26.70	26.23 (−1.7)	27.61 (3.4)	25.85 (−3.1)	26.39 (−1.1)	26.14 (−2.0)	0.924[a]
MCHC (g/dl)	32.47	31.39 (−3.3)	33.58 (3.4)	31.90 (−1.7)	32.45 (−0.6)	31.92 (−1.6)	0.932[a]
RDW_CV (%)	14.14	14.14 (0.0)	14.20 (0.4)	15.02 (6.2)	14.63 (3.4)	14.76 (4.3)	0.486[b]
RDW_SD (fL)	32.38	32.38 (0.0)	33.55 (3.6)	31.76 (−1.9)	32.14 (−0.7)	30.17 (−6.8)	0.756[b]
Sickle cell trait donor blood							
RBC ($\times10^{12}$/L)	4.75	4.06 (−14.5)	3.58 (−24.6)	3.57 (−24.8)	3.56 (−25.0)	3.49 (−26.5)	0.016[a]
Hb (g/dl)	14.45	12.84 (−11.1)	12.47 (−13.7)	11.47 (−20.6)	11.57 (− 19.9)	11.43 (−20.8)	0.002[a]
HCT (%)	39.96	36.75 (−8.0)	33.34 (−16.5)	33.29 (−16.7)	32.55 (− 18.5)	33.22 (− 16.8)	0.005[a]
MCV (fL)	82.54	86.71 (5.0)	82.02 (−0.6)	81.27 (−1.5)	82.03 (− 0.61)	82.95 (0.4)	0.573[a]
MCH (pg)	30.36	30.29 (−0.2)	30.39 (0.3)	28.54 (−5.9)	29.12 (−4.0)	28.43 (−6.3)	0.424[a]
MCHC (g/dl)	36.75	34.99 (−4.7)	37.08 (0.9)	34.96 (− 4.8)	35.50 (−3.4)	34.30 (−6.6)	0.001[a]
RDW_CV (%)	14.75	14.75 (0.0)	14.91 (1.0)	15.30 (3.7)	15.03 (1.8)	23.68 (60.5)	0.518[b]
RDW_SD (fL)	35.59	35.59 (0.0)	36.54 (2.6)	33.80 (5.0)	34.06 (4.2)	31.83 (10.5)	0.082[b]
Asymptomatic malaria donor blood							
RBC ($\times10^{12}$/L)	5.00	4.48 (−10.4)	4.02 (−19.6)	4.00 (−20.0)	3.96 (−20.8)	3.72 (−25.6)	0.001[*,a]
Hb (g/dl)	14.73	13.06 (−11.3)	12.12 (−17.7)	11.82 (− 19.7)	11.98 (− 18.6)	11.53 (−21.7)	0.001[*,a]
HCT (%)	42.72	38.83 (−9.1)	34.04 (−20.3)	34.32 (− 19.6)	34.33 (−19.6)	33.38 (−21.8)	0.001[*,a]
MCV (fL)	89.15	87.66 (−1.6)	82.04 (−7.9)	81.81 (−8.2)	82.68 (−7.2)	83.31 (−6.5)	0.067[a]
MCH (pg)	30.85	29.42 (−4.6)	29.66 (−3.8)	28.13 (−8.8)	29.20 (−5.3)	29.15 (−5.5)	0.320[a]
MCHC (g/dl)	35.48	33.57 (−5.3)	36.22 (2.0)	34.45 (2.9)	35.38 (−0.2)	35.01 (−1.3)	0.002[b]
RDW_CV (%)	14.81	14.81 (0.0)	15.80 (6.6)	16.39 (10.6)	16.16 (9.1)	16.26 (9.7)	0.024[a]
RDW_SD (fL)	36.53	36.53 (0.0)	35.75 (−2.1)	33.82 (−7.4)	34.49 (−5.5)	34.49 (−5.5)	0.267[a]

Abbreviations: *RBC* = Red blood cells, *Hb* = Haemoglobin, *HCT* = Haematocrit, *MCV* = Mean cell volume, *MCH* = Mean cell haemoglobin, *MCHC* = Mean cell haemoglobin concentration, *RDW_CV* = Red cell distribution width coefficient of variation, *RDW_SD* = Red cell distribution width standard deviation, *L* = Litre, *fL* = Fentolitre, *pg* = picogram

[*]*p* values less than 0.001; [a]*p*-value determined by one-way ANOVA; [b]*p*-value determined by Kruskal-Wallis H test

LDH levels were significantly higher in asymptomatic malaria blood donor group compared to respective values in the other blood donor groups. Additionally, although baseline plasma potassium levels were comparable in all blood donor groups, weekly plasma potassium levels were respectively higher in asymptomatic malaria or SCT blood donor group compared to sickle cell and malaria negative blood donor group. Moreover, plasma sodium and chloride significantly decreased in the asymptomatic malaria group compared to the other groups.

Discussion

Preservation and long term storage of red blood cells is essential for continuous supply of safe blood for clinical use [24]. Previous studies have found deleterious storage effect on blood cell morphology and functions [31–33]. This study found similar trend of storage lesion in whole blood stored up to 5 weeks but the changes were more pronounced in blood collected from sickle cell trait (SCT) donors or donors infected asymptomatically with malaria parasites. In the three groups, gradual reduction in total white cells and neutrophils and progressive increase in lymphocytes were observed; a phenomenon that was previously observed by Adias [24]. This observation probably can be due to cell loss and cytotoxic effect of histamine and cytokines released by neutrophils [34]. TWBC, neutrophils and eosinophils cells lost were more evident in the SCT or asymptomatic malaria positive stored blood than sickle cell and malaria negative blood. It was observed that lymphocytes to eosinophils,

Table 3 Platelet and platelet indices storages changes in donor blood

	Baseline Mean	Week 1 Mean (%Δ)	Week 2 Mean (%Δ)	Week 3 Mean (%Δ)	Week 4 Mean (%Δ)	Week 5 Mean (%Δ)	F	*P*-value
Sickle cell and malaria negative donor blood								
Plt (×10^9/L)	224.10	199.55(10.9)	171.10(23.6)	162.60(27.4)	167.40(25.3)	139.30(37.8)	4.09	0.003
MPV (fL)	8.45	9.05(7.1)	9.93(17.5)	9.71(14.9)	9.17(8.5)	10.10(19.5)	8.18	0.001*
PDW (fL)	12.74	12.41(2.5)	13.93(9.3)	13.00(2.0)	11.98(5.9)	13.63(6.9)	1.00	0.425
PCT (%)	0.18	0.16(11.1)	0.17(5.5)	0.15(16.6)	0.15(16.6)	0.13(27.7)	1.09	0.374
P_LCR (%)	18.15	20.11(10.7)	21.86(20.4)	22.15(22.0)	19.21(5.8)	24.18(33.2)	1.24	0.304
Sickle cell trait donor blood								
Plt (×10^9/L)	225.90	214.10(5.2)	185.20(18.0)	189.40(16.1)	207.80(8.0)	167.61(25.8)	1.25	0.301
MPV (fL)	8.69	8.53(1.8)	9.83(13.1)	9.78(12.5)	9.83(13.1)	10.45(20.2)	3.85	0.005
PDW (fL)	12.31	12.03(2.2)	13.89(12.8)	13.75(11.6)	13.72(11.4)	15.54(26.2)	1.55	0.189
PCT (%)	0.19	0.19(0.0)	0.18(5.2)	0.18(5.2)	0.20(5.2)	0.18(5.2)	0.31	0.903
P_LCR (%)	16.62	16.19(2.5)	20.02(20.4)	21.65(30.2)	20.35(22.4)	24.28(46.0)	2.09	0.080
Asymptomatic malaria donor blood								
Plt (×10^9/L)	191.90	141.30(26.3)	132.70(30.8)	118.40(38.3)	106.80(44.3)	96.10(49.9)	7.47	0.001*
MPV (fL)	8.59	8.59(0.0)	9.87(14.9)	9.93(15.6)	9.10(5.9)	10.19(18.6)	2.52	0.040
PDW (fL)	13.90	13.90(0.0)	14.28(2.7)	14.75(6.1)	12.25(11.8)	15.98(14.9)	1.49	0.208
PCT (%)	0.15	0.15(0.0)	0.16(6.6)	0.15(0.0)	0.16(6.6)	0.14(6.6)	0.41	0.835
P_LCR (%)	19.48	19.48((0.0)	22.19(13.9)	22.17(13.8)	21.40(9.8)	26.89(38.0)	1.33	0.265

Abbreviations: *Plt* = Platelets, *PMV* = Mean platelet volume, *PDW*=Platelet distribution width, *PCT* = Plateletcrit, *P_LCR* = Platelet large cell ratio
**p* values less than 0.001

monocytes, basophils and neutrophils ratios were elevated in the three groups but in all cases significant elevations occurred in SCT and malaria positive donor blood. Insignificant elevations were observed in SCT/malaria negative blood. Elevation in LER, LMR, LBR and LNR values occurred as a result of progressive elevations in mean lymphocytes percentages and reduction in mean absolute eosinophils, monocytes, basophils and neutrophils. This predisposes blood recipients to bacterial invasion and increased proliferation of pathogenic bacterial

Table 4 Storage related changes in leucocyte ratios

Leukocyte ratio	Baseline Mean	Week 1 Mean(%Δ)	Week 2 Mean(%Δ)	Week 3 Mean(%Δ)	Week 4 Mean(%Δ)	Week 5 Mean(%Δ)	F	*P*-value
Sickle cell and malaria negative donor blood								
LER	19.8	20.6(4.0)	20.3(2.5)	21.2(7.1)	22.5(13.6)	23.9(20.7)	2.36	0.052
LMR	9.7	10.0(3.1)	9.0(7.2)	8.7(10.3)	10.2(5.2)	10.0(3.1)	0.42	0.828
LBR	184	205(11.4)	128(30.4)	130(29.3)	150(18.5)	149(19.0)	0.34	0.882
LNR	0.73	0.83(13.7)	1.12(53.4)	1.17(60.3)	1.33(82.2)	1.88(157.5)	1.44	0.222
Sickle cell trait donor blood								
LER	11.8	18.4(55.9)	26.8(127.1)	36.1(205.9)	38.5(226.3)	32.8(178.0)	5.16	0.001*
LMR	12.3	13.1(6.5)	14.2(15.4)	16.9(37.4)	22.4(82.1)	13.9(13.0)	1.95	0.100
LBR	198	177(10.6)	141(28.8)	169(14.6)	183(7.6)	169(14.6)	0.73	0.602
LNR	0.79	1.02(29.1)	1.42(79.8)	2.22(181.0)	2.83(258.2)	3.23(308.8)	4.53	0.001
Asymptomatic malaria donor blood								
LER	6.8	9.2(35.3)	19.3(183.8)	19.0(179.4)	23.0(238.2)	41.8(514.7)	4.46	0.001
LMR	5.9	8.7(47.5)	10.6(79.7)	11.3(91.5)	10.6(79.7)	10.8(83.1)	2.07	0.083
LBR	79	99(25.3)	127(60.8)	175(121.5)	181(129.1)	199(151.9)	5.11	0.001*
LNR	0.32	0.56(75.0)	1.07(234.4)	1.42(343.7)	1.27(296.9)	1.72(437.5)	10.9	0.001*

Abbreviations: *LER*-lymphocytes-to-eosinophils ratio, *LMR*-lymphocytes-to-monocytes ratio, *LBR*-lymphocytes-to-basophils ratio, *LPR*-lymphocyte-to-platelets ratio, *LNR*-lymphocytes-to-neutrophils ratio
**p*-value less than 0.001

Table 5 Analysis of haemolytic and biochemical parameters in donor blood stored for baseline, week 1, week 3 and week 5

Haemolytic parameters	Baseline Mean	Week 1 Mean (%Δ)	Week 3 Mean (%Δ)	Week 5 Mean (%Δ)	*P*-value
Sickle cell and malaria negative donor blood					
Plasma Hb (g/dl)	0.00	0.10	0.11(9.1)[c]	0.21(52.4)[c]	0.001[*,a]
% Haemolysis	0.00	0.52	0.75(30.7)[c]	1.44(63.9)[c]	0.001[*,a]
LDH (U/L)	199.40	319.20 (60.1)	428.00 (114.6)	522.70 (162.1)	0.001[*,a]
Potassium (mmol/L)	4.14	5.65 (56.5)	7.72 (86.5)	10.03(142.3)	0.001[*,b]
Sodium (mmol/L)	137.94	134.52 (−2.5)	130.00 (−5.7)	126.33 (−8.4)	0.001[*,a]
Chloride (mmol/L)	98.66	89.06 (−3.5)	84.98 (−13.9)	83.55 (−15.3)	0.001[*,b]
Sickle cell trait donor blood					
Plasma Hb (g/dl)	0.00	0.24	0.37(35.1)[c]	0.46(47.8)[c]	0.001[*,b]
% Haemolysis	0.00	1.16	2.08(44.2)[c]	2.62(55.7)[c]	0.001[*,a]
LDH (U/L)	207.10	329.20 (59.0)	491.60 (137.4)	610.40 (194.7)	0.001[*,a]
Potassium (mmol/L)	4.27	6.95 (62.8)	12.14 (184.3)	20.58 (382.0)	0.001[*,a]
Sodium (mmol/L)	139.51	136.74 (−2.0)	133.67 (−4.2)	130.35 (−6.5)	0.001[*,a]
Chloride (mmol/L)	99.63	90.77 (−8.9)	83.99 (− 15.7)	78.50 (−21.2)	0.001[*,b]
Asymptomatic malaria donor blood					
Plasma Hb (g/dl)	0.00	0.22	0.26(15.4)[c]	0.32(31.3)[c]	0.001[*,a]
% Haemolysis	0.00	1.00	1.46(31.5)[c]	1.90(47.3)[c]	0.001[*,a]
LDH (U/L)	192.30	418.70 (117.7)	596.60 (210.4)	806.70 (319.5)	0.001[*,b]
Potassium (mmol/L)	4.38	8.38 (91.3)	11.66 (166.2)	15.01 (242.7)	0.001[*,b]
Sodium (mmol/L)	140.72	135.17 (−3.9)	130.16 (−7.5)	125.60 (−10.0)	0.001[*,a]
Chloride (mmol/L)	100.62	91.00 (−9.6)	85.71 (−14.8)	79.21 (−21.3)	0.001[*,a]

Abbreviations: *LDH* = Lactate dehydrogenase, *SD* = Standard deviation, *Hb* = Haemoglobin
[*]*p* values less than 0.001, [a]*p*-value determined by Kruskal-Wallis H test, [b]*p*-value determined by one-way ANOVA, [c] %Δ calculated with respect to week 1 mean values

[35, 36]. Fever is a common symptom of sepsis [37]. Donor blood with high LER, LMR, LBR and LNR could cause pathogen induced acute or delayed febrile reactions in recipients with low leukocyte count.

In sickle cell and malaria negative group, red blood cells were relatively stable during storage but in the SCT or asymptomatic malaria donor group, there were significant reduction in red blood cells, haemoglobin and haematocrit. These haematological changes corresponded with gradual increases in plasma haemoglobin due to increased red cell breakdown as well as gradual elevation of potassium ions and lactate dehydrogenase during storage. These observations could be as a result of haemoglobin S erythrocytes fragility subsequent to polymerization of haemoglobin S and reduced deformability and loss of red cell elasticity during storage due to low oxygen tension and low pH storage medium [38–40] on the one hand, as well as metabolically active intra-erythrocytic *Plasmodium* parasites could account for these haematological changes. Malaria parasites have been found to be viable in stored blood for at least the first 14 days [41]. When one malaria parasite per microliter of blood is found, that converts to about 500,000 red cells parasitized in a unit of blood [42]. These viable parasites are enough to cause significant haematological derangement in the blood of an infected healthy donor during storage. One of the goals of haemo-transfusion is to restore tissue oxygenation [43]. Stored blood from SCT and asymptomatic malaria donors may develop storage lesions over time due to polymerization of haemoglobin S in SCT donor blood, loss of deformability and increased osmotic fragility which could compromise their haemorheological properties and oxygen binding and delivery capacity [44, 45].

Storage of blood collected from SCT and asymptomatic malaria donors were significantly associated with red cell lysis and elevated plasma haemoglobin. On day of blood collection, donor plasma was free of haemoglobin as well as insignificant differences in potassium, sodium, LDH and chloride in all the donor groups. However at week 1, plasma haemoglobin was 2.4 times higher in SCT donor blood and 2.2 higher in asymptomatic malaria blood compared to sickle cell and malaria negative group. At week 3, plasma haemoglobin was 3.36 times and 2.36 times higher in SCT and asymptomatic malaria donor blood respectively, and at week 5, plasma haemoglobin was 2.2 times higher in SCT and 1.5 higher in asymptomatic malaria group. Excess plasma haemoglobin increased over time in the SCT and

Table 6 ANOVA analysis of inter-donor category biochemical and haemolytic parameters

Parameters	Sickle cell/malaria negative donors Mean ± SD	Sickle cell trait donors Mean ± SD	Asymptomatic malaria donors Mean ± SD	F	*P*-value
Baseline					
Plasma Hb	0.00	0.00	0.00		
% haemolysis	0.00	0.00	0.00		
LDH (U/L)	202.45 ± 20.51	202.90 ± 18.91	173.20 ± 63.74	1.76	0.188
Potassium (mmol/L)	4.15 ± 0.70	4.22 ± 0.71	4.01 ± 1.50	0.39	0.681
Sodium (mmol/L)	138.44 ± 2.40	139.52 ± 2.54	126.37 ± 44.53	3.16	0.057
Chloride (mmol/L)	98.78 ± 1.66	99.88 ± 1.78	90.37 ± 31.87	2.68	0.085
Week 1					
Plasma Hb	0.10 ± 0.00	0.25 ± 0.13	0.20 ± 0.09	23.6	0.001*
% haemolysis	0.51 ± 0.05	1.12 ± 0.27	1.01 ± 0.35	20.7	0.001*
LDH (U/L)	318.36 ± 29.30	346.00 ± 78.68	370.90 ± 137.89	14.6	0.001*
Potassium (mmol/L)	5.54 ± 0.41	7.02 ± 1.15	8.46 ± 0.75	33.6	0.001*
Sodium (mmol/L)	134.90 ± 3.06	136.95 ± 2.88	121.09 ± 42.80	1.16	0.326
Chloride (mmol/L)	89.60 ± 3.12	90.53 ± 4.19	81.74 ± 28.74	1.47	0.246
Week 3					
Plasma Hb	0.11 ± 0.03	0.39 ± 0.12	0.23 ± 0.11	22.2	0.001*
% haemolysis	0.76 ± 0.35	2.21 ± 0.62	1.37 ± 0.41	17.3	0.001*
LDH (U/L)	436.36 ± 46.31	491.10 ± 47.17	605.77 ± 61.98	33.0	0.001*
Potassium (mmol/L)	8.05 ± 1.39	12.02 ± 1.61	11.83 ± 1.47	40.3	0.001*
Sodium (mmol/L)	130.88 ± 4.23	133.45 ± 3.42	129.00 ± 3.51	3.74	0.035
Chloride (mmol/L)	85.61 ± 3.91	83.37 ± 3.44	85.37 ± 2.85	0.73	0.487
Week 5					
Plasma Hb	0.20 ± 0.04	0.48 ± 0.19	0.28 ± 0.14	8.84	0.001*
% haemolysis	1.46 ± 0.51	2.75 ± 1.00	1.78 ± 0.65	4.48	0.001*
LDH (U/L)	536.09 ± 58.71	631.90 ± 109.29	798.00 ± 64.38	13.0	0.001*
Potassium (mmol/L)	11.35 ± 4.46	19.48 ± 2.86	15.18 ± 1.98	8.25	0.001*
Sodium (mmol/L)	127.64 ± 6.00	129.62 ± 5.17	124.73 ± 4.79	9.70	0.001*
Chloride (mmol/L)	84.27 ± 4.29	77.81 ± 4.31	78.61 ± 3.44	1.22	0.309

Abbreviations: *LDH* = Lactate dehydrogenase, *SD* = Standard deviation, *Hb* = Haemoglobin
**p*-values less than 0.001

the asymptomatic malaria donor groups. At week 1, the percentage haemolysis in the SCT and asymptomatic malaria was more than the permissible level of 0.8%. Blood with % haemolysis of 0.8% is not recommended for clinical use [30]. Excess haemoglobin has been found to have negative influence on the intravascular nitric oxide (NO) metabolism after transfusion. Plasma haemoglobin has been found to be a potent scavenger of NO, the most important endogenous vasodilator. In view of this, transfusing blood with high concentration of plasma haemoglobin could decrease NO bioavailability, decreased organ perfusion, increased organ injury [46, 47] and increased mortality in patients with sepsis [48]. Patients with organ failure and patients with septic shock may worsen their condition when transfused with blood with high plasma haemoglobin content. Potassium increased in the SCT and asymptomatic malaria groups and continued till their respective levels were 4.8 and 3.4 times higher than the baseline at week 5, a factor far more than was observed in the sickle cell/malaria negative group. It is recommended to include malaria and sickle cells screening into donor screening protocols to prevent potassium and free haemoglobin overload. In addition, the clinical impact of transmitting malaria to the recipient, albeit asymptomatic in the donor, merits consideration with recommendations to prevent such transmissions [49].

Conclusion

Storage of SCT and malaria infected blood affected all the cell lines. At week 1, total white blood cells, neutrophils, red cells, haemoglobin and haematocrit began to fall significantly in SCT and asymptomatic donor blood.

Significant elevation plasma haemoglobin, increase in % haemolysis above the permissible level of 0.8% and potassium elevation above the upper reference range for Ghanaian adults (5.2 mmol/L) [50] were observed. Significant reduction in red blood cells coupled with significant elevations in plasma haemoglobin, intracellular potassium and lactate dehydrogenase can led to the conclusion that significant number of red cells haemolysis in the experimental set up. This assumption was confirmed by steady elevation of % haemolysis over the storage weeks.

Limitations of the study

Malaria parasites were not quantified in the infected blood units. The analysis did not take into consideration the blood group and Rhesus phenotypes of the study units. The gender of the blood donors was unknown. Haemoglobin S was not quantified in the sickle cell trait donor blood.

Abbreviations

2,3 BPG: 2,3-biphosphoglycerate; ANOVA: One-way analysis of variance; ATP: Adenosine triphosphate; Bas: Basophils; CPDA: Citrate Phosphate Dextrose Adenine; Eos: Eosinophils; fL: Fentoliter; GHS: Ghana Health Service; Hb: Haemoglobin; HCT: Haematocrit; LBR: Lymphocytes-to-basophils ratio; LER: Lymphocytes-to-eosinophils ratio; LMR: Lymphocytes-to-monocytes ratio; LNR: Lymphocytes-to-neutrophils ratio; Lymp: Lymphocytes; MCH: Mean cell haemoglobin; MCHC: Mean cell haemoglobin concentration; MCV: Mean cell volume; Mon: Monocytes; NBSG: National Blood Service Ghana; Neut: Neutrophils; P_LCR: Platelet large cell ratio; PCT: Plateletcrit; PDW: Platelet distribution width; pg: pictogram; Plt: Platelets; PMV: Mean platelet volume; RBC: Red blood cells; RDW_CV: Red cell distribution width coefficient of variation; RDW_SD: Red cell distribution width standard deviation; SCT: Sickle cell trait; SD: Standard deviation; SSA: sub-Saharan Africa; TTIs: Transfusion transmitted infections; TWBC: Total white blood cell

Acknowledgements

The authors are thankful to the management and staff of National blood service, Ghana for collaborating with us in implementing the study. We are also grateful to Linda Baafi (Ga West Municipal Hospital Laboratory) for her voluntary participation in performing the biochemical analysis. Finally we are grateful to the National Malaria Control Programme Ghana for supplying us with malaria rapid diagnostic test kits.

Funding

The research was 100% funded by the corresponding author.

Authors' contributions

AE, AP, EYA, AOD conceived, designed the study, collected the data, performed and validated the laboratory findings and drafted the manuscript. TDE performed the statistical analysis. All authors read and approved the final manuscript.

Competing interests

The authors declare that they have no competing interests.

Author details

[1]Department of Biomedical Sciences, School of Allied Health Sciences, University of Cape Coast, Cape Coast, Ghana. [2]School of Public Health, University of Ghana, Legon, Accra, Ghana. [3]Department of Medical Laboratory Technology, University of Cape Coast, Cape Coast, Ghana.

References

1. Desai M, ter Kuile FO, Nosten F, McGready R, Asamoa K, Brabin B, Newman RD. Epidemiology and burden of malaria in pregnancy. Lancet Infect Dis. 2007;7(2):93–104.
2. Belizario VY, Saul A, Bustos MD, Lansang MA, Pasay CJ, Gatton M, Salazar NP. Field epidemiological studies on malaria in a low endemic area in the Philippines. Acta Trop. 1997;63:241–56.
3. Roucher C, Rogier C, Dieye-Ba F, Sokhna C, Tall A, Trape J-F. Changing malaria epidemiology and diagnostic criteria for *Plasmodium falciparum* clinical malaria. PLoS One. 2012;7:e46188.
4. da Silva-Nunes M, Ferreira MU. Clinical spectrum of uncomplicated malaria in semi-immune Amazonians: beyond the 'symptomatic' vs 'asymptomatic' dichotomy. Memorias Do Instituto Oswaldo Cruz. 2007;102(3):341–7.
5. Harris I, Sharrock WW, Bain LM, et al. A large proportion of asymptomatic *Plasmodium* infections with low and sub-microscopic parasite densities in the low transmission setting of Temotu Province, Solomon Islands: challenges for malaria diagnostics in an elimination setting. Malar J. 2010;9:254.
6. Hoyer S, Nguon S, Kim S, Habib N, Khim N, Sum S, et al. Focused screening and treatment (FSAT): a PCR-based strategy to detect malaria parasite carriers and contain drug resistant *P. falciparum*, Pailin, Cambodia. PLoS One. 2012;7(10):e45797.
7. Owusu-Ofori A, Gadzo G, Bates I. Transfusion-transmitted malaria: donor prevalence of parasitaemia and a survey of healthcare workers knowledge and practices in a district hospital in Ghana. Malar J. 2016;15:234–41.
8. Mogtomo ML, Fomekong SL, Kuate HF, Ngane AN. Screening of infectious microorganisms in blood banks in Douala (1995-2004). Sante. 2009;19:3–8.
9. Diop S, Ndiaye M, Seck M, Knight B, Jambou R, Sarr A, Dieye TN, Toure AO, Thiam D, Diakhate L. Prevention of transfusion transmitted malaria in endemic area. Clinical and biological transfusion. 2009;16:454–9.
10. Kinde-Gazard OJ, Gnahoui I, Massougbodji A. The risk of malaria transmission by blood transfusion at Cotonou, Benin. Cahiers Sante. 2000; 10(6):389–92.
11. Oladeinde BH, Omoregie R, Osakue EO, Onaiwu TO. Asymptomatic malaria among blood donors in Benin City Nigeria. Iranian J Parasitol. 2014;9(3):415–22.
12. Aguiar KM, Maia CN. Prevalence of hemoglobin S in blood donors at the Hemocentro regional in the town of Montes Claros. Minas Gerais RBAC. 2011;43(4):284–7.
13. Antwi-Baffour S, Asare RO, Adjei JK, Kyeremeh R, Adjei DN. Prevalence of hemoglobin S trait among blood donors: a cross-sectional study. BMC Res Notes. 2015;8:583.
14. Omotade OO, Kayode CM, Falade SL, Ikpeme S, Adeyemo AA, Akinkugbe FM. Routine screening for sickle cell haemoglobinopathy by electrophoresis in an infant welfare clinic. West Afr J Med. 1998;17:91–4.
15. Tubman VN, Marshall R, Jallah W. Newborn screening for sickle cell disease in Liberia: a pilot study. Pediatr Blood Cancer. 2016;63:671–6.
16. Ndeezi G, Kiyaga C, Hernandez AG, Munube D, Howard TA, Ssewanyana I, Nsungwa J, Kiguli S, Ndugwa CM, Ware RE, Aceng JR. Burden of sickle cell trait and disease in the Uganda sickle surveillance study (US3): a cross-sectional study. Lancet Global Health. 2016;4:e195–200.
17. Ama V, Kengne AP, Nansseu NJ, Nouthe B, Sobngwi E. Would sickle cell trait influences the metabolic control in sub-Saharan individuals with T2D? Diabet Med. 2012;29:334–7.

18. Elguero E, Delicat-Loembet LM, Rougeron V, Arnathau C, Roche B, Becquart P, Gonzalez JP, Nkoghe D, Sica L, Leroy EM, Durand P, Ayala FJ, Ollomo B, Renaud F, Prugnolle F. Malaria continues to select for sickle cell trait in Central Africa. Proc Natl Acad Sci U S A. 2015;112:7051–4.
19. Grignani C, Iamamoto C, Goncalves T, Mashima D, et al. Prevalence of hemoglobin AS among blood donors from Londrina - Parana. RBAC. 2006; 38(4):259–62.
20. Goncalves LB, Duarte EHG, Cabral MD. Prevalence of hemoglobin S in blood donors in the hospital Dr. Agostinho Neto, Praia City – Cape Verde. Sci J Public Health. 2015;3(5):600–4.
21. Garba N, Danladi SB, Abubakar HB, Ahmad SG, Gwarzo MY. Distribution of Haemoglobin variants, ABO and Rh blood groups in blood donors attending Aminu Kano teaching hospital. Clin Med J. 2016;2(2):20–4.
22. Adu P, Simpong DL, Takyi G, Ephraim RKD. Glucose-6-phosphate dehydrogenase deficiency and sickle cell trait among prospective blood donors: a cross-sectional study in Berekum, Ghana. Adv Haematol. 2016; https://doi.org/10.1155/2016/7302912.
23. Ghartimagar D. Rational clinical use of blood and blood products – a summary. J Pathol Nepal. 2017;7:1111–7.
24. Adias TC, Moore-Igwe B, Jeremiah ZA. Storage related Haematological and biochemical changes of CPDA-1 whole blood in a resource limited setting. J Blood Disorders Transf. 2012;3:124. https://doi.org/10.4172/2155-9864.1000124.
25. Cheesbrough M. Blood transfusion practice: blood donation and storage of blood, district laboratory practice in tropical countries. Low price edition. Cambridge Universal Press. 2002;2:352–3.
26. Koch CG, Figueroa PI, Li L, et al. Red blood cell storage: how long is too long? Ann Thorac Surg. 2013;96(5):1894–9.
27. Bonaventura J. Clinical implications of the loss of vasoactive nitric oxide during red blood cell storage. Proc Natl Acad Sci U S A. 2007;104:19165–6.
28. Spinella PC, Sparrow RL, Hess JR, et al. Properties of stored red blood cells: understanding immune and vascular reactivity. Transfusion. 2011;51(4):894–900.
29. WHO. Guidelines on assessing donor suitability for blood donation. World Health Organization 2012. http://www.who.int/iris/handle/10665/76724. Assessed 7 Aug 2018.
30. Sawant RB, Jathar SK, Rajadhyaksha SB, Kadam PT. Red cell hemolysis during processing and storage. Asian J Transfus Sci. 2007;1(2):47–51.
31. Koch CG, Li L, Sessler DI, Figueroa P, Hoeltge GA, et al. Duration of red-cell storage and complications after cardiac surgery. N Engl J Med. 2008;358: 1229–39.
32. van de Watering L. Red cell storage and prognosis. Vox Sang. 2011;100:36–45.
33. Hess JR. Red cell changes during storage. Transfus Apher Sci. 2010;43:51–9.
34. Hess JR. An update on solutions for red cell storage. Vox Sang. 2006;91:13–9.
35. Antoniadou A, Giamarellou H. Fever of unknown origin in febrile leukopenia. Infect Dis Clin N Am. 2007;21(4):1055–90.
36. Friese CR. Chemotherapy-induced neutropenia: important new data to guide nursing assessment and management. Cancer Ther Support Care. 2006;4(2):21–5.
37. Schortgen F. Fever in sepsis. Minerva Anestesiol. 2012;78(11):1254–64.
38. Brandao MM, Saad O, Cezar CL, Fontes A, Costa FF, Barjas-Castro ML. Elastic properties of stored red blood cells from sickle trait donor units. Int J Transfusion Med. 2003. https://doi.org/10.1046/j.1423-0410.2003.00344.x.
39. Noguchi CT, Torchia DA, Schechter AN. Polymerization of hemoglobin in sickle cell trait erythrocytes and lysate. J Biol Chem. 1981;256:4168–71.
40. Helzlsouer KJ, Hayden FG, Rogol AD. Severe metabolic complications in a cross country runner with sickle cell trait. JAMA. 1983;249:777–9.
41. Kitchen AD, Chiodini PL. Malaria and blood transfusion. Vox Sang. 2006; 90(2):77–84.
42. Owusu-Ofori AK, Betson M, Parry CM, Stothard R, Bates I. Transfusion-transmitted malaria in Ghana. Clin Infect Dis. 2013;56(12):1735–41.
43. Raat NJ, Ince C. Oxygenating the microcirculation: the perspective from blood transfusion and blood storage. Vox Sang. 2007;93:12–8.
44. Kim-Shapiro DB, Lee J, Gladwin GT. Storage lesions: role of red blood cell breakdown. Transfusion. 2011;51:844–51.
45. Aubron C, Nichol A, Cooper DJ, Bellomo R. Age of red blood cells and transfusion in critically ill patients. Ann Intensive Care. 2013. https://doi.org/10.1186/2110-5820-3-2.
46. Donadee C, Raat NJ, Kanias T, Tejero J, Lee JS, Kelley EE, Zhao X, Liu C, Reynolds H, Azarov I, Frizzell S, Meyer EM, Donnenberg AD, Qu L, Triulzi D, Kim-Shapiro DB, Gladwin MT. Nitric oxide scavenging by red blood cell microparticles and cell-free hemoglobin as a mechanism for the red cell storage lesion. Circulation. 2011;26:465–76.
47. Minneci PC, Deans KJ, Zhi H, Yuen PS, Star RA, Banks SM, Schechter AN, Natanson C, Gladwin MT, Solomon SB. Hemolysis-associated endothelial dysfunction mediated by accelerated NO inactivation by decompartmentalized oxyhemoglobin. J Clin Invest. 2005;115:3409–17.
48. Adamzic M, Hamburger T, Petrat F, Peters J, de Groot H, Hartmann M. Free hemoglobin concentration in severe sepsis: methods of measurement and prediction of outcome. Crit Care. 2012. https://doi.org/10.1186/cc11425.
49. Infectious disease testing for blood transfusions. NIH Consensus Panel on Infectious Disease Testing for blood transfusions. JAMA. 1995;274(17):1374–9.
50. Dosoo DK, Adu-Gyasi D, Kwara E, Ocran J, Osei-Kwakye, et al. Haematological and biochemical reference values for healthy adults in the middle belt of Ghana. PLoS ONE. 2012;7(4):e36308. https://doi.org/10.1371/journal.pone.0036308.

Adapting medical guidelines to be patient-centered using a patient-driven process for individuals with sickle cell disease and their caregivers

Robert Michael Cronin[1,2,3*], Tilicia L. Mayo-Gamble[4], Sarah-Jo Stimpson[5], Sherif M. Badawy[6], Lori E. Crosby[7], Jeannie Byrd[5], Emmanuel J. Volanakis[5], Adetola A. Kassim[8], Jean L. Raphael[9], Velma M. Murry[10] and Michael R. DeBaun[5]

Abstract

Background: Evidence-based guidelines for sickle cell disease (SCD) health maintenance and management have been developed for primary health care providers, but not for individuals with SCD. To improve the quality of care delivered to individuals with SCD and their caregivers, the main purposes of this study were to: (1) understand the desire for patient-centered guidelines among the SCD community; and (2) adapt guideline material to be patient-centered using community-engagement strategies involving health care providers, community -based organizations, and individuals with the disease.

Methods: From May–December 2016, a volunteer sample of 107 individuals with SCD and their caregivers gave feedback at community forums ($n = 64$) and community listening sessions ($n = 43$) about technology use for health information and desire for SCD-related guidelines. A team of community research partners consisting of community stakeholders, individuals living with SCD, and providers and researchers (experts) in SCD at nine institutions adapted guidelines to be patient-centered based on the following criteria: (1) understandable, (2) actionable, and (3) useful.

Results: In community forums (n = 64), almost all participants (91%) wanted direct access to the content of the guidelines. Participants wanted guidelines in more than one format including paper (73%) and mobile devices (79%). Guidelines were adapted to be patient-centered. After multiple iterations of feedback, 100% of participants said the guidelines were understandable, most (88%) said they were actionable, and everyone (100%) would use these adapted guidelines to discuss their medical care with their health care providers.

Conclusions: Individuals with SCD and their caregivers want access to guidelines through multiple channels, including technology. Guidelines written for health care providers can be adapted to be patient-centered using Community-engaged research involving providers and patients. These patient-centered guidelines provide a framework for patients to discuss their medical care with their health care providers.

Keywords: Sickle cell disease, Clinical practice guidelines, Patient-centered, Community-engaged research, Technology, Patient decision making, Qualitative methods

* Correspondence: robert.cronin@vanderbilt.edu
[1]Department of Biomedical Informatics, Vanderbilt University Medical Center, 2525 West End Blvd., Suite 1475, Nashville, TN 37232, USA
[2]Department of Internal Medicine, Vanderbilt University Medical Center, Nashville, TN, USA
Full list of author information is available at the end of the article

Background

Sickle cell disease (SCD) is an inherited disorder of hemoglobin affecting over 100,000 Americans, many of whom are poor and minorities [1–4]. SCD causes severe complications and has a substantial impact on both the population of affected individuals and the utilization of health care services in the United States; adults with SCD average 197,000 emergency room visits per year, and the lifetime costs of care for the average sickle cell patient are estimated at $900,000 by the age of 45 [4–6]. The primary care of adults with SCD is largely guided by the 2014 Evidence -Based Management of Sickle Cell Disease: Expert Panel Report. This report used the GRADE method to define and create evidence-based guidelines [7], and informs health care providers' approaches to screening to prevent diseases or complications of chronic diseases, selecting treatments, monitoring and preventing complications, educating about disease, and counseling for individuals with SCD [8]. Recognizing the importance of disseminating the guidelines and given the ubiquitous access to information technology [9, 10], provider-facing mobile health (mHealth) applications (apps) [11] and telemedicine interventions have been developed to educate providers about SCD guidelines [9, 10, 12]. However, to date no national strategy has been developed to make these SCD-related guidelines; hereafter, referred to as *guidelines*, patient-centered.

We define guidelines to be patient-centered if they are designed to be concordant with the patient's values and preferences, and would allow them to have an active dialog with their health care providers about their health care [13]. To ensure these patient-centered guidelines are concordant with patient's values, needs, and preferences, the guidelines needed to be: (1) provided at a health literacy level they can understand; (2) actionable, as using these guidelines effectively requires an active dialog with their health care provider about specific action items in their health care; and (3) a document that they could access and would use as a reference for their medical care. Developing educational material such as patient-centered guidelines can improve disease-specific knowledge [14–20]. Low SCD-specific knowledge is considered a modifiable risk factor associated with substantial negative impact on health outcomes and higher acute health care utilization among individuals with SCD [21–23]. Adapting guidelines to be patient-centered can engage individuals with SCD and their families, thereby having the potential to improve SCD-specific knowledge and decrease health care utilization.

Clinical practice guidelines are written for health care providers, and there is increasing interest in creating a guideline version for patients and their caregivers [24–28]. In SCD, these guidelines have been created for providers but not for patients. In addition, these guidelines are not always actionable for patients. The guidelines do not have action items that patients can follow to help with self-management or preventive measures they can discuss with their provider, thereby limiting their ability to engage in their own care. To improve the quality of care delivered to individuals with SCD and their caregivers, we developed a novel recursive process to create a single set of patient-centered guidelines using community-engaged research in a rare disease, SCD, where guidelines and high-quality evidence have been created for providers. Community-engaged research involves creating a partnership with community members, organizational representatives, health care providers, and researchers where all contributions are equal, shared decision making occurs, and everyone has ownership of the entire research process [29]. Community-engaged research is different than community-based participatory research as community-based participatory research is defined by working with an organization, which serves as a community partner who actively participates in the research. [30–34]. Community-engaged research engages the community to give input on the research questions, but does not necessarily partner with the community in the research process. The aims of this study were to use community-engaged research strategies [35–38] to: (1) explore the research question about if the SCD community wants access to these SCD-related guidelines and how they would want to access them, and (2) to adapt provider-centered guidelines to be patient-centered for the SCD community to improve productive discussions with a prepared, proactive practice team.

Methods

The engagement process

Using community-engaged strategies to include the SCD community through community-engaged research is crucial in developing patient-centered guidelines. These patient-centered guidelines need to be useful to providers as well as to individuals with SCD and their caregivers. Community-based organization partners (Sickle Cell Disease Association of America (SCDAA) and Sickle Cell Foundation of Tennessee (SCFT)) guided the process of community-engaged research and served as a conduit between health care providers, researchers and individuals with SCD. Through our partnership, we implemented several different community-engaged research strategies: (1) three community forums, (2) four community listening sessions, (3) weekly teleconferences, and (4) a two-day in person meeting. The iterative process to adapt the guidelines occurred from May 2016 to December 2016 (Fig. 1). The details of each strategy are discussed in the sections below.

The engagement process started with a needs assessment at the Vanderbilt University's annual SCD retreat

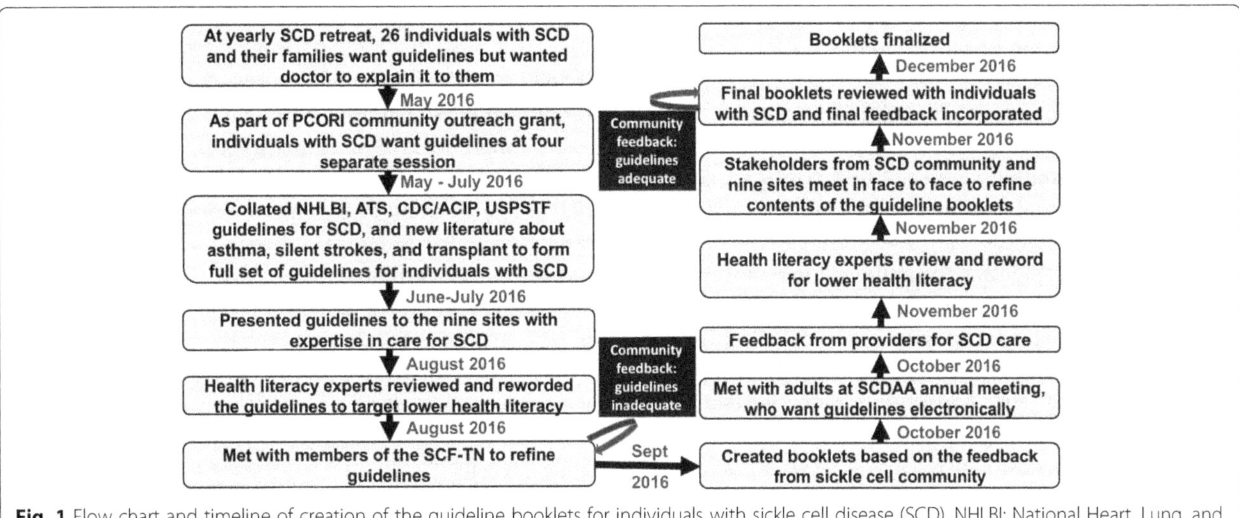

Fig. 1 Flow chart and timeline of creation of the guideline booklets for individuals with sickle cell disease (SCD). NHLBI: National Heart, Lung, and Blood Institute; ATS: American Thoracic Society; CDC: Centers for Disease Control; ACIP: Advisory Committee of Immunization Practices

community forum. This needs assessment aimed to discover whether the SCD community (individuals with the disease, parents of children with disease) wanted guidelines. Once the needs assessment was completed, and the SCD community expressed desire for guidelines during this community forum, a series of weekly teleconferences commenced.

The objective of these weekly teleconferences was to include providers and community representatives in an effort to curate guidelines so they would be acceptable to both providers at SCD centers across the United States, as well as individuals with the disease. Guidelines that are acceptable to providers and patients could allow for improved joint decision making.

These weekly teleconferences, attended by community-based organization leadership and experts in the care of SCD from across the country at nine academic institutions, were held over a six-month period. These experts in SCD included hematologists, primary care providers, psychologists, researchers, and nurse case managers. All of these experts provided care for individuals with SCD. The teleconferences allowed community-based organization leadership to give insight from the SCD community perspective with these experts in SCD present. During these teleconferences, experts in SCD and community-based organization leaders reviewed and curated a set of guidelines from (1) the 2014 "Evidence -Based Management of Sickle Cell Disease: Expert Panel Report" guidelines, (2) the American Thoracic Society guidelines about pulmonary hypertension for SCD, (3) the United States Preventative Services Task Force, (4) the Advisory Committee on Immunization Practices, and (5) recent randomized controlled trial evidence about asthma and silent strokes [39–41]. At the conclusion of these meetings, a set of guidelines was agreed upon that health care providers could use in the care for individuals with SCD. Once this set of guidelines was agreed upon by the SCD experts and community-based organization leadership, these guidelines were refined to be understandable for patients through a discussion with the health literacy experts at Vanderbilt University Medical Center. The health literacy experts gave recommendations on language that reduced the reading level to the 5th–7th grade reading level using the Flesch–Kincaid readability tests, and substituted medical jargon with layman's language.

Now with a curated, more understandable, acceptable set of SCD guidelines, the community-based organization leadership recommended more community involvement to get a patient perspective, and make them useful to the community. This advice prompted implementation of community engagement strategies. These community engagement strategies included community forums and community listening sessions, which served as a continuation of the needs assessment as well as a platform to review guideline content. These strategies allowed for community feedback about the content's understandability, actionability, and usability. The engagement strategies are described in detail below.

After feedback was obtained, another iteration of the cycle was required, where the SCD experts and community-based organization leadership discussed the revised content, health literacy experts reviewed and modified these updates to make the content understandable at a 5th–7th grade literacy level, and the SCD community provided feedback (Fig. 1). The process concluded with a two-day in-person meeting held at Vanderbilt University Medical Center to allow for face-to-face discussion among all members of the research team (experts in SCD care, leadership from the community-based organizations, and individuals with SCD and their caregivers). During this face-to-face meeting, Guideline booklets were reviewed and feedback was incorporated.

Recruitment methods for community forums and community listening sessions:

A convenience sampling was used to recruit participants for the community forums and community listening sessions. The effectiveness of these strategies is demonstrated in studies eliciting community input on an area of importance for the community not previously described [42–44]. The researchers elected to implement both community forums and community listening sessions to provide an opportunity for feedback in research-led and community-led environments. The participants for the community forums were attendees of the Vanderbilt University's annual SCD retreat that took place in central Tennessee, the SCDAA annual meeting held in Baltimore, and the SCFT monthly meeting held in Nashville. Participants were either individuals with SCD or caregivers of individuals with SCD. The participants at the Vanderbilt University's annual SCD retreat were individuals that are cared for at the Vanderbilt Meharry Sickle Cell Center for Excellence. These individuals were invited to participate in a weekend of camaraderie and an educational session about guidelines. Participants at the annual SCDAA meeting included a group of adolescents and young adults with SCD that were attending the annual meeting. This group was invited to come to a session discussing the guidelines as part of the itinerary of the meeting. Participants from the SCFT community forums were invited to be a part of their monthly meetings that took place in Nashville.

Community listening sessions were facilitated by a trained representative from the SCFT. Participants for the community listening sessions were individuals with SCD and their caregivers ($n = 43$) in two urban and two rural communities throughout three regions (West, Middle, and East) in Tennessee. Participants were recruited via email distribution through the SCFT. Interested participants were then invited to attend a scheduled session held in a community setting. Sessions lasted approximately 1.5 h each. The sessions were audio-recorded and notes were scribed. All sessions were commercially transcribed and used verbatim for analysis.

Community forums and community listening sessions:
Community forums

Community forums were planned for individuals with SCD and their caregivers to explore the research question about desire to access guidelines and then to adapt the guidelines to be patient-centered. Similar to other studies, these forums were led by researcher staff. The forum started with multiple-choice questions to explore our research question about if individuals with SCD and their caregivers wanted access to the SCD-related guidelines, and then how they would want to access these guidelines. Other questions included respondent demographics and perceptions of impact of guideline usage on personal health. Individuals with SCD, their caregivers, or both used response clickers, remote control-like devices, to submit anonymous responses to straw poll surveys about information technology and guidelines. The responses to the multiple-choice answers were evaluated with quantitative methods described below.

After the multiple-choice questions were completed, these meetings focused on guideline content and what changes should be made to make them patient-driven. Qualitative feedback was recorded by participants and the research team on guideline booklets and collected by the research team at the end of the session. Respondents voluntarily attended the community forums and contributed data through participation in the audience response activity.

Community listening sessions

Community listening sessions ($n = 4$) are a qualitative method of obtaining feedback that allows individuals to express their views on an issue in a more wide-ranging manner [45]. These sessions were different from the community forums as they were led by trained representatives from the SCFT and not researchers, and allowed qualitative feedback about a range of issues (e.g., disease management, nutrition, and provider interaction) including patient-centered guidelines.

Data analysis for community forums

For quantitative data, descriptive statistical methods and tests were used to summarize demographics and responses to community forum multiple-choice questions. Continuous variables were summarized and tabulated in terms of totals and percentages. Fisher's exact tests were performed to determine differences in: (1) the demographics of the different community forums, (2) question responses among the different community forums, and (3) channels that respondents wanted the guidelines to be communicated. Statistical tests were performed using R version 3.2.2 [46]. P-values of < 0.05 were considered significant.

For qualitative data, the participants were asked about the importance of each point brought up and if more than one person agreed in the importance of the point, the point was recorded by the research team. After conclusion of the community forums, all points recorded were reviewed by the research team and the team conducted a thematic analysis from the data obtained and explored common themes across group responses using grounded theory [47, 48].

Qualitative data analysis for community listening sessions

An inductive, qualitative content analysis approach was used to analyze the data from the community listening sessions. Members of the research team trained in qualitative data analysis reviewed these data and conducted a thematic analysis. Common themes across participant responses were explored using grounded theory [47, 48].

Ethical aspects

Participants were informed that their responses would be used for quality improvement purposes, such as the development and implementation of an information technology system for communicating guideline information. Informed consent was waived for this IRB-exempt, HIPAA-compliant, retrospective review of prospectively acquired quality improvement data. The Vanderbilt University Medical Center IRB approved this work.

Results

Individuals with SCD and their caregivers used technology, wanted to know about guidelines and were interested in having the guideline educational material delivered in different ways

A total of 64 individuals with SCD and their caregivers were included in the community forums. There were more adults and caregivers who participated in the sessions than children and adolescents (Table 1). The majority of participants at the SCD retreat were caregivers, and at the SCDAA and SCFT were adults. The groups had significantly different demographics ($p < 0.01$).

In the first community forum (SCD retreat, $n = 27$), 25 of 27 participants (93%) wanted to know what the guidelines were, providing strong motivation to proceed with the effort to adapt the SCD guidelines. Among the 64 participants pooled from all four venues, over half (58%) knew what a medical guideline was, and 91% would want to know what the content of the guidelines are (Table 2). A majority of individuals with SCD and their caregivers wanted the guidelines to be available in multiple formats, but only 44% want them on a patient portal ($p < 0.01$) (Table 2). The responses to questions were significantly different for using apps for the health of someone with SCD ($p = 0.01$), wanting the guidelines on the patient portal ($p < 0.01$), and wanting the guidelines in a mobile app ($p = 0.03$).

Individuals with SCD used technologies at different rates to find health information or to track their health. A large majority of participants used their smartphones and cell phones for texting (95 and 98%, respectively). More than half used email and social media for their health (65 and 61% respectively), but less than half used smartphone health apps (47%). The apps that were most commonly used included various patient portal apps and the VOICE crisis alert app [49].

In the community listening sessions ($n = 4$), the major themes from respondents ($n = 43$) included: (1) a desire for guidelines and educational material from physicians on how to manage their disease; (2) a need for information on how to access the guidelines; and (3) a desire to learn more about how to use the guidelines to communicate with health care providers. Respondents, who had accessed the existing guidelines, also expressed that the educational material is written at a level that they cannot understand.

Guideline content was modified by input from many different members of the SCD community, including individuals with SCD and their caregivers

Adapting the SCD guidelines was an iterative process. Health literacy experts from the Vanderbilt Effective Health Communication Core edited the original guidelines based on grade-level metrics. The edited guidelines were brought back to the SCD community for comment. The main themes that developed from the SCD community included: (1) creating more explanations for medical concepts; (2) streamlining the format and organization of the information; (3) identifying which content was actionable; and (4) using more visual representations of the content. They recommended that the guidelines could be "made more actionable" and described the initial version as "too wordy". Some examples of specific changes from these themes are presented in Table 3. The community members also had additional ideas for future sections of the guidelines booklet including: (1) a section on aging with SCD; (2) a section on overall healthy living, including diet, exercise, and other general concepts about how to live a healthy life with SCD; and (3) a section on preventing complications including issues like high altitudes, cold, heat, dehydration, and other anticipatory care.

Table 1 Demographics of SCD and caregivers who participated in the community sessions. Fisher's exact test was used to determine the *p*-value of differences between the different forums and age groups

	Age less than 15	Age = 15–25	Age older than 25	Caregivers	*p*-value
Sickle Cell Retreat	0	0	1	26	< 0.01
Sickle Cell Disease Association of America	2	9	15	0	
Sickle Cell Foundation of Tennessee	1	1	9	0	

Table 2 Responses to questions asked at the different community forums. An 'x' means the question was not asked in that forum. Fisher's exact test was used to calculate the p-value

Question	Response	SCD retreat (n = 27)	SCDAA (*n* = 26)	SCFT (*n* = 11)	*p*-value
Do you have a smart phone like a Samsung, iPhone, Android?	Yes	25	24	10	0.39
	No	2	0	1	
Do you use your phone for text messaging?	Yes	27	23	10	0.56
	No	0	1	0	
Do you use email for the health of someone with SCD?	Yes	x	14	8	0.43
	No	x	10	2	
Do you use social media like Facebook, Twitter or Instagram for the health of someone with SCD?	Yes	x	15	5	0.25
	No	x	6	6	
Do you use mobile apps for your health?	Yes	13	10	7	0.42
	No	14	15	4	
Do you use apps for the health of someone with SCD?	Yes	8	15	7	0.01
	No	19	6	4	
Do you know what a medical guideline is?	Yes	x	11	8	0.24
	No	x	10	2	
Would you want to know what these guidelines are?	Yes	25	18	10	1
	No	2	1	0	
Would you feel you could provide better care to the family member with sickle cell if you knew what the guidelines were?	Yes	20	19	9	0.14
	No	7	1	1	
Would you want your doctor or nurse explain the content of the guidelines to you?	Yes	25	17	10	1
	No	2	2	1	
Would you want a paper copy of the guidelines?	Yes	20	16	8	1
	No	7	5	3	
Would you want to receive text messages about the guidelines (short ones daily)?	Yes	22	15	7	0.77
	No	4	2	2	
Would you want the guidelines available on your patient portal?	Yes	x	6	9	< 0.01
	No	x	18	1	
Would you want guidelines in Facebook/Instagram/Twitter?	Yes	25	17	7	0.1
	No	2	7	2	
Would you want guidelines in mobile app?	Yes	17	13	10	0.03
	No	8	11	0	
Would you want guidelines in app over Facebook?	Yes	x	19	9	1
	No	x	3	1	
Facebook to communicate about guidelines and other things	Yes	25	x	x	x
	No	2	x	x	

Feedback was incorporated and another version of the guidelines booklet was developed. After this iterative process was completed two times, only minor changes were recommended, which resulted in the final version of the guidelines booklet. Some examples of changes made because of feedback from the SCD community included: (1) creating actionable checkboxes for items that individuals with SCD and their caregivers can take action, (2) having examples of forms such as pain action plans, (3) including more bullet points with shorter sentences, (4) explaining more medical concepts such as pulmonary hypertension, and (5) organizing booklets into the following major sections: Staying Well; Treating Sickle Cell Disease, Managing Sickle Cell Complications, and Other Conditions that can Affect Sickle Cell Disease (Table 4). At the end of the feedback, 100% of participants said the

Table 3 Themes and examples of specific feedback about initial content of guidelines

Themes	Examples of feedback
Creating more explanations for medical concepts	"There was still a bit of medical jargon in there that either needs to be removed, or there should be a definitions and examples page"
	"For drugs, [it] would be nice to have definition, examples, side effects ([especially] Hydroxyurea)"
	"I would want symptoms, or what do we mean by 'gallstones' or 'discomfort'"
	"Also, [we] want more about why SCD causes this or affects this, that these complications happen over years"
Streamlining the format and organization of the information	"Categories need to be better laid out, for example, by age would be better"
	"More small sentences and bullet points, not long paragraphs"
	"Remove all the 'if you are XX age' ... and make content only appear in certain sections by age"
	"There is too much information that may not be relevant to a person at their [current] age, and they would just want relevant information [filter by their age]"
	"Some things were repetitive like vaso-occlusive episode, and there should be a definition for the section, but then just call the episode a 'pain crisis'"
	"Combine depression screening, or at least make [the recommendations] by age, and again, less wording, more bullet points"
Identifying which content was actionable	"Make the verbiage more actionable, for example, if you don't have a pain action plan – get a pain action plan"
	"I can't tell what is actionable [in these guidelines]"
Using more visual representations of the content	"I would like a vaccine schedule in the content and more pictures"
	"We need more pictures"

guidelines were understandable, 88% said the guidelines were actionable, 90% would use these guidelines to keep track of their SCD, and 100% would use these guidelines to discuss their medical care with their providers. Consistent with feedback from participants, the future goal will be to provide widespread access to this version of the guidelines via a paper-based version and via incorporation into an mHealth app to the SCD community and other SCD centers [50, 51].

Discussion

As evidence -based medical guidelines become standard for practicing medicine [52] and are applied as metrics for quality of care [53], individuals affected by the disease should be partners in adapting and implementing such guidelines. To our knowledge this is the first application of community-engaged research principles in SCD to modify established evidence -based guidelines and current best evidence to make them more directly useful for individuals with SCD, and their caregivers to use with health care providers. Over a six-month period, the process weighed input from all stakeholders equally (individuals with SCD their caregivers, and SCD experts involving SCD health care providers) including SCD community-based organizations. The process started with understanding if the SCD community members (individuals with the disease, parents of children with disease, and leaders of community-based organizations for SCD) wanted usable guidelines and how the SCD community wanted access to the guidelines. In an iterative process that included a multidisciplinary team of SCD experts, health literacy experts, and the SCD community, published evidence -based SCD guidelines were transformed into a version that is patient-centered. To be patient-centered, the guidelines were adapted to be understandable, actionable, accessible, and useful for individuals with SCD and their caregivers. This patient-centered guideline booklet was agreed upon by SCD health care providers from across the United States and rated as widely acceptable by SCD community members, making it a feasible tool for use by health care providers and individuals with SCD and caregivers in making shared decisions about their care. The booklet also has the potential to engage and activate patients and improve their *SCD-specific knowledge*. Engaged and activated patients have better health outcomes including better diabetes control, less depression, more preventive cancer screening tests for women (Pap smear and mammography); and lower costly utilization (emergency department visit or hospitalization) [54, 55]. Improving *SCD-specific knowledge* can lower annual rates of emergency department utilization and hospitalizations in individuals with SCD [21].

Limited literature exists to describe a process of adapting and "translating" clinical practice guidelines to become more patient-centered. Knowledge of clinical practice guidelines among patients is low and there is a growing desire for patients and their care providers to embrace and have the knowledge of these guidelines [56–58], similar to our findings in SCD. Engaging patients in clinical guideline development and review has also been described [25, 59–61]. Some of these studies

Table 4 Examples of strong SCD NHLBI recommendation and evidence for individuals with SCD according to the NHLBI guidelines and recent randomized controlled trials. Boxes denote action items an individual can take based on the NHLBI guidelines.

Provider Guidelines	First version of Patient-Centered Guidelines	Patient-Centered Guidelines after iterative process described in Fig. 1
Use an individualized prescribing and monitoring protocol (written by the patient's SCD clinician) or an SCD-specific protocol whenever possible to promote rapid, effective, and safe analgesic management and resolution of the vaso-occlusive crisis in children and adults (Pain action plan)	Sometimes blocked blood vessels can cause a sickle crisis, which involves severe pain. In order to help you quickly and safely during these crises, talk to your SCD doctor about creating a set of rules specific to your needs. Include rules about getting medication, and how often your doctor will check in with you.	What can be done at home to manage the pain? • A pain action plan describes how to manage sickle cell pain at home. Action plans should be used as soon as the pain starts. An example of a pain action plan can be found in *Forms*. □ Ask your health care provider about creating a written pain action plan that works for you. • Call your health care provider if the pain does not get better, or gets worse even though you are using your pain action plan.
Treat avascular necrosis with analgesics and consult physical therapy and orthopedic departments for assessment and follow-up	If you experience discomfort caused by your bones not getting enough blood supply, sometimes called avascular necrosis, talk to your doctor about taking pain medications. Your doctor may recommend you see physical therapy and orthopedic doctors.	What is the treatment for avascular necrosis? • Treatment options depend on how much the joint is affected. □ Talk with your health care provider about sending you for physical therapy to make the muscles around the joint stronger and more flexible. □ Talk with your health care provider about ways other than medication to manage your pain: • Using heat, such as a warm compress, warm bath, or a heating pad • Gently massaging the area that hurts • Doing something to distract you from the pain like listening to music, drawing, watching TV, or writing in a journal • Doing deep breathing and relaxation exercises □ If approaches without medications do not help, talk with your health care provider about medications to control the pain. □ A special health care provider (orthopedic surgeon) may see you for additional evaluation and treatment. Sometimes surgery is needed if other treatments do not work.
In infants 9 months of age or older, in children, in adolescents, and in adults with SCA, offer treatment with hydroxyurea regardless of clinical severity to reduce complications (e.g., pain, dactylitis, ACS, anemia) related to SCD	If your child with SCD is between 9 months old and 18 years old, check with his or her doctor about using the drug hydroxyurea to try to lessen complications of SCD. Examples of complications include pain, finger/toe swelling and redness, and low red blood cell count.	What is Hydroxyurea? • Hydroxyurea is a medication that increases the amount of fetal hemoglobin in red blood cells. Fetal hemoglobin helps to keep the red blood cells from sickling. • Hydroxyurea is not a cure for sickle cell disease, but it may help *decrease* many of the complications of the disease, including: Anemia Pain episodes Episodes of acute chest syndrome The need for blood transfusions Long hospital stays • In adults, some studies have found that hydroxyurea helps you live longer. Who should take hydroxyurea? • Talk with your health care provider about hydroxyurea if: □ You have sickle cell anemia (type SS or sickle beta thalassemia zero) □ You have sickle cell disease (type SC or sickle beta thalassemia plus) and have pain or other sickle cell complications that affect your ability to do your daily activities or that affects your quality of life.

Table 4 Examples of strong SCD NHLBI recommendation and evidence for individuals with SCD according to the NHLBI guidelines and recent randomized controlled trials. Boxes denote action items an individual can take based on the NHLBI guidelines. *(Continued)*

Provider Guidelines	First version of Patient-Centered Guidelines	Patient-Centered Guidelines after iterative process described in Fig. 1
No definition in guidelines	Not included in the first version	What is pulmonary hypertension? • Pulmonary hypertension is more common in people with sickle cell disease than in people without sickle cell disease. • Your heart is made up of two pump systems. The right side of your heart pumps blood to your lungs to pick up oxygen. The left side of your heart pumps blood to the rest of your body. • Blood pressure measured with a cuff on your arm is measuring the pressure it takes to pump blood to your body. High blood pressure is called hypertension. • The pressure it takes to pump blood to your lungs can also be measured. High blood pressure here is called pulmonary hypertension.

described the following potential strategies that mirror our community-engaged research approach: including patient input, having appropriate stakeholders at the table (e.g., consumer stakeholders), and convening multiple meetings with sufficient time. By utilizing these strategies, we were able to mitigate barriers previously described to create patient-centered guidelines including: difficulty understanding the discussion or content, resisting patient input by healthcare providers, allowing a dialog among patients, caregivers, community-based organizations, and health care providers, and having sufficient time for discussion.

Few examples of patient-centered guidelines exist in the literature today, and most of those examples are from the United Kingdom and Europe [61–66]. Description of how guidelines were adapted for patients was limited to a few studies, all outside of the United States [62–64]. These studies, like ours, used experts and patients to modify the wording of guidelines to be more patient-centered, while maintaining original meaning [62, 63]. Our study included community-based organizations in addition to patients, and used an iterative process to arrive at a final version, where these prior studies did not use community-based organizations in the process and finalized their patient-centered guidelines during or after only a single meeting of all stakeholders. While most studies used lay language to explain complex medical terminology, Kiltz et al. described keeping some original scientific language, as modifying them did not improve understanding of the concept. Our finalized booklets also kept some scientific language, such as "pulmonary hypertension", "hydroxyurea", and "sickle cell beta thalassemia", for the same reasons. Similar to our study, other studies mentioned a list of ideas that patients desired to be included in the next update of the guidelines. Another article by the Scottish Intercollegiate Guidelines Network (SIGN) group demonstrated that the value and usefulness of the patient-centered guideline was based on how it informed the public, linked information to actions, and empowered people in interacting with their healthcare providers [67]. Our findings were similar, with the desire for actionable content and information that was clear and understandable. We also found that individuals with SCD had a desire to know how to stay well when having their disease, and wanted a wellness section. The only manuscript about patient-centered U.S. guidelines was McClure's adaptation of clinical practice guidelines for people with cancer [66]. These guidelines were adapted from the National Comprehensive Cancer Network (NCCN) clinical practice guidelines that provide diagnosis, evaluation, and treatment options about people's cancer [66, 68]. Our work does not explain the methods of adaptation or if and how people and communities with cancer were engaged in the adaptation of the guidelines. Our study expanded upon previous literature by describing the methods of how to create patient-centered guidelines using community-engaged research for U.S. guidelines on SCD, and illuminated the importance of input from the SCD community into the adaptation of existing clinical guidelines to be most understandable, actionable, accessible, and useful for them.

In the initial three meetings with the community, a majority of individuals with SCD and their caregivers could not define a medical guideline, but almost all participants wanted the guidelines to be available to them once they understood what a guideline was. The SCD community wanted the guidelines available in multiple formats, with an overwhelming majority wanting them to be explained by a health care provider, and about 70% wanting them in paper and electronic formats. Patient portals were distinctly less appealing, with less than half wanting to access the guidelines in this way.

In our prior work, we demonstrated that individuals with SCD and their caregivers want to access technology when asked: "How would you prefer to be contacted to learn about potential research studies?" [69] The results of the community-engaged research project confirm that technology is emerging as a preferred medium for individuals with SCD and their caregivers to learn about their care, specifically evidence -based guidelines. However, individuals with SCD and their caregivers are unsure of the optimal technology for tracking and managing their health. This health care technology gap in the SCD community will make Meaningful Use governmental regulations that focus on the use of health technologies to promote improved outcomes in patients, difficult to implement [70]. As a result of the government mandate, many health care systems and providers are using patient portals to meet these Meaningful Use regulations [71], which is in contrast to what individuals with SCD and their caregivers wanted to access guidelines. Further work is required to further describe and develop ways to address this health care technology gap.

Community involvement in translating the evidence-based guidelines from documents intended for health care providers into patient-accessible content was of paramount importance. After the family retreat, the participants demonstrated their desire to have access to guidelines. The process started with the expertise of SCD providers across the country to curate the guidelines into the essential knowledge content that health care providers would use to care for individuals with SCD. As previous literature has demonstrated, educational material for SCD is often developed at too high of a reading level [72]. Therefore, our next step was to work with a health literacy expert team to make the language more accessible; however, when we approached the community with the adapted guidelines, the community could not extract meaningful content and did not yet find the guidelines useful. This community input led to a set of improvements including changing the format of the guidelines from dense paragraphs translated from the original medical documents into a digestible set of explanatory points, and adding action items that could easily be used by the SCD community. The iterative process allowed all groups to converge on a guideline booklet that was factual, comprehensive, patient-centered, actionable, and most importantly, one that individuals with SCD and their caregivers would want to use in their discussions with health care providers.

There were several limitations to our community-engaged research approach. Our data collection strategy did not allow for subgroup analysis (i.e., how many people selected each multiple-choice option) across the population. However, we do not believe this limitation significantly impacted our results as for most study findings and guideline adaptations (i.e. should we have guidelines, should the guidelines have a paper format) there were no substantial alternate findings or opinions. Further, we elected to use a clicker system to increase the likelihood of honest feedback from the self-selected groups that participated in the community forums. We realize that the health care providers participating in this project may not be representative of SCD health care providers across the country. To limit biases, we deliberately selected published evidence-based guidelines or new published evidence to determine what evidence -based guidelines should be included and presented to caregivers. Specific topics that were included in our booklet but not the NHLBI guidelines were depression screening, role of hematopoietic stem cell transplant for cure, screening for silent strokes, and screening for asthma. While we obtained feedback from the national SCDAA meeting where individuals with SCD from around the United States meet, our results may not generalize to the broader population of individuals living with SCD or their caregivers. Finally, we have not evaluated uptake of using the guidelines by patients and providers; however, this is an active area of research for our group and 100% of individuals with SCD and caregivers state they would like to use these guidelines.

The emphasis of providing the guidelines for care in SCD has been directed toward health care providers. SCD experts have developed an mHealth apps for health care providers to increase the adoption of the 2014 guidelines [11]. Others have created educational programs using telemedicine to educate providers about these guidelines [12]. However, to date no national strategy has been developed to make these guidelines patient-centered, accessible and comprehensible for individuals with SCD.

We undertook this activity as an extension of Vanderbilt's Sickle Cell Center of Excellence approach of providing individuals with SCD and their caregivers with evidence -based knowledge and action items to improve their overall care and satisfaction with the care [73]. This work describes a community-engaged process that will aid in the adaptation of provider-centered guidelines for individuals and caregivers of a hematologic disease to become informed and activated. This patient-driven approach resulted in a guideline booklet that the SCD community found useful and would want to use for productive discussions with a prepared, proactive practice team [74]. As guidelines continue to evolve, this patient-driven process will be useful for adapting future evidence-based care recommendations to be patient-centered, comprehensible, and accessible. Next steps include evaluating these guidelines and their ability to activate individuals with SCD, improve *SCD-specific knowledge*, and decrease acute health care utilization.

Conclusions

In this study, we engaged the community using community-engaged research strategies and found that individuals with SCD and their caregivers wanted access to the same SCD guidelines relied on by health care providers, and wanted these guidelines through multiple channels, including technology. Based on these positive results, we used community-engaged research involving health care providers, community-based organizations, and individuals with SCD, to adapt guideline material for the SCD community. The adapted patient-centered guidelines have the potential to improve the SCD community's knowledge of their SCD, and serve as a conduit for productive discussions with a prepared, proactive practice team. The approach presented in this manuscript is potentially generalizable to adapting guidelines in other diseases designed for providers, to be patient-centered.

Abbreviations

SCD: Sickle cell disease; SCDAA: Sickle Cell Disease Association of America; SCFT: Sickle Cell Foundation of Tennessee

Acknowledgements

We would like to thank the experts of the nine institutions (UCSF Benioff Children's Hospitals Oakland and San Francisco (Marsha Treadwell); Boston Medical Center (Patricia Kavanagh, Amy Sobota); Duke University (Nirmish Shah); Washington University School of Medicine–St Louis (Allison King); Cincinnati Children's Hospital Medical Center (Karen Kalinyak); Texas Children's Hospital (Gladstone Airewele); Ann and Robert H. Lurie Children's Hospital of Chicago (Alexis Thompson); St. Jude Children's Research Hospital and Methodist Comprehensive Sickle Cell Center (Jane Hankins, Jerlym Porter, Pat Adams-Graves); and Vanderbilt University Medical Center (Karina Wilkerson), the Effective Health Communication Core at the Vanderbilt University Medical Center, the Sickle Cell Foundation of Tennessee (Trevor Thompson, Alexis Gorden), and the Sickle Cell Disease Association of America (Sonja Banks, Sonya Ross). The Vanderbilt University Medical Center IRB approved this work.

Funding

This research was funded by grants patient centered outcomes research institute (PCORI) Number Clinical Data Research Network (CDRN) 1501–26498, and the National Institutes of Health - National Center for Advancing Translational Sciences grant #UL1TR000445 and the National Heart, Lung, And Blood Institute under Award Number K23HL141447 funded this work. The funding bodies did not have any involvement in the design of this study or in the collection, analysis, and interpretation of data or in writing of the manuscript.

Authors' contributions

All authors listed have contributed sufficiently to the project to be included as authors, and all those who are qualified to be authors are listed in the author byline. RMC, TLM, JB, EJV, AAK, VMM, and MD were involved with the conception and design of the study. RMC, TLM, SS, SMB, LEC, JLR, VMM, and MD were involved in data collection. RMC, TLM, SMB, LEC, JB, EJV, AAK, JLR, VMM, and MD were involved with the analysis of the study. All authors were involved with the writing and editing the manuscript. All authors meet conditions: 1) substantial contributions to conception and design, acquisition of data, or analysis and interpretation of data; 2) drafting the article or revising it critically for important intellectual content; and 3) final approval of the version to be published. I, as the corresponding author, confirm full access to all aspects of the research and writing process, and take final responsibility for the paper.

Competing interests

All authors declare that no conflict of interest, financial or other, exists. The manuscript represents valid work; neither this manuscript nor one with substantially similar content under my authorship has been published or is being considered for publication elsewhere (except as described in the manuscript submission); and copies of any closely related manuscripts are enclosed in the manuscript submission; and, I agree to allow the corresponding author to serve as the primary correspondent with the editorial office and to review and sign off on the final proofs prior to publication.

Author details

[1]Department of Biomedical Informatics, Vanderbilt University Medical Center, 2525 West End Blvd., Suite 1475, Nashville, TN 37232, USA. [2]Department of Internal Medicine, Vanderbilt University Medical Center, Nashville, TN, USA. [3]Department of Pediatrics, Vanderbilt University Medical Center, Nashville, TN, USA. [4]Department of Family and Community Medicine, Meharry Medical College, Nashville, TN, USA. [5]Department of Pediatrics, Division of Hematology/Oncology, Vanderbilt-Meharry Center for Excellence in Sickle Cell Disease, Vanderbilt University Medical Center, Nashville, TN, USA. [6]Department of Pediatrics, Division of Hematology, Oncology and Stem Cell Transplant, Ann & Robert H. Lurie Children's Hospital of Chicago, Northwestern University Feinberg School of Medicine, Chicago, IL, USA. [7]Division of Behavioral Medicine, Department of Pediatrics, Cincinnati Children's Hospital Medical Center and the University of Cincinnati, College of Medicine, Cincinnati, OH, USA. [8]Department of Medicine, Division of Hematology/Oncology, Vanderbilt-Meharry Center for Excellence in Sickle Cell Disease, Vanderbilt University Medical Center, Nashville, TN, USA. [9]Department of Pediatrics, Section of Hematology-Oncology and Section of Academic General Pediatrics, Baylor College of Medicine, Houston, TX, USA. [10]Department of Human & Organizational Development, Vanderbilt University, Nashville, TN, USA.

References

1. Brousseau DC, Panepinto JA, Nimmer M, Hoffmann RG. The number of people with sickle-cell disease in the United States: national and state estimates. Am J Hematol. 2010;85(1):77–8.
2. Mvundura M, Amendah D, Kavanagh PL, Sprinz PG, Grosse SD. Health care utilization and expenditures for privately and publicly insured children with sickle cell disease in the United States. Pediatr Blood Cancer. 2009;53(4):642–6.
3. Steiner CA, Miller JL. Sickle cell disease patients in US hospitals, 2004. 2006.
4. Yusuf HR, Atrash HK, Grosse SD, Parker CS, Grant AM. Emergency department visits made by patients with sickle cell disease: a descriptive study, 1999-2007. Am J Prev Med. 2010;38(4 Suppl):S536–41. https://doi.org/10.1016/j.amepre.2010.01.001.
5. Dunlop RJ, Bennett KC. Pain management for sickle cell disease. Cochrane Database Syst Rev. 2006;2:CD003350. https://doi.org/10.1002/14651858.CD003350.pub2.
6. Kauf TL, Coates TD, Huazhi L, Mody-Patel N, Hartzema AG. The cost of health care for children and adults with sickle cell disease. Am J Hematol. 2009;84(6):323–7 https://doi.org/10.1002/ajh.21408.
7. Guyatt GH, Oxman AD, Vist GE, et al. GRADE: an emerging consensus on rating quality of evidence and strength of recommendations. BMJ. 2008; 336(7650):924–6. https://doi.org/10.1136/bmj.39489.470347.AD.
8. Yawn BP, Buchanan GR, Afenyi-Annan AN, et al. Management of sickle cell disease: summary of the 2014 evidence-based report by expert panel members. JAMA. 2014;312(10):1033–48. https://doi.org/10.1001/jama.2014.10517.
9. Pew Research Center, April, 2015. "The Smartphone Difference" Available at: http://www.pewinternet.org/2015/04/01/us-smartphone-use-in-2015/.
10. Research PI. Mobile Fact Sheet. In: Pew Internet Research. 2017. http://www.pewinternet.org/fact-sheet/mobile/. Accessed March 10 2018.
11. Lunyera J, Jonassaint C, Jonassaint J, Shah N. Attitudes of primary care physicians toward sickle cell disease care, guidelines, and Comanaging hydroxyurea with a specialist. J Prim Care Community Health. 2016; https://doi.org/10.1177/2150131916662969.
12. Shook LM, Farrell CB, Kalinyak KA, et al. Translating sickle cell guidelines into practice for primary care providers with project ECHO. Med Educ Online. 2016;21:33616. https://doi.org/10.3402/meo.v21.33616.

13. Epstein RM, Franks P, Fiscella K, et al. Measuring patient-centered communication in patient–physician consultations: theoretical and practical issues. Soc Sci Med. 2005;61(7):1516–28.
14. Barry MM, D'Eath M, Sixsmith J. Interventions for improving population health literacy: insights from a rapid review of the evidence. J Health Commun. 2013; 18(12):1507–22. https://doi.org/10.1080/10810730.2013.840699.
15. Car J, Lang B, Colledge A, Ung C, Majeed A. Interventions for enhancing consumers' online health literacy. Cochrane Database Syst Rev. 2011;(6): Cd007092. https://doi.org/10.1002/14651858.CD007092.pub2.
16. Clement S, Ibrahim S, Crichton N, Wolf M, Rowlands G. Complex interventions to improve the health of people with limited literacy: a systematic review. Patient Educ Couns. 2009;75(3):340–51. https://doi.org/10.1016/j.pec.2009.01.008.
17. DeWalt DA, Hink A. Health literacy and child health outcomes: a systematic review of the literature. Pediatrics. 2009;124(Suppl 3):S265–74. https://doi.org/10.1542/peds.2009-1162B.
18. Pignone M, DeWalt DA, Sheridan S, Berkman N, Lohr KN. Interventions to improve health outcomes for patients with low literacy. A systematic review. J Gen Intern Med. 2005;20(2):185–92. https://doi.org/10.1111/j.1525-1497.2005.40208.x.
19. Schaefer CT. Integrated review of health literacy interventions. Orthop Nurs. 2008;27(5):302–17. https://doi.org/10.1097/01.nor.0000337283.55670.75.
20. Dennis S, Williams A, Taggart J, et al. Which providers can bridge the health literacy gap in lifestyle risk factor modification education: a systematic review and narrative synthesis. BMC Fam Pract. 2012;13:44. https://doi.org/10.1186/1471-2296-13-44.
21. Carden MA, Newlin J, Smith W, Sisler I. Health literacy and disease-specific knowledge of caregivers for children with sickle cell disease. Pediatr Hematol Oncol. 2016;33(2):121–33. https://doi.org/10.3109/08880018.2016.1147108.
22. Molter BL, Abrahamson K. Self-efficacy, transition, and patient outcomes in the sickle cell disease population. Pain Manag Nurs. 2015;16(3):418–24. https://doi.org/10.1016/j.pmn.2014.06.001.
23. Broome ME, Maikler V, Kelber S, Bailey P, Lea G. An intervention to increase coping and reduce health care utilization for school-age children and adolescents with sickle cell disease. J Natl Black Nurses Assoc. 2001;12(2):6–14.
24. Loudon K, Santesso N, Callaghan M, et al. Patient and public attitudes to and awareness of clinical practice guidelines: a systematic review with thematic and narrative syntheses. BMC Health Serv Res. 2014;14:321. https://doi.org/10.1186/1472-6963-14-321.
25. Roman BR, Feingold J. Patient-centered guideline development: best practices can improve the quality and impact of guidelines. Otolaryngology Head Neck Surg 2014; 151(4):530–532. doi:https://doi.org/10.1177/0194599814544878.
26. Sawyer KN, Brown F, Christensen R, Damino C, Newman MM, Kurz MC. Surviving sudden cardiac arrest: a pilot qualitative survey study of survivors. Ther Hypothermia Temp Manag. 2016;6(2):76–84. https://doi.org/10.1089/ther.2015.0031.
27. Gonzalez MG, Kelly KN, Dozier AM, et al. Patient perspectives on transitions of surgical care: examining the complexities and interdependencies of care. Qual Health Res. 2017;27(12):1856–69. https://doi.org/10.1177/1049732317704406.
28. Hurtado-de-Mendoza D, Loaiza-Bonilla A, Bonilla-Reyes PA, Tinoco G, Cardio-Oncology AR. Cancer therapy-related cardiovascular complications in a molecular targeted era: new concepts and perspectives. Cureus. 2017;9(5): e1258. https://doi.org/10.7759/cureus.1258.
29. Israel BA, Schulz AJ, Parker EA, Becker AB. Review of community-based research: assessing partnership approaches to improve public health. Annu Rev Public Health. 1998;19:173–202. https://doi.org/10.1146/annurev.publhealth.19.1.173.
30. Mikesell L, Bromley E, Khodyakov D. Ethical community-engaged research: a literature review. Am J Public Health. 2013;103(12):e7–e14. https://doi.org/10.2105/AJPH.2013.301605.
31. Fialkowski MK, DeBaryshe B, Bersamin A, et al. A community engagement process identifies environmental priorities to prevent early childhood obesity: the Children's healthy living (CHL) program for remote underserved populations in the US affiliated Pacific Islands, Hawaii and Alaska. Matern Child Health J. 2014;18(10):2261–74. https://doi.org/10.1007/s10995-013-1353-3.
32. Ahmed SM, Palermo AG. Community engagement in research: frameworks for education and peer review. Am J Public Health. 2010;100(8):1380–7. https://doi.org/10.2105/AJPH.2009.178137.
33. Khodyakov D, Mikesell L, Schraiber R, Booth M, Bromley E. On using ethical principles of community-engaged research in translational science. Transl Res. 2016;171:52–62 e1. https://doi.org/10.1016/j.trsl.2015.12.008.
34. Joosten YA, Israel TL, Williams NA, et al. Community engagement studios: a structured approach to obtaining meaningful input from stakeholders to inform research. Acad Med. 2015;90(12):1646–50. https://doi.org/10.1097/ACM.0000000000000794.
35. Jones L, Wells K. Strategies for academic and clinician engagement in community-participatory partnered research. JAMA. 2007;297(4):407–10. https://doi.org/10.1001/jama.297.4.407.
36. Jones L, Meade B, Forge N, et al. Begin your partnership: the process of engagement. Ethn Dis. 2009;19(4 Suppl 6) S6–8-16
37. Jones L, Wells K, Norris K, Meade B, Koegel P. The vision, valley, and victory of community engagement. Ethn Dis. 2009;19(4 Suppl 6):S6. -3-7
38. Wells K, Jones L. "research" in community-partnered, participatory research. JAMA. 2009;302(3):320–1. https://doi.org/10.1001/jama.2009.1033.
39. DeBaun MR, Kirkham FJ. Central nervous system complications and management in sickle cell disease. Blood. 2016;127(7):829–38. https://doi.org/10.1182/blood-2015-09-618579.
40. Bernaudin F, Verlhac S, Arnaud C, et al. Long-term treatment follow-up of children with sickle cell disease monitored with abnormal transcranial Doppler velocities. Blood. 2016;127(14):1814–22. https://doi.org/10.1182/blood-2015-10-675231.
41. An P, Barron-Casella EA, Strunk RC, Hamilton RG, Casella JF, DeBaun MR. Elevation of IgE in children with sickle cell disease is associated with doctor diagnosis of asthma and increased morbidity. J Allergy Clin Immunol. 2011; 127(6):1440–6. https://doi.org/10.1016/j.jaci.2010.12.1114.
42. Gonzalez-Guarda RM, Diaz EG, Cummings AM. A community forum to assess the needs and preferences for domestic violence prevention targeting Hispanics. Hisp Health Care Int. 2012;10(1):18–27. https://doi.org/10.1891/1540-4153.10.1.18.
43. Erves JC, Mayo-Gamble TL, Malin-Fair A, et al. Needs, priorities, and recommendations for engaging underrepresented populations in clinical research: a community perspective. J Community Health. 2017;42(3):472–80. https://doi.org/10.1007/s10900-016-0279-2.
44. Development UoKWGfCHa. Community Tool Box: Community Assessment. 2015. http://ctb.ku.edu/en/table-of-contents/assessment. Accessed Nov 9, 2017 2017.
45. Erves JC, Mayo-Gamble TL, Malin-Fair A, et al. Needs, priorities, and recommendations for engaging underrepresented populations in clinical research: a community perspective. J Community Health. 2016:1–9.
46. Team RCD. R: A language and environment for statistical computing. R foundation for statistical computing. Vienna Austria; 2005.
47. Patton MQ. Qualitative evaluation and research methods: SAGE publications, inc; 1990.
48. Starks H, Trinidad SB. Choose your method: a comparison of phenomenology, discourse analysis, and grounded theory. Qual Health Res. 2007;17(10):1372–80. https://doi.org/10.1177/1049732307307031.
49. VOICE Crisis Alert on the App Store. @AppStore. 2017. https://itunes.apple.com/us/app/voice-crisis-alert/id860311098?mt=8. Accessed March 20, 2017 2017.
50. Badawy SM, Thompson AA, Liem RI. Technology access and smartphone app preferences for medication adherence in adolescents and young adults with sickle cell disease. Pediatr Blood Cancer. 2016; https://doi.org/10.1002/pbc.25905.
51. Shah N, Jonassaint J, De Castro L. Patients welcome the sickle cell disease mobile application to record symptoms via technology (SMART). Hemoglobin. 2014;38(2):99–103. https://doi.org/10.3109/03630269.2014.880716.
52. Steinberg E, Greenfield S, Wolman DM, Mancher M, Graham R. Clinical practice guidelines we can trust: National Academies Press. Washington, D.C: The National Academies Press; 2011.
53. Williams SC, Schmaltz SP, Morton DJ, Koss RG, Loeb JM. Quality of care in US hospitals as reflected by standardized measures, 2002–2004. N Engl J Med. 2005;353(3):255–64.
54. Hibbard JH, Greene J. What the evidence shows about patient activation: better health outcomes and care experiences; fewer data on costs. Health Aff (Millwood). 2013;32(2):207–14. https://doi.org/10.1377/hlthaff.2012.1061.

55. Greene J, Hibbard JH, Sacks R, Overton V, Parrotta CD. When patient activation levels change, health outcomes and costs change, too. Health Aff. 2015;34(3):431–7.
56. Julian S, Rashid A, Baker R, Szczepura A, Habiba M. Attitudes of women with menstrual disorders to the use of clinical guidelines in their care. Fam Pract. 2010;27(2):205–11. https://doi.org/10.1093/fampra/cmp090.
57. Liira H, Saarelma O, Callaghan M, et al. Patients, health information, and guidelines: a focus-group study. Scand J Prim Health Care. 2015;33(3):212–9. https://doi.org/10.3109/02813432.2015.1067517.
58. Fearns N, Kelly J, Callaghan M, et al. What do patients and the public know about clinical practice guidelines and what do they want from them? A qualitative study. BMC Health Serv Res. 2016;16:74. https://doi.org/10.1186/s12913-016-1319-4.
59. Armstrong MJ, Mullins CD, Gronseth GS, Gagliardi AR. Recommendations for patient engagement in guideline development panels: a qualitative focus group study of guideline-naive patients. PLoS One. 2017;12(3):e0174329. https://doi.org/10.1371/journal.pone.0174329.
60. Pittens CA, Vonk Noordegraaf A, van Veen SC, Anema JR, Huirne JA, Broerse JE. The involvement of gynaecological patients in the development of a clinical guideline for resumption of (work) activities in the Netherlands. Health Expect. 2015;18(5):1397–412. https://doi.org/10.1111/hex.12121.
61. Franx G, Niesink P, Swinkels J, Burgers J, Wensing M, Grol R. Ten years of multidisciplinary mental health guidelines in the Netherlands. Int Rev Psychiatry. 2011;23(4):371–8. https://doi.org/10.3109/09540261.2011.606538.
62. Kiltz U, van der Heijde D, Mielants H, Feldtkeller E, Braun J. ASAS/EULAR recommendations for the management of ankylosing spondylitis: the patient version. Ann Rheum Dis. 2009;68(9):1381–6. https://doi.org/10.1136/ard.2008.096073.
63. de Wit MP, Smolen JS, Gossec L, van der Heijde DM. Treating rheumatoid arthritis to target: the patient version of the international recommendations. Ann Rheum Dis. 2011;70(6):891–5. https://doi.org/10.1136/ard.2010.146662.
64. Hauser W, Bernardy K, Wang H, Kopp I. Methodological fundamentals of the development of the guideline. Schmerz. 2012;26(3):232–46. https://doi.org/10.1007/s00482-012-1189-6.
65. Santesso N, Morgano GP, Jack SM, et al. Dissemination of clinical practice guidelines: a content analysis of patient versions. Med Decis Making. 2016; 36(6):692–702. https://doi.org/10.1177/0272989x16644427.
66. McClure JS. Informing patients: translating the NCCN guidelines. J Natl Compr Cancer Netw. 2011;9(Suppl 3):S4–5.
67. Fearns N, Graham K, Johnston G, Service D. Improving the user experience of patient versions of clinical guidelines: user testing of a Scottish intercollegiate guideline network (SIGN) patient version. BMC Health Serv Res. 2016;16:37. https://doi.org/10.1186/s12913-016-1287-8.
68. Network NCC. NCCN guidelines for patients. 2017. https://www.nccn.org/patients/guidelines/cancers.aspx.
69. Cronin RM, Hankins JS, Adams-Graves P, et al. Barriers and facilitators to research participation among adults, and parents of children with sickle cell disease: a trans-regional survey. Am J Hematol. 2016; https://doi.org/10.1002/ajh.24483.
70. Blumenthal D, Tavenner M. The "meaningful use" regulation for electronic health records. N Engl J Med. 2010;363(6):501–4. https://doi.org/10.1056/NEJMp1006114.
71. Shapochka A. Providers turn to portals to meet patient demand, meaningful use. J AHIMA. 2012. Available from: http://journal.ahima.org/2012/08/23/providers-turn-to-portals-to-meet-patient-demand-meaningful-use. [cited 2014 Sep 30].
72. McClure E, Ng J, Vitzthum K, Rudd R. A mismatch between patient education materials about sickle cell disease and the literacy level of their intended audience. Prev Chronic Dis. 2016;13:E64. https://doi.org/10.5888/pcd13.150478.
73. Bodenheimer T, Wagner EH, Grumbach K. Improving primary care for patients with chronic illness: the chronic care model, part 2. JAMA. 2002; 288(15):1909–14.
74. Coleman EA, Grothaus LC, Sandhu N, Wagner EH. Chronic care clinics: a randomized controlled trial of a new model of primary care for frail older adults. J Am Geriatr Soc. 1999;47(7):775–83.

Permissions

All chapters in this book were first published in HEMATOLOGY, by BioMed Central; hereby published with permission under the Creative Commons Attribution License or equivalent. Every chapter published in this book has been scrutinized by our experts. Their significance has been extensively debated. The topics covered herein carry significant findings which will fuel the growth of the discipline. They may even be implemented as practical applications or may be referred to as a beginning point for another development.

The contributors of this book come from diverse backgrounds, making this book a truly international effort. This book will bring forth new frontiers with its revolutionizing research information and detailed analysis of the nascent developments around the world.

We would like to thank all the contributing authors for lending their expertise to make the book truly unique. They have played a crucial role in the development of this book. Without their invaluable contributions this book wouldn't have been possible. They have made vital efforts to compile up to date information on the varied aspects of this subject to make this book a valuable addition to the collection of many professionals and students.

This book was conceptualized with the vision of imparting up-to-date information and advanced data in this field. To ensure the same, a matchless editorial board was set up. Every individual on the board went through rigorous rounds of assessment to prove their worth. After which they invested a large part of their time researching and compiling the most relevant data for our readers.

The editorial board has been involved in producing this book since its inception. They have spent rigorous hours researching and exploring the diverse topics which have resulted in the successful publishing of this book. They have passed on their knowledge of decades through this book. To expedite this challenging task, the publisher supported the team at every step. A small team of assistant editors was also appointed to further simplify the editing procedure and attain best results for the readers.

Apart from the editorial board, the designing team has also invested a significant amount of their time in understanding the subject and creating the most relevant covers. They scrutinized every image to scout for the most suitable representation of the subject and create an appropriate cover for the book.

The publishing team has been an ardent support to the editorial, designing and production team. Their endless efforts to recruit the best for this project, has resulted in the accomplishment of this book. They are a veteran in the field of academics and their pool of knowledge is as vast as their experience in printing. Their expertise and guidance has proved useful at every step. Their uncompromising quality standards have made this book an exceptional effort. Their encouragement from time to time has been an inspiration for everyone.

The publisher and the editorial board hope that this book will prove to be a valuable piece of knowledge for researchers, students, practitioners and scholars across the globe.

List of Contributors

Maya M. Mahajan, Betty Cheng, Ashley I. Beyer, Usha S. Mulvaney, Matt B. Wilkinson and Marina E. Fomin
Blood Systems Research Institute, 270 Masonic Ave., San Francisco, CA, USA

Marcus O. Muench
Blood Systems Research Institute, 270 Masonic Ave., San Francisco, CA, USA
Department of Laboratory Medicine, University of California, San Francisco, CA, USA

Olorunfemi Emmanuel Amoran and Temitope Kuponiyi
Department of Community Medicine and Primary Care, Olabisi Onabanjo University Teaching Hospital, Sagamu, Nigeria

Ahmed Babatunde Jimoh
State Hospital Ala, Sagamu, Nigeria

Omotola Ojo
Department of Heamatology, College of Health Sciences, Olabisi Onabanjo University Teaching Hospital, Sagamu, Nigeria

R. Marchi
Centro de Medicina Experimental, Laboratorio Biología del Desarrollo de la Hemostasia, Instituto Venezolano de Investigaciones Científicas, Caracas, República Bolivariana de Venezuela

O. Castillo
Centro de Medicina Experimental, Laboratorio Biología del Desarrollo de la Hemostasia, Instituto Venezolano de Investigaciones Científicas, Caracas, República Bolivariana de Venezuela
Universidad de Carabobo, Escuela de Bioanálisis (Sede Aragua), Maracay, República Bolivariana de Venezuela

H. Rojas
Instituto de Inmunología, Universidad Central de Venezuela, Caracas, República Bolivariana de Venezuela
Laboratorio de Fisiología Celular, Centro de Biofísica y Bioquímica, Instituto Venezolano de Investigaciones Científicas, Caracas, República Bolivariana de Venezuela

Z. Domínguez
Instituto de Medicina Experimental, Universidad Central de Venezuela, Caracas, República Bolivariana de Venezuela

E. Anglés-Cano
Inserm UMR_S 1140, Faculté de Pharmacie, Paris, France
Université Paris Descartes, Sorbonne Paris Cité, Paris, France

F. Ménard and G. E. Rivard
CHU Sainte-Justine, Montréal, Canada

J. St-Louis
CHU Sainte-Justine, Montréal, Canada
Hôpital Maisonneuve-Rosemont, Montreal, Canada

D. J. Urajnik
3Laurentian University, Sudbury, Canada

N. L. Young
Laurentian University, Sudbury, Canada
Hospital for Sick Children, Toronto, Canada

S. Cloutier
Hôpital de l'Enfant-Jésus, Quebec city, Canada

B. Ritchie
University of Alberta, Edmonton, Canada

R. J. Klaassen
Children's Hospital of Eastern Ontario, Ottawa, Canada

M. Warner
McGill University Health Centre, Montréal, Canada

V. Blanchette
University of Toronto, Toronto, Canada
Hospital for Sick Children, Toronto, Canada

William E. Strauss, Naomi V. Dahl, Zhu Li, Gloria Lau and Lee F. Allen
AMAG Pharmaceuticals, Inc., 1100 Winter Street, Waltham, MA 02451, USA

Michelle Sholzberg
Division of Hematology, Department of Medicine and Department of Laboratory Medicine and Pathobiology, St. Michael's Hospital, University of Toronto, 30 Bond Street, Room 2-007G Core Lab, Carter Wing, Toronto, ON M5B-1 W8, Canada

Katerina Pavenski
Division of Hematology, Department of Medicine and Department of Laboratory Medicine and Pathobiology St. Michael's Hospital, University of Toronto, Toronto, Ontario, Canada

Nadine Shehata
Departments of Medicine and Laboratory Medicine and Pathobiology, Mount Sinai Hospital, University of Toronto, Toronto, ON, Canada

Christine Cserti-Gazdewich
Department of Laboratory Medicine and Pathobiology, University Health Network, University of Toronto, Toronto, ON, Canada

Yulia Lin
Department of Clinical Pathology, Sunnybrook Health Sciences Centre; and Department of Laboratory Medicine and Pathobiology, University of Toronto, Toronto, ON, Canada

Vincent S. Verla
Department of Internal Medicine and Pediatrics, Faculty of Health Sciences, University of Buea, Buea, Cameroon

Anne M. Andong
Department of Internal Medicine and Pediatrics, Faculty of Health Sciences, University of Buea, Buea, Cameroon
Health and Human Development (2HD) Research Network, Douala, Cameroon

Simeon-Pierre Choukem
Department of Internal Medicine and Pediatrics, Faculty of Health Sciences, University of Buea, Buea, Cameroon
Health and Human Development (2HD) Research Network, Douala, Cameroon
Department of Internal Medicine, Douala General Hospital, Douala, Cameroon

Daniel Nebongo and Yannick Mboue-Djieka
Health and Human Development (2HD) Research Network, Douala, Cameroon

Eveline D. T. Ngouadjeu
Faculty of Medicine and Pharmaceutical Sciences, University of Douala, Douala, Cameroon
Department of Internal Medicine, Douala General Hospital, Douala, Cameroon

Cavin E. Bekolo
Ministry of Public Health, Centre Medical d'Arrondissement de Bare, Nkongsamba, Cameroon

C Sekaggya, D Nalwanga, A Von Braun, R Nakijoba, A Kambugu, M Lamorde and B Castelnuovo
Infectious Diseases Institute, College of Health Sciences, Makerere University, Kampala, Uganda

J Fehr
Division of Infectious Diseases and Infection Control, University Hospital Zurich, University of Zurich, Zurich, Switzerland

Ismail Dragon Legason
School of Postgraduate Studies, Uganda Christian University, Mukono, Uganda

John Banson Barugahare
School of Postgraduate Studies, Uganda Christian University, Mukono, Uganda
Faculty of Science and Education, Busitema University, Tororo, Uganda

Alex Atiku
Kuluva Hospital, Arua, Uganda

Ronald Ssenyonga
School of Public Health, Makerere College of Health Sciences, Kampala, Uganda

Peter Olupot-Olupot
Faculty of Health Sciences, Busitema University, Mbale, Uganda

Sabrina Peters, Christian Junghanss, Anne Knueppel, Hugo Murua Escobar, Catrin Roolf, Gudrun Knuebel, Anett Sekora, Mathias Freund and Sandra Lange
1Department of Hematology, Oncology, Palliative Medicine, Division of Medicine, University of Rostock, Ernst-Heydemann-Str. 6, 18057 Rostock, Germany

Iris Lindner
Institute of Legal Medicine, Division of Medicine, University of Rostock, St.-Georg-Str. 108, 18055 Rostock, Germany

Ludwig Jonas
Electron Microscopic Centre, Division of Medicine, University of Rostock, Strempelstr. 14, 18057 Rostock, Germany

Eyuel Kassa and Bamlaku Enawgaw
Department of Hematology and Immunohematology, School of Biomedical and Laboratory Sciences, College of Medicine and Health Sciences (CMHS), University of Gondar (UOG), Gondar, Ethiopia

Aschalew Gelaw and Baye Gelaw
Department of Medical Microbiology, School of Biomedical and Laboratory Sciences, College of Medicine and Health Sciences, University of Gondar, Gondar, Ethiopia

Emily M. Teshome and Andrew M. Prentice
MRCG Keneba at MRC Unit The Gambia, Banjul, The Gambia
MRC International Nutrition Group, Faculty of Epidemiology and Population Heath, London School of Hygiene and Tropical Medicine, Keppel Street, London WC1E7HT, UK

Hans Verhoef
MRCG Keneba at MRC Unit The Gambia, Banjul, The Gambia
MRC International Nutrition Group, Faculty of Epidemiology and Population Heath, London School of Hygiene and Tropical Medicine, Keppel Street, London WC1E7HT, UK
Division of Human Nutrition and Cell Biology and Immunology Group, Wageningen University, 6700 AA Wageningen, The Netherlands

Ayşe Y. Demir
Meander Medical Centre, Laboratory for Clinical Chemistry, Maatweg 3, 3813 TZ, Amersfoort, Netherlands

Pauline E.A. Andang'o
School of Public Health and Community Development, Maseno University, Private Bag, Maseno, Kenya

Abibatou Sall, Awa Oumar Touré, Fatimata Bintou Sall, Moussa Ndour, Abdoulaye Sène, Blaise Félix Faye, Moussa Seck, Macoura Gadji, Tandakha Ndiaye Dièye and Saliou Diop
Hematology, Cheikh Anta Diop University, Dakar, Senegal

Seynabou Fall
Hematology, Aristide Le Dantec Hospital, Dakar, Senegal

Claire Mathiot
Curie Institute, Paris, France

Sophie Reynaud
Hematology, University Hospital, Nice, France

Martine Raphaël
University Paris XI, Paris, France

Marloe Prince, Charles J. Glueck, Parth Shah, Ashwin Kumar, Michael Goldenberg, Matan Rothschild, Nasim Motayar, Vybhav Jetty, Kevin Lee and Ping Wang
From the Internal Medicine Residency Program, Cholesterol, Metabolism, and Thrombosis Center of the Jewish Hospital of Cincinnati, 2135 Dana Avenue, Suite 430, Cincinnati, OH 45207, USA

Tsion Sahle
Department of Clinical Laboratory, Gambella Hospital, Gambella, Ethiopia

Tilahun Yemane and Lealem Gedefaw
Department of Medical Laboratory Science and Pathology, Jimma University, Jimma, Ethiopia

Martha L. Louzada, Anargyros Xenocostas, Ian H. Chin-Yee and Leonard Minuk
Department of Medicine, Division of Hematology, London, ON, Canada
University of Western Ontario, London, ON, Canada

Alejandro Lazo-Langner
Department of Medicine, Division of Hematology, London, ON, Canada
University of Western Ontario, London, ON, Canada
Department of Epidemiology and Biostatistics, London, ON, Canada

Cyrus C. Hsia
Department of Medicine, Division of Hematology, London, ON, Canada
University of Western Ontario, London, ON, Canada
London Health Sciences Centre, Department of Medicine, Division of Hematology. Rm E6-219A, Victoria Hospital, 800 Commissioners Road E., London, ON N6A 5W9, Canada

Fatimah Al-Ani
University of Western Ontario, London, ON, Canada

Fiona Ralley
University of Western Ontario, London, ON, Canada
Department of Anesthesia and Perioperative Medicine, London, ON, Canada

Janet Martin and Sarah E. Connelly
University of Western Ontario, London, ON, Canada
Department of Pharmacy, London Health Sciences Centre, London, ON, Canada

Hawley Kunz
KBRwyle, 2400 NASA Parkway, Houston, TX 77058, USA

Heather Quiriarte
Louisiana State University, Baton Rouge, Louisiana 70803, USA

Richard J. Simpson
University of Houston, 4800 Calhoun Rd, Houston, TX 77004, USA

Robert Ploutz-Snyder
University of Michigan School of Nursing, 400 North Ingalls Building, Ann Arbor, MI 48109, USA

Kathleen McMonigal, Clarence Sams and Brian Crucian
NASA Johnson Space Center, 2101 E NASA Parkway, Houston, TX 77058, USA

Sara Aljarad and Ameen Suliman
Department of Hematology, Al Mouwasat University Hospital, Damascus, Syria

Ziad Aljarad
Department of Gastroenterology, Aleppo University Hospital, Aleppo, Syria

Ahmad Alhamid and Ahmad Sankari Tarabishi
Medical student, Faculty of Medicine, University of Aleppo, Aleppo, Syria

Berhanu Elfu Feleke
Department of Epidemiology and Biostatistics, University of Bahir Dar, Bahir Dar, Ethiopia

Teferi Elfu Feleke
Departement of pediatrics, saint paulose hospital, Addis Ababa, Ethiopia

Andrea Kühnl, David Cunningham, Margaret Hutka, Hamoun Rozati, Federica Morano, Irene Chong, Angela Gillbanks, Michelle Harris, Tracey Murray and Ian Chau
Department of Medicine, Royal Marsden NHS Foundation Trust, Downs Road, Sutton, Surrey SM2 5PT, UK

Clare Peckitt
Department of Computing, Royal Marsden NHS Foundation Trust, London, Surrey, UK

Andrew Wotherspoon
Department of Histopathology, Royal Marsden NHS Foundation Trust, London, Surrey, UK

Zelalem Teklemariam, Habtamu Mitiku and Fitsum Weldegebreal
College of Health and Medical Sciences, Department of Medical Laboratory Sciences, Haramaya University, Harar, Ethiopia

Roman M. Shapiro
Department of Medicine, Western University, London, ON, Canada

Alejandro Lazo-Langner
Department of Medicine, Division of Hematology, Western University, London, ON, Canada
Department of Epidemiology and Biostatistics, Western University, London, ON, Canada
Hematology Division, London Health Sciences Centre, 800 Commissioners Rd E, Rm E6-216A, London, ON N6A 5W9, Canada

Akueté Yvon Segbena and Irénée Kueviakoe
CHU Campus, Lomé, Togo

Aldiouma Guindo, Dapa A. Diallo and Pierre Guindo
Centre de Recherche et Lutte contre la Drépanocytose, 03 BP: 186 BKO 03, Point G, Commune III, Bamako, Mali

Romain Buono, Gregory Guernec and Valériane Leroy
Inserm UMR 1027, Epidémiologie et analyses en santé publique : risques, maladies chroniques et handicaps, Université Paul Sabatier Toulouse 3, Faculté de Médecine Purpan, 37 Allées Jules Guesde, 31073 Toulouse Cedex 7, France

Mouhoudine Yerima
Département de Santé Publique, Université de Lomé, Lome, Togo

Emilie Lauressergues and Aude Mondeilh
Pierre Fabre Foundation, Lavaur, France

Valentina Picot
Mérieux Foundation, Lyon, France

Angesom Gebreweld
Department of Medical Laboratory Science, College of Medicine and Health Science, Wollo University, Dessie, Ethiopia

Delayehu Bekele
Department of Obstetrics and Gynecology, Saint Paul's Hospital Millennium Medical College, Addis Ababa, Ethiopia

Aster Tsegaye
School of Medical Laboratory Science, College of Health science, Addis Ababa University, Addis Ababa, Ethiopia

Ayenew Negesse and Habtamu Temesgen
Department of Human Nutrition and Food Sciences, College of Health Science, Debre Markos University, Debre Markos, Ethiopia

Temesgen Getaneh
Department of Midwifery, College of Health Science, Debre Markos University, Debre Markos, Ethiopia

Tesfahun Taddege
Ethiopia Field Epidemiology and Laboratory Training Program (EFELTP) Resident, University of Go0.1ndar, Gondar, Ethiopia

Dube Jara
Department of Public Health, College of Health Science Debre Markos University, Debre Markos, Ethiopia
School of Public Health, College of Health Science, Addis Ababa University, Addis Ababa, Ethiopia

Zeleke Abebaw
Department of Health Informatics, University of Gondar, Gondar, Ethiopia

Tamirat Edie Fekene and Leja Hamza Juhar
Department of internal medicine, College of Public Health and Medical Sciences, Jimma University, Jimma, Ethiopia

Chernet Hailu Mengesha
Department of Epidemiology, Jimma University, Jimma, Ethiopia

Dawit Kibru Worku
Department of Internal Medicine, Bahir Dar University, -79 Bahir Dar, Ethiopia

Sabuj Kanti Mistry, Fatema Tuz Jhohura, Fouzia Khanam, Fahmida Akter, Safayet Khan, Md Belal Hossain and Mahfuzar Rahman
Research and Evaluation Division, BRAC, BRAC Centre, 75 Mohakhali, Dhaka 1212, Bangladesh

Kaosar Afsana and Md Raisul Haque
Health, Nutrition and Population Programme, BRAC, BRAC Centre, 75 Mohakhali, Dhaka 1212, Bangladesh

Fakir Md Yunus
College of Pharmacy and Nutrition, The University of Saskatchewan, 104 Clinic Place, Saskatoon, SK S7N 2Z4, Canada

Enoch Aninagyei, Alexander Egyir-Yawson and Desmond Omane Acheampong
Department of Biomedical Sciences, School of Allied Health Sciences, University of Cape Coast, Cape Coast, Ghana

Emmanuel Tetteh Doku
School of Public Health, University of Ghana, Legon, Accra, Ghana

Patrick Adu
Department of Medical Laboratory Technology, University of Cape Coast, Cape Coast, Ghana

Robert Michael Cronin
Department of Biomedical Informatics, Vanderbilt University Medical Center, 2525 West End Blvd., Suite 1475, Nashville, TN 37232, USA
Department of Internal Medicine, Vanderbilt University Medical Center, Nashville, TN, USA
Department of Pediatrics, Vanderbilt University Medical Center, Nashville, TN, USA

Tilicia L. Mayo-Gamble
Department of Family and Community Medicine, Meharry Medical College, Nashville, TN, USA

Sarah-Jo Stimpson, Jeannie Byrd, Emmanuel J. Volanakis and Michael R. DeBaun
Department of Pediatrics, Division of Hematology/ Oncology, Vanderbilt-Meharry Center for Excellence in Sickle Cell Disease, Vanderbilt University Medical Center, Nashville, TN, USA

Sherif M. Badawy
Department of Pediatrics, Division of Hematology, Oncology and Stem Cell Transplant, Ann and Robert H. Lurie Children's Hospital of Chicago, Northwestern University Feinberg School of Medicine, Chicago, IL, USA

Lori E. Crosby
Division of Behavioral Medicine, Department of Pediatrics, Cincinnati Children's Hospital Medical Center and the University of Cincinnati, College of Medicine, Cincinnati, OH, USA

Adetola A. Kassim
Department of Medicine, Division of Hematology/ Oncology, Vanderbilt-Meharry Center for Excellence in Sickle Cell Disease, Vanderbilt University Medical Center, Nashville, TN, USA

Jean L. Raphael
Department of Pediatrics, Section of Hematology-Oncology and Section of Academic General Pediatrics, Baylor College of Medicine, Houston, TX, USA

Velma M. Murry
Department of Human and Organizational Development, Vanderbilt University, Nashville, TN, USA

Index

www.ingramcontent.com/pod-product-compliance
Lightning Source LLC
Chambersburg PA
CBHW061312190326
41458CB00011B/3784
* 9 7 8 1 6 3 2 4 2 6 7 5 8 *